AF443116

Cancer Treatment and Research

Volume 157

Series Editor
Steven T. Rosen

For further volumes, go to
http://www.springer.com/series/5808

Gary H. Lyman · David C. Dale
Editors

Hematopoietic Growth Factors in Oncology

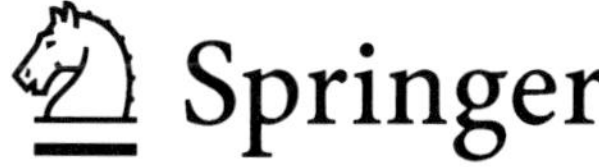 Springer

Editors
Gary H. Lyman, MD, MPH
Duke University and the Duke
  Comprehensive Cancer Center
Durham, NC 27705, USA

David C. Dale, MD
Department of Medicine
University of Washington
Seattle, WA 98195, USA

ISSN 0927-3042
ISBN 978-1-4419-7072-5   e-ISBN 978-1-4419-7073-2
DOI 10.1007/978-1-4419-7073-2
Springer New York Dordrecht Heidelberg London

Library of Congress Control Number: 2010938328

Printed on acid-free paper

Springer is part of Springer Science+Business Media (www.springer.com)

*To Nancy Thomasson for her outstanding
assistance with manuscript processing and
to my dedicated wife and companion, Nicole,
and sons Stephen and Christopher.*

–Gary H. Lyman

*To my excellent staff, especially, Audrey
Anna Bolyard, Elin Rodger, and Laurie
Steele, and my devoted wife, Rose Marie.*

–David C. Dale

Preface

Without doubt, we are living in the most exciting of times in the history of clinical medicine especially in the realm of cancer research and treatment. The rate at which scientific progress has occurred and is being translated into improved medical diagnostics and therapeutics is breathtaking. Our improved understanding of basic molecular biology and genetics has presented cancer researchers and clinicians with a staggering array of therapeutic targets and novel therapeutic modalities. At this moment in time, we can only stand in awe at what the future almost certainly holds in store for future victims of this often devastating disease. However, as important as promising new and often novel cancer therapies have been, progress in our ability to effectively and safely support patients through cancer treatment has been equally exciting and groundbreaking often built as well upon the foundation laid by advances in molecular biology and genetics.

Among the barriers to the optimal delivery of systemic cancer therapies, hematologic toxicity arising from the myelosuppressive effects of most cytotoxic cancer treatments remains the lead cause of treatment-related complications including neutropenia, anemia, and thrombocytopenia. Such "cytopenias" result in frequent, serious, and potentially life-threatening complications including a wide range of bacterial, fungal, and parasitic infections, hemorrhagic complications as well as clinically significant fatigue. In addition, the risk or occurrence of such complications also often result in limitations to the full delivery of effective and potentially curative systemic chemotherapy while, at the same time, compromise quality of life and increase costs associated with the care of cancer patients. Many of the most exciting novel and targeted cancer therapies are, in fact, most effective when combined with traditional cytotoxic and myelosuppressive chemotherapy. Likewise, complications of cancer treatment are often exacerbated by our multidisciplinary and combined modality efforts to improve long-term survival and cure among cancer patients.

Supportive care efforts including the appropriate and timely use of empiric broad-spectrum antibiotics in patients with fever and neutropenia and selective blood transfusions in patients with severe anemia and thrombocytopenia greatly improved early efforts to deliver antineoplastic chemotherapy. However, improved understanding of hematopoiesis and the factors that control the proliferation and morphologic and functional differentiation of hematopoietic lineages has provided insights and opportunities for reducing the complications associated with myelosuppression and other disorders resulting in neutropenia, anemia, or thrombocytopenia. This improved understanding coupled with outstanding advances in recombinant DNA technology has resulted in the development and clinical validation of a number of hematopoietic growth factors.

Hematopoietic Growth Factors in Oncology represents the latest in a series of texts in the Cancer Treatment and Research series edited by Dr. Steven T. Rosen. This volume brings under a single cover a discussion of the early discoveries, extensive preclinical and clinical investigation, and the validation of these efforts through the successful clinical extension of these discoveries into clinical hematology and oncology practice improving the treatment and quality of life of countless patients. As Editors, we have been extremely fortunate to have engaged in this project some of the world's leading investigators and authorities on both the science and the clinical application of the hematopoietic growth factors. We want to extend our very sincere thanks to this outstanding representation of investigators who have assisted us in assembling this comprehensive repository of information on the development and clinical application of these agents.

The text begins with an outstanding review of the biologic, physiologic, and pharmacologic underpinnings of the discoveries, laboratory studies, and early preclinical and clinical development of the hematopoietic growth factors from some of the actual pioneers in these fundamental studies. While the anticipation around development of early-acting hematopoietic growth factors has not been fully realized, developments in granulocyte colony-stimulating factors, the erythropoietic-stimulating agents, and the thrombopoietin factors have in many ways exceeded the expectations of many. The next three parts in this book then highlight the further clinical development and application of the three major categories of the hematopoietic growth factors, by individuals involved in both the pivotal studies and extended clinical trials that have further defined the efficacy and safety of these agents. Current recommendations for clinical application of the hematopoietic growth factors based on practice guidelines from major professional organizations are presented along with the evidence synthesis available on both efficacy and safety. While we are constantly made aware of the need to balance efficacy and safety, the emergence of the erythroid-stimulating agents, the myeloid growth factors as well as the new thrombopoietic agents have had a great impact on the supportive care of patients with cancer.

In the final part of this volume, a number of very important special considerations regarding the use of the hematopoietic growth factors are discussed including their often controversial role in management of patients with acute leukemia and the myelodysplastic syndromes, their efficacy and toxicity in older cancer patients, and the cost and cost-effectiveness of these agents in the prevention and treatment of hematologic complications exemplified by the use of G-CSF for the prevention of febrile neutropenia in patients receiving cancer chemotherapy. The authors emphasize that any comprehensive evaluation of benefits, harms and costs must consider not only the immediate reduction in risk of neutropenic complications in patients receiving cancer chemotherapy but also the potential long-term effects on disease control and survival when treatment intensity is sustained or enhanced with the adjunctive use of the myeloid growth factors.

In total, this represents the most comprehensive compilation available of pre-clinical and clinical experience related to the development, validation, and clinical application of the hematopoietic growth factors. The editors share the perspective of the individual authors that no aspect of cancer care deserves more attention as well as further clinical research than the treatment and prevention of life-threatening complications of cancer treatment. We recognize and share the excitement and anticipation of all hematologists and oncologists arising from the multitude of diagnostic and therapeutic breakthroughs of the past two decades. At the same time, we also recognize the importance of the many supportive care efforts enabling the optimal management of patients including the optimal delivery of modern cancer therapy while improving the quality of life of patients with cancer and other blood disorders throughout the course of their illness. Optimal clinical outcomes for each patient in the most complete sense remains the primary goal of all hematologists and oncologists as it is for other healthcare providers. The availability of advanced supportive care measures including the hematopoietic growth factors utilized in a rational, effective, and cost-effective fashion will further enhance these goals and bring us closer to that ultimate goal of optimal patient care.

<table>
<tr><td>Durham, NC</td><td>Gary H. Lyman</td></tr>
<tr><td>Seattle, WA</td><td>David C. Dale</td></tr>
</table>

Contents

Part III   The Erythroid-Stimulating Agents

Part IV   The Thrombopoietic Agents

Part V   Special Considerations

Contributors

Lodovico Balducci Oncology Program, H. Lee Moffitt Cancer Center and Research Institute, Tampa, FL 33612, USA, lodovico.balducci@moffitt.org

Julia Bohlius Institute of Social and Preventive Medicine, University of Bern, Bern, Switzerland, jbohlius@ispm.unibe.ch

James B. Bussel Division of Pediatric Hematology–Oncology, Department of Pediatrics in Obstetrics and Gynecology and in Medicine, Weill Cornell Medical College, New York Presbyterian Hospital, Weill Cornell Medical Center, New York, NY 10044, USA, jbussel@med.cornell.edu

David Cella Department of Medical Social Sciences, Prevention and Control, Robert H. Lurie Comprehensive Cancer Center, Northwestern University, Chicago, IL 60611, USA, d-cella@northwestern.edu

David C. Dale Department of Medicine, University of Washington, Seattle, WA 98195, USA, dcdale@u.washington.edu

Adi Eldar-Lissai Associate, Analysis Group, Inc., Boston, MA 02199, USA, aeldar-lissai@analysisgroup.com

Steve Elliott Department of Hematology, Amgen, Inc., Thousand Oaks, CA 91320, USA, selliott@amgen.com

David T. Eton Department of Health Sciences Research, Division of Healthcare Policy & Research, Mayo Clinic, Rochester, MN, 55905 USA, eton.david@mayo.edu

Olga Frankfurt Division of Hematology and Oncology, Feinberg School of Medicine, Robert H. Lurie Comprehensive Care Cancer, Northwestern University, Chicago, IL 60611, USA, o-frankfurt@northwestern.edu

Arnold Ganser Department of Hematology, Hemostasis, Oncology, and Stem Cell Transplantation, Hannover Medical School, Hannover, Germany 30625, ganser.arnold@mh-hannover.de

John A. Glaspy Division of Hematology and Oncology, Department of Medicine, David Geffen School of Medicine – UCLA, Los Angeles, CA 90095, USA, jglaspy@mednet.ucla.edu

Michael Heuser Department of Hematology, Hemostasis, Oncology, and Stem Cell Transplantation, Hannover Medical School, 30625 Hannover, Germany, heuser.michael@mh-hannover.de

Dieter Hoelzer Onkologikum Frankfurt am Museumsufer, 60596 Frankfurt, Germany, hoelzer@em.uni-frankfurt.de

Jessica Malone Kleiner University of Rochester School of Medicine and Dentistry, Rochester, NY 14621, USA, jessica.kleiner@usoncology.com

Rami Komrokji H Lee Moffitt Cancer Center and Research Institute, Tampa, FL 33612, USA, rami.komrokji@moffitt.org

Nicole M. Kuderer Duke University School of Medicine, Durham, NC 27705, USA, nicole.kuderer@duke.edu

David J. Kuter Hematology Division, Massachusetts General Hospital, Boston, MA 02114, USA, kuter.david@mgh.harvard.edu

Alan E. Lichtin Department of Medicine, Cleveland Clinic Lerner College of Medicine, Cleveland, OH 44195, USA; Taussig Cancer Center, Cleveland Clinic Health Systems, Cleveland, OH 44195, USA, lichtia@ccf.org

Alan F. List Department of Malignant Hematology, H. Lee Moffitt Cancer Center and Research Institute, Tampa, FL 33612 USA, alan.list@moffitt.org

Gary H. Lyman Duke University and the Duke Comprehensive Cancer Center, Durham, NC 27705, USA, gary.lyman@duke.edu

Graham Molineux Amgen, Inc., Thousand Oaks, CA 91320, USA, graham@amgen.com

Jose Ortega Department of Hematology and Medical Oncology, H. Lee Moffitt Cancer Center and Research Institute, Tampa, FL 33612, USA, jose.ortega@moffitt.org

Mariana P. Pinheiro Division of Pediatric Hematology-Oncology, Weill Cornell Medical Center, Weill Cornell Medical College, New York Presbyterian Hospital, New York, NY 10044, USA, map2053@med.cornell.edu

Charles A. Schiffer Division of Hematology/Oncology, Karmanos Cancer Institute, Wayne State University School of Medicine, Detroit, MI 48201, USA, schiffer@karmanos.org

Michelle Shayne Division of Hematology/Oncology, University of Rochester, Rochester, NY 14607, USA, michelle.shayne@urmc.rochester.edu

Stephen J. Szilvassy Hematology/Oncology Research Therapeutic Area, Amgen, Inc., Thousand Oaks, CA 91320, USA, sszilvas@amgen.com

Martin S. Tallman Memorial Sloan Kettering Cancer Center, Weill Cornell Medical College, New York, NY, m-tallman@northwestern.edu

Thomy Tonia Institute of Social and Preventive Medicine, University of Bern, Switzerland, ttonia@ispm.unibe.ch

Jason Valent Division of Hematology/Oncology, Karmanos Cancer Institute, Wayne State University, Detroit, MI 48201, USA, valentjs@hotmail.com

Ping Wei Department of Hematology, Amgen, Inc., Thousand Oaks, CA 91320, USA, pwei@amgen.com

Karl Welte Department of Molecular Hematopoiesis, Kinderklinik, Medizinische Hochschule, Hannover, Germany, welte.karl.h@mh-hannover.de

Part I
Background: Biology, Physiology, and Pharmacology

Chapter 1
Introduction to the Hematopoietic Growth Factors

Gary H. Lyman and David C. Dale

Background

The hematopoietic growth factors (HGFs) are an important class of biologic molecules which augment production and functional maturation of hematopoietic cells. As shown in Fig. 1.1, endogenous production of HGFs modulates a wide variety of both hematopoietic and nonhematopoietic cells derived from the myeloid stem cell including progenitor and precursor cells and more functionally mature cells. Clinically, recombinant or mimetic forms of these cytokines are utilized to reduce the severity and duration of hematologic complications resulting from impairment of granulocytopoiesis, erythropoiesis, or thrombopoiesis. The primary therapeutic goal of these agents clinically is to reduce the risk and severity of complications such as infection, fatigue, and bleeding. In addition, their appropriate use may enable the safe delivery of effective myelosuppressive cancer chemotherapy and treatment potentially enhancing long-term disease control and curability. This volume presents both the early history as well as the current status of the hematopoietic growth factors including their biology, physiology, and pharmacology as well as their clinical application in enhancing hematopoiesis in clinical conditions associated with granulocytopenia, anemia, and thrombocytopenia. The first five chapters summarize in considerable detail the underlying biology, physiology, and pharmacology of the hematopoietic growth factors including the early-acting molecules as well as the granulocyte colony-stimulating factors, the erythropoiesis-stimulating agents, and the thrombopoietic factors (Table 1.1). The next three parts of the volume consider in much greater detail the clinical application including efficacy and safety considerations of each class of the hematopoietic growth factors, respectively. The final part of this book addresses a few very important but often circumvented issues around the use of these agents including their role in the management of the

G.H. Lyman (✉)
Duke University and the Duke Comprehensive Cancer Center, Durham, NC 27705, USA
e-mail: gary.lyman@duke.edu

G.H. Lyman, D.C. Dale (eds.), *Hematopoietic Growth Factors in Oncology*,
Cancer Treatment and Research 157, DOI 10.1007/978-1-4419-7073-2_1,
© Springer Science+Business Media, LLC 2011

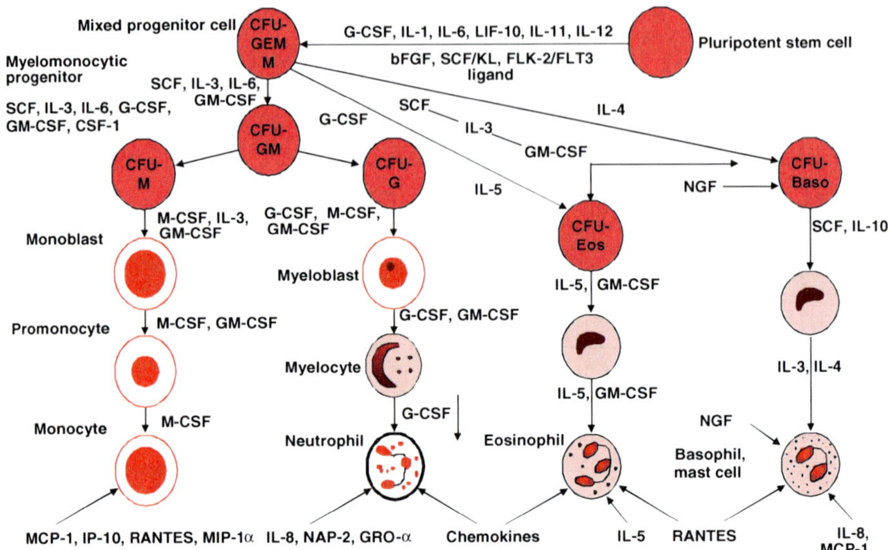

Fig. 1.1 Representation of myeloid hematopoietic differentiation. Cytokines capable of stimulating specific cells are listed below such cells [27]. (BFU-E, burst-forming unit, erythroid; CFU-GEMM, colony-forming unit granulocyte–erythrocyte–megakaryocyte macrophage; CFU-GM, colony-forming unit granulocyte–macrophage; EPO, erythropoietin; G-CSF, granulocyte colony-stimulating factor; GM-CSF, granulocyte–macrophage colony-stimulating factor; IL, interleukin; M-CSF, macrophage colony-stimulating factor; SCF, stem cell factor; TPO, thrombopoietin.)

myeloid malignancies and the myelodysplastic syndromes as well as their use in elderly patients where hematopoietic reserves are often reduced. Finally, important economic considerations related to the application of the colony-stimulating factors in the prevention of febrile neutropenia in patients receiving cancer chemotherapy are discussed.

Early-Acting Hematopoietic Growth Factors

Early studies revealed that certain glycoproteins are capable of supporting the formation of hematopoietic colonies when present in culture with bone marrow cells [1, 2]. Subsequently, the genes encoding granulocyte colony-stimulating factor (G-CSF), granulocyte–macrophage colony-stimulating factor (GM-CSF), and interleukin-3 (IL-3) were cloned and recombinant forms of these molecules were developed using recombinant DNA technology [3]. Subsequent studies suggested that certain HGFs exhibit early actions raising the promise that a true "stem cell factor" would be identified that would prove both biologically illuminating and clinically valuable in the management of a broad range of hematopoietic disorders. As interesting and intensively studied as these molecules continue to be, it is quite remarkable, as pointed out by Steve Szilvassy in the next chapter, that some 25 years

Table 1.1   Hematopoietic growth factors

Cytokine	Other names	Generic names	Expression vector	Brand names	No. of amino acids	Human chromosome location	Normal endogenous sources
G-CSF	Granulocyte colony-stimulating factor	Filgrastim	*E. coli* CHO	Neupogen (Amgen)	174	17	Monocytes/macrophages, fibroblasts, endothelial cells, keratinocytes
		Pegfilgrastim	*E. coli*	Neulasta (Amgen)			
		Lenograstim		Granocyte (Chugai)			
GM-CSF	Granulocyte–macrophage colony-stimulating factor	Sargramostim	Yeast	Leukine (Immunex)	127	5	T lymphocytes, monocytes/macrophages, fibroblasts, endothelial cells, osteoblasts, epithelial cells
		Molgramostim	*E. coli*	Leucomax (Schering)			
		Regramostim	CHO				
EPO	Erythropoietin	Epoetin-α	CHO	Epogen (Amgen)	165	7	Renal cells, hepatocytes
		Epoetin-α	CHO	Procrit/Eprex (Ortho)			
		Epoetin-β	CHO	NeoRecormon (Roche)			
		Darbepoetin-α	CHO	Aranesp (Amgen)			
IL-11	Interleukin-11	Oprelvekin	*E. coli*	Neumega (Genetics Institute)	178	19	Stromal fibroblasts, trophoblasts
SCF	Stem cell factor, steel factor, mast cell growth factor, c-kit ligand	Ancestim	*E. coli*	Stemgen (Amgen)	165	12	Endothelial cells, fibroblasts, circulating mononuclears, bone marrow stromal cells
TPO	Thrombopoietin, megakaryocyte growth and development factor				332	3	Liver, kidney

CHO, Chinese hamster ovary cells; CSF, colony-stimulating factor.

following the discovery of the first cytokine demonstrating activity on hematopoietic stem cells, none have demonstrated value other than as potentiators of later-acting cell line-specific progenitors or precursors. Nonetheless, the recent development of novel mpl ligands such as romiplostim and eltrombopag, which may activate key transcriptional and developmental pathways, suggests that the potential utility of the early-acting factors may still yield interesting and therapeutically important strategies.

The Colony-Stimulating Factors

G-CSF, with the ability to induce granulocyte differentiation of a myelomonocytic leukemia cell line, was first identified in the serum of mice [4, 5]. G-CSF is produced endogenously by monocytes, macrophages, endothelial cells, fibroblasts, and mesenchymal cells as well as marrow stromal cells while the G-CSF receptor is expressed on mature neutrophils and their precursors. G-CSF is essential for normal neutrophil production and function, acting on late myeloid progenitors and leading to increase cell proliferation, reduced marrow transit time and differentiation and functional maturation of neutrophils. Pegfilgrastim, a recombinant G-CSF too large for renal clearance, is associated with a long half-life while retaining biological activity enhancing neutrophil proliferation and morphologic and functional differentiation. Following receptor saturation, the predominant neutrophil-dependent clearance of pegfilgrastim during the period of neutropenia enables once per cycle dosing in patients receiving cancer chemotherapy with potentially greater efficacy [6]. GM-CSF was first identified in 1977 with human GM-CSF purified shortly thereafter [7, 8]. GM-CSF is produced by monocytes, macrophages, fibroblasts, and endothelial cells [9, 10]. While apparently having minimal role in normal hematopoiesis under steady-state conditions, GM-CSF gene knock-out mice exhibit normal hematopoiesis suggesting that it has minimal role in leukocytosis in the steady-state situation. GM-CSF not only stimulates the survival and functional activity of neutrophils, macrophages, monocytes, and eosinophils but is also a potent stimulator of dendritic cells that are fundamental to the primary immune response [9–11]. In Chapter 3 of this volume, Graham Molineux reviews the identification of this class of cytokines along with the development and biological and pharmacologic characterization of the recombinant formulations. Also discussed in that chapter is the recent development of biosimilars or follow-on biologic versions of G-CSF which have already been approved in Europe and are soon to be considered in the United States. The role of G-CSF in the management of patients with cyclic and chronic neutropenia is fully discussed in Chapter 6 by David Dale. The remaining chapters on the Colony-Stimulating Factors focus on the primary clinical utility of these agents in the management of patients receiving cancer chemotherapy. In Chapter 7, Gary Lyman summarizes the clinical development and application of the colony-stimulating factors in clinical oncology while in Chapter 8, Nicole Kuderer presents a pivotal systematic review and meta-analysis of the published randomized controlled trials of G-CSF for primary prophylaxis of febrile neutropenia in solid tumor and lymphoma patients receiving conventional cancer chemotherapy. In Chapter 9, Gary Lyman and Jessica Kleiner review and contrast the major clinical practice guidelines for the use of the myeloid growth factors in patients receiving systemic chemotherapy. To round out the section on the colony-stimulating factors in Chapter 10, Gary Lyman and Nicole Kuderer then present a recently completed systematic review and meta-analysis of randomized controlled trials of cancer chemotherapy with and without G-CSF support addressing the risk of acute myeloid leukemia or myelodysplastic syndrome as well as all-cause mortality.

The Erythropoiesis-Stimulating Agents

The primary endogenous regulator of red cell production is the glycoprotein erythropoietin which is principally produced in the peritubular interstitial cells and regulated by an oxygen sensor. The recombinant erythropoiesis-stimulating agent (ESA), epoetin alfa, and the hypergycosylated recombinant erythropoietin, darbepoetin alfa, are available in the United States while epoetin beta is available outside of the United States. As summarized in Chapter 4 by Steve Elliott, darbepoetin results from the addition of two N-glycosylation sites resulting in a substantial increase in molecular weight and prolonged circulation due to protection from metabolic degradation [12, 13]. The efficacious effects of the ESAs include proliferation and differentiation of erythroid progenitors to mature functional erythrocytes.

Anemia in cancer patients is often the result of multiple factors including cancer stage, renal toxicity, and treatment with radiation and chemotherapy. As summarized by David Eton and David Cella in Chapter 11, anemia in cancer patients has measurable and significant effects on quality of life as well as costs. Due to paradoxical elevations of endogenous erythropoietin (EPO) concentrations, inappropriately low as well as high ESA concentrations have been reported following chemotherapy [14–16]. Treatment with intravenous iron has been shown to improve hemoglobin response to recombinant ESAs in cancer patients [17].

In Chapter 12, John Glaspy discusses the results of major randomized controlled trials of the ESAs in patients with cancer. Summarizing an exhaustive Cochrane meta-analysis of the ESAs, Julia Bohlius highlights the efficacy as well as toxicity associated with these agents in Chapter 13. Wrapping up this section on the ESAs, in Chapter 14 Alan Lichtin reviews the major clinical practice guidelines for the use of the ESAs from the American Society of Clinical Oncology (ASCO), the European Organization for Research and Treatment of Cancer (EORTC), and the National Comprehensive Cancer Network (NCCN).

The Thrombopoietic Agents

The pluripotent stem cell gives rise to the early mixed myeloid progenitor which then leads to the megakaryocyte–erythroid (MK) progenitor. c-Kit ligand or stem cell factor acts at very early stages stimulating progenitor cell division and differentiation into the MK lineage. The latter may, in turn, give rise to either progenitors of the erythroid or megakaryocyte line. Thrombopoietin, initially identified in 1994, is the primary regulator of thrombopoiesis, stimulating the growth and maturation of MK progenitor cells into mature megakaryocytes [18–20]. Thrombopoietin (TPO) is a 332-amino acid glycoprotein produced primarily in the liver with its effects mediated through a receptor on megakaryocytes and platelets [21]. In addition, in vitro and animal studies suggest that interleukin-11 (IL-11) directly stimulates megakaryocytes. In healthy individuals, 10^{11} platelets are released from megakaryocytes daily [22].

Due to the associated risk of life-threatening hemorrhage, severe thrombocytopenia associated with immune platelet destruction, bone marrow failure, or exposure to myelosuppressive agents has been treated urgently with platelet transfusions. The current status of platelet transfusion for cancer-associated thrombocytopenia including benefits and harms is summarized by Charles Schiffer and Jason Valent in Chapter 15. Recombinant IL-11 was the first cytokine approved for the prevention of chemotherapy-induced thrombocytopenia based on clinical trials demonstrating a reduction in the risk of chemotherapy-induced thrombocytopenia [23, 24]. Romiplostim was the first thrombopoietin receptor agonist approved by the US Food and Drug Administration (FDA) for the treatment of thrombocytopenia in patients with chronic immune thrombocytopenic purpura (ITP) poorly responsive to corticosteroids, immunoglobulins, or splenectomy. Romiplostim is a recombinant fusion protein with two thrombopoietin-binding domains covalently bound to the Fc domain of a human IgG molecule [25]. The preclinical experience and clinical development of romiplostim is summarized by David Kuter in Chapter 16. The FDA subsequently approved a selective small molecule, nonpeptide agonist of the thrombopoietin receptor, eltrombopag, which promotes proliferation and differentiation of progenitors into committed megakaryocyte precursors [26]. As eltrombopag is only known to be active in humans and chimpanzees, available preclinical data on this agent are limited. In Chapter 17, Mariana Pinheiro and James Bussel summarize the clinical experience with eltrombopag including several large randomized controlled trials. Although a reversible increase of bone marrow reticulin or even collagen has not been associated with any long-term hematological consequences, it is the subject of ongoing studies for both agents.

The final part of this volume addresses a number of special issues relevant to the HGFs including their utilization in patients with acute leukemia and the myelodysplastic syndromes as well as their efficacy and safety in elderly cancer patients and ever-present question around the cost and cost effectiveness of these agents in clinical practice. The presence of receptors for myeloid growth factors on the surface of a substantial proportion of myeloid leukemia cells has raised concerns about their efficacy and safety in treatment of patients with myeloid malignancies or premalignant conditions. Nevertheless, a growing body of evidence suggests that these agents do have a role to play in cancer treatment and supportive. In Chapters 18 and 19, Olga Frankfurt and Martin Tallman and Michael Heuser, Arnold Ganser, and Dieter Hoelzer, respectively, review the extensive literature on the use of HGFs in patients with acute leukemia. While the clinical evidence reviewed is consistent, bringing together the combined expertise of two of the world's leading research groups on this topic provides considerable depth and breadth of understanding to this particular topic. The myelodysplastic syndromes represent hematopoietic stem cell malignancies associated with impaired hematopoietic maturation in the bone marrow and progressive cytopenias as well as a high risk of developing acute myeloid leukemia (AML). In Chapter 20, Jose Ortega, Rami Komrokji, and Alan List review the available clinical data on the use of the HGFs in patients with the myelodysplastic syndromes. Hematopoietic reserves decline and myelosuppression associated with cytotoxic chemotherapy increases with advancing age. Nonetheless, elderly patients with cancer respond to treatment and supportive care measures in a fashion similar to that of younger individuals. In Chapter 21, Michelle Shayne and Lodovico Balducci review the supporting evidence and current recommendations for the clinical use of HGFs in older cancer patients. Although the science and clinical application of these important molecules have dominated the attention of researchers, clinicians, patients, and regulators, the cost of the HGFs has also garnered considerable attention in recent years. In an era of rapidly increasing healthcare costs and healthcare reform, the economics of cancer patient care including that of supportive or adjunctive agents such as the HGFs must be considered along with the efficacy and safety of this important new class of cancer therapeutics. In the final chapter of this volume, Adi Eldar-Lisai and Gary Lyman review issues related to the cost and cost effectiveness of the HGFs using G-CSF as an illustration of the clinical and economic issues that need to be considered.

Since the early biologic discoveries demonstrating the presence of circulating factors exerting a stimulating and modulating effect on hematopoiesis from the earliest stem cells to their mature functional end products, rapid advances in understanding as well as technology have made the HGFs some of the most interesting and important advances in medicine in the past few decades. As the role for recombinant and small molecular forms of these agents continues to be defined and expanded, the impact on cancer patient care and clinical outcomes has grown rapidly as well. This volume represents a detailed summary of the history and current state-of-the-art of this increasingly important repertoire of therapeutic and prophylactic agents designed to further improve the efficacy and safety of cancer treatment and supportive care.

References

1. Metcalf D. Studies on colony formation in vitro by mouse bone marrow cells. I. Continuous cluster formation and relation of clusters to colonies. J Cell Physiol. 1969;74:323–32.
2. Metcalf D, Foster R. Bone marrow colony-stimulating activity of serum from mice with viral-induced leukemia. J Natl Cancer Inst. 1967;39:1235–45.
3. Clark SC, Kamen R. The human hematopoietic colony-stimulating factors. Science. 1987;236:1229–37.
4. Burgess AW, Metcalf D. Characterization of a serum factor stimulating the differentiation of myelomonocytic leukemic cells. Int J Cancer. 1980;26:647–54.
5. Moore MA. G-CSF: its relationship to leukemia differentiation-inducing activity and other hemopoietic regulators. J Cell Physiol Suppl. 1982;1:53–64.

6. Molineux G. The design and development of pegfilgrastim (PEG-rmetHuG-CSF, Neulasta). Curr Pharm Des. 2004;10:1235–44.
7. Burgess AW, Camakaris J, Metcalf D. Purification and properties of colony-stimulating factor from mouse lung-conditioned medium. J Biol Chem. 1977;252:1998–2003.
8. Gough NM, Gough J, Metcalf D, et al. Molecular cloning of cDNA encoding a murine haematopoietic growth regulator, granulocyte–macrophage colony stimulating factor. Nature. 1984;309:763–7.
9. Bagby G, Heinrich M. Growth factors, cytokines, and the control of hematopoiesis. In: Hoffman R, Shattil SJ, editors. Haematology basic principles and practice. Philadelphia, PA: Churchill Livingstone; 2000. pp. 154–202.
10. Moore M. Colony stimulating factors: basic principles and preclinical studies. In: Rosenberg S, editor. Principles and practice of the biologic therapy of cancer. Philadelphia, PA: Lippincott Williams & Wilkins; 2000. pp. 113–40.
11. Demir G, Klein HO, Tuzuner N. Low dose daily rhGM-CSF application activates monocytes and dendritic cells in vivo. Leuk Res. 2003;27:1105–8.
12. Elliott S, Lorenzini T, Asher S, et al. Enhancement of therapeutic protein in vivo activities through glycoengineering. Nat Biotechnol. 2003;21:414–21.
13. Allon M, Kleinman K, Walczyk M, et al. Pharmacokinetics and pharmacodynamics of darbepoetin alfa and epoetin in patients undergoing dialysis. Clin Pharmacol Ther. 2002;72:546–55.
14. Birgegard G, Wide L, Simonsson B. Marked erythropoietin increase before fall in Hb after treatment with cytostatic drugs suggests mechanism other than anaemia for stimulation. Br J Haematol. 1989;72:462–6.
15. Smith DH, Goldwasser E, Vokes EE. Serum immunoerythropoietin levels in patients with cancer receiving cisplatin-based chemotherapy. Cancer. 1991;68:1101–5.
16. Schapira L, Antin JH, Ransil BJ, et al. Serum erythropoietin levels in patients receiving intensive chemotherapy and radiotherapy. Blood. 1990;76:2354–9.
17. Auerbach M, Ballard H, Trout JR, et al. Intravenous iron optimizes the response to recombinant human erythropoietin in cancer patients with chemotherapy-related anemia: a multicenter, open-label, randomized trial. J Clin Oncol. 2004;22:1301–7.
18. Douglas VK, Tallman MS, Cripe LD, et al. Thrombopoietin administered during induction chemotherapy to patients with acute myeloid leukemia induces transient morphologic changes that may resemble chronic myeloproliferative disorders. Am J Clin Pathol. 2002;117:844–50.
19. Vadhan-Raj S. Recombinant human thrombopoietin: clinical experience and in vivo biology. Semin Hematol. 1998;35:261–8.
20. Vadhan-Raj S. Clinical experience with recombinant human thrombopoietin in chemotherapy-induced thrombocytopenia. Semin Hematol. 2000;37:28–34.
21. Nurden AT, Viallard JF, Nurden P. New-generation drugs that stimulate platelet production in chronic immune thrombocytopenic purpura. Lancet. 2009;373:1562–9.
22. Deutsch VR, Tomer A. Megakaryocyte development and platelet production. Br J Haematol. 2006;134:453–66.
23. Gordon MS, McCaskill-Stevens WJ, Battiato LA, et al. A phase I trial of recombinant human interleukin-11 (neumega rhIL-11 growth factor) in women with breast cancer receiving chemotherapy. Blood. 1996;87:3615–24.
24. Isaacs C, Robert NJ, Bailey FA, et al. Randomized placebo-controlled study of recombinant human interleukin-11 to prevent chemotherapy-induced thrombocytopenia in patients with breast cancer receiving dose-intensive cyclophosphamide and doxorubicin. J Clin Oncol. 1997;15:3368–77.
25. Wang B, Nichol JL, Sullivan JT. Pharmacodynamics and pharmacokinetics of AMG 531, a novel thrombopoietin receptor ligand. Clin Pharmacol Ther. 2004;76:628–38.
26. Jenkins JM, Williams D, Deng Y, et al. Phase 1 clinical study of eltrombopag, an oral, nonpeptide thrombopoietin receptor agonist. Blood. 2007;109:4739–41.
27. Abboud CN, Liesveld JL. Granulopoiesis and monocytopoiesis. In: Hoffman R, et al., editors. Hematology: basic principles and practice. 2nd ed. New York, NY: Churchill Livingstone; 1995. p. 258.

Chapter 2
Early-Acting Hematopoietic Growth Factors: Biology and Clinical Experience

Stephen J. Szilvassy

Abstract Secreted protein growth factors that stimulate the self-renewal, proliferation, and differentiation of the most primitive stem cells are among the most biologically interesting molecules and at least theoretically have diverse applications in the evolving field of regenerative medicine. Among this class of regulators, the early-acting hematopoietic growth factors and their cellular targets are perhaps the best characterized and serve as a paradigm for manipulating other stem cell based tissues. This chapter reviews the preclinical knowledge accumulated over ~40 years, since the discovery of the first such growth factor, and the clinical applications of those that, upon testing in humans, ultimately gained regulatory approval for the treatment of various hematological diseases.

Introduction

Blood comprises many cell types that carry out highly specialized functions such as transporting oxygen to tissues and combating infection via both cell-based and humoral mechanisms. The production of blood, or hematopoiesis, is one of the most well-studied physiological processes and serves as a paradigm for other adult stem cell systems and the regulation of self-renewing tissues. During steady-state hematopoiesis in humans, approximately 200 billion new erythrocytes, 100 billion leukocytes, and 100 billion platelets are produced each day to replace those lost through natural aging processes. In response to hematological stress (e.g., hypoxia, infection), the numbers of a particular type of blood cell required to meet physiological demands can expand rapidly by >tenfold. This remarkable capacity for lineage-specific expansion while maintaining the appropriate balance of blood cell types resides in a hierarchy of hematopoietic stem and progenitor cells that are found

S.J. Szilvassy (✉)
Hematology/Oncology Research Therapeutic Area, Amgen Inc., Thousand Oaks, CA 91320, USA
e-mail: sszilvas@amgen.com

G.H. Lyman, D.C. Dale (eds.), *Hematopoietic Growth Factors in Oncology*,
Cancer Treatment and Research 157, DOI 10.1007/978-1-4419-7073-2_2,
© Springer Science+Business Media, LLC 2011

mainly in the bone marrow (BM). At the origin of this hierarchy lies a comparatively rare population of ~50 million pluripotent hematopoietic stem cells (HSCs) [1]. HSCs are normally quiescent or cycle very slowly. When stimulated to proliferate, they undergo a series of asymmetric cell divisions and fate decisions during which they gradually lose the potential to execute one or more developmental options. This leads to the generation of a heterogeneous pool of multipotent, tripotent, bipotent, and ultimately unipotent progenitor cells that are committed to differentiate into one of the eight lineages of morphologically identifiable cells in the peripheral blood. In addition to their extensive capacity for proliferation and multilineage differentiation, HSCs have the ability to self-renew thus preventing exhaustion of the stem cell pool and ensuring that an adequate supply of blood cells can be produced for the lifetime of the individual.

At the level of each individual stem or progenitor cell, the probability of executing any one of these developmental options, or of dying by apoptosis, is tightly regulated by a network of glycoprotein hormones known as the hematopoietic growth factors (HGFs). HGFs exhibit a general hierarchical organization in their actions that mirrors that of the cellular elements of the hematopoietic system. However, there is considerable overlap in target cell populations and some cytokines that were originally thought to act only on lineage-committed progenitor cells or their progeny are now known to have multiple levels of activity, including on the most primitive HSCs (e.g., thrombopoietin; TPO). Conversely, some factors that were initially thought to act only on multipotential cells were found to stimulate the proliferation of mature cells (e.g., stem cell factor; SCF). Thus, pleiotropy and redundancy have emerged as dominant themes.

Most HGFs are produced by macrophages, fibroblasts, osteoblasts, and endothelial cells that comprise the BM microenvironment. These so-called stromal cells also express adhesion molecules that serve to physically retain stem and progenitor cells within "niches," thus co-localizing them with factors that regulate the earliest events in their development. The action of HGFs to promote proliferation and differentiation is balanced by that of various inhibitory factors that attenuate the proliferation response once physiological demand is satisfied. The opposing activities of these positive and negative regulators on various cell types can be further modulated in a concentration-dependent manner and depending on the context in which they are presented to the target cell, i.e., either alone or in combination with other cytokines, and whether the growth factor is secreted or bound to the surface of stromal cells.

Since the regulatory approval and commercial launch of the first recombinant human (rHu) HGFs in the early-mid-1990s, several such agents have been administered to millions of patients. Much attention has been focused on the late-acting cytokines such as erythropoietin (EPO), granulocyte colony-stimulating factor (G-CSF), and TPO because these have proven to be most useful for the treatment of different cytopenias. Comparatively little attention has been given to early-acting factors as these have in general not made a large therapeutic impact or proven to be as commercially successful. Moreover, discovery of the "holy grail" of experimental hematology, the putative stem cell-specific self-renewal factor, has remained elusive (indeed current evidence suggests it may not exist at all). Nevertheless, early-acting HGFs, defined herein as cytokines with actions on multipotential cells, exhibit an array of interesting activities and their therapeutic utility remains to be fully explored. In this chapter, the biology of the most well-characterized early-acting HGFs will be reviewed with particular emphasis on those that have been investigated in the clinic.

Stem Cell Factor (SCF)

The history of the discovery of SCF originates early in the last century with the description of the dominant White spotting (*W*) locus in mice. Mice bearing any of the ~20 allelic variants of the *W* gene exhibit multiple defects including macrocytic anemia [2]. The identification of another mutation, designated Steel (*Sl*), with a virtually identical phenotype but localized to a different chromosome led to the hypothesis that these loci may represent a receptor/ligand pair. Confirmation of his hypothesis was obtained in 1988, when two groups simultaneously showed that the *W* locus encoded a tyrosine kinase receptor, c-kit, with the same general structure as the receptors for macrophage colony-stimulating factor (M-CSF), Flt3 ligand (Flt3L), and platelet-derived growth factor [3, 4]. This ignited a vigorous race to identify the cognate ligand that culminated with the cloning of the mouse, rat, and human SCF genes simultaneously by three groups in 1990 [5–7]. Though named differently by each team, SCF (c-kit ligand [KL], steel factor, or mast cell growth factor [MGF]) was found to be a 248 amino acid type I transmembrane protein that also undergoes proteolytic cleavage to generate a ~165 amino acid secreted ligand, both of which are biologically active [5, 6, 8]. Alternative mRNA splicing appears to be an additional mechanism for producing soluble or membrane-bound forms of SCF. The ratio of these isoforms differs between tissues, but the physiological relevance of this phenomenon is unknown. Cell-bound SCF is required for normal development since mice bearing the Steel-Dickie (*Sl^d*) mutation that eliminates only this form of the factor exhibit several developmental abnormalities [9]. Moreover, when cDNAs encoding either form of human SCF were transfected into *Sl/Sl* stromal cells, the membrane-bound form of SCF was better able to support human hematopoietic cells in vitro than secreted SCF [10]. The amino acid sequences of the mouse and human proteins are 82% identical, but while murine SCF is fully active on human cells, human SCF is ~1,000-fold less active on rodent cells than murine SCF [6]. Native SCF is glycosylated [11]. The recombinant human protein produced for clinical studies in *Escherichia coli* (see below) is non-glycosylated but identical to the native amino acid sequence except for the presence of an N-terminal methionine (met).

SCF (together with Flt3L discussed below) exemplifies a distinct group of early-acting HGFs that have little or no growth-promoting activity as single agents, but which selectively promote the survival of primitive hematopoietic cells including stem cells with long-term repopulating ability [12, 13]. However, SCF can synergize with most other HGFs in vitro to directly enhance stem and progenitor cell proliferation [14–16]. In such cultures, SCF increases the number and size of the colonies produced, but their composition typically reflects the later-acting lineage-associated cytokines that are present. In vivo administration of recombinant SCF to *Sl/Sl^d* mice ameliorates their anemia, which reappears upon cessation of treatment. The number of granulocytes, monocytes, platelets, and lymphocytes also increases above normal levels [17]. Early after administration of SCF to normal mice, circulating neutrophil counts increase modestly and primitive clonogenic cells are mobilized to the peripheral blood from which they redistribute to peripheral sites such as the spleen [18]. BM stem and progenitor cells also begin to proliferate so that their numbers may be greatly expanded after ~2 weeks. These effects are much more pronounced when SCF is combined with G-CSF, resulting in greater than additive increases in circulating neutrophils and enhanced mobilization of stem/progenitor cells that are capable of rescuing mice, dogs, and non-human primates from lethal irradiation [19–21]. Mast cells are the most dependent on SCF for their survival, proliferation, maturation, and function. SCF increases mast cell numbers in *Sl* (but not *W*) mutant mice as well as in normal rodents and non-human primates [22].

Based on these preclinical data, clinical development of r-metHuSCF (ancestim, STEMGEN®) focused on its use in combination with r-metHuG-CSF (filgrastim, NEUPOGEN®) to optimally mobilize hematopoietic stem and progenitor cells for transplantation after myeloablative therapy in cancer patients. Results of these clinical studies have been reviewed in detail [23]. Briefly, in phase I/II studies of patients with breast cancer, non-Hodgkin's lymphoma, and ovarian cancer, 5 μg/kg/day rHuSCF as a single agent did not induce significant mobilization. However, when combined with r-metHuG-CSF, r-metHuSCF improved apheresis yields by twofold to threefold. The numbers of circulating $CD34^+$ cells and in vitro colony-forming cells (CFCs) then returned to pretreatment levels usually within 4–7 days after cessation of treatment. In the pivotal phase III trial, a greater proportion of breast cancer patients treated with 20 μg/kg/day r-metHuSCF plus 10 μg/kg/day filgrastim achieved the target yield of 5×10^6 $CD34^+$ cells/kg for autologous transplantation than did patients treated with filgrastim alone (63% vs. 47%) [24] (Fig. 2.1). The improved mobilization with r-metHuSCF plus r-metHuG-CSF resulted in a statistically significant reduction in the number of aphereses required to collect the target number of peripheral blood stem/progenitor cells (median 4 vs. ≥ 6) and increased the number of patients for which a sufficient graft could be collected, compared to mobilization with r-metHuG-CSF alone. These clinical findings led to approval of STEMGEN® in Canada, Australia, and New Zealand as a co-administration with filgrastim for hematopoietic stem and progenitor cell mobilization. Consistent with the collateral effects of SCF in stimulating mast cell proliferation and degranulation, all patients require prophylactic administration of H1 and H2 antihistamines and a bronchodilator to ameliorate systemic anaphylactoid reactions.

In addition to stem cell mobilization, SCF has demonstrated utility in ex vivo expansion. Addition of SCF to cultures containing interleukin (IL)-3, IL-6, IL-11, TPO, granulocyte-macrophage colony-stimulating factor (GM-CSF), and other cytokines enhances the survival, proliferation, and differentiation of $CD34^+CD38^-$

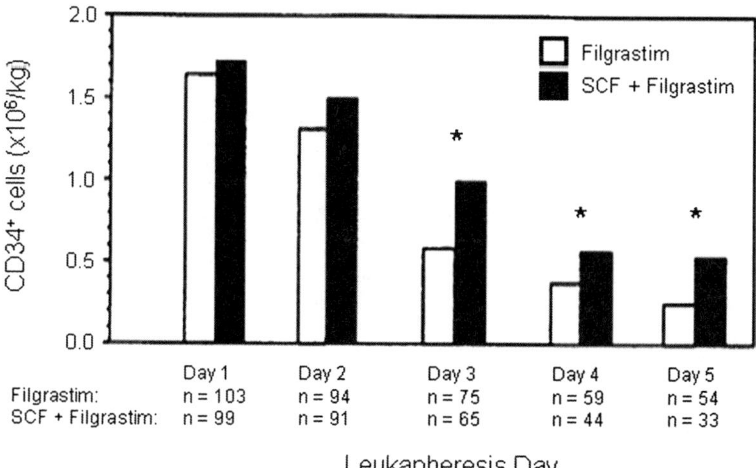

Fig. 2.1 SCF enhances the mobilization of hematopoietic cells by G-CSF. Shown is the median CD34$^+$ cell yield on each day of leukapheresis in patients mobilized with 10 μg/kg/day rHuG-CSF (filgrastim) alone or together with 20 μg/kg/day rHuSCF. Leukapheresis was started on day 5 after growth factor treatment (indicated as day 1) until the cumulative CD34$^+$ cell yield reached ≥5 × 10^6/kg or a maximum of 5 leukaphereses. Reproduced with permission from Ref. [24]

candidate HSCs, long-term culture-initiating cells (LTC-IC), and stem cells with long-term repopulating ability [25–27]. Expanded hematopoietic cells have been used to accelerate the rate of hematopoietic reconstitution after transplantation [28, 29] and to support repetitive cycles of high-dose chemotherapy thus eliminating the need for additional BM harvests or leukaphereses [30]. Ex vivo expansion may also extend the application of umbilical cord blood stem cell transplantation to adult patients for whom the number of HSCs in a typical cord blood unit is often insufficient to facilitate engraftment or enable the purging from autologous stem cell preparations of contaminating tumor cells that can contribute to disease relapse following transplantation. Finally, SCF is being used extensively in the developing field of gene therapy where it offers an advantage over late-acting HGFs in better preserving the engraftment potential of the targeted stem cells during their infection with viral vectors in vitro.

Flt3 Ligand (Flt3L)

Like SCF, the discovery of Flt3L began with the identification of its receptor, fms-like tyrosine kinase 3 or flt3 [31]. Murine flt3 was used as a probe to identify the murine [32, 33] and human [33, 34] ligands, which were found to be 72% identical at the amino acid level. Flt3L has many features in common with SCF. Like SCF, Flt3L is a type I transmembrane glycoprotein, the mature form of which is composed of 209 amino acids in man. The membrane-bound isoform is predominant and biologically active, though like SCF, rare alternative isoforms resulting from alternative splicing have been reported and an active soluble protein is produced by proteolytic cleavage [32]. The form of rHuFlt3L used in clinical studies described below is truncated (153 aa) and glycosylated with a molecular weight of 18–29 kDa. Unlike SCF, Flt3L does not exhibit any species specificity and human Flt3L is equally potent on rodent, rabbit, and non-human primate cells.

Flt3L is produced at highest levels in the BM and expression is further upregulated by conditions that damage the HSC compartment (e.g., radiation). Although SCF and Flt3L overlap considerably in their biological actions, there are notable differences. For example, murine long-term repopulating HSCs are c-kit$^+$ but flt3-negative and upregulate the receptor only upon activation and maturation [35]. However, in a rare example of differences between the mouse and human hematopoietic systems, human HSCs capable of engrafting immunodeficient mice are flt3$^+$ [36, 37]. Expression of flt3 is then progressively downregulated during myeloid differentiation and is shut off completely prior to erythroid commitment. Flt3 is also absent on mast cells so it does not exhibit the anaphylactic effects of SCF in vivo. Similar to SCF, as a single agent Flt3L promotes the survival rather than proliferation of HSCs but synergizes with virtually all the other HGFs, including SCF, to enhance their activities [38–40]. However, when directly compared to SCF as a supplement to otherwise identical cytokine combinations, Flt3L is often less potent, generating slightly fewer and smaller colonies than those observed with SCF-containing cocktails. This is consistent with the absence of Flt3 on more primitive clonogenic cells, at least in mice, as discussed above.

In vivo administration of rHuFlt3L results in the expansion of hematopoietic progenitor populations in the BM and their mobilization into the blood [41]. Stem cell mobilization induced by G-CSF is increased ∼fivefold by co-administration of Flt3L, and mobilized stem/progenitor cells retain the ability to reconstitute hematopoiesis after transplantation [42]. Injection of Flt3L into mice also increases the number of immature B cells, monocytes, and natural killer (NK) cells in the BM and blood and induces the appearance of dendritic cells (DCs) in the spleen and secondary lymphoid tissues. The expansion of DCs is particularly significant as these cells are among the most efficient at presenting processed antigens to cytotoxic T cells (CTL), resulting in their activation and proliferation to mediate antitumor and antiviral immune responses. DCs have been used as vaccine vectors for cancer and infectious diseases, but success is limited by their low abundance in peripheral blood and lymphoid tissues. Administration of Flt3L has beneficial effects in preclinical cancer models [43, 44], but maximal efficacy is probably limited by the fact that the DCs generated by Flt3L alone are immature [45]. Combination therapy with CD40 ligand (CD40L), a potent inducer of DC maturation that is required to promote the development and expansion of antigen-specific CTL, has been shown to significantly improve antitumor immunity [46] (Fig. 2.2).

Based on these preclinical data, clinical studies were conducted to assess the ability of Flt3L to improve the yield of stem/progenitor cells for stem cell mobilization,

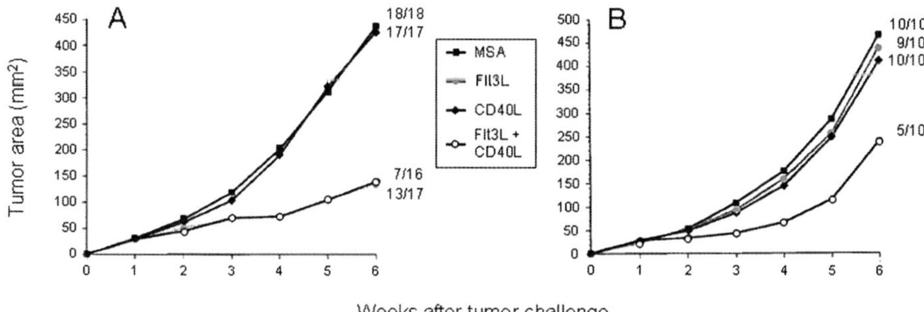

Fig. 2.2 Combination treatment with Flt3L and CD40L inhibits the growth of murine tumors in vivo. **Panel a**: C57BL/6 mice were transplanted 5×10^5 B10.2 sarcoma cells and treated for 19 days with mouse serum albumin (MSA; 0.1 μg/day), Flt3L (10 μg/day), CD40L (10–30 μg/day), or a combination of Flt3L (10 μg/day) and CD40L (10–30 μg/day). Treatments were started on the same day as the tumor cell inoculations. **Panel b**: C3H/HeN mice were transplanted 5×10^5 '87' sarcoma cells and treated with mouse serum albumin (MSA; 0.1 μg/day), Flt3L (10 μg/day), CD40L (10 μg/day), or a combination of Flt3L and CD40L (each at 10 μg/day). Treatments were started on the day after tumor cell inoculation, except for CD40L either alone or in combination with Flt3L, which began 7 days after the initiation of MSA or Flt3L treatment. Mice were treated until day 20. The number of tumor-bearing mice as a fraction of all animals per treatment group is indicated for the last time point. Reproduced with permission from Ref. [46]

as a stand-alone immunotherapeutic agent for cancer patients or as an adjuvant for cancer or infectious diseases. As in animals, administration of Flt3L alone induced dose-dependent increases in circulating neutrophils, monocytes, CD34⁺ cells, B cells, and plasmacytoid and conventional DCs. Combining Flt3L with r-metHuG-CSF (NEUPOGEN®) or rHuGM-CSF (sargramostim, LEUKINE®) resulted in increased stem cell mobilization in "hard to mobilize" patients with non-Hodgkin's lymphoma (NHL) but had limited effects in "easy to mobilize" patients with breast cancer. When combined with chemotherapy in patients with hormone-refractory prostate cancer, NHL, or metastatic melanoma, Flt3L treatment led to increased numbers of monocytes and DCs in the peripheral blood. However, there was no effect on tumor response rates perhaps, as noted in preclinical studies, because the DCs that were generated in vivo were immature. In numerous studies in which Flt3L was tested in the vaccine adjuvant setting, it did not augment antigenicity when delivered in vivo prior to the vaccine. However, intriguing results were noted in one study when Flt3L was used to stimulate DC expansion in vivo, from which a vaccine was prepared ex vivo [47]. In this study, 12 patients were administered Flt3L at different dosing schedules to expand DCs prior to collection of peripheral blood cells, which were then primed with tumor antigen in culture. Following reinfusion of tumor antigen-primed DCs, seven patients developed tumor-specific CTL and five patients had their tumors regress though they did not receive any other cancer treatment during this time (Fig. 2.3). Although CTL activity after vaccination did not correlate directly with clinical responses, both the percent and fold expansion of vaccine-induced CD8⁺ T cells did.

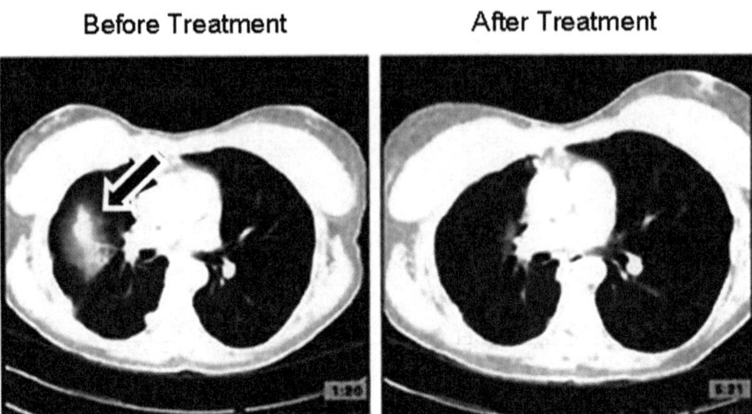

Fig. 2.3 Tumor regression in a cancer patient treated with a DC vaccine generated ex vivo following in vivo treatment with Flt3L. Computed tomography scans were performed within 1 month before the first DC vaccination (*left*) and 4 months after the final DC vaccination (*right*) in a patient with progressive metastatic colorectal cancer. A growing lung metastasis (*black arrow* in *left* scan) and malignant pleural effusion (not shown) that were evident before vaccination completely resolved after treatment. Reproduced with permission from Ref. [47]

For now, clinical development of rHuFlt3L has been discontinued, but preclinical research continues in earnest. Recently, Flt3L was included among a list of 12 agents with the greatest potential to cure cancer by a National Cancer Institute workshop [48]. In addition to the uses described above, other applications of Flt3L (as with SCF) include gene therapy to improve HSC transduction efficiency with viral vectors and ex vivo expansion. The recent finding that common lymphoid progenitors (CLPs), but not HSCs or common myeloid progenitors (CMPs), are reduced ~tenfold in Flt3L knock-out mice [49] suggests its potential utility in driving CLP expansion as a means to accelerate the typically slow rate of lymphoid reconstitution that follows allogeneic transplantation in particular or as a prophylactic therapy for infection in neonates or the elderly who often have dampened immunity. The promise of this agent remains high, and there is an obvious need for further studies.

Thrombopoietin (TPO)

TPO is the seminal regulator of megakaryocyte differentiation and platelet production that is constitutively produced mainly in the liver. TPO was first postulated to exist in 1958 [50], well before the gene was cloned by five groups simultaneously in 1994 [51–55]. Purified recombinant TPO was confirmed to be the ligand for the orphan cytokine receptor, c-mpl (the cellular homolog of the myeloproliferative leukemia virus oncogene, v-mpl), whose expression is restricted to primitive hematopoietic cells, megakaryocytes, and platelets. Human TPO comprises a total of 332 amino acids and nearly half of its ~70 kDa mass is contributed by N-linked and O-linked carbohydrates [52–54]. Sugars are attached predominantly to the 181 amino acid C-terminal domain that lacks any sequence similarity to other HGFs and serves to enhance secretion of the protein from producer cells [56]. An N-terminal domain of 153 amino acids has some sequence similarity to EPO and is sufficient for biological activity in vitro [53]. The basic biology of TPO, its late-acting effects on megakaryocytopoiesis, and the clinical development of rHuTPO and second-generation mpl ligands (e.g., romiplostim, Nplate$^{®}$) for the treatment of thrombocytopenia are described in detail elsewhere in this volume. I will focus here on the early actions of TPO on primitive HSCs, which have only recently been described in mechanistic detail and have not as yet been exploited for therapeutic purposes.

The effect of TPO on non-megakaryocytic lineages was obvious from early studies characterizing *TPO*-deficient and *c-mpl*-deficient mice. As expected, both knock-out strains had reduced numbers of megakaryocytic progenitor cells (CFU-Mk) in the BM and spleen, a lower average ploidy of surviving megakaryocytes, and ~85% fewer circulating platelets. Significantly, however, the number of mul-tipotential and committed myeloid and erythroid progenitors in the BM, spleen, and peripheral blood was also reduced [57, 58], suggesting that TPO exerts either direct or indirect actions on multipotential stem cells. This was supported by studies demonstrating that administration of recombinant TPO or megakaryocyte growth and development factor (MGDF, a non-glycosylated and truncated version of TPO that is covalently conjugated to polyethylene glycol [PEG] to enhance the stability of the molecule) to normal or myelosuppressed mice resulted in the expansion of CFU-GM and BFU-E (as well as CFU-Mk) and reduced the sever-ity of chemotherapy-induced or radiation-induced leukopenia and anemia [59, 60]. TPO was shown to act directly in single cell cultures of highly enriched murine long-term repopulating HSCs. In combination with other early-acting HGFs (e.g., SCF, Flt3L, IL-3, IL-6), TPO enhanced HSC survival, accelerated the timing of the first cell division, and synergistically increased the number and size of multilin-eage colonies [61–64]. Solar et al. [65] found that ~50–70% of murine fetal liver AA4.1^{+}Sca-1^{+}c-kit^{+} cells, murine BM-derived Sca-1^{+}c-kit^{+}Lin^{-} cells, and human BM CD34^{+}CD38^{-} cells expressed the c-mpl protein. As shown in Table 2.1 for human stem cells, when these were fractionated into mpl^{-} and mpl^{+} populations, essentially all of the HSCs able to reconstitute hematopoiesis in vivo were recovered in the mpl^{+} fraction [65].

The molecular mechanisms underlying these actions of TPO on HSCs are begin-ning to be deciphered (Fig. 2.4). TPO was recently shown to modulate HoxB4 and HoxA9, members of a homeodomain-containing family of transcription factors that are expressed at high levels in HSCs and are critical for self-renewal. The level of HoxB4 mRNA is ~threefold lower in mouse stem cells (Sca-1^{+}c-kit^{+}Gr-1^{-}) from *TPO*$^{-/-}$ vs. wild-type mice. TPO increases HoxB4 mRNA levels in a p38-dependent manner in a cell line engineered to express human *c-mpl* [66]. TPO also induces the importation of HoxA9 into the nucleus, in this case without altering overall levels, where it can physically associate with the co-factor MEIS1 (myeloid ecotropic viral integration site 1) whose expression is also increased by TPO [67].

Table 2.1 Human hematopoietic stem cells with in vivo repopulating ability express the TPO receptor (c-mpl)

Cell phenotype	Study no.	No. of mice engrafted	Donor HLA/CD34 (%)	Donor HLA/CD33 (%)	Donor HLA/CD19 (%)
CD34+CD38−	1	3/5	8.4 ± 2.8	14.3 ± 5.3	64.2 ± 11.3
CD34+CD38−c-mpl+	1	5/5	22.7 ± 5.7	18.9 ± 3.6	67.6 ± 2.5
CD34+CD38−c-mpl−	1	1/4	4.2	12.5	18.9
CD34+CD38−	2	3/5	7.9 ± 1.2	17.7 ± 4.2	48.5 ± 3.3
CD34+CD38−c-mpl+	2	4/5	27.8 ± 3.5	12.9 ± 4.9	59.3 ± 9.6
CD34+CD38−c-mpl−	2	1/5	1.8	5.6	5.9

Immunodeficient *scid/scid* mice were implanted with human fetal bone marrow fragments and then injected with 3×10^4 adult bone marrow-derived CD34+CD38− hematopoietic stem cells that had been separated into c-mpl− or c-mpl+ fractions by fluorescence-activated cell sorting. The progeny of transplanted human HSCs was distinguished from cells comprising the human fetal bone graft and host mouse cells by expression of a donor-specific human leukocyte antigen (HLA). In contrast to c-mpl− cells that contributed rarely to only low levels to hematopoiesis, c-mpl+ HSCs could regenerate large numbers of stem/progenitor (HLA/CD34), myeloid (HLA/CD33), and B lymphoid cells in the majority of transplanted recipients. Reproduced with permission from Ref. [65].

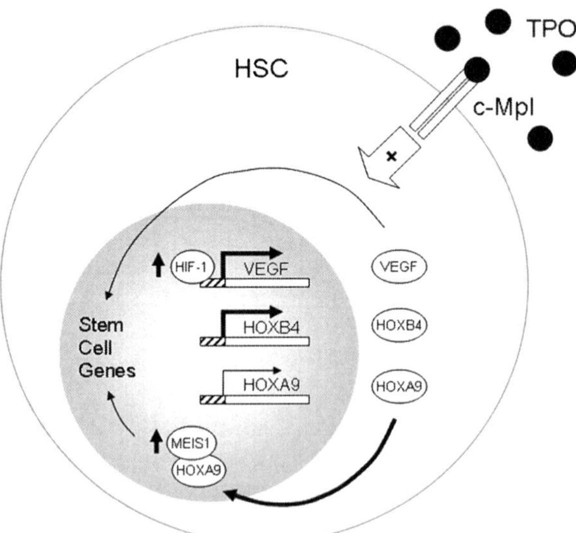

Fig. 2.4 TPO stimulates an intracellular circuit to promote the survival and proliferation of hematopoietic stem cells. TPO binding to its cell surface receptor, c-mpl, initiates signals that increase transcription of VEGF (through enhanced synthesis and stabilization of HIF-α) and HOXB4. Nuclear import of HOXA9 protein is also enhanced facilitating its interaction with MEIS1, transcription of which is also stimulated by TPO. Together these signals increase the expression of diverse "stemness" genes that play key roles in HSC development

Finally, TPO increases the synthesis and stabilization of hypoxia-inducible factor (HIF)-1α, the primary transcription factor responsible for expression of vascular endothelial growth factor (VEGF), which in addition to being the principal regulator of blood vessel formation, also controls HSC survival and repopulating potential through an intracellular autocrine loop [68]. This is consistent with the fact that compared to other tissues, under physiological conditions the marrow is somewhat hypoxic, and exposure of human HSCs to low oxygen tension in vitro leads to an increase in HIF-1 expression and in vivo repopulating ability [69]. Enriched HSCs from $TPO^{-/-}$ mice express ~fivefold lower levels of VEGF mRNA than wild-type mice but VEGF expression can be induced by TPO [70]. Pharmacologic blockade of VEGF receptor kinase activity in cultures of single BM stem cells significantly reduced the ability of TPO to promote their survival and proliferation in vitro [70]. Taken together, these findings paint a complex picture of TPOs action on HSCs and provide an interesting example of how a secreted HGF can modulate stem cell development by influencing the production of an array of transcription factors.

Leukemia Inhibitory Factor (LIF)

LIF was originally named for its ability to induce differentiation and suppress proliferation of a murine myeloid leukemia cell line, M1. However, with the breadth of activities that have now been ascribed to LIF [71], the most interesting of which are arguably outside of the hematopoietic system, it is somewhat misleading to refer to this hormone as a hematopoietic growth factor, at least in the same vane as the other cytokines described herein and elsewhere in this volume. Mice harboring only one or no intact copies of the *LIF* gene do have reduced numbers of hematopoietic progenitor cells, proportional to *LIF* copy number and which can be normalized by administration of recombinant LIF, but the number of circulating erythrocytes, leukocytes, and platelets is normal. Furthermore, $LIF^{-/-}$ BM and spleen cells exhibit normal hematopoietic repopulating ability in vivo, indicating that LIF is not required for the maintenance of primitive HSCs [72]. Thus while LIF can act directly on lineage-committed progenitors and differentiated cells as described below, more primitive HSCs do not express LIF receptors [73] and LIFs action on these cells appears to be indirect.

Structurally, LIF is similar to many other HGFs, comprised of a single 4-α-helix polypeptide chain of 179 amino acids with ~79% sequence identity between mouse and human proteins [74]. Human LIF acts on mouse, non-human primate, and human cells, but murine LIF is species-restricted in its action. The molecule is heavily glycosylated, resulting in a molecular mass ranging from 38 to 67 kDa, but this is not required for biological activity in vivo. LIF mRNA is transcribed in multiple organs, but of most relevance to its hematopoietic actions, LIF protein is produced by a variety of BM mesenchymal and immune system cells, including fibroblasts, monocytes/macrophages, endothelial cells, and activated T cells, among others [75]. It is thought to be produced constitutively in many tissues but can be upregulated by other cytokines (e.g., IL-1, IL-6, IL-8, and tumor necrosis factor

[TNF]-α) as part of a generalized pro-inflammatory response. The primary form of the protein is secreted, but like SCF and Flt3L, an immobilized form that associates with the extracellular matrix can be generated by alternative splicing [76]. LIF is not normally detected in the serum, due to its sequestration by circulating soluble LIF receptors. This serves to restrict LIFs action to local sites of production and helps explain how such a pleiotropic factor can elicit unique responses in different organs without simultaneous effects on other tissues.

As a single agent, LIF does not stimulate progenitors of any hematopoietic lineage. In combination with other cytokines, LIF also has no effects on in vitro colony-forming cells, with the exception of augmenting proliferation of murine megakaryocytic progenitors stimulated with IL-3 [77] and late-stage myeloid progenitors (CFU-GM, CFU-M) stimulated with IL-3, GM-CSF, M-CSF, and SCF [78]. However, addition of LIF to stromal cell-based cultures significantly improves the maintenance of HSCs with competitive long-term in vivo repopulating ability [79]. LIF appears to act indirectly because alone it does not support the proliferation of enriched HSCs in stroma-free cultures. Rather, LIF induces the expression of multiple HGFs (IL-1, IL-2, and IL-6; G-CSF and GM-CSF; transforming growth factors; SCF; and LIF itself), of which IL-6 and SCF have been shown to be able to substitute for LIF in stimulating stem cell proliferation [79].

The first study of LIFs actions in vivo employed mice that were chronically exposed to high levels by transplanting them with a LIF-producing hematopoietic cell line. These animals died relatively rapidly of a syndrome characterized by diverse hematopoietic and non-hematopoietic abnormalities, again highlighting the pleiotropic nature of this molecule [80, 81]. In subsequent studies in which purified recombinant protein was injected into mice to more carefully control the exposure profile, LIF stimulated a rise in megakaryocyte and platelet numbers and a tenfold increase in megakaryocytic progenitor cells in the spleen that peaked after 7–10 days [82]. Notably, the half-life of injected LIF was extremely short (<1 h), most likely due to clearance of the molecule by binding to circulating LIF receptors as described above. LIF was studied intensively in mice and non-human primates to identify a potential therapeutic use in HSC transplantation or amelioration of chemotherapy-induced thrombocytopenia (CIT). It is worth remembering that at this time TPO had only recently been cloned and studies to evaluate its clinical utility had not yet been completed so the therapeutic value of other thrombopoietic agents was of great interest. In non-myelosuppressed mice, as little as 0.2 μg/day rHuLIF increased platelet counts, but at tenfold higher doses this was associated with remarkable body weight loss. In carboplatin-treated mice, 4 μg/day rHuLIF beginning 24 h after chemotherapy stimulated the recovery of platelet counts beginning on day 5 [83]. Recombinant HuLIF also stimulated the expansion of hematopoietic progenitor cells in vivo and resulted in significantly faster recovery of circulating platelets and leukocytes when BM from LIF-treated mice was transplanted into lethally irradiated syngeneic hosts [84]. In rhesus monkeys, rHuLIF dose-dependently increased platelet counts with peak levels of ~twofold above normal observed on day 11 after treatment [85]. This effect was similar to that elicited by rHuIL-6, which was also being evaluated as a thrombopoietic drug at that time, but considerably less than that obtained with rHuTPO. LIF did not induce changes in leukocyte counts or the number of progenitor cells in the peripheral blood.

Recombinant HuLIF (emfilermin) was studied in a phase I clinical trial to promote platelet recovery in patients with advanced cancer [86]. As observed previously in animals, the half-life of rHuLIF in humans was very short (1–5 h). Two patients who were injected with 4 μg/kg rHuLIF three times daily for 7 days, but who had not received chemotherapy or any other HGFs, exhibited >tenfold increases in CFU-GM and BFU-E and a three or eightfold increase in CFU-Mk numbers in the peripheral blood. Circulating platelet levels in these patients increased 1.5-fold and 2-fold. The hematological actions of emfilermin were more apparent in the chemotherapy setting where it was administered for 7 days beginning on the day before or for 14 days beginning on the day after chemotherapy. In such patients, platelets recovered to baseline levels earlier and the neutrophil nadir was less severe at doses of ≥4 μg/kg/day of rHuLIF (Fig. 2.5) [86]. These modest hematological effects were accompanied by dose-limiting toxicities of hypotension and rigors. Clinical development of emfilermin has been halted so any potential future therapeutic applications of rHuLIF await the outcome of ongoing research.

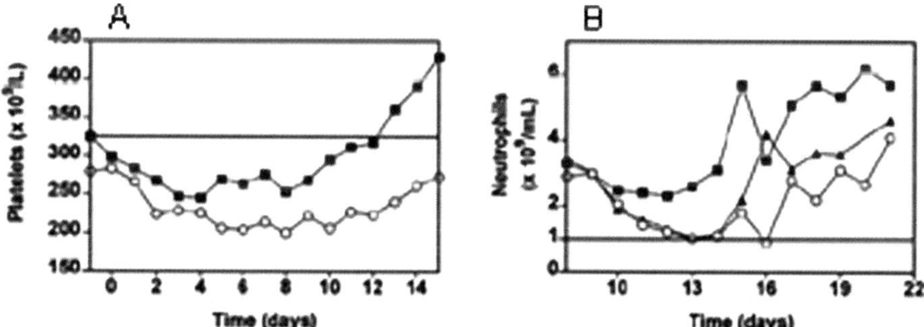

Fig. 2.5 Exposure to IL-3 *in vivo* abrogates the re-transplantation potential of human hematopoietic stem cells. Panel A: Human cord blood CD34+ cells (10⁵/mouse) were transplanted into immunodeficient *NOD/SCID* mice together with 5×10⁶ rat fibroblasts that were stably transfected with either a control vector (Rat-1) or a vector containing the human IL-3 gene (Rat-IL-3). Injection of the latter cells resulted in the presence of 3-5 ng/ml HuIL-3 in the mouse peripheral blood. Six to 9 weeks later the proportion of human cells (%HLA-I+) of hematopoietic origin (%CD45+) in the BM, and their contribution to T (CD2) and B (CD19) lymphoid, myeloid (CD14, CD33), and stem/progenitor (CD34, CD38) cell compartments was determined by flow cytometry. The data show that co-injection of IL-3-producing fibroblasts increased the level of human cell chimerism in primary recipients. Panel B: Six weeks after primary transplantation, BM cells were re-transplanted into secondary *NOD/SCID* mice (107/mouse) and the level of human cell engraftment observed 6-9 weeks later was analyzed as above. Despite the superior level of human cell engraftment observed in primary mice containing Rat-IL-3 cells, this was not maintained in secondary animals, indicating that HSCs were depleted during their prior exposure to IL-3 *in vivo*. Reproduced with permission from Nitsche *et al.* Stem Cells. 2003;21:236–244

Interleukin-3 (IL-3, Multi-CSF)

Murine interleukin IL-3 has the distinction of being the first hematopoietic cytokine that was cloned (in 1984) [87], followed shortly thereafter by the cloning of human IL-3 [88]. The 140 amino acid sequence of human and murine IL-3 is only 29% identical and they exhibit no species cross-reactivity in their actions. As with most HGFs, native IL-3 is glycosylated resulting in a molecular weight of the human factor of 23–30 kDa, but the carbohydrate component is not necessary for biological activity. One of many names originally assigned to this cytokine was "multi-CSF" because it exhibits an exceptionally broad range of proliferative effects on myeloid, erythroid, and megakaryocytic progenitors, eosinophils, mast cells, and multipotential stem cells. Given this polyfunctionality, it was surprising that *IL-3* knock-out mice exhibit no abnormalities in steady-state hematopoiesis [89] but this provides another example of the redundancy which characterizes many of the hematopoietic regulators. IL-3 is produced by activated T cells and various stromal cell populations such as monocytes/macrophages and mast cells in vitro. It is the primary component of "conditioned medium" that was used by early experimental hematologists to stimulate the proliferation of myeloid colony-forming cells before purified recombinant HGFs were widely available. Because IL-3 has been available for study so long, the literature describing its effects on hematopoietic cells is vast. Focusing here on its early actions on HSCs simplifies the survey, but reveals striking contradictions in the data as to whether IL-3 amplifies or depletes long-term hematopoietic repopulating ability [90]. Differences in the results of in vitro studies performed by different laboratories depend largely on the presence of serum in the culture system, which is generally (but not universally) deleterious to IL-3-stimulated HSC self-renewal. In serum-free cultures of highly enriched human and murine HSCs, the addition of IL-3 to optimized HGF cocktails can increase the yield of total cells and hematopoietic progenitors by >tenfold and long-term repopulating HSCs by ~threefold [91]. However, this effect in vitro is completely eliminated by the addition of serum. Definitive proof of the exhausting effect of IL-3 on long-term repopulating HSCs in vivo was provided by Nitsche et al. [92] who transplanted human CD34$^+$ cord blood cells into immunodeficient mice with or without a rat fibroblast cell line engineered to express human IL-3. Mice co-transplanted with IL-3-expressing fibroblasts were reconstituted to a higher level by human cells than mice injected with CD34$^+$ CB cells alone. However, when BM from these primary recipients was re-transplanted into secondary mice, human chimerism was virtually completely lost (Fig. 2.6), indicating that repopulating HSCs were depleted during their residence in the primary hosts where they were exposed to high levels of IL-3. This effect on long-term repopulating HSCs contrasts with that on more mature progenitor cells such as spleen colony-forming units (CFU-S), which expand >25-fold in animals perfused with IL-3 [93]. Expansion of the progenitor compartment is accompanied by moderate increases in the number of circulating neutrophils, eosinophils, monocytes, erythrocyte precursors, and particularly mast cells. This prompted investigation of the use of IL-3 to enhance hematological recovery in humans.

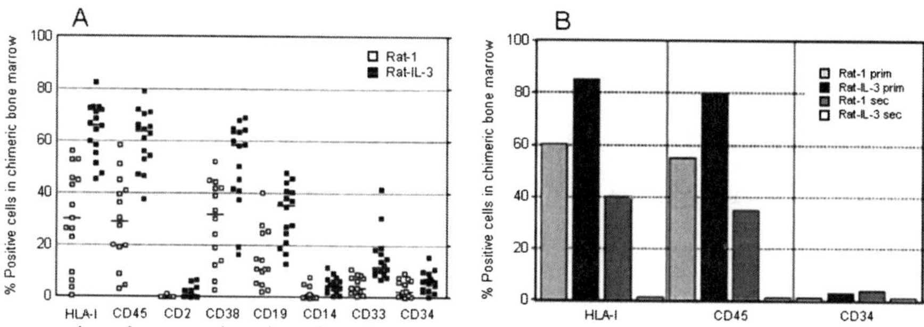

Fig. 2.6 Exposure to IL-3 in vivo abrogates the re-transplantation potential of human hematopoietic stem cells. **Panel a**: Human cord blood CD34$^+$ cells (10^5/mouse) were transplanted into immunodeficient *NOD/SCID* mice together with 5 × 10^6 rat fibroblasts that were stably transfected with either a control vector (Rat-1) or a vector containing the human *IL-3* gene (Rat-IL-3). Injection of the latter cells resulted in the presence of 3–5 ng/mL HuIL-3 in the mouse peripheral blood. Six to nine weeks later the proportion of human cells (%HLA-I$^+$) of hematopoietic origin (%CD45$^+$) in the BM, and their contribution to T (CD2) and B (CD19) lymphoid, myeloid (CD14, CD33), and stem/progenitor (CD34, CD38) cell compartments was determined by flow cytometry. The data show that co-injection of IL-3-producing fibroblasts increased the level of human cell chimerism in primary recipients. **Panel b**: Six weeks after primary transplantation, BM cells were re-transplanted into secondary *NOD/SCID* mice (10^7/mouse) and the level of human cell engraftment observed 6–9 weeks later was analyzed as above. Despite the superior level of human cell engraftment observed in primary mice containing Rat-IL-3 cells, this was not maintained in secondary animals, indicating that HSCs were depleted during their prior exposure to IL-3 in vivo. Reproduced with permission from Ref. [92]

A broad clinical development program was conducted throughout the 1990s to assess the therapeutic potential of human IL-3. Initial results of some phase I/II trials were promising, indicating that subcutaneous administration of 5–10 μg/kg rHuIL-3 daily for 5–10 days in patients with various types of cancer either alone or as an adjunct to stem cell transplantation reduced chemotherapy delays in dose-intensive treatment regimens and induced faster regeneration of neutrophils and platelets [94]. However, these early data were not supported by larger phase III studies of IL-3 alone or in combination with other cytokines (e.g. G-CSF, GM-CSF) to enhance hematopoiesis following cancer therapy or in patients with myelodysplastic syndrome (MDS). This experience precipitated a period of particularly innovative research to produce novel synthetic cytokines that exhibited greater biological activity than native IL-3 but with fewer inflammatory side effects [94]. Thus were created Synthokine (SC-55494 or daniplestim), a potent IL-3 receptor agonist [95], and an array of hybrid factors wherein the *IL-3* gene was fused to genes encoding GM-CSF (PIXY321 or Pixykine) [96], G-CSF (Myelopoietin [MPO] or Leridistim) [97], TPO (Promegapoietin-1 or PMP) [98], or insulin-like growth factor (compound 406) [99]. These too were evaluated in vitro for their ability to increase the expansion of myeloid and megakaryocytic progenitor cells, in vivo in non-human primates and humans for their ability to mobilize hematopoietic stem/progenitor cells for transplantation, and as supportive care agents to promote hematological reconstitution following chemotherapy or radiation-induced myelo-suppression. Many proved moderately effective but were ultimately abandoned in favor of r-metHuG-CSF (filgrastim, NEUPOGEN®), rHuGM-CSF (sargramostim, LEUKINE®), and rHuEPO (epoetin alfa, EPOGEN®), which exhibited more desirable pharmacodynamic properties as discussed elsewhere in this volume and which have now been used in millions of patients for the treatment of neutropenia and anemia.

Summary

From the first studies demonstrating that certain HGFs exhibit early actions that reach to the apex of the hematopoietic hierarchy, and exemplified by the naming of c-kit ligand as "stem cell factor," scientists and clinicians have had high hopes for the therapeutic value of early-acting hematopoietins. It is therefore notable that 25 years after the discovery of the first cytokine with demonstrated actions on HSCs, none have proven to be revolutionizing medicines despite some utility as potentiators of the action of later-acting lineage-specific growth factors. This lack of clinical and commercial success underscores the reality that patients with cancer, MDS, and congenital or treatment-related cytopenias do not in fact succumb to their diseases because they harbor inadequate numbers of HSCs, even though the genetic lesion that led to disease may have in some cases originated in this cell compartment. Rather, patients die because of functional or quantitative deficiencies in the end products of stem cell proliferation and differentiation, namely mature erythrocytes, granulocytes, and platelets. Thus it is the HGFs that drive these later stages of hematopoiesis that have proven more clinically useful. Defective stem cell self-renewal is not in itself a terminal condition though molecules that enhance HSC replication without simultaneous differentiation may eventually find utility in niche therapies such as ex vivo expansion. Even for these applications, various intracellular signaling proteins and stem cell transcription factors (e.g., Wnt 3A, HOXB4) that have now been expressed in stable form and used as soluble factors have proven more effective than conventional early-acting HGFs, at least in an experimental setting. This is certainly not to imply that the early-acting HGFs are uninteresting or not worthy of additional study. LIF is critical for the maintenance of embryonic stem cell lines in vitro and will continue to play an important albeit supportive role in the burgeoning field of stem cell therapy and tissue engineering. In the nascent discipline of immunotherapy, Flt3L remains untested in humans under optimal conditions in which it is employed together with dendritic cell maturation factors. Finally, novel mpl ligands such as Nplate® (romiplostim) and Promacta® (eltrombopag), a non-peptidyl molecule, have also only recently been approved and these agents may, like TPO, activate key transcriptional and developmental pathways in early stem cells. Thus in many ways the potential utility of the early-acting factors is just beginning to be explored as the field of stem cell biology reaches its zenith – the next decade may yield interesting surprises.

References

1. Szilvassy SJ. The biology of hematopoietic stem cells. Arch Med Res. 2003;34:446–60.
2. Russell ES. Hereditary anemias of the mouse: a review for geneticists. Adv Genet. 1979;20:357–459.
3. Chabot B, Stephenson DA, Chapman VM, et al. The proto-oncogene *c-kit* encoding a transmembrane tyrosine kinase receptor maps to the mouse *W* locus. Nature. 1988;335:88–9.
4. Geissler EN, Ryan MA, Houseman DE. The dominant-white spotting (*W*) locus of the mouse encodes the *c-kit* proto-oncogene. Cell. 1988;55:185–92.
5. Huang E, Nocka K, Beier DR, et al. The hematopoietic growth factor KL is encoded by the *Sl* locus and is the ligand of the *c-kit* receptor, the gene product of the *W*locus. Cell. 1990;63:225–33.
6. Martin FH, Suggs SV, Langley KE, et al. Primary structure and functional expression of rat and human stem cell factor cDNAs. Cell. 1990;63:203–11.
7. Williams DE, Eisenman J, Baird A, et al. Identification of a ligand for the *c-kit* proto-oncogene. Cell. 1990;63:167–74.
8. Anderson DM, Lyman SD, Baird A, et al. Molecular cloning of mast cell growth factor, a hematopoietin that is active in both membrane bound and soluble forms. Cell. 1990;63:235–43.
9. Brannan CI, Lyman SD, Williams DE, et al. Steel–Dickie mutation encodes a c-kit ligand lacking transmembrane and cytoplasmic domains. Proc Natal Acad Sci USA. 1991;88:4671–4.
10. Toksoz D, Zsebo KM, Smith KA, et al. Support of human hematopoiesis in long-term bone marrow cultures by murine stromal cells selectively expressing the membrane-bound and secreted forms of the human homolog of the steel gene product, stem cell factor. Proc Natal Acad Sci USA. 1992;89.7350–4.
11. Zsebo KM, Wypych J, McNiece IK, et al. Identification, purification, and biological characterization of hematopoietic stem cell factor from buffalo rat liver-conditioned medium. Cell. 1990;63:195–201.
12. Li CL, Johnson GR. Stem cell factor enhances the survival but not the self-renewal of murine hematopoietic long-term repopulating cells. Blood. 1994;84:408–14.
13. Keller JR, Ortiz M, Ruscetti FW. Steel factor (c-kit ligand) promotes the survival of hematopoietic stem/progenitor cells in the absence of cell division. Blood. 1995;86:1757–64.
14. McNiece IK, Langley KE, Zsebo KM. Recombinant human stem cell factor synergizes with GM-CSF, G-CSF, IL-3 and Epo to stimulate human progenitor cells of the myeloid and the erythroid lineages. Blood. 1991;19:226–31.
15. Kobayashi M, Laver JH, Kato T, et al. Thrombopoietin supports proliferation of human primitive hematopoietic cells in synergy with steel factor and/or interleukin-3. Blood. 1996;88:429–36.
16. Bernstein ID, Andrews RG, Zsebo KM. Recombinant human stem cell factor enhances the formation of colonies by CD34$^+$ and CD34$^+$Lin$^-$ cells, and the generation of colony-forming cell progeny from CD34$^+$Lin$^-$ cells cultured with interleukin-3, granulocyte colony-stimulating factor, or granulocyte–macrophage colony-stimulating factor. Exp Hematol. 1991;77:2316–21.
17. Zsebo KM, Williams DA, Geissler EN, et al. Stem cell factor is encoded at the *Sl* locus of the mouse and is the ligand for the *c-kit* tyrosine kinase receptor. Cell. 1990;63:213–24.
18. Molineux G, Migdalska A, Szmitkowski M, et al. The effects on hematopoiesis of recombinant stem cell factor (ligand for *c-kit*) administered in vivo to mice either alone or in combination with granulocyte colony-stimulating factor. Blood. 1991;78:961–6.
19. Yan X-Q, Briddell R, Hartley C, et al. Mobilization of long-term hematopoietic reconstituting cells in mice by the combination of stem cell factor plus granulocyte colony-stimulating factor. Blood. 1994;84:795–9.

20. de Revel T, Appelbaum FR, Storb R, et al. Effects of granulocyte colony-stimulating factor and stem cell factor, alone and in combination, on the mobilization of peripheral blood cells that engraft lethally irradiated dogs. Blood. 1994;83:3795–9.
21. Andrews RG, Briddell RA, Knitter GH, et al. Rapid engraftment by peripheral blood progenitor cells mobilized by recombinant human stem cell factor and recombinant human granulocyte colony-stimulating factor in nonhuman primates. Blood. 1995;85:15–20.
22. Nocka K, Buck J, Levi E, et al. Candidate ligand for the c-kit transmembrane kinase receptor: KL, a fibroblast derived growth factor stimulates mast cells and erythroid progenitors. EMBO J. 1990;9:3287–94.
23. Lacerna L Jr, Sheridan WP, Basser R, et al. Stem cell factor. In: Ho AD, Haas R, Champlin RE, editors. Hematopoietic stem cell transplantation. New York, NY: Marcel Dekker Inc; 2000. pp. 31–46.
24. Shpall EJ, Wheeler CA, Turner SA, et al. A randomized phase 3 study of peripheral blood progenitor cell mobilization with stem cell factor and filgrastim in high-risk breast cancer patients. Blood. 1999;93:2491–501.
25. Brandt J, Briddell RA, Srour EF, et al. Role of *c-kit* ligand in the expansion of human hematopoietic progenitor cells. Blood. 1992;79:634–41.
26. Holyoake TL, Freshney MG, McNair L, et al. Ex vivo expansion with stem cell factor and interleukin-11 augments both short-term recovery post-transplant and the ability to serially transplant marrow. Blood. 1996;87:4589–95.
27. Möhle R, Kanz L. Hematopoietic growth factors for hematopoietic stem cell mobilization and expansion. Semin Hematol. 2007;44:193–202.
28. McNiece IM, Jones R, Bearman SI, et al. Ex vivo expanded peripheral blood progenitor cells provide rapid neutrophils recovery after high-dose chemotherapy in patients with breast cancer. Blood. 2000;96:3001–7.
29. Prince HM, Simmons PJ, Whitty G, et al. Improved haematopoietic recovery following transplantation with ex vivo-expanded mobilized blood cells. Br J Haematol. 2004;126: 536–45.
30. Brugger W, Heimfeld S, Berenson RJ, et al. Reconstitution of hematopoiesis after high-dose chemotherapy by autologous progenitor cells generated ex vivo. N Engl J Med. 1995;333:283–7.
31. Rosnet O, Marchetto S, deLapeyriere O, et al. Murine *flt3*, a gene encoding a novel tyrosine kinase receptor of the PDGFR/CSF1R family. Oncogene. 1991;6:1641–50.
32. Lyman SD, James L, Vanden Bos T, et al. Molecular cloning of a ligand for the flt3/flk-2 tyrosine kinase receptor: a proliferative factor for primitive hematopoietic cells. Cell. 1993;75:1157–67.
33. Hannum C, Culpepper J, Campbell D, et al. Ligand for flt3/flk2 receptor tyrosine kinase regulates growth of haematopoietic stem cells and is encoded by variant RNAs. Nature. 1994;368:643–8.
34. Lyman SD, James L, Johnson L, et al. Cloning of the human homologue of the murine flt3 ligand: a growth factor for early hematopoietic progenitor cells. Blood. 1994;83:2795–801.
35. Christensen JL, Weissman IL. Flk-2 is a marker in hematopoietic stem cell differentiation: a simple method to isolate long-term stem cells. Proc Natl Acad Sci USA. 2001;98: 14541–6.
36. Sitnicka E, Buza-Vidas N, Larsson S, et al. Human CD34[+] hematopoietic stem cells capable of multilineage engrafting NOD/SCID mice express flt3: distinct flt3 and c-kit expression and response patterns on mouse and candidate human hematopoietic stem cells. Blood. 2003;102:881–6.
37. Kikushige Y, Yoshimoto G, Miyamoto T, et al. Human flt3 is expressed at the hematopoietic stem cell and the granulocyte/macrophage progenitor stages to maintain cell survival. J Immunol. 2008;180:7358–67.
38. Rasko JEJ, Metcalf D, Rossner MT, et al. The flt3/flk-2 ligand: receptor distribution and action on murine haemopoietic cell survival and proliferation. Leukemia. 1995;9:2058–66.

39. Jacobsen SEW, Okkenhaug C, Myklebust J, et al. The FLT3L potently and directly stimulates the growth and expansion of primitive murine bone marrow progenitor cells in vitro: synergistic actions with interleukin (IL) 11, IL-12, and other hematopoietic growth factors. J Exp Med. 1995;181:1357–63.

40. Broxmeyer HE, Lu L, Cooper S, et al. Flt3 ligand stimulates/costimulates the growth of myeloid stem/progenitor cells. Exp Hematol. 1995;23:1121–9.

41. Brasel K, McKenna HJ, Morrissey PJ, et al. Hematologic effects of flt3 ligand in vivo in mice. Blood. 1996;88:2004–12.

42. Molineux G, McCrea C, Yan XQ, et al. Flt-3 ligand synergizes with granulocyte colony-stimulating factor to increase neutrophils numbers and to mobilize peripheral blood stem cells with long-term repopulating potential. Blood. 1997;89:3998–4004.

43. Lynch DH, Andreasen A, Maraskovsky E, et al. Flt3 ligand induces tumor regression and antitumor immune responses in vivo. Nat Med. 1997;3:625–31.

44. Esche C, Subbotin VM, Maliszewski C, et al. FLT3 ligand administration inhibits tumor growth in murine melanoma and lymphoma. Cancer Res. 1998;58:380–3.

45. Reber AJ, Ashour AE, Robinson SN, et al. Flt3 ligand bioactivity and pharmacology in neoplasia. Curr Drug Targets – Immune Endocr Metabol Disord. 2004;4:149–57.

46. Borges L, Miller RE, Jones J, et al. Synergistic action of fms-like tyrosine kinase 3 ligand and CD40 ligand in the induction of dendritic cells and generation of antitumor immunity in vivo. J Immunol. 1999;163:1289–97.

47. Fong L, Hou Y, Rivas A, et al. Altered peptide ligand vaccination with Flt3 ligand expanded dendritic cells for tumor immunotherapy. Proc Natl Acad Sci USA. 2001;98:8809–14.

48. Cheever MA. Twelve immunotherapy drugs that could cure cancers. Immunol Rev. 2008;222:357–68.

49. Sitnicka E, Bryder D, Theilgaard-Mönch K, et al. Key role of flt3 ligand in regulation of the common lymphoid progenitor but not in maintenance of the hematopoietic stem cell pool. Immunity. 2002;17:463–72.

50. Keleman E, Cserhati I, Tanos B. Demonstration of some properties of human thrombopoietin in thrombocythaemic sera. Acta Haematologica. 1958;20:350–5.

51. Kato T, Ogami K, Shimada Y, et al. Purification and characterization of thrombopoietin. J Biochem. 1995;118:229–36.

52. Bartley TD, Bogenberger J, Hunt P, et al. Identification and cloning of a megakaryocyte growth and development factor that is a ligand for the cytokine receptor Mpl. Cell. 1994;77:1117–24.

53. de Sauvage FJ, Hass PE, Spencer SD, et al. Stimulation of megakaryocytopoiesis and thrombopoiesis by the c-Mpl ligand. Nature. 1994;369:533–8.

54. Lok S, Kaushansky K, Holly RD, et al. Cloning and expression of murine thrombopoietin cDNA and stimulation of platelet production in vivo. Nature. 1994;369:565–8.

55. Kuter DJ, Beeler DL, Rosenberg RD. The purification of megapoietin: a physiological regulator of megakaryocyte growth and platelet production. Proc Natl Acad Sci USA. 1994;91:11104–8.

56. Linden HM, Kaushansky K. The glycan domain of thrombopoietin enhances its secretion. Biochemistry. 2000;39:3044–51.

57. Alexander WS, Roberts AW, Nicola NA, et al. Deficiencies in progenitor cells of multiple hematopoietic lineages and effective megakaryocytopoiesis in mice lacking the thrombopoietin receptor c-mpl. Blood. 1996;87:2162–70.

58. Carver-Moore K, Broxmeyer HE, Luoh S-M, et al. Low levels of erythroid and myeloid progenitors in thrombopoietin- and c-mpl-deficient mice. Blood. 1996;88:803–8.

59. Kaushansky K, Lin N, Grossmann A, et al. Thrombopoietin expands erythroid, granulocyte–macrophage, and megakaryocytic progenitor cells in normal and myelosuppressed mice. Exp Hematol. 1996;24:265–9.

60. Hokom MM, Lacey D, Kinstler OB, et al. Pegylated megakaryocyte growth and development factor abrogates the lethal thrombocytopenia associated with carboplatin and irradiation in mice. Blood. 1995;86:4486–92.

61. Sitnicka E, Lin N, Priestley GV, et al. The effect of thrombopoietin on the proliferation and differentiation of murine hematopoietic stem cells. Blood. 1996;87:4998–5005.
62. Ku H, Yonemura Y, Kaushansky K, et al. Thrombopoietin, the ligand for the mpl receptor, synergizes with steel factor and other early acting cytokines in supporting proliferation of primitive hematopoietic progenitors in mice. Blood. 1996;87:4544–51.
63. Borge OJ, Ramsfjell V, Veiby OP, et al. Thrombopoietin, but not erythropoietin promotes viability and inhibits apoptosis of multipotent murine hematopoietic progenitor cells in vitro. Blood. 1996;88:2859–70.
64. Matsunaga T, Kato T, Miyazaki H, et al. Thrombopoietin promotes the survival of murine hematopoietic long-term reconstituting cells: comparison with the effects of Flt3/Flk-2 ligand and interleukin-6. Blood. 1998;92:452–61.
65. Solar GP, Kerr WG, Zeigler FC, et al. Role of c-mpl in early hematopoiesis. Blood. 1998;92:4–10.
66. Kirito K, Fox N, Kaushansky K. Thrombopoietin stimulates *Hoxb4* expression: an explanation for the favorable effects of TPO on hematopoietic stem cells. Blood. 2003;102:3172–8.
67. Kirito K, Fox N, Kaushansky K. Thrombopoietin induces HOXA9 nuclear transport in immature hematopoietic cells: potential mechanism by which the hormone favorably affects hematopoietic stem cells. Mol Cell Biol. 2004;24:6751–62.
68. Gerber HP, Malik AK, Solar GP, et al. VEGF regulates haematopoietic stem cell survival by an internal autocrine loop mechanism. Nature. 2002;417:954–8.
69. Danet GH, Pan Y, Luongo JL, et al. Expansion of human SCID-repopulating cells under hypoxic conditions. J Clin Invest. 2003;112:126–35.
70. Kirito K, Fox N, Komatsu N, et al. Thrombopoietin enhances expression of vascular endothelial growth factor (VEGF) in primitive hematopoietic cells through induction of HIF-1a. Blood. 2005;105:4258–63.
71. Metcalf D. The unsolved enigmas of leukemia inhibitory factor. Stem Cells. 2003;21:5–14.
72. Escary J-L, Perreau J, Duménil D, et al. Leukaemia inhibitory factor is necessary for maintenance of haematopoietic stem cells and thymocyte stimulation. Nature. 1993;363:361–4.
73. McKinstry WJ, Li C-L, Rasko JEJ, et al. Cytokine receptor expression on hematopoietic stem and progenitor cells. Blood. 1997;89:65–71.
74. Gough NM, Gearing DP, King JA, et al. Molecular cloning and expression of the human homologue of the murine gene encoding myeloid leukemia-inhibitory factor. Proc Natal Acad Sci USA. 1988;85:2623–7.
75. Chodorowska G, Glowacka A, Tomczyk M. Leukemia inhibitory factor (LIF) and its biological activity. Ann Univ Mariae Curie Sklodowska Med. 2004;59:189–93.
76. Rathjen PD, Toth S, Willis A, et al. Differentiation inhibiting activity is produced in matrix-associated and diffusible forms that are generated by alternate promoter usage. Cell. 1990;62:1105–14.
77. Metcalf D, Hilton D, Nicola NA. Leukemia inhibitory factor can potentiate murine megakaryocyte production in vitro. Blood. 1991;77:2150–3.
78. Keller JR, Gooya JM, Ruscetti FW. Direct synergistic effects of leukemia inhibitory factor on hematopoietic progenitor cell growth: comparison with other hematopoietins that use the gp130 receptor subunit. Blood. 1996;88:863–9.
79. Szilvassy SJ, Weller KP, Lin W, et al. Leukemia inhibitory factor upregulates cytokine expression by a murine stromal cell line enabling the maintenance of highly enriched competitive repopulating stem cells. Blood. 1996;87:4618–28.
80. Metcalf D, Gearing DP. Fatal syndrome in mice engrafted with cells producing high levels of the leukemia inhibitory factor. Proc Natl Acad Sci USA. 1989;86:5948–52.
81. Metcalf D, Gearing DP. A myelosclerotic syndrome in mice engrafted with cells producing high levels of leukemia inhibitory factor (LIF). Leukemia. 1989;3:847–52.
82. Metcalf D, Nicola NA, Gearing DP. Effects of injected leukemia inhibitory factor on hematopoietic and other tissues in mice. Blood. 1990;76:50–6.

83. Akiyama Y, Kikuchi Y, Matsuzaki J, et al. Protective effect of recombinant human leukemia inhibitory factor against thrombocytopenia in carboplatin-treated mice. Jpn J Cancer Res. 1997;88:584–9.
84. Pruijt JFM, Lindley IJD, Heemskerk DPM, et al. Leukemia inhibitory factor induces in vivo expansion of bone marrow progenitor cells that accelerate hematopoietic reconstitution but do not enhance radioprotection in lethally irradiated mice. Stem Cells. 1997;15: 50–55.
85. Mayer P, Geissler K, Ward M, et al. Recombinant human leukemia inhibitory factor induces acute phase proteins and raises the blood platelet counts in nonhuman primates. Blood. 1993;81:3226–33.
86. Gunawardana DH, Basser RL, Davis ID, et al. A phase I study of recombinant human leukemia inhibitory factor in patients with advanced cancer. Clin Cancer Res. 2003;9: 2056–65.
87. Fung MC, Hapel AJ, Ymer S, et al. Molecular cloning of cDNA for murine interleukin-3. Nature. 1984;307:233–7.
88. Yang YC, Ciarletta AB, Temple PA, et al. Human interleukin 3 multi-colony-stimulating factor identification by expression cloning of a novel hematopoietic growth factor related to murine interleukin 3. Cell. 1986;47:3–10.
89. Mach N, Lantz CS, Galli SJ, et al. Involvement of interleukin-3 in delayed-type hypersensitivity. Blood. 1998;91:778–83.
90. Ivanovic Z. Interleukin-3 and ex vivo maintenance of hematopoietic stem cells: facts and controversies. Eur Cytokine Netw. 2004;15:6–13.
91. Bryder D, Jacobsen SEW. Interleukin-3 supports expansion of long-term multilineage repopulating activity after multiple stem cell divisions in vitro. Blood. 2000;96:1748–55.
92. Nitsche A, Junghahn I, Thulke S, et al. Interleukin-3 promotes proliferation and differentiation of human hematopoietic stem cells but reduces their repopulation potential in NOD/SCID mice. Stem Cells. 2003;21:236–44.
93. Kindler V, Thorens B, Vassalli P. In vivo effect of murine recombinant interleukin 3 on early hematopoietic progenitors. Eur J Immunol. 1987;17:1511–14.
94. Mangi MH, Newland AC. Interleukin-3 in hematology and oncology: current state of knowledge and future directions. Cytokines Cell Mol Ther. 1999;5:87–95.
95. Ahmed N, Khokher MA, Hassan HT. Synthetic cytokines containing interleukin-3 exert potent megakaryocytic activity. Haematologica. 2000;30:167–76.
96. Vadhan-Raj S. PIXY321 (GM-CSF/IL-3 fusion protein): biology and early clinical development. Stem Cells. 1994;12:253–61.
97. Nabholtz J-M, Cantin J, Chang J, et al. Phase III trial comparing granulocyte colony-stimulating factor to leridistim in breast cancer patients treated with docetaxel/doxorubicin/cyclophosphamide: results of the BCIRG 004 trial. Clin Breast Cancer. 2002;3:268–75.
98. Farese AM, Smith WG, Giri JG, et al. Promegapoietin-1a, an engineered chimeric IL-3 and mpl-L receptor agonist, stimulates hematopoietic recovery in conventional and abbreviated schedules following radiation-induced myelosuppression in nonhuman primates. Stem Cells. 2001;19:329–38.
99. Difalco MR, Dufresne L, Congote LF. Efficacy of an insulin-like growth factor-interleukin-3 fusion protein in reversing the hematopoietic toxicity associated with azidothymidine in mice. J Pharmacol Exp Ther. 1998;284:449–54.

Chapter 3
Granulocyte Colony-Stimulating Factors

Graham Molineux

The Discovery of G-CSF

Despite the first recognition of red cells in the blood by the Dutch scientist Jan Swammerdam around 1658 and the first description of the shape of erythrocytes by his acquaintance Antoni van Leeuwenhoek in 1695, the colorless cellular component of the blood remained unrecognized until 1843. At this time "white globules" were identified in the blood simultaneously by Gabriel Andral and William Addison (working in France and Scotland, respectively) and shown to be associated with disease. Addison, for instance, recognized pus cells as being blood cells that had passed out of the circulation to the site of infection [1]. Leukemia was described in the intervening years but it was 1879 before Paul Ehrlich published his method for staining blood films. This was the birth of the blood "differential" and the recognition that leukocytes (from the Greek *leukos* meaning white and *kytos* meaning cell) are in some way associated with infectious disease.

Leukocytosis has been associated with infection, especially with pyrogenic organisms, for many years and leukocyte counts in excess of 12,000–20,000/mm^3 are not uncommon. The majority of immune effector cells generated in such circumstances are granulocytes and granulocyte colony-stimulating factor (G-CSF) is the major regulator of the leukocyte subgroup of neutrophilic granulocytes or neutrophils. Neutrophils are essential in innate immunity especially in the context of bacterial infections and this role is emphasized in individuals who, through congenital or acquired means, have neutrophil deficiency and who are at critical risk of lethal infections.

Even in the basal state, leukocytes are produced at an impressive pace; in the average adult approximately one billion neutrophils per kilogram body weight per day are both released from the bone marrow and lost from the blood, maintaining a normal count in the range of 3,000/mm^3. As implied by the increased circulating

G. Molineux (✉)
Amgen Inc., Thousand Oaks, CA 93021, USA
e-mail: graham@amgen.com

G.H. Lyman, D.C. Dale (eds.), *Hematopoietic Growth Factors in Oncology*,
Cancer Treatment and Research 157, DOI 10.1007/978-1-4419-7073-2_3,
© Springer Science+Business Media, LLC 2011

numbers in infection, the production rate can be accelerated many fold as needs arise.

The hematopoietic cells of the bone marrow can normally sustain without pause the almost overwhelming number of blood cells required throughout the lifespan of an individual, as well as maintaining the appropriate balance between the distinct types of blood cells recognized for the last 150 years. The numbers are satisfied by proliferation within a hierarchy of increasingly specialized cells sustained at the most primitive level by a small population of self-renewing hematopoietic stem cells. These stem and progenitor cells are under the control of both fixed (microenvironental or "stromal") elements and hormone-like circulating proteins. Our understanding of the interaction between the fixed and humoral elements and the blood-forming cells continues to evolve, but direct and controlled manipulation of the fixed elements remains elusive to date. In contrast, the humoral factors or hematopoietic growth factors (in which can be included colony-stimulating factors, cytokines, and interleukins) have proven more readily exploitable, particularly as a result of the pioneering work done at the Walter and Eliza Hall Institute of Medical Research in Melbourne, Australia.

The myeloid hematopoietic growth factors, and G-CSF among them, owe their discovery to the development of in vitro colony-forming cell assays pioneered in the 1960s [2, 3]. The clonal growth of bone marrow cells in these systems relies upon the addition of exogenous proteinaceous materials obtained from either tissues, body fluids or medium "conditioned" by other cells. Starting in the late 1960s and continuing through the 1970s the seminal work to purify these "colony-stimulating factors" or CSFs resulted in the first myeloid regulator to be purified to homogeneity. Purified first from human urine and then from medium conditioned by a cell line, this factor was named CSF-1 though is now widely referred to as macrophage CSF or M-CSF [4]. This was followed by purification of granulocyte–macrophage CSF or GM-CSF from medium conditioned by mouse lung cells in 1977 [5], later to be cloned in 1984 [6]. The first purification of murine granulocyte CSF or G-CSF was published in 1983 [7] and at the time its modest ability to stimulate the growth of small colonies of only a single cell lineage led to it being considered the least interesting of the three myeloid factors known at that time [8].

The purification and cloning of human G-CSF used similar assay procedures involving in vitro colony growth and differentiation of a leukemic cell line to purify and identify an activity from medium conditioned by a bladder carcinoma cell line [9, 10].

Cloning G-CSF

Two splice variants of G-CSF were originally described [11, 12], one with the familiar 174 amino acid sequence and the other with a 3 amino acid insert between residues 32 and 33 which was less active. Recombinant G-CSF (filgrastim, NEUPOGEN®, metHuG-CSF) is 175 amino acids which includes an N-terminal methionine typical of proteins expressed in *Escherichia coli*. It is this form that entered clinical trials in humans and was approved for administration to patients in the United States in 1991 [13–16]. A second Chinese hamster ovary (CHO) cell derived form (lacking the N-terminal methionine of filgrastim but post-translationally modified during expression to include a carbohydrate component) was also approved for human use in Europe in 1993 (lenograstim, Granocyte®). G-CSF was first administered to patients for the treatment of cancer chemotherapy-induced neutropenia and the prevention of associated infections. Since its initial approval for that indication, G-CSF has been recommended for use after bone marrow transplantation, for treatment of severe congenital neutropenia, and for support of patients with AIDS, acute leukemia, aplastic anemia, and myelodysplastic syndromes. It has also been used to mobilize repopulating stem cells to the blood of both cancer patients and normal donors – an unexpected benefit which was not imagined in the early days of development [17].

Native G-CSF

Biochemically identical G-CSF can be produced by many tissues [18] and substantial amounts are detectable in the circulation after challenge with bacteria or bacterial products [19]. The nature of the control of G-CSF production in steady-state conditions or in infection remains unclear.

The organization of the G-CSF (*CSF3*) gene is described as five mRNA-encoding exons and four introns [11] on human chromosome 17q21–q22 [20] and production of the mature protein appears to be controlled at the levels of both transcription and translation [21, 22]. Bacterial lipopolysaccharide, IL-1β, and TNFα are all known to upregulate G-CSF production [23]. However, these may not be the only signals for production as myelosuppression in the absence of signs of infection also raises G-CSF levels in patients [24].

The G-CSF promoter is known to have the capacity to bind NF-κB p65 and EBPβ [25], transcription factors that are also known to be involved in numerous inflammatory responses. Emerging data suggest that interleukin-17 (IL-17, a product of Th17 T lymphocytes) may be part of the inflammatory response mechanism by which G-CSF levels are controlled [26]. Tissue-infiltrating neutrophils appear to depress IL-23 secretion, one of the main stimuli for IL-17 production [27]. Thus it may be the case that the absence of neutrophils in a tissue results in high levels of IL-23 production. This in turn promotes the secretion of IL-17 which then can promote G-CSF production, neutropoiesis, and a return to normal tissue neutrophil numbers.

The structure of G-CSF has been determined by high resolution X-ray crystallography [28] and, in common with other members of the type 1 cytokine family, was found to comprise four antiparallel α helices in an "up–up–down–down" structure with a short helix between the first and second of these structures. The first ten amino acid residues are optional for activity [29], but the two disulfide bonds (between residues 37–43 and 65–75) are essential [30]. Natural or mammalian cell-derived recombinant G-CSF has a single O-linked glycosylation site at threonine-133 [31], but the form produced in *E. coli* which lacks this structure is fully active.

G-CSF Receptor

G-CSF receptor (G-CSFR, also know as CD114) is a member of the type 1 cytokine receptor family and is encoded by a single gene on human chromosome 17q21 [32]. A number of splice variants have been described but their function and relevance remain unclear. The extracellular C-terminal domain comprises a cytokine receptor homology (CRH) region, an IgG-like domain, and three fibronectin type III-like domains. The intracellular portion of the receptor is somewhat atypical of the family. Close to the cell membrane are two regions of homology with the erythropoietin receptor (EPO-R) and gp130 and the intervening region appears to be responsible for Jak2 binding and the transduction of the proliferative signal; the receptor itself has no intrinsic signaling function [33]. The extreme intracellular N-terminal portion of the receptor appears to be responsible for transducing signals related to differentiation and mature cell functioning [34–36] and deletions of this region have been associated with leukemic transformation in patients with congenital neutropenias [37, 38].

G-CSFR has been demonstrated on myeloid cells, platelets, and some lymphoid leukemia cells as well as normal B and T cells [39–46] using a variety of techniques from biotinylated G-CSF binding to mRNA detection and antibody binding.

G-CSF has been proposed to bind to G-CSFR in the ratio 2:2 [47] – similar to the interaction of IL-6 with its receptor. The interaction of G-CSF with G-CSFR is mainly through two regions within the CRH and Ig-like domains of the receptor and two sites on different helices of the G-CSF molecule. This results in two G-CSF molecules forming an "X"-like bridge between two adjacent G-CSFR molecules which in turn rearranges the receptor pair into the appropriate configuration to initiate signaling through a number of intracellular signaling cascades including familiar components of not only the Jak2/Stat3 pathway, but also the PI3 Kinase/Akt and Shc/Ras/MAP kinase pathways. There are in addition negative intracellular signaling elements such as SOCS3 and SHIP that probably attenuate the effects of ligand binding. Though most studies focus on a single candidate signaling pathway, in all likelihood activation of G-CSFR provokes a number of interconnected intracellular events some of which are recognized, some of which await elucidation, but which in concert result in self-limited proliferation and activation signals (see, e.g., Ref. [48]).

The Biology of G-CSF

Numerous model systems have been created to explain the role that G-CSF plays in normal biology. These exploit either the over-production or removal of G-CSF in animals or the deletion of its receptor. Taken together all of the data confirm that:

1. G-CSF is the major regulator of neutrophil production and activity.
2. G-CSF-driven processes do not account for all neutrophil production.

3. There is good evidence that G-CSF has a single receptor and that that receptor has but a single ligand.

Using a retroviral vector carrying G-CSF cDNA, murine bone marrow cells were made to over-express G-CSF and then transplanted into irradiated recipient mice [49]. In this manner long-term expression of G-CSF was observed for up to 30 weeks. Treated animals showed a marked granulocytosis, infiltration of many tissues with neutrophils, and progenitor cell expansion in many non-marrow sites. The marrow was remarkably normal and the mice suffered no overall untoward effects, including the absence of neoplasia. Though driving over-production through marrow cells undoubtedly fulfilled the experimental objective of chronic exposure to G-CSF, it is not clear whether local production in the marrow provided a physiological representation of the role played by the endogenous ligand. In an alternative approach Yamada et al. [50] created a G-CSF transgenic mouse. Like the retroviral/transplant mouse this animal also produced a huge excess of G-CSF. The consequences were not too dissimilar to the work described above and observations included neutrophilia, progenitor mobilization, tissue infiltration with leukocytes, and in addition a notable lymphocytosis. In contrast there was also now an excess of progenitor cells in the bone marrow. Thus there were some minor differences between the observations in the different sets of mice, but in general the picture was one of excessive neutrophil production, some shift in progenitor number and localization, and some off-target (non-myeloid) effects which may have been peculiar to the specific model. An important finding was that there were few deleterious changes even in the face of these spectacular hematological values. No neoplasia, signs of gross inflammation, or other effects secondary to neutrophilia. Repeated injection of the recombinant protein produced similar effects [51, 52] but now the observations included an apparent suppression of erythropoiesis, an observation that was followed up in detail later [53] but one that has yet to be reproduced in humans.

In the opposite approach the G-CSF gene was disrupted to produce a G-CSF knockout (KO) mouse [54]. These animals had a 70–80% reduction in circulating neutrophil numbers and an impaired ability to resolve bacterial infections which was corrected upon injecting G-CSF. They also had some changes in monocyte parameters especially as the mice aged, perhaps emphasizing an effect on this closely related lineage of hematopoietic cells. In another approach to the same question, mice were made immune to G-CSF by administering to them G-CSF conjugated to highly immunogenic materials such as keyhole limpet hemocyanin (KLH) or ovalbumin [55]. High titers of anti-G-CSF antibodies effectively neutralized circulating G-CSF in these animals and resulted in a phenotype almost identical to the G-CSF knockout mouse [54]. In both settings a residual 20–30% of basal neutrophil numbers remained, suggesting a G-CSF-independent mechanism for generating at least a minority of neutrophils. Those remaining neutrophils, however, seemed less effective in dealing with bacteria. These data suggest that G-CSF has a partially redundant role in baseline neutrophil production but an essential role in mature neutrophil activity. Overlap in functions exists between many of the myeloid cytokines and these deletion studies need to be considered in the context of the other redundant players in the system [56].

G-CSF receptor knockout mice were made by homologous recombination and shown to be broadly similar to animals in which the ligand had been deleted [57]. These animals still produced the residual 20% or so of normal neutrophils seen in the G-CSF KO or autoimmune mice, but had lower numbers of circulating cells resulting from reduced expansion of myeloid populations in the bone marrow and excessive apoptosis of neutrophilic precursor cells. These mice also have decreased progenitor numbers in the bone marrow. Interestingly, a largely inexplicable effect on monocyte biology was also noted when G-CSFR$^{-/-}$ cells or mice were exposed to high levels of G-CSF. At baseline and in contrast to the ligand-deficient mice that exhibit monocytopenia, the receptor knockouts have a modest monocytosis, which is unaffected by treatment with exogenous G-CSF, However, G-CSFR$^{-/-}$ cells treated ex vivo with both IL-6 and G-CSF showed a monocyte reaction to G-CSF. Thus it remains possible that an alternate receptor exists for G-CSF.

Despite the presence of G-CSFR on various blood cell lineages discussed above, there appears to be little consequence for these cell types when G-CSFR is disrupted. Importantly, there are also no untoward effects in other, non-hematopoietic tissues such as vascular, cardiac, or neural tissues suggesting that G-CSF does not play an essential role in organ systems other than blood cell development. There are many emerging and widely documented effects of G-CSF on lymphocytes, dendritic cells, and immune effector cells, some of which may be direct.

In general the findings aggregated from the various deletion and over-expression studies are consistent with a role for G-CSF mainly, though not entirely exclusively, limited to neutrophil production and mature cell function. Little evidence has emerged that neither alternate receptors exist for G-CSF, nor that alternative ligands work through G-CSFR.

The Cellular Targets of G-CSF

One hundred and twenty billion neutrophils are produced each day in an adult to balance the loss through normal cellular aging mechanisms. This prodigious rate of production is maintained by low circulating levels of G-CSF – in fact when G-CSF is normally present at such low levels it is difficult to detect in plasma [58]. In conditions such as infection, complicated pregnancy, neutropenia, and aplastic anemia circulating levels may be substantially higher – over 100,000 pg/mL (e.g., Ref. [59]).

It has been shown that the absence of G-CSF affects an increase in the susceptibility of neutrophilic precursors to apoptosis, or programmed cell death [57]. The bone marrow of G-CSFR$^{-/-}$ mice was found to have normal cellularity, progenitor numbers were down only slightly, and recognizable neutrophilic cells were normal except metamyelocytes and band/segmented neutrophils. These are relatively mature cells in comparison to progenitors, yet it is the progenitor cells that proliferate and differentiate in vitro in response to G-CSF. In the presence of G-CSF, the appropriate progenitors will survive and proliferate, but in order to see band and segmented neutrophils that typically comprise the colonies generated by these progenitors in culture, the intermediate myeloblasts and promyelocytes must also survive, proliferate, and differentiate. So this is where G-CSF might be expected to have the majority of its effects. This proved to be correct in both mice and humans. It has been shown [60] that the primary target of G-CSF is the promyelocyte/myeloblast population and that the accelerated neutrophil production observed under the influence of injected G-CSF can be accounted for by the accelerated emigration of neutrophils from the marrow to the blood and the insertion of a modest number of extra amplification divisions (less than 2) into their cell cycle history. In addition, it was documented by both Lord and others [57, 61] that monocyte production is impacted by G-CSF, by unknown mechanisms. The modified form of G-CSF, pegfilgrastim, introduced below and which represents a quite different pharmacokinetic/exposure profile to NEUPOGEN® has, perhaps surprisingly, similar effects on neutrophil production kinetics [62].

Skeletal pain has been associated with G-CSF administration since the earliest trials [13]. Though a number of explanations have been offered, a complete explanation of the phenomenon is still not readily to hand. There are a number of observations that suggest G-CSF has effects in bone which include actions upon both (bone forming) osteoblasts and (bone destroying) osteoclasts. In attempting to unravel the mechanism of progenitor cell mobilization, it was found that markers of bone formation were reduced and markers of bone resorption markedly increased [63] in association with G-CSF administration in mice. Inhibiting the resorption phase with bisphophonate (pamidronate) did not affect the primary pharmacodynamic response (i.e., progenitor mobilization), but eliminated markers of excessive bone destruction. In children with SCN treated for extended periods with G-CSF, osteoporosis has been repeatedly noted, but initial questions were raised over whether this is linked to G-CSF administration or is a natural feature of the disease [64, 65]. Takahashi et al. have shown excessive bone turnover in association with G-CSF exposure in otherwise normal mice [66] arguing that G-CSF alone may account for the bone loss. At least one study links the turnover of bone, in this case osteoblast activity, with bone pain [67], though it has also been suggested this is not a direct effect [68]. Thus it is well established that bone biology is profoundly affected by G-CSF. The osteoclast effects are at least compatible with the documented effects on monocyte production [69] and the ability of monocytic cells to develop osteoclast-like properties [70].

Control of bone pain associated with G-CSF is normally acceptable with acetaminophen or rarely opioids. There is a popular belief that the antihistamine loratadine (Claritin®) can help control the pain. This does not appear to result from any systematic study of the issue and may be based on a report that astemizole, a withdrawn antihistamine, was suggested to help with bone pain in a case report of a patient with breast cancer who was receiving taxol as antitumor chemotherapy with G-CSF support. The duration of pain was, perhaps coincidentally, associated with the duration of G-CSF administration [71].

PK/PD Relationship

The pharmacodynamic response to G-CSF administration is comparable irrespective of whether it is administered intravenously [14, 16], subcutaneously [72], or intramuscularly [73]. Subcutaneously administered material is rapidly absorbed and detectable in the plasma.

G-CSF is a relatively small protein and can be rapidly cleared by the kidneys. Renal elimination is a linear process in that the loss of G-CSF by this route is related to its concentration in the plasma; the higher the concentration, the more G-CSF is lost this way. However, overall G-CSF clearance is, in general, non-linear. The reason for this is that G-CSF is among several hematopoietic cytokines whose clearance is mediated, at least in part, by the cellular products of its action, in this case neutrophils. This was illustrated a number of years ago when the half-life of G-CSF was shown to be 4.7 h in the absence of neutrophils, but less than 2 h when the ANC was higher. This mechanism further advances a paradigm created by the seminal work of Richard Stanley with M-CSF [74]. This combination of dual clearance mechanisms results in (1) the necessity for multiple injections of exogenous G-CSF to obtain a substantial pharmacodynamic effect and (2) accelerated clearance of G-CSF as neutrophil numbers increase. Understanding these elements led to the development of pegfilgrastim which is discussed in more detail below.

Available Preparations of G-CSF

Different forms of recombinant human G-CSF are available in different countries from different manufacturers. Filgrastim (NEUPOGEN®, Amgen, Inc.), lenograstim (Granocyte®, Chugai Pharmaceutical Co. Ltd), and KW-2228 (Nartograstim®) (Kyowa-Hakko Kogyo Co.) are the dominant forms but have been recently joined by variant G-CSFs described more fully below.

Filgrastim (NEUPOGEN®)

Native G-CSF is a 204 amino acid glycoprotein including a 30 amino acid signal sequence that is removed from the secreted form. Recombinant methionyl G-CSF (r-metHuG-CSF) is a 175 amino acid protein produced in *E. coli*. This version has an additional N-terminal methionine to aid stability in the bacterial expression system. Due to its bacterial origin it also lacks the O-linked carbohydrate on threonine-133 of the natural protein [31], but retains all five cysteines typical of the human sequence (at positions 17, 36, 42, 64, and 74 – the murine version lacks Cys-17). The latter four of these cysteines contribute to disulfide bonds which stabilize the structure as four antiparallel helices [75].

Lenograstim (Granocyte®)

Though the gene is the same as that expressed in *E. coli* to make filgrastim, the mammalian expression system (CHO cells) used to make lenograstim does not require the extra methionine and so the final molecule consists of the 174 amino acids of the natural sequence [31]. The O-linked carbohydrate chain is also present in this form of G-CSF.

The function of this carbohydrate is unclear; it has been proposed to inhibit proteolytic degradation and aggregation and increase serum half-life [76]. Though the in vitro activity of glycosylated rHuG-CSF has been suggested to be greater than the non-glycosylated form, the activity in vivo is similar to the bacterially synthesized form in all respects [77–82]. So the role of the additional carbohydrate remains unclear.

KW-2228 (Nartograstim®)

A useful technique in drug distribution studies is to attach a radioactive tracer (often ^{125}I) to molecules in order to track their dissemination in the body or to examine receptor interactions. However, G-CSF, particularly the recombinant form, is a notoriously difficult molecule to radio-iodinate. KW-2228 is a version of G-CSF in which the peptide sequence has been changed to allow the attachment of radioactive iodine [83]. The amino acid substitutions were Thr-1, Leu-3, Gly-4, Pro-5, and Cys-17 for Ala, Thr, Tyr, Arg, and Ser, respectively (as noted above, Cys-17 is absent from murine G-CSF). The mutein was found to be active and capable of binding to G-CSF receptors [29, 83, 84] and clinical studies have demonstrated its value in chemotherapy-induced neutropenia [85]. Preclinical studies in primates have also compared KW-2228 with both lenograstim (glycosylated rHuG-CSF) and filgrastim (r-metHuG-CSF) and found all three preparations to have identical pharmacokinetic properties [81].

G-CSF Follow-On Biologics

Since the 2006 expiry of the patent for NEUPOGEN® in the EU, numerous "follow-on biologic" (FOB), "biosimilar," or "subsequent entry" versions of G-CSF have entered the European regulatory framework and two gained approval for clinical use in 2008. The first, which had previously only been available in Lithuania under the name Grasalva, is now more broadly marketed under a number of different names; Ratiograstim® (filgrastim) from Ratiopharm GmbH, Biograstim® (filgrastim) from CT Arzneimittel GmbH, and Tevagrastim® (filgrastim) from Teva Generics GmbH. The second G-CSF, from Novartis' generics division Sandoz has two names; Zarzio and filgrastim-Hexal (Hexal is owned by Sandoz). The abbreviated approval process for these drugs in the EU was based on comparison with a reference product (usually NEUPOGEN®) and the guidelines called for assessment of comparability in relatively small studies. For example, Tevagrastim was approved based on the following clinical studies:

1. A cross-over pharmacokinetics study with 24–26 healthy volunteers in each arm and single doses of 5 or 10 μg/kg with a 2-week washout period.
2. A bioequivalence study of PK and PD with 34–36 normal volunteers in each arm at doses of 5 or 10 μg/kg administered either SC or IV.
3. A study of efficacy (duration of severe neutropenia), safety and PK in patients receiving chemotherapy for breast cancer: 133 received tevagrastim (5 μg/kg), 129 received NEUPOGEN® (5 μg/kg), and 58 received placebo. Patients were dosed for between 5 and 14 days until absolute neutrophil counts (ANCs) reached $\geq 10 \times 10^9$/L for up to four cycles of chemotherapy.
4. Two non-placebo controlled studies of safety with efficacy and PK data collected in patients receiving chemotherapy for lung cancer or non-Hodgkin's lymphoma: 148 lung cancer patients received tevagrastim compared to 77 treated with NEUPOGEN®, and 55 lymphoma patients received tevagrastim compared to 29 who received NEUPOGEN®.

Thus approval was based upon treatment of only approximately 200 normal volunteers and around 350 cancer-chemotherapy patients with tevagrastim [86]. Interestingly, other uses of NEUPOGEN® such as mobilization of hematopoietic stem/progenitor cells have been assumed to also be comparable despite potentially different underlying biological processes.

In addition to these European FOBs there exist approximately (numbers vary) 20 Chinese and 7 other Asian formulations of G-CSF many of which have substantial clinical history and some of which could conceivably become available in the West through commercial partnerships. A framework for regulatory approval of FOBs in the United States is still under consideration, but the 2005 EU issued guidance that includes product-specific guidelines and the European experience may hold some clues as to what might be expected.

Pegfilgrastim (Neulasta®)

Approved for clinical use in the United States in 2002, pegfilgrastim is the only second generation G-CSF available for use in patients. It results from the covalent addition of a 20-kDa polyethylene glycol moiety to the N-terminal methionine of the 175 amino acid *E. coli*-derived peptide familiar as filgrastim. This derivative conjugate is larger than the parent molecule, more resistant to proteolytic degradation, and appropriate for fixed (non-body weight dependent) dosing.

To date, the only known binding site of pegfilgrastim is the conventional G-CSF receptor, so the biological effects of pegfilgrastim are in general the same as the parent molecule. Where the two agents differ is in the unique pharmacokinetic properties of pegfilgrastim [87]. The size of the molecule has been increased sufficiently by the conjugation to PEG to avoid renal elimination. The only remaining known mechanism of clearance is via neutrophils – the same cells that are the product of the drug's action. This has the effect of yielding a drug which is "automated" in its action. Once administered to a neutropenic patient it remains in the circulation, prompting rapid neutrophil recovery, until that recovery progresses to the point where the drug is cleared by those very same cells. Though this end-cell-mediated clearance is a feature of several hematopoietic cytokines, this is the only example of a drug specifically designed to use this principle to offer a superior therapeutic.

A G-CSF preparation suitable for pulmonary delivery has been developed but gained littler traction to date [88]. Similarly, G-CSF can be administered rectally [89] and PEGylated forms at least can be administered via the GI tract [90] (though not orally). These approaches have yet to gain any broad application. Indeed, other than the development of pegfilgrastim, the pharmaceutical manipulation of the G-CSF axis has been relatively stationary for some years. A small molecule mimetic was published in 1998 [91, 92] but seemed to activate only the murine receptor. In addition at least one antibody which activates G-CSFR has been patented, but further details are not available.

Clinical Use of G-CSF

Neutropenia Management

Neutropenia is dangerous no matter how it is caused – iatrogenic or congenital, because of the central role neutrophils play in host defense. The most appealing use of recombinant G-CSF might be as a type of hormone replacement where levels of the endogenous cytokine are low. As mentioned above, G-CSF is an "emergency" cytokine and though its absence in mice reduces neutrophil counts to only 20–30% of normal, the mice live a normal lifespan unless challenged with infection, to which they more rapidly succumb than their G-CSF (or G-CSFR) wild-type counterparts. The most frequent cause of iatrogenic neutropenia is treatment with the relatively non-selective agents of conventional cancer chemotherapy. Recognition of the unmet medical need in this circumstance led to the first clinical trials of G-CSF in the 1980s [15, 17]. However, cancer patients will in general launch their own G-CSF response to the neutropenia caused by chemotherapy, so why does exogenous G-CSF provide any benefit? The answers, it would seem, lie in both early and generous supplementation of the endogenous response.

Basal G-CSF levels are less than 30 pg/mL in plasma and peak at around 100 pg/mL 16 days after chemotherapy [93]. However, patients injected with filgrastim starting 24 h after chemotherapy attain levels exceeding 100 pg/mL from day 3 onward (it may have been earlier, but this was the first day measured) and peak levels around 10,000 pg/mL were noted on days 11–12. These G-CSF levels provoked recovery of neutrophil numbers to over 5,000/μL by day 17, a significant improvement compared to three untreated patients (who relied on the endogenous G-CSF response) among whom only one had attained this neutrophil count by day 23, one recovered later than this and another who never reached this level over the total observation period. So high G-CSF concentrations provided early were effective, but which was the more important component, the high concentration or the early provision? In the same study the authors also undertook two more creative scheduling studies – one in which G-CSF dosing was initiated on the first day of documented neutropenia and a second regimen in which G-CSF dosing was begun on day 8.

All regimens were more effective than relying on endogenous G-CSF. Prophylactic administration starting one day after chemotherapy resulted in the shortest duration of severe neutropenia, but paradoxically also resulted in the lowest neutrophil count at nadir. The delayed start (beginning at day 8) and the reactive (starting when neutropenia was noted) regimens were also effective, but not as effective (in terms of the duration of severe neutropenia) as the next-day regimen. It would appear therefore that early provision is an important component, but the importance of the high plasma concentration is a question that is difficult to address in patients. At the heart of the difficulty is the short half-life of G-CSF. The pharmacokinetics are discussed above but it is notable that delivering G-CSF via a pump (which sustains a more constant plasma level) was more effective (as measured by rise in ANC) than repeated SC injection [94]. Subcutaneous or intravenous injection results in very high plasma concentration (C_{max}), higher than would be expected from a pump of the type described. Perhaps the C_{max} is less important than the duration of "coverage" during which time the plasma concentration is above a minimally effective threshold. Such a model is widely appreciated for EPO [95] and recognition of this issue has led to the development of a modified form of G-CSF with improved therapeutic performance [87]. To summarize therefore, it appears that the most beneficial manner studied to date by which to administer G-CSF would be to provide sufficient drug to attain an effective plasma level 24 h after chemotherapy and to maintain that level until a suitable response is noted.

Other than its use in the management of neutropenia, G-CSF has been shown to offer further opportunities in settings as diverse as peripheral blood progenitor cell (PBPC) mobilization, immune modulation, and the repair of diverse tissues.

Hematopoietic Cell Mobilization

PBPC mobilization, sometimes somewhat imprecisely referred to as "stem cell" mobilization, has become a mainstay of clinical practice in regenerating bone marrow damaged either by disease or by chemotherapy. In essence the cells that reside within the bone marrow and that function in the early stages of the hematopoietic hierarchy can be made to emigrate from the bone marrow to the blood under the influence of G-CSF, there to be more easily collected and processed for transplantation. G-CSF is not unique in its ability to mobilize PBPC and agents as diverse as dextran, anti-VLA-4 antibodies, metalloproteinase inhibitors, IL-8, GM-CSF, small molecule or antibody inhibitors of chemokines or chemokine receptors (e.g., CXCR4), chemotherapeutic drugs and early-acting growth factors like stem cell factor (SCF, STEMGEN®), and Flt-3 ligand have all been shown to mobilize PBPC to one degree or another and on timescales ranging from 30 min [96, 97] to 4–5 days [98]. The mechanism of mobilization has attracted a lot of study over the 20 years it has been a recognized phenomenon. Over several days administration, G-CSF creates a highly proteolytic environment [99] in the bone marrow which is thought to degrade the proteins (via neutrophil-derived enzyme products like elasase and cathepsin G) that tether progenitor cells in the marrow milieu. The candidate tethers are numerous, as are the suggested effector molecules, but it would seem that the interaction between stromal cell-derived factor-1 (SDF-1, CXCL12) and CXCR4, its receptor and the target of AMD3100, plerixafor, Mozobil™ [97], is among the more prominent. Once relocated to the blood, PBPC can be collected by leukapheresis and purified on the basis of their cell surface expression of CD34 or CD133, though in some circumstances the concentration of primitive hematopoietic cells may be high enough that blood itself is an appropriate source of engrafting cells without the need for further concentration [100]. Once transplanted, mobilized PBPC performs well, possibly better than cells harvested directly from the bone marrow, though overarching statements cannot be made as agreement is not complete and different circumstances may be better suited to one source material than the other.

Though chronic graft-versus-host disease (GvHD) remains an issue with allogeneic PBPC grafts, in some circumstances acute GvHD is less of a problem than might be expected especially considering the number of transferred T cells. There may even be an advantage in terms of reduced risk of disease relapse mediated by a graft-versus-tumor effect. There seems little doubt that the immune cells transferred along with a G-CSF-mobilized PBPC product perform differently than T cells from a non-G-CSF-treated donor. Candidate mechanisms for this effect include the action of G-CSF on polarization of T cells toward a $T_{H}2$ phenotype, modulation of T_{reg} activity, and effects on antigen-presenting cells and NK cells. The exploitation of these effects remains a subject of active investigation but what would appear to be emerging is that the use of G-CSF in a PBPC donor can reduce the incidence of mild-to-moderate acute GvHD, while retaining the graft-versus-tumor effect. The consequences of the use of G-CSF in the transplant recipient differ substantially depending on whether the graft received was bone marrow from a naïve donor or PBPC from a G-CSF-treated donor. It would seem that the benign or even beneficial effects of donor cell exposure to G-CSF can be safely supplemented with recipient G-CSF treatment to accelerate engraftment, but post-transplant administration of G-CSF to a bone marrow recipient naïve to G-CSF exposure may present a greater risk of GvHD and a reduction in overall survival.

Tissue Repair

A quite different application of G-CSF in mobilizing cells for the repair of non-hematopoietic tissues is represented by early experiments to regenerate cardiac, brain, and other cells damaged by events such as ischemia. In general, the hypotheses around potential mechanisms of action can be categorized as follows:

1. G-CSF can mobilize hematopoietic stem cells which contribute directly to tissue repair, i.e., G-CSF-mobilized stem cells can migrate to and adopt ("transdifferentiate" into) the phenotypic, morphological, and functional properties of cardiomyocytes, neural cells, pancreatic islet cells, etc.

2. G-CSF can act directly on non-hematopoietic cells already resident in the target tissue and encourage their contribution to tissue repair, e.g., cardiomyocyte precursor cells.
3. G-CSF may mobilize endothelial progenitor cells that contribute directly to vascularization of the target tissue, thereby promoting improved tissue repair by cells found either in situ or migrating from a remote site.
4. G-CSF may cause cells to emigrate to the site of tissue injury, where they contribute indirectly to tissue repair by producing secondary factors, e.g., a G-CSF-mobilized cell may produce cytokines such as VEGF that encourage revascularization and repair of the target tissue.

Whether any or all of these various hypotheses are substantiated by definitive data is still the subject of active debate. Mechanisms such as cell fusion have been shown to explain some findings, while immunomodulation may explain some others. Of greater concern is that despite the lack of any consistent hypothesis related to mechanism of action, a number of clinical studies have been undertaken in attempts to exploit any potential therapeutic value of G-CSF in stroke, heart attacks, peripheral vascular disease, liver disease, traumatic nerve damage, and others. Reviewing the entire data set is beyond the scope of this work, but excellent reviews have been prepared by Klocke et al. [101] and Vertesaljai et al. [102]. Many of the outstanding issues were discussed by Kurdi et al. [103, 104] and it remains true to say that many of these remain unresolved today. For instance how and when to dose G-CSF (compare the seminal Orlic [105] pre/post-dosing paradigm with low dose, post-MI dosing [106]), whether mesenchymal stem cells are players [107], whether immunomodulation plays a role [108], and whether the effective cells originate from the bone marrow or cardiac tissue [109] have only been further clouded by more recent findings. Most importantly, it is still not clear whether an overall benefit is conferred upon patients by G-CSF treatment via objective measures of response [110–113].

Future Considerations

The main deployment of G-CSF remains the treatment of cancer chemotherapy-induced neutropenia. Cancer chemotherapy is, however, a moving target with new agents and combinations of agents continually being approved. Some of the newer cancer therapeutics work by attacking the blood supply of tumors through antagonism of either VEGF (vascular endothelial growth factor) or its receptor. The most prominent of these anti-angiogenic agents is bevacizumab (Avastin®). Treatment with bevacizumab can increase the incidence of neutropenic sepsis in patients [114]. As this would typically be treated using exogenous G-CSF, some of the mechanisms discussed above in the context of tissue repair invoke the possibility that G-CSF may provide pro-angiogenic signals. So is there a conflict? In preclinical cancer models it was shown that bone marrow-derived $CD11b^+Gr-1^+$ myeloid cells localize in tumors that are resistant to an anti-VEGF antibody (a mouse reactive reagent used as a surrogate for bevacizumab, which does not cross-species well) and that elimination of this cell population could restore the tumors sensitivity to anti-VEGF treatment [115]. This observation was complemented by the identification of another VEGF family member, Bv8 [116, 117], as a key mediator of the pro-angiogenic effects of these myeloid cells. The particular myeloid cell in question here is one that has been recognized for some time as part of the inflammatory milieu around neoplastic lesions, the so-called myeloid-derived suppressor cell or MDSC [118, 119]. Several features of the cell remain unclear, not least of which is whether it actually exists in humans, but perhaps an equally important question is whether this cell type might survive in vivo in the chemotherapy setting. If it does not, as suggested by at least one study [115], then the potential pro-angiogenic effects of a G-CSF-stimulated cell type on the efficacy of bevacizumab in human cancer is largely moot since both G-CSF and bevacizumab are only used in combination with chemotherapy. A well-designed clinical study maybe required to address the question of the potential interaction between G-CSF and bevacizumab.

References

1. Hajdu SI. The discovery of blood cells. Ann Clin Lab Sci. 2003;33:237–8.
2. Pluznik DH, Sachs L. The cloning of normal "mast" cells in tissue culture. J Cell Physiol. 1965;66:319–24.
3. Bradley TR, Metcalf D. The growth of mouse bone marrow cells in vitro. Aust J Exp Biol Med Sci. 1966;44:287–99.
4. Stanley ER, Heard PM. Factors regulating macrophage production and growth purification and some properties of the colony stimulating factor from medium conditioned by mouse l neoplastic fibroblast cells. J Biol Chem. 1977;252:4305–12.
5. Burgess AW, Camakaris J, Purification MD. Properties of colony stimulating factor from mouse lung conditioned medium. J Biol Chem. 1977;252:1998–2003.
6. Gough NM, Gough J, Metcalf D, et al. Molecular cloning of cDNA encoding a murine haematopoietic growth regulator, granulocyte–macrophage colony stimulating factor. Nature. 1984;309:763–7.
7. Nicola NA, Metcalf D, Matsumoto M, Johnson GR. Purification of a factor inducing differentiation in murine myelomonocytic leukemia cells. Identification as granulocyte colony-stimulating factor. J Biol Chem. 1983;258:9017–23.
8. Metcalf D. Hematopoietic cytokines. Blood. 2008;111:485–91.
9. Souza LM, Boone TC, Gabrilove J, et al. Recombinant human granulocyte colony-stimulating factor: effects on normal and leukemic myeloid cells. Science. 1986;232:61–5.
10. Welte K, Platzer E, Lu L, et al. Purification and biochemical characterization of human pluripotent hematopoietic colony-stimulating factor. Proc Natl Acad Sci USA. 1985;82:1526–30.
11. Nagata S, Tsuchiya M, Asano S, et al. Molecular cloning and expression of cDNA for human granulocyte colony-stimulating factor. Nature. 1986;319:415–18.
12. Zsebo KM, Cohen AM, Murdock DC, et al. Recombinant human granulocyte colony stimulating factor: molecular and biological characterization. Immunobiology. 1986;172:175–84.
13. Morstyn G, Campbell L, Souza LM, et al. Effect of granulocyte colony stimulating factor on neutropenia induced by cytotoxic chemotherapy. Lancet. 1988;1:667–72.
14. Gabrilove JL, Jakubowski A, Fain K, et al. Phase I study of granulocyte colony-stimulating factor in patients with transitional cell carcinoma of the urothelium. J Clin Invest. 1988;82:1454–61.

15. Bronchud MH, Scarffe JH, Thatcher N, et al. Phase I/II study of recombinant human granulocyte colony-stimulating factor in patients receiving intensive chemotherapy for small cell lung cancer. Br J Cancer. 1987;56:809–13.

16. Gabrilove JL, Jakubowski A, Scher H, et al. Effect of granulocyte colony-stimulating factor on neutropenia and associated morbidity due to chemotherapy for transitional-cell carcinoma of the urothelium. N Engl J Med. 1988;318:1414–22.

17. Welte K, Gabrilove J, Bronchud MH, et al. Filgrastim (r-metHuG-CSF) – the first 10 years. Blood. 1996;88:1907–29.

18. Nicola NA, Biochemical MD. Properties of differentiation factors for murine myelo monocytic leukemic cells in organ conditioned media separation from colony stimulating factors. J Cell Physiol. 1981;109:253–64.

19. Cheers C, Haigh AM, Kelso A, et al. Production of colony-stimulating factors (CSFs) during infection: separate determinations of macrophage-, granulocyte-, granulocyte–macrophage-, and multi-CSFs. Infect Immun. 1988;56:247–51.

20. Tweardy DJ, Cannizzaro LA, Palumbo AP, et al. Molecular cloning and characterization of a complementary DNA for human granulocyte colony-stimulating factor (G-CSF) from a glioblastoma multiforme cell line and localization of the G-CSF gene to chromosome band 17q21. Cytogenet Cell Genet. 1987;46.

21. Ernst TJ, Ritchie AR, Demetri GD, Griffin JD. Regulation of granulocyte- and monocyte-colony stimulating factor mRNA levels in human blood monocytes is mediated primarily at a post-transcriptional level. J Biol Chem. 1989;264:5700–3.

22. Falkenburg JH, Harrington MA, de Paus RA, et al. Differential transcriptional and posttranscriptional regulation of gene expression of the colony-stimulating factors by interleukin-1 and fetal bovine serum in murine fibroblasts. Blood. 1991;78:658–65.

23. Demetri GD, Griffin JD. Granulocyte colony-stimulating factor and its receptor. Blood. 1991;78:2791–808.

24. Miksits K, Beyer J, Siegert W. Serum concentrations of G-CSF during high-dose chemotherapy with autologous stem cell rescue. Bone Marrow Transplant. 1993;11:375–7.

25. Dunn SM, Coles LS, Lang RK, et al. Requirement for nuclear factor (NF)-kappa B p65 and NF-interleukin-6 binding elements in the tumor necrosis factor response region of the granulocyte colony-stimulating factor promoter. Blood. 1994;83:2469–79.

26. Ye P, Rodriguez FH, Kanaly S, et al. Requirement of interleukin 17 receptor signaling for lung CXC chemokine and granulocyte colony-stimulating factor expression, neutrophil recruitment, and host defense. J Exp Med. 2001;194:519–27.

27. Langrish CL, Chen Y, Blumenschein WM, et al. IL-23 drives a pathogenic T cell population that induces autoimmune inflammation. J Exp Med. 2005;201:233–40.

28. Hill CP, Osslund TD, Eisenberg D. The structure of granulocyte-colony-stimulating factor and its relationship to other growth factors. Proc Natl Acad Sci USA. 1993;90:5167–71.

29. Okabe M, Asano M, Kuga T, et al. In vitro and in vivo hematopoietic effect of mutant human granulocyte colony-stimulating factor. [see comments]. Blood. 1990;75:1788–93.

30. Lu HS, Clogston CL, Narhi LO, et al. Folding and oxidation of recombinant human granulocyte colony stimulating factor produced in *Escherichia coli* characterization of the disulfide-reduced intermediates and cysteine–serine analogs. J Biol Chem. 1992;267:8770–7.

31. Kubota N, Orita T, Hattori K, et al. Structural characterization of natural and recombinant human granulocyte colony-stimulating factors. J Biochem. 1990;107:486–92.

32. Boulay J-L, O'Shea JJ, Paul WE. Molecular phylogeny within type 1 cytokines and their cognate receptors. Immunity. 2003;19:159–63.

33. Barge RM, de Koning JP, Pouwels K, et al. Tryptophan 650 of human granulocyte colony-stimulating factor (G-CSF) receptor, implicated in the activation of JAK2, is also required for G-CSF-mediated activation of signaling complexes of the p21ras route. Blood. 1996;87:2148–53.

34. Dong F, van Buitenen C, Pouwels K, et al. Distinct cytoplasmic regions of the human granulocyte colony-stimulating factor receptor involved in induction of proliferation and maturation. Mol Cell Biol. 1993;13:7774–81.
35. Fukunaga R, Ishizaka-Ikeda E, Nagata S. Growth and differentiation signals mediated by different regions in the cytoplasmic domain of granulocyte colony-stimulating factor receptor. Cell. 1993;74:1079–87.
36. Santini V, Scappini B, Indik ZK, et al. The carboxy-terminal region of the granulocyte colony-stimulating factor receptor transduces a phagocytic signal. Blood. 2003;101: 4615–22.
37. Dong F, Brynes RK, Tidow N, et al. Mutations in the gene for the granulocyte colony-stimulating-factor receptor in patients with acute myeloid leukemia preceded by severe congenital neutropenia. N Engl J Med. 1995;333:487–93.
38. Dong F, Dale DC, Bonilla MA, et al. Mutations in the granulocyte colony-stimulating factor receptor gene in patients with severe congenital neutropenia. Leukemia. 1997;11:120–5.
39. Budel LM, Touw IP, Delwel R, Lowenberg B. Granulocyte colony-stimulating factor receptors in human acute myelocytic leukemia. Blood. 1989;74:2668–73.
40. Hanazono Y, Hosoi T, Kuwaki T, et al. Structural analysis of the receptors for granulocyte colony-stimulating factor on neutrophils. Exp Hematol. 1990;18:1097–103.
41. Khwaja A, Carver J, Jones HM, et al. Expression and dynamic modulation of the human granulocyte colony-stimulating factor receptor in immature and differentiated myeloid cells. Br J Haematol. 1993;85:254–9.
42. Shimoda K, Okamura S, Harada N, et al. Identification of a functional receptor for granulocyte colony-stimulating factor on platelets. J Clin Invest. 1993;91:1310–13.
43. Corcione A, Corrias MV, Daniele S, et al. Expression of granulocyte colony-stimulating factor and granulocyte colony-stimulating factor receptor genes in partially overlapping monoclonal B-cell populations from chronic lymphocytic leukemia patients. Blood. 1996;87:2861–9.
44. Matsushita K, Arima N. Involvement of granulocyte colony-stimulating factor in proliferation of adult T-cell leukemia cells. Leuk Lymphoma. 1998;31:295–304.
45. Boneberg EM, Hareng L, Gantner F, et al. Human monocytes express functional receptors for granulocyte colony-stimulating factor that mediate suppression of monokines and interferon-gamma. Blood. 2000;95:270–6.
46. Morikawa K, Morikawa S, Nakamura M, Miyawaki T. Characterization of granulocyte colony-stimulating factor receptor expressed on human lymphocytes. Br J Haematol. 2002;118:296–304.
47. Layton JE, Hall NE. The interaction of G-CSF with its receptor. Front Biosci. 2006;11: 3181–9.
48. Roberts AW. G-CSF: a key regulator of neutrophil production, but that's not all! Growth Factors. 2005;23:33–41.
49. Chang JM, Metcalf D, Gonda TJ, Johnson GR. Long-term exposure to retrovirally expressed granulocyte-colony-stimulating factor induces a nonneoplastic granulocytic and progenitor cell hyperplasia without tissue damage in mice. J Clin Invest. 1989;84:1488–96.
50. Yamada T, Kaneko H, Iizuka K, et al. Elevation of lymphocyte and hematopoietic stem cell numbers in mice transgenic for human granulocyte. Lab Invest. 1996;74:384–94.
51. Pojda Z, Molineux G, Dexter TM. Hemopoietic effects of short-term in vivo treatment of mice with various doses of rhG-CSF. Exp Hematol. 1990;18:27–31.
52. Cronkite EP, Bullis J, Pappas N, Shimosaka AS. In-vivo G-CSF induces anemia thrombopenia and hemopoiesis in fatty marrow. Exp Hematol. 1990;18.
53. de Haan G, Engel C, Dontje B, et al. Mutual inhibition of murine erythropoiesis and granulopoiesis during combined erythropoietin, granulocyte colony-stimulating factor, and stem cell factor administration: in vivo interactions and dose–response surfaces. Blood. 1994;84:4157–63.

54. Lieschke GJ, Grail D, Hodgson G, et al. Mice lacking granulocyte colony-stimulating factor have chronic neutropenia, granulocyte and macrophage progenitor cell deficiency, and impaired neutrophil mobilization. Blood. 1994;84:1737–46.

55. Coccia M, Hartley C, Sutherland W, et al. Neutropenia in a novel anti-mG-CSF autoantibody mouse model. Exp Hematol. 2000;28.

56. Lieschke GJ. CSF-deficient mice – what have they taught us? Ciba Found Symp. 1997;204:60–74.

57. Liu F, Wu HY, Wesselschmidt R, et al. Impaired production and increased apoptosis of neutrophils in granulocyte colony-stimulating factor receptor-deficient mice. Immunity. 1996;5:491–501.

58. Cebon J, Layton JE, Maher D, Morstyn G. Endogenous haemopoietic growth factors in neutropenia and infection. Br J Haematol. 1994;86:265–74.

59. Barth E, Fischer G, Schneider EM, et al. Peaks of endogenous G-CSF serum concentrations are followed by an increase in respiratory burst activity of granulocytes in patients with septic shock. Cytokine. 2002;17:275–84.

60. Lord BI. Myeloid cell kinetics in response to haemopoietic growth factors. Baillieres Clin Haematol. 1992;5:533–50.

61. Lord BI, Molineux G, Pojda Z, et al. Myeloid cell kinetics in mice treated with recombinant interleukin-3, granulocyte colony-stimulating factor (CSF), or granulocyte–macrophage CSF in vivo. Blood. 1991;77:2154–9.

62. Lord BI, Woolford LW, Molineux G. Kinetics of neutrophil production following filgrastim SD/01. Exp Hematol. 2000;28.

63. Takamatsu Y, Simmons PJ, Moore RJ, et al. Osteoclast-mediated bone resorption is stimulated during short-term administration of granulocyte colony-stimulating factor but is not responsible for hematopoietic progenitor cell mobilization. Blood. 1998;1.

64. Simon M, Lengfelder E, Reiter S, Hehlmann R. Osteoporosis in severe congenital neutropenia: inherent to the disease or a sequela of G-CSF treatment? Am J Hematol. 1996;52:127.

65. Dale DC, Cottle TE, Fier CJ, et al. Severe chronic neutropenia: treatment and follow-up of patients in the Severe Chronic Neutropenia International Registry. Am J Hematol. 2003;72:82–93.

66. Takahashi T, Wada T, Mori M, et al. Overexpression of the granulocyte colony-stimulating factor gene leads to osteoporosis in mice. Lab Invest. 1996;74:827–34.

67. Froberg MK, Garg UC, Stroncek DF, et al. Changes in serum osteocalcin and bone-specific alkaline phosphatase are associated with bone pain in donors receiving granulocyte-colony-stimulating factor for peripheral blood stem and progenitor cell collection. Transfusion. 1999;39:410–14.

68. Semerad CL, Christopher MJ, Liu F, et al. G-CSF potently inhibits osteoblast activity and CXCL12 mRNA expression in the bone marrow. Blood. 2005;106:3020–7.

69. Lord BI, Molineux G, Chang J, et al. Hemopoietic cell kinetics in mice and humans during treatment in-vivo with hemopoietic growth factors. Exp Hematol. 1990;18.

70. Faust J, Lacey DL, Hunt P, et al. Osteoclast markers accumulate on cells developing from human peripheral blood mononuclear precursors. J Cell Biochem. 1999;72:67–80.

71. Gudi R, Krishnamurthy M, Pachter BR. Astemizole in the treatment of granulocyte colony-stimulating factor-induced bone pain. [see comment]. Ann Intern Med. 1995;123:236–7.

72. Morstyn G, Campbell L, Lieschke G, et al. Treatment of chemotherapy-induced neutropenia by subcutaneously administered granulocyte colony-stimulating factor with optimization of dose and duration of therapy. J Clin Oncol. 1989;7:1554–62.

73. Di Leo A, Bajetta E, Nole F, et al. The intramuscular administration of granulocyte colony-stimulating factor as an adjunct to chemotherapy in pretreated ovarian cancer patients: an Italian Trials in Medical Oncology (ITMO) Group Pilot Study. Br J Cancer. 1994;69:961–6.

74. Bartocci A, Mastrogiannis DS, Migliorati G, et al. Macrophages specifically regulate the concentration of their own growth factor in the circulation. Proc Natl Acad Sci USA. 1987;84:6179–83.

75. Zink T, Ross A, Luers K, et al. Structure and dynamics of the human granulocyte colony-stimulating factor determined by NMR spectroscopy: loop mobility in a four-helix-bundle protein. Biochemistry. 1994;33:8453–63.
76. Ono M. Physicochemical and biochemical characteristics of glycosylated recombinant human granulocyte colony stimulating factor (lenograstim). Eur J Cancer. 1994;30A(Suppl-11).
77. Nissen C. Glycosylation of recombinant human granulocyte colony stimulating factor: implications for stability and potency. Eur J Cancer. 1994;30A(Suppl-4).
78. Pedrazzoli P, Gibelli N, Pavesi L, et al. Effects of glycosylated and non-glycosylated G-CSFs, alone and in combination with other cytokines, on the growth of human progenitor cells. Anticancer Res. 1996;16:1781–5.
79. Mire-Sluis AR, Das RG, Thorpe R. The international standard for granulocyte colony stimulating factor (G-CSF). Evaluation in an international collaborative study. Participants of the collaborative study. J Immunol Methods. 1995;179:117–26.
80. Querol S, Cancelas JA, Amat L, et al. Effect of glycosylation of recombinant human granulocytic colony-stimulating factor on expansion cultures of umbilical cord blood CD34$^+$ cells. Haematologica. 1999;84:493–8.
81. Tanaka H, Tanaka Y, Shinagawa K, et al. Three types of recombinant human granulocyte colony-stimulating factor have equivalent biological activities in monkeys. Cytokine. 1997;9:360–9.
82. Bonig H, Silbermann S, Weller S, et al. Glycosylated vs non-glycosylated granulocyte colony-stimulating factor (G-CSF) – results of a prospective randomised monocentre study. Bone Marrow Transplant. 2001;28:259–64.
83. Uzumaki H, Okabe T, Sasaki N, et al. Identification and characterization of receptors for granulocyte colony-stimulating factor on human placenta and trophoblastic cells. Proc Natl Acad Sci USA. 1989;86:9323–6.
84. Piao YF, Okabe T. Receptor binding of human granulocyte colony-stimulating factor to the blast cells of myeloid leukemia. Cancer Res. 1990;50:1671–4.
85. Togawa A, Mizoguchi H, Toyama K, et al. Clinical evaluation of rhG-CSF in patients with neutropenia induced by chemotherapy for multiple myeloma. [Japanese]. Rinsho Ketsueki – Jpn J Clin Hematol. 2000;41:115–22.
86. Agency EM. Assessment report for Tevagrastim. 2008. http://www.emea.europa.eu/humandocs/PDFs/EPAR/tevagrastim/H-827-en6.pdf
87. Molineux G, Kinstler O, Briddell B, et al. A new form of filgrastim with sustained duration in vivo and enhanced ability to mobilize PBPC in both mice and humans. Exp Hematol. 1999;27:1724–34.
88. Niven RW, Prestrelski SJ, Treuheit MJ, et al. Protein nebulization II. Stabilization of G-CSF to air-jet nebulization and the role of protectants. Int J Pharm (Amsterdam). 1996;127:191–201.
89. Watanabe Y, Kiriyama M, Oe J, et al. Pharmacodynamic activity (leukopoietic effect) of recombinant human granulocyte colony-stimulating factor (rhG-CSF) after rectal administration in rabbits with leukopenia induced by cyclophosphamide. Biol Pharm Bull. 1996;19:1064–7.
90. Jensen-Pippo KE, Whitcomb KL, Deprince RB, et al. Enternal bioavailability of human granulocyte colony stimulating factor conjugated with poly(ethylene glycol). Pharm Res (New York). 1996;13:102–7.
91. Tian SS, Lamb P, King AG, et al. A small, nonpeptidyl mimic of granulocyte-colony-stimulating factor [see comments]. Science. 1998;281:257–9.
92. Doyle ML, Tian S-S, Miller SG, et al. Selective binding and oligomerization of the murine granulocyte colony-stimulating factor receptor by a low molecular weight, nonpeptidyl ligand. J Biol Chem. 2003;278:9426–34.
93. Takatani H, Soda H, Fukuda M, et al. Levels of recombinant human granulocyte colony-stimulating factor in serum are inversely correlated with circulating neutrophil counts. Antimicrob Agents Chemother. 1996;40:988–91.

94. Furuya H, Wakayama T, Ohguni S, et al. Effect of continuous subcutaneous administration of a small dose of granulocyte colony stimulating factor (G-CSF) by the use of a portable infusion pump in patients with non-Hodgkin's lymphoma receiving chemotherapy. Int J Hematol. 1995;61:123–9.
95. Besarab A, Flaharty KK, Erslev AJ, et al. Clinical pharmacology and economics of recombinant human erythropoietin in end-stage renal disease: the case for subcutaneous administration. J Am Soc Nephrol. 1992;2:1405–16.
96. Laterveer L, Lindley IJD, Hamilton MS, et al. Interleukin-8 induces rapid mobilization of hematopoietic stem cells with radioprotective capacity and long-term myelolymphoid repopulating ability. Blood. 1995;85:2269–75.
97. Liles WC, Broxmeyer HE, Rodger E, et al. Mobilization of hematopoietic progenitor cells in healthy volunteers by AMD3100, a CXCR4 antagonist. Blood. 2003;102:2728–30.
98. Duhrsen U, Villeval JL, Boyd J, et al. Effects of recombinant human granulocyte colony-stimulating factor on hematopoietic progenitor cells in cancer patients. Blood. 1988;72:2074–81.
99. Lévesque J-P, Hendy J, Takamatsu Y, et al. Mobilization by either cyclophosphamide or granulocyte colony-stimulating factor transforms the bone marrow into a highly proteolytic environment. Exp Hematol. 2002;30:440–9.
100. Woll PJ, Thatcher N, Lomax L, et al. Use of hematopoietic progenitors in whole blood to support dose-dense chemotherapy: a randomized phase II trial in small-cell lung cancer patients. J Clin Oncol. 2001;19:712–19.
101. Klocke R, Kuhlmann MT, Scobioala S, et al. Granulocyte colony-stimulating factor (G-CSF) for cardio- and cerebrovascular regenerative applications. Curr Med Chem. 2008;15:968–77.
102. Vertesaljai M, Piroth Z, Fontos G, et al. Drugs, gene transfer, signaling factors: a bench to bedside approach to myocardial stem cell therapy. Heart Fail Rev. 2008;13:227–44.
103. Kurdi M, Booz GW. G-CSF-based stem cell therapy for the heart – unresolved issues. Part B: stem cells, engraftment, transdifferentiation, and bioengineering. Congest Heart Fail. 2007;13:347–51.
104. Kurdi M, Booz GWG-. CSF-based stem cell therapy for the heart-unresolved issues. Part A: paracrine actions, mobilization, and delivery. Congest Heart Fail. 2007;13:221–7.
105. Orlic D, Kajstura J, Chimenti S, et al. Bone marrow cells regenerate infarcted myocardium. [see comments]. Nature. 2001;410:701–5.
106. Okada H, Takemura G, Li Y, et al. Effect of a long-term treatment with a low-dose granulocyte colony-stimulating factor on post-infarction process in the heart. J Cell Mol Med. 2008;12:1272–83.
107. Tatsumi K, Otani H, Sato D, et al. Granulocyte-colony stimulating factor increases donor mesenchymal stem cells in bone marrow and their mobilization into peripheral circulation but does not repair dystrophic heart after bone marrow transplantation. Circ J. 2008;72:1351–8.
108. Liang HL, Yi DH, Zheng QJ, et al. Improvement of heart allograft acceptability associated with recruitment of CD4$^+$CD25$^+$ T cells in peripheral blood by recipient treatment with granulocyte colony-stimulating factor. Transplant Proc. 2008;40:1604–11.
109. Brunner S, Huber BC, Fischer R, et al. G-CSF treatment after myocardial infarction: impact on bone marrow-derived vs cardiac progenitor cells. Exp Hematol. 2008;36:695–702.
110. Zohlnhofer D, Ott I, Mehilli J, et al. Stem cell mobilization by granulocyte colony-stimulating factor in patients with acute myocardial infarction: a randomized controlled trial. [see comment]. JAMA. 2006;295:1003–10.
111. Ripa RS, Jorgensen E, Wang Y, et al. Stem cell mobilization induced by subcutaneous granulocyte-colony stimulating factor to improve cardiac regeneration after acute ST-elevation myocardial infarction: result of the double-blind, randomized, placebo-controlled stem cells in myocardial infarction (STEMMI) trial. [see comment]. Circulation. 2006;113:1983–92.

112. Erbs S, Linke A, Schachinger V, et al. Restoration of microvascular function in the infarct-related artery by intracoronary transplantation of bone marrow progenitor cells in patients with acute myocardial infarction: the Doppler Substudy of the Reinfusion of Enriched Progenitor Cells and Infarct Remodeling in Acute Myocardial Infarction (REPAIR-AMI) trial. [reprint in Nat Clin Pract Cardiovasc Med. 2008 Feb;5(2):78–9; PMID: 17984996]. Circulation. 2007;116:366–74.

113. Ince H, Petzsch M, Kleine HD, et al. Preservation from left ventricular remodeling by front-integrated revascularization and stem cell liberation in evolving acute myocardial infarction by use of granulocyte-colony-stimulating factor (FIRSTLINE-AMI). [see comment]. Circulation. 2005;112:3097–106.

114. Cohen MH, Gootenberg J, Keegan P, Pazdur R. FDA drug approval summary: bevacizumab (Avastin) plus Carboplatin and Paclitaxel as first-line treatment of advanced/metastatic recurrent nonsquamous non-small cell lung cancer. Oncologist. 2007;12:713–18.

115. Shojaei F, Wu X, Malik AK, et al. Tumor refractoriness to anti-VEGF treatment is mediated by $CD11b^+Gr1^+$ myeloid cells. Nat Biotechnol. 2007;25:911–20.

116. Shojaei F, Wu X, Zhong C, et al. Bv8 regulates myeloid-cell-dependent tumour angiogenesis. Nature. 2007;450:825–31.

117. Shojaei F, Wu X, Qu X, et al. G-CSF-initiated myeloid cell mobilization and angiogenesis mediate tumor refractoriness to anti-VEGF therapy in mouse models. Proc Natl Acad Sci USA. 2009;106:6742–7.

118. Movahedi K, Guilliams M, Van den Bossche J, et al. Identification of discrete tumor-induced myeloid-derived suppressor cell subpopulations with distinct T cell-suppressive activity. Blood. 2008;111:4233–44.

119 Umemura N, Saio M, Suwa T, et al. Tumor-infiltrating myeloid-derived suppressor cells are pleiotropic-inflamed monocytes/macrophages that bear M1- and M2-type characteristics. J Leukoc Biol. 2008;83:1136–44.

Chapter 4
Erythropoiesis-Stimulating Agents

Steve Elliott

Abstract Erythropoiesis is the process whereby erythroid progenitor cells differentiate and divide, resulting in increased numbers of red blood cells (RBCs). RBCs contain hemoglobin, the main oxygen carrying component in blood. The large number of RBCs found in blood is required to support the prodigious consumption of oxygen by tissues as they undergo oxygen-dependent processes. Erythropoietin is a hormone that when it binds and activates Epo receptors resident on the surface of cells results in stimulation of erythropoiesis. Successful cloning of the *EPO* gene allowed for the first time production of recombinant human erythropoietin and other erythropoiesis stimulating agents (ESAs), which are used to treat anemia in patients. In this chapter, the control of Epo levels and erythropoiesis, the various forms of ESAs used commercially, and their physical and biological properties are discussed.

Introduction

Erythropoietin (Epo) is a late-acting growth factor, so named because of early studies suggesting it had a singular effect on stimulation of red blood cell formation (erythropoiesis). Epo functions by binding and activating an Epo receptor expressed on the surface of committed erythroid progenitor cells resulting in their proliferation and differentiation. This elegant process results in formation of enucleated hemoglobin-containing red blood cells (RBCs) that are released into the circulation where they can bind oxygen in the lungs and deliver it to tissues with a high oxygen demand, e.g., brain or working muscles.

Successful cloning of the *EPO* gene in the 1980s [1, 2] allowed the commercial production of recombinant human erythropoietin (rHuEpo). The utility of rHuEpo in treating anemia (low hemoglobin [Hb] levels) was explored in patients with chronic

S. Elliott (✉)
Department of Hematology, Amgen, Inc., Thousand Oaks, CA 91320, USA
e-mail: selliott@amgen.com

G.H. Lyman, D.C. Dale (eds.), *Hematopoietic Growth Factors in Oncology*,
Cancer Treatment and Research 157, DOI 10.1007/978-1-4419-7073-2_4,
© Springer Science+Business Media, LLC 2011

kidney disease (CKD), anemia of cancer (AoC), chemotherapy-induced anemia (CIA), and anemia of inflammation such as rheumatoid arthritis. It was also studied in patients scheduled for major surgery who were expected to require blood transfusions. rHuEpo (e.g., epoetin alfa) has been approved for use in humans and is currently used primarily to treat anemia associated with CKD and CIA.

This review will examine the structure, function, and regulation of Epo production, mechanisms affecting clearance of Epo, erythropoiesis, various forms of ESAs, and the data suggesting Epo has effects on other biological processes beyond erythropoiesis.

Hemoglobin, Erythropoietin, and Erythropoiesis

Red Blood Cells and Hemoglobin

RBCs in humans represent 40–45% of total blood volume and 99% of all circulating cells. In a healthy person with roughly 5 L of blood, this represents approximately 2.5×10^{13} cells. RBCs are long-lived with a lifespan of approximately 100–120 days [3]. The daily loss of RBCs, approximately 0.8–1.0% of the total, is matched by a prodigious production capacity of $\sim 2.5 \times 10^{11}$ cells/day [4]. Hb residing within mature RBCs is the primary oxygen-binding component and constitutes 99% of the cytosolic protein [5]. Iron residing within hemoglobin (2.5 g) represents the major component of total body iron (3–4 g) and levels are tightly regulated [6]. These high levels of iron, hemoglobin, and RBCs are consistent with the importance of maintaining oxygen homeostasis in the body.

Hb is a tetrameric protein with each subunit containing a tightly associated nonprotein heme iron. In human adults the major form of Hb is hemoglobin A, consisting of two α and two β (beta) subunits. The affinity of O_2 for Hb in RBCs is increased with low temperature, low CO_2, and low 2,3 DPG as occurring in lungs. Affinity is reduced by increases in body temperature, hydrogen ion, 2,3-diphosphoglycerate, or carbon dioxide concentration (the Bohr effect) under conditions where O_2 levels are low, such as working muscles. Therefore, in muscles that are consuming O_2 and generating CO_2 and lactic acid, O_2 is released from Hb [7].

Erythropoietin

As O_2 levels decrease with exercise, blood loss, anemia, or change in concentration of oxygen in breathed air, the breathing rate, heart rate, and adjustments in O_2-carrying capacity are made to meet the demand. One mechanism to increase O_2-carrying capacity is to increase hemoglobin levels by stimulating formation of increased numbers of Hb-containing RBCs through increases in erythropoietin

(Epo) levels which stimulates erythropoiesis. Epo is a circulating glycosylated protein hormone that is the primary regulator of RBC formation. Endogenous Epo (eEpo) is synthesized primarily in the kidney, although it is also made at lower levels in other tissues such as liver and brain [8–12].

Endogenous Epo in humans is transcribed as a 1.6–2-kb mRNA [2] and translated into a 193 amino acid precursor [1, 13]. During transit through the secretory apparatus, the 27 amino acid signal peptide and C-terminal arginine are removed and carbohydrate chains are added to three N-linked glycosylation sites and the one O-linked glycosylation site [13, 14]. The secreted protein contains 165 amino acids with approximately 40% of the mass composed of carbohydrate. The structure of rHuEpo is a compact globular bundle, which contains four alfa-helices in a characteristic 4-helix bundle, a topology shared with other growth factors [15, 16] (Fig. 4.1).

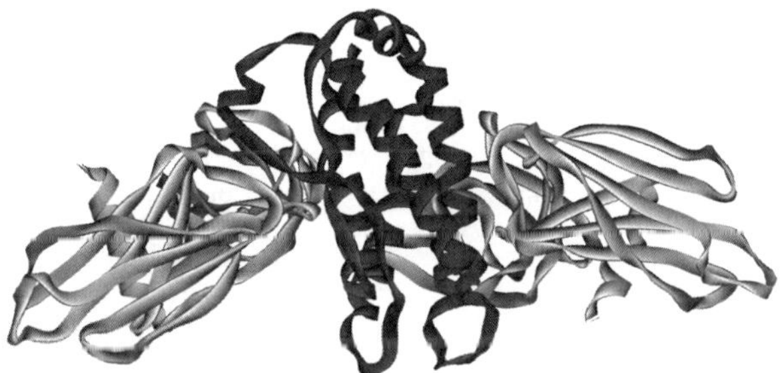

Fig. 4.1 Structure of an Epo:EpoR complex. The *top view* (*ribbon diagram*) of the crystal structure shows Epo (*gray*) bound to the extracellular domains of two EpoRs (*dark gray*). Two different surfaces of Epo bind to similar regions of EpoR resulting in high- and low-affinity binding sites. The "cross-linked" EpoR is activated resulting in downstream signaling

Erythropoiesis

RBC production (erythropoiesis) is a result of an elegant proliferation and differentiation pathway (Fig. 4.2). Early hematopoietic progenitor cells residing primarily in the bone marrow differentiate in the presence of an early growth factor such as SCF, IL-3, or GM-CSF [17] into burst-forming unit erythroid (BFUe) and then into colony-forming unit (CFUe) cells [18, 19]. BFUe cells acquire responsiveness to and become dependent on Epo as they differentiate into the CFUe stage [17, 20]. Further differentiation of CFUe cells results in molecular and physical changes and the immature "blast" cells become proerythroblasts, and finally, erythroblasts. These cells begin to take up iron and show increased synthesis and accumulation of Hb. The late-stage erythroblasts discharge their nucleus (enucleation), resulting in reticulocytes that are released into the circulation. After several days, reticulin (ribosomal RNA and associated material) declines resulting in mature, circulating RBCs.

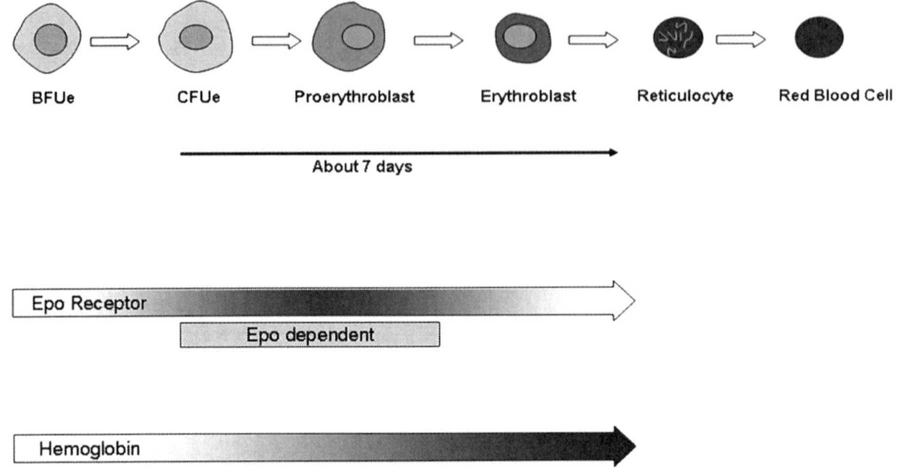

Fig. 4.2 Erythropoiesis. The schematic diagram shows the differentiation of erythroid progenitor cells. BFUe (burst-forming unit erythroid) cells differentiate in blood islands in the bone marrow into CFUe (colony-forming unit erythroid) and ultimately into reticulocytes that are released into the circulation. The process involves increased synthesis of EpoR and hemoglobin

Epo Receptor and Its Activation

The mechanism by which Epo stimulates erythropoiesis has been the subject of considerable investigation. Radiolabeled Epo was shown to bind to a "receptor" expressed on the surface of erythroid cells. The gene encoding the Epo receptor was identified by expression cloning and found to be a single gene with no apparent homologs [21, 22]. The human *EPOR* gene encodes a 508 aa protein which following removal of the 24 aa signal peptide results in a 484 aa protein with a molecular weight of approximately 52.7 kDa [23]. Addition of an N-linked carbohydrate chain results in a secreted protein with a calculated size of 56–57 kDa which is comparable to the size of mature EpoR determined by Western immunoblotting ($\sim$59 kDa) [23].

In early studies, EpoR transcripts were detected by Northern analysis in bone marrow or spleen with none detected in heart, kidney, liver, or brain [24]. This is consistent with [125I]Epo-binding studies which also suggested that high-level expression of EpoR is normally restricted to cells of the erythroid lineage [24–28]. Reticulocytes and circulating RBCs do not express EpoR [29–31].

While other components may mediate affinity to Epo or aid in signal transduction, current evidence suggests that the activation of EpoR is initiated by a direct interaction of a single Epo molecule with two EpoRs via high- and low-affinity binding sites effectively "cross-linking" them (Fig. 4.1). The binding and cross-linking by Epo induces a conformational change thereby bringing together two separate regions on the transmembrane and intracellular regions of the receptor. Activation results in cross-phosphorylation of EpoR and Jak2 which is followed by activation of the downstream STAT5, MAP kinase, and PI3 kinase/Akt pathways [32].

Following stimulation of signal transduction, negative regulators of EpoR, including Src homology region 2 domain-containing phosphatase 1 (SHP-1) and suppressor of cytokine signaling proteins SOCS-1 and SOCS-2, downmodulate responses [33, 34].

Normal circulating levels of Epo in humans are approximately 5 pM, substantially below the kDa of the Epo:EpoR interaction indicating that only a fraction of the EpoR is Epo bound but this level of binding is sufficient to maintain erythropoiesis at a rate that will maintain RBC levels. Lower Epo receptor occupancy results in apoptosis of precursor cells (post-CFUe stage) [35].

Epo responsive erythroid cells express 300–1,100 high-affinity ($\sim$100 pM) surface EpoR/cell [1, 2, 34]. The half-maximal response to Epo of CFUe cells is achieved when approximately 7% of their cell surface-expressed EpoR are bound by Epo suggesting approximately 70 surface EpoR are bound by Epo at this Epo concentration [9]. These observations indicate that a single Epo–EpoR binding event is insufficient for stimulation of complete differentiation of erythroid precursors. Instead, adequate concentrations of Epo must be present during the entire process to ensure survival and proliferation of the cells.

Acquired Epo responsiveness appears to require a threshold amount of EpoR expression and Epo binding. This notion is consistent with a number of observations. EpoR mRNA and surface EpoR protein expression increase up to the normoblast stage of cell differentiation followed by a rapid decline thereafter (Fig. 4.2) and this timing is associated with acquired Epo responsiveness [29, 31, 36]. Mice with haploinsufficiency containing only one functional allele of EpoR have lower EpoR levels and decreased hematocrit. Colony formation using cells recovered from these animals requires higher Epo concentrations compared to control animals [37]. BFUe cells which show minimal response to Epo [17, 38, 39] acquire Epo-dependent growth following forced over-expression of EpoR [26]. Similarly forced over-expression of EpoR in various leukemic cell lines will make them dependent on Epo for growth or survival [40–43]. HEL cells express low but detectable levels of EpoR on their cell surface [31] but these cells show increased STAT5 phosphorylation if EpoR levels are increased by forced over-expression of EpoR [44].

Expression of EpoR is necessary but not sufficient for Epo responsiveness. OCIM1 cells are an immortalized cell line derived from a patient with erythroleukemia [45]. These cells express EpoR on their surface at levels comparable to that found on Epo responsive erythroid precursor cells but they do not respond to Epo. Functional EpoR was cloned from OCIM1 cells [22], indicating the lack of Epo responsiveness was not due to mutations in EpoR. While forced expression of EpoR in some cell types (32D, FDCP1, and BaF3) results in acquisition of Epo responsiveness [40–43], this was not true of forced over-expression in other cell types such as NIH-3T3 or CTLL2 suggesting they lack positive factors or over-express negative factors [46–48]. A subline of EpoR CTLL2-transfected cells was initially nonresponsive but became dependent on Epo following selection for growth on Epo. Both the subline and the original transfected cells expressed similar levels of surface EpoR and both expressed Jak2, but Epo induced Jak2 phosphorylation only in the subline [48–51] indicating the JAK-2 to STAT5 pathway was present but could not be activated.

Erythropoiesis-Stimulating Agents (ESAs)

Endogenous Epo and rHuEpo

Recombinant HuEpo was initially used for the treatment of anemia associated with chronic kidney disease. It is also indicated for cancer patients who have CIA. According to a number of studies rHuEpo is well tolerated, can correct and maintain hemoglobin levels, and reduce the likelihood of transfusions when used according to guidelines [52–58].

Epoetin alfa, the first commercialized rHuEpo (Epogen®, Procrit®, Eprex®), is a 165 amino acid glycoprotein with an average molecular weight of 30,400 Da. As is eEpo, epoetin alfa is a heavily glycosylated protein containing N-linked and O-linked complex carbohydrates with over >50 different forms described [59–61]. There is also a natural variation in charge due to the presence of a variable number of sialic acids (up to four) on each of the three N-linked carbohydrate chains and up to two sialic acids on the single O-linked carbohydrate chain.

Endogenous Epo and rHuEpo have the same amino acid sequence but are not identical to each other [62, 63]. This is because eEpo is a complex biological produced by specialized cells that are impacted by forces unique to the body, including a complex interaction of circulating growth factors, nutrients, and particular cell–cell interactions. The circulating eEpo is then subject to differential clearance of the various glycoforms. It is not possible to duplicate these processes in a manufacturing setting. Some of the resulting differences have been described. For example, endogenous Epo has sialic acid attached to galactose in NeuAcα2→6 or 2→3 linkages. Chinese hamster ovary (CHO) cells are frequently used to manufacture rHuEpo and because these cells lack a sialotransferase with NeuAcα2→6 activity only NeuAcα2→3 linkages are present in rHuEpo made from these cells [64]. rHuEpo made in CHO cells but not eEpo can contain traces of *N*-glycolylneuraminic acid in addition to the typical Neu5Ac found in urinary Epo [65, 66]. rHuEpo can also be made in other cell types where NGNA was also found. Endogenous Epo has a substantially higher content of sulfate on the attached carbohydrate compared to rHuEpo. Thus eEpo can be considerably more negative (acidic) than rHuEpo [67, 68] and this difference has been exploited to detect abuse of rHuEpo in athletes [63].

Follow-on Biologics

Glycosylation of proteins may impact properties such as binding affinity for cognate ligands, resistance to proteolytic degradation, and physical properties such as stability and solubility, and these can affect product quality as well as clearance, efficacy, and safety [69–73]. Changes in cell lines, minor changes in growth conditions or manufacturing processes, can affect the final ESA product characteristics including the microheterogeneity of glycoforms. It is not possible for another manufacturer to match exactly the product profile of the innovator. Thus, the term "generic" is not used to describe rHuEpo molecules made by different manufacturers. Instead, the descriptors "follow-on biologics" or FOBS, "biosimilars" or "biosimilar biopharmaceuticals" are used [74].

The inherent difficulties in matching product characteristics and the demand that biosimilars have similar efficacy and safety to the innovator products [75, 76] have slowed approval of biosimilar rHuEpos because they require more oversight in the drug approval process [75–77]. In contrast to vaccines, whose efficacy depends on the ability to stimulate protective immunity in hosts, the safety and efficacy of recombinant biopharmaceutical proteins depends in part on their biochemical and immunochemical similarity to the corresponding endogenous proteins. These features help to optimize therapeutic activity of the recombinant proteins while minimizing their potential immunogenicity [78–81]. Neutralizing Abs should they form may cause or contribute to certain immunopathologies, such as Ab-mediated pure red cell aplasia (PRCA) in patients treated with ESAs [82, 83]. Antibody-mediated PRCA is a serious hematologic condition characterized by the onset, following a period of successful therapy, of severe ESA-resistant anemia that most often resolves only after cessation of ESA therapy and intervention with immuno-suppressive agents [84]. The sudden appearance in 1999 of increased number of patients who presented with antibody-mediated PRCA was associated with changes in manufacturing processes of Eprex thereby highlighting the potential adverse consequence of manufacturing differences on product safety of FOBs [81, 82].

rHuEpo FOBs are also manufactured and distributed in countries where less oversight on drug manufacturing results in significant product quality and in structural differences from epoetins distributed in the United States and EU [85–87]. These ESAs can vary considerably from each other and from marketed epoetins manufactured in the United States and EU in labeling, drug content, and specific activity. There may also be considerable lot-to-lot variability. There have been reports that some patients administered with these ESAs have presented with antibody-mediated PRCA [88].

In addition to differences in product characteristics, there is also confusion about naming conventions of newer rHuEpo molecules. Following the introduction of the first epoetin alfa a second was approved in the EU (Recormon/Neorecormon Roche Diagnostics GmbH, Mannheim, Germany) and was given the name epoetin beta. It has the same amino acid sequence as epoetin alfa manufactured by Amgen, Inc. with some minor differences in the microheterogeneity in the attached carbohydrate. Other epoetins followed with different Greek names. Epoetin omega, produced in baby hamster kidney cells, differed somewhat from epoetin alfa and beta in the glycosylation profile [89]. However, this agent is distributed only in South Africa. Dynepo (epoetin delta) was manufactured by Shire Pharmaceutical Contracts Ltd, Hampshire, UK and was approved in Europe for the treatment of anemia in adult patients with chronic renal failure, but as of December 2008 was withdrawn from the market. Other ESA biosimilars are being introduced in the EU: Silapro/Retacrit (epoetin zeta). However, Abseamed/Binocrit/Hexal is marketed as an "epoetin alfa" as are some epoetins manufactured in countries outside the United States and EU.

Darbepoetin Alfa

Aranesp® (darbepoetin alfa; Amgen, Inc.) is manufactured in the United States and marketed in Europe, the United States, Australia, Canada, and others. Aranesp® is a novel hyperglycosylated rHuEpo analog with five amino acid changes that compared to epoetin alfa contain two additional N-linked glycosylation sites resulting in the attachment of two additional carbohydrate chains for a total of five [90]. Aranesp® has the same mechanism of action as rHuEpo, stimulating of erythropoiesis through activation of the Epo receptor (EpoR). However, Darbepoetin alfa has increased in vivo potency [69, 90, 91] due to a threefold longer serum half-life and mean residence time than epoetin alfa [91, 92]. The longer serum half-life allows for more convenient modes of administration, including extended dosing intervals with a similar efficacy and safety profile to epoetin alfa.

Other ESAs

Mircera® (methoxy polyethylene glycol-epoetin beta) is epoetin beta with a covalent attachment to the peptide backbone of a linear methoxy polyethylene glycol (PEG), resulting in approximately a doubling in size compared to epoetin alfa (30.4 vs 60 kDa) [13, 93]. PEG-epoetin beta has a prolonged elimination half-life in patients with CKD, approximately 134 h [94]. Mircera® is approved for the treatment of anemia associated with CKD in Europe.

Hematide is a nonnaturally occurring Epo dipeptide mimetic that binds to the Epo receptor in a manner similar to rHuEpo, thereby activating it [95, 96]. The dipeptide was pegylated resulting in a longer serum half-life and it is currently in clinical development.

Control of Circulating Epo Levels

Synthesis of eEpo

In adult mammals, Epo is expressed in liver hepatocytes [9] and in interstitial fibroblast-like cells in the kidney which are uniquely located adjacent to kidney tubular cells where they can sense changes in oxygen levels and rapidly and robustly respond [8, 97]. In anemic subjects, circulating Epo levels were inversely proportional to Hb levels which in severe cases of anemia were increased up to 1,000-fold [98]. In isolated nuclei from kidneys from hypoxic vs normal animals, Epo mRNA levels increased substantially with hypoxia (reduced O_2) in a short time-frame (2–4 h) [99] and rapidly declined following introduction of normal O_2 levels. The increased Epo production was due to a logarithmic increase in the number of cells producing Epo in the renal cortex of bled mice as the degree of hypoxia increased and not to the rate/cell in these cells which appeared constant [10]. The increased response to hypoxia is blunted if Epo-producing cells are lost (e.g., due to kidney disease) or have compromised ability to sense reduced O_2 levels explaining the anemia associated with progressive kidney disease.

The mechanism by which hypoxia upregulates Epo production is now partially understood. Hypoxia inducible factor (HIF) is a transcription factor that binds to a hypoxia response element (HRE) found in certain genes thereby stimulating mRNA synthesis from them [100, 101]. Homologs of HIF (HIF-1α, HIF-2α, HIF-3α) each form a heterodimer composed of an oxygen-sensitive HIFα and a constitutive HIF-1β [102]. HIF-2α is thought to play the dominant role in regulation of *EPO* gene transcription. HIF is expressed constitutively but its levels are controlled by rapid O_2-dependent degradation. Degradation of HIF-α is triggered when it is hydroxylated at specific prolines within an oxygen degradation domain by an O_2-dependent enzyme, HIF-prolyl hydroxylase; HIF-PH [103–106]. Such hydroxylation triggers an association of the hydroxylated HIF with the von Hippel-Lindau protein (VHL), which promotes ligation with ubiquitin and subsequent degradation by the proteasome [106–108]. Thus at low levels of O_2, HIF accumulates due to reduced activity of HIF-PH, resulting in increased eEpo synthesis. At increased O_2 tension, however, HIF levels decline rapidly due to increased HIF-PH activity (within minutes) resulting in a rapid halt in Epo synthesis.

Control of Epo Levels – Clearance

In adult and pediatric patients with CKD, the elimination half-life of epoetin alfa administered intravenously (IV) ranged from 4 to 13 h [109], similar to that reported for eEpo (5 h) [110]. Subcutaneous (SC) administration resulted in slower absorption, with peak plasma levels achieved after 5–24 h. Peak plasma levels were lower than that observed with IV administration (5–10%) with an apparent extended $t_{1/2}$ (~20–25 h) [111, 112]. This clearance profile is known as "flip–flop pharmacokinetics" [113], where the rate of absorption is slower than the rate of elimination. In the case of rHuEpo, absorption is rate limiting and the increased apparent half-life after SC dosing reflects the absorption rather than elimination rate.

Bioavailability estimates for SC rHuEpo range from about 20 to 40%, suggesting a substantial loss of material during transport from the interstitial space to the lymphatic system and blood [109]. The pharmacokinetic (pk) characteristics of rHuEpo in healthy volunteers appear similar or comparable to those in several other populations, including chronic kidney disease, liver cirrhosis, and myelodysplastic syndrome patients.

In contrast to rHuEpo, darbepoetin alfa has an extended serum half-life [91]. Following IV administration in hemodialysis patients, the serum half-life of darbepoetin alfa was roughly threefold longer than that observed with epoetin alfa (25 vs 8.5 h) [92]. With SC administration, darbepoetin alfa concentrations peaked at 34–58 h post-dose and the serum half-life was extended approximately twofold compared to IV administration. A later study that examined pk parameters in CKD patients following SC administration at extended times reported a mean terminal serum half-life of 70 h [114]. The mean terminal half-life of darbepoetin alfa administered SC in cancer patients treated with chemotherapy was also approximately 70 h [115] and was comparable in pediatric patients with CIA [116].

The mean $t_{1/2}$ of PEG-epoetin beta was 134 h in patients receiving peritoneal dialysis when administered IV [94]. Unlike rHuEpo and darbepoetin alfa, the terminal half-life when administered SC was similar; PEG-epoetin beta did not display "flip–flop" pharmacokinetics. Bioavailability of PEG-epoetin beta was 52% suggesting that IV administration may be the more efficient route.

The mechanism by which ESAs are cleared has been studied. Clearance of ESAs was first thought to be mediated primarily by liver hepatocytes through an asialo-glycoprotein receptor (ASGR) [117, 118] or through the kidney [63, 119]. But these conclusions were not supported by other studies [120–122]. Binding of Epo to EpoR can lead to cellular internalization and degradation [123, 124] suggesting that Epo receptor-mediated uptake and metabolism may affect clearance. An engineered rHuEpo analog (NM385) that was devoid of detectable receptor binding but retained similar structure and carbohydrate content to rHuEpo was constructed and its clearance properties were examined [125]. In rodents NM385 had a slightly longer terminal half-life but similar clearance compared with rHuEpo, suggesting that ESAs may be cleared to some degree through this pathway but this may not be the only or dominant one.

Other studies suggested clearance may be via metabolism in tissue. Indeed, the lymphatic system is thought to play an important role in the reduced bioavailability after subcutaneous administration of proteins [126]. Degraded, but little intact, darbepoetin alfa was found in tissues following administration to rats suggesting that darbepoetin distributed to tissue where it was degraded [127, 128]. Thus clearance of Epo may occur by diffusion from the blood to the interstitium where metabolism occurs, such as by cells involved in the reticuloendothelial scavenging pathway or lymphatic system.

PEGylated epoetin beta and darbepoetin alfa have reduced receptor-binding activity suggesting that the effect of PEG and additional carbohydrate on clearance may be due to reduced Epo receptor-mediated endocytosis and degradation. However, PEGylated rHuEpo and PEGylated NM385 (that lacks receptor-binding activity) both had similar clearance properties [125], suggesting that EpoR-mediated clearance is minimally impacted by hyperglycosylation or PEGylation. Hyperglycosylated and PEGylated ESAs have other biophysical characteristics such as increased hydrodynamic size. Thus a more likely possibility is that these ESAs have larger hydrodynamic size that reduces transport from the blood to the interstitial fluid where degradation takes place.

Pharmacodynamics

In cell culture with hematopoietic cells obtained from bone marrow or peripheral blood, there is an increase in number of colonies that grow in semisolid medium with increasing concentration of Epo. The rate of growth of individual cells appears relatively constant indicating that increasing concentrations of Epo support growth and survival of increasing numbers of progenitor cells. At concentrations above approximately 1 unit/mL, no additional colony growth occurs [69]. Normal circulating levels of Epo are $\sim$10–30 mU/mL [129]. In healthy subjects, this level is sufficient to produce enough RBCs to maintain a normal hematocrit and increased Epo concentrations result in an increase in rate of erythropoiesis [69, 130, 131].

In patients with CKD, production of erythropoietin is impaired, and this is the primary cause of their anemia [52, 130]. "Replacement therapy" by administration of ESAs can stimulate erythropoiesis and raise hemoglobin levels in these patients. The rate of hematocrit increase varies among patients and is dependent upon the dose of epoetin alfa, within a therapeutic range of approximately 50–300 U/kg 3 times weekly. A greater biologic response is not typically observed at higher doses [130]. Other factors affecting the rate and extent of response include availability of iron stores, the baseline hematocrit, and the presence of concurrent medical problems.

Patients with cancer also can have anemia either due to the disease itself or due to the effects of chemotherapy. In these patients, the level of circulating Epo is insufficient for the degree of anemia. The response in these patients to rHuEpo varies and incomplete response is attributed to insufficient iron levels or to the inhibition of erythropoiesis caused by elevated levels of inflammatory cytokines that inhibit erythropoiesis [132, 133].

RHuEpo administered to CKD patients showed a modest increase in the rate of erythropoiesis with increasing doses of Epo ($\sim$fourfold) [130]. However, this change was relatively small compared to the changes in circulating Epo concentrations that occur with severe anemia ($\sim$1,000-fold increase) [129]. Indeed, administration of rHuEpo to animals can result in peak serum concentrations that are substantially above that associated with maximal rates of erythropoiesis, yet at high doses there is a dose-dependent increase in final Hb levels. These observations indicate that Epo concentration level per se is not the primary driver of enhanced erythropoiesis in this setting. Instead, the magnitude of increase in RBC concentration is primarily controlled by the length of time Epo concentrations are maintained at higher levels, and increased starting concentrations of Epo result in a prolonged time that concentration is above a threshold. Darbepoetin alfa, a novel ESA with a prolonged serum half-life that has increased in vivo potency compared to faster clearing ESAs, exploits this association [69, 90].

The effect on hematocrit of rHuEpo administration is prolonged compared to the exposure time of ESAs due to the disproportionate relationship between rHuEpo serum half-life and RBC lifespan. Administration of rHuEpo results in circulating levels above baseline that can last for 2–4 days. This time period is comparable to the lifespan of reticulocytes ($t_{1/2}=1$–5 days) [134, 135] but short compared to the lifespan of RBCs (100–120 days) [3]. Thus, a short duration of increased rHuEpo exposure results in a prolonged increase in RBC concentration. This observation is exploited in clinical settings where intermittent dosing schedules can increase or maintain Hb levels for extended time periods. Dose and dosing schedule are determined according to both pk–PD parameters as well as patient and physician practice patterns. For example, patients on hemodialysis present to the clinic 2–3 times/week and may be dosed on each visit with an ESA.

In patients with CIA, administration of rHuEpo is typically 2–3 times/week or 1 time/week according to pk and PD parameters. However in this setting, patients typically present to the clinic on a 3–4 week schedule which is the time between chemotherapy sessions. Darbepoetin alfa with an extended serum half-life is indicated for reduced frequency of administration compared to epoetin alfa allowing ESA administration to more closely match office visits.

Nonhematopoietic Effects of Epo

ESAs were reported to promote proliferation or survival of nonhematopoietic cells and show benefit to various ischemic insults in organs such as heart, kidney, and brain. The effect was reportedly due to an interaction of Epo with Epo receptors expressed on those cells [136]. The possibility that nonhematopoietic tumor cells expressed EpoR and responded to Epo raised concerns about the use of ESAs in patients with cancer [137]. While these proposals have its proponents, the hypothesis is controversial.

EpoR mRNA was detected in nonerythroid tissues using sensitive RT-PCR methodologies. The significance of this observation is unclear because most RT-PCR experiments were nonquantitative, and those that were quantitative showed that EpoR expression in nonhematopoietic cells ranged from 10-fold to 1,000-fold lower than in cells known to bind or respond to Epo [24, 28, 138–141]. The studies that reportedly detected EpoR protein in nonhematopoietic cells were based largely on antibodies that were shown to be nonspecific; they did not distinguish between EpoR positive and negative cells in IHC experiments and the EpoR protein in Western immunoblotting experiments was often misidentified [23, 138, 142–144].

The possibility that Epo affected growth or survival of nonerythroid hematopoietic cells is inconsistent with the minimal change in circulating nonerythroid cell counts when Epo was administered to normal animals and humans [145, 146]. Furthermore, mice that were engineered to express EpoR exclusively in hematopoietic cells showed normal size and development [147]. The notion that rHuEpo promoted survival of ischemic insult in the brain was not fully supported by pk studies showing that rHuEpo was poorly transported into the brain [148, 149]. Some studies using in vitro cell culture systems showed putative activation of signaling, stimulation of in vitro proliferation, or increased survival of tumor cells or cell lines following ESA addition. However, the effects were generally modest, were compromised by methodological issues, and many studies from other investigators demonstrated no effect of ESAs [138, 150, 151]. Studies examining growth-promoting activity of tumor cells by ESAs in animal models almost universally saw either no effect or reported a decrease in tumor cell growth in the ESA arm of the studies [151].

The tissue protective effects reportedly due to ESA administration may be indirect. For example, Katavetin argued that the beneficial effect of ESA administration was not explained by a reduction in apoptosis due to EpoR activation by ESAs but alternatively due to a decrease in oxidative stress [152]. Thus the enhanced erythropoiesis due to ESA administration may reduce oxidative stress through increased mobilization of iron from tissues into the erythron [153]. Additional work is necessary in this area to test and confirm the various hypotheses.

Conclusion

Before the availability of rHuEpo, the methods to treat anemia were limited to transfusion with its associated problems, or administered iron or steroids which were largely ineffective by themselves. The cloning of the Epo gene allowed commercial production of rHuEpo and new ways to treat patients with anemia. Second generation molecules with a longer serum half-life, such as darbepoetin alfa, were discovered and developed providing additional physician and patient convenience. Experiments with rHuEpo also allowed an enhanced understanding of anemia, the mechanisms by which Epo functions and how Epo levels are controlled through both synthesis of Epo and its clearance. Scientists continue to provide advances which should provide increased understanding of these processes and further advance our ability to treat patients.

References

1. Lin FK, Suggs S, Lin CH, et al. Cloning and expression of the human erythropoietin gene. Proc Natl Acad Sci USA. 1985;82:7580–4.
2. Jacobs K, Shoemaker C, Rudersdorf R, et al. Isolation and characterization of genomic and cDNA clones of human erythropoietin. Nature. 1985;313:806–10.
3. Smith JA. Exercise, training and red blood cell turnover. Sports Med. 1995;19:9–31.
4. Elliott S, Pham E, Macdougall IC. Erythropoietins: a common mechanism of action. Exp Hematol. 2008;36:1573–84.
5. Hebbel RP, Eaton JW. Pathobiology of heme interaction with the erythrocyte membrane. Semin Hematol. 1989;26:136–49.
6. Ganz T. Iron homeostasis: fitting the puzzle pieces together. Cell Metab. 2008;7:288–90.
7. Elliott S. Erythropoiesis-stimulating agents and other methods to enhance oxygen transport. Br J Pharmacol. 2008;154:529–41.
8. Koury ST, Bondurant MC, Koury MJ. Localization of erythropoietin synthesizing cells in murine kidneys by in situ hybridization. Blood. 1988;71:524–7.
9. Koury ST, Bondurant MC, Koury MJ, Semenza GL. Localization of cells producing erythropoietin in murine liver by in situ hybridization. Blood. 1991;77:2497–503.
10. Koury ST, Koury MJ, Bondurant MC, Caro J, Graber SE. Quantitation of erythropoietin-producing cells in kidneys of mice by in situ hybridization: correlation with hematocrit, renal erythropoietin mRNA, and serum erythropoietin concentration. Blood. 1989;74:645–51.

11. Lacombe C, Da Silva JL, Bruneval P, et al. Peritubular cells are the site of erythropoietin synthesis in the murine hypoxic kidney. J Clin Invest. 1988;81:620–3.
12. Maxwell PH, Osmond MK, Pugh CW, et al. Identification of the renal erythropoietin-producing cells using transgenic mice. Kidney Int. 1993;44:1149–62.
13. Lai PH, Everett R, Wang FF, Arakawa T, Goldwasser E. Structural characterization of human erythropoietin. J Biol Chem. 1986;261:3116–21.
14. Browne JK, Cohen AM, Egrie JC, et al. Erythropoietin: gene cloning, protein structure, and biological properties. Cold Spring Harb Symp Quant Biol. 1986;51:693–702.
15. Syed RS, Reid SW, Li C, et al. Efficiency of signalling through cytokine receptors depends critically on receptor orientation. Nature. 1998;395:511–16.
16. Cheetham JC, Smith DM, Aoki KH, et al. NMR structure of human erythropoietin and a comparison with its receptor bound conformation. Nat Struct Biol. 1998;5:861–6.
17. Mitjavila MT, Natazawa M, Brignaschi P, et al. Effects of five recombinant hematopoietic growth factors on enriched human erythroid progenitors in serum-replaced cultures. J Cell Physiol. 1989;138:617–23.
18. Uoshima N, Ozawa M, Kimura S, et al. Changes in c-Kit expression and effects of SCF during differentiation of human erythroid progenitor cells. Br J Haematol. 1995;91:30–6.
19. Broudy VC, Lin N, Zsebo KM, et al. Isolation and characterization of a monoclonal antibody that recognizes the human c-kit receptor. Blood. 1992;79:338–46.
20. Wu H, Liu X, Jaenisch R, Lodish HF. Generation of committed erythroid BFU-E and CFU-E progenitors does not require erythropoietin or the erythropoietin receptor. Cell. 1995;83:59–67.
21. Winkelmann JC, Penny LA, Deaven LL, Forget BG, Jenkins RB. The gene for the human erythropoietin receptor: analysis of the coding sequence and assignment to chromosome 19p. Blood. 1990;76:24–30.
22. Jones SS, D'Andrea AD, Haines LL, Wong GG. Human erythropoietin receptor: cloning, expression, and biologic characterization. Blood. 1990;76:31–5.
23. Elliott S, Busse L, Bass MB, et al. Anti-Epo receptor antibodies do not predict Epo receptor expression. Blood. 2006;107:1892–5.
24. Liu ZY, Chin K, Noguchi CT. Tissue specific expression of human erythropoietin receptor in transgenic mice. Dev Biol. 1994;166:159–69.
25. Wognum AW, Lansdorp PM, Humphries RK, Krystal G. Detection and isolation of the erythropoietin receptor using biotinylated erythropoietin. Blood. 1990;76:697–705.
26. McArthur GA, Longmore GD, Klingler K, Johnson GR. Lineage-restricted recruitment of immature hematopoietic progenitor cells in response to Epo after normal hematopoietic cell transfection with EpoR. Exp Hematol. 1995;23:645–54.
27. Ashihara E, Vannucchi AM, Migliaccio G, Migliaccio AR. Growth factor receptor expression during in vitro differentiation of partially purified populations containing murine stem cells. J Cell Physiol. 1997;171:343–56.
28. Billia F, Barbara M, McEwen J, Trevisan M, Iscove NN. Resolution of pluripotential intermediates in murine hematopoietic differentiation by global complementary DNA amplification from single cells: confirmation of assignments by expression profiling of cytokine receptor transcripts. Blood. 2001;97:2257–68.
29. Broudy VC, Lin N, Brice M, Nakamoto B, Papayannopoulou T. Erythropoietin receptor characteristics on primary human erythroid cells. Blood. 1991;77:2583–90.
30. Sawada K, Krantz SB, Kans JS, et al. Purification of human erythroid colony-forming units and demonstration of specific binding of erythropoietin. J Clin Invest. 1987;80:357–66.
31. Fraser JK, Lin FK, Berridge MV. Expression of high affinity receptors for erythropoietin on human bone marrow cells and on the human erythroleukemic cell line, HEL. Exp Hematol. 1988;16:836–42.
32. Wojchowski DM, Gregory RC, Miller CP, Pandit AK, Pircher TJ. Signal transduction in the erythropoietin receptor system. Exp Cell Res. 1999;253:143–56.
33. Jegalian AG, Wu H. Differential roles of SOCS family members in EpoR signal transduction. J Interferon Cytokine Res. 2002;22:853–60.

34. Minoo P, Zadeh MM, Rottapel R, Lebrun JJ, Ali S. A novel SHP-1/Grb2-dependent mechanism of negative regulation of cytokine-receptor signaling: contribution of SHP-1 C-terminal tyrosines in cytokine signaling. Blood. 2004;103:1398–407.
35. Koury MJ, Bondurant MC. Erythropoietin retards DNA breakdown and prevents programmed death in erythroid progenitor cells. Science. 1990;248:378–81.
36. Mayeux P, Billat C, Jacquot R. The erythropoietin receptor of rat erythroid progenitor cells – characterization and affinity cross-linkage. J Biol Chem. 1987;262:13985–90.
37. Jegalian AG, Acurio A, Dranoff G, Wu H. Erythropoietin receptor haploinsufficiency and in vivo interplay with granulocyte–macrophage colony-stimulating factor and interleukin 3. Blood. 2002;99:2603–5.
38. Migliaccio AR, Jiang Y, Migliaccio G, et al. Transcriptional and posttranscriptional regulation of the expression of the erythropoietin receptor gene in human erythropoietin-responsive cell lines. Blood. 1993;82:3760–9.
39. Migliaccio G, Migliaccio AR, Visser JW. Synergism between erythropoietin and interleukin-3 in the induction of hematopoietic stem cell proliferation and erythroid burst colony formation. Blood. 1988;72:944–51.
40. Migliaccio AR, Migliaccio G, D'Andrea A, et al. Response to erythropoietin in erythroid subclones of the factor-dependent cell line 32D is determined by translocation of the erythropoietin receptor to the cell surface. Proc Natl Acad Sci USA. 1991;88:11086–90.
41. Santucci MA, Pierce JH, Zannini S, et al. Erythropoietin increases the radioresistance of a clonal hematopoietic progenitor cell line expressing a transgene for the erythropoietin receptor. Stem Cells. 1994;12:506–13.
42. Wang Y, Kayman SC, Li JP, Pinter A. Erythropoietin receptor (EpoR)-dependent mitogenicity of spleen focus-forming virus correlates with viral pathogenicity and processing of env protein but not with formation of gp52–EpoR complexes in the endoplasmic reticulum. J Virol. 1993;67:1322–7.
43. Gobert S, Chretien S, Gouilleux F, et al. Identification of tyrosine residues within the intracellular domain of the erythropoietin receptor crucial for STAT5 activation. EMBO J. 1996;15:2434–41.
44. Binder C, Lafayette A, Archibeque I, et al. Optimization and utilization of the SureFire phospho-STAT5 assay for a cell-based screening campaign. Assay Drug Dev Technol. 2008;6:27–37.
45. Broudy VC, Lin N, Egrie J, et al. Identification of the receptor for erythropoietin on human and murine erythroleukemia cells and modulation by phorbol ester and dimethyl sulfoxide. Proc Natl Acad Sci USA. 1988;85:6513–17.
46. Longmore GD, Lodish HF. An activating mutation in the murine erythropoietin receptor induces erythroleukemia in mice: a cytokine receptor superfamily oncogene. Cell. 1991;67:1089–102.
47. Sakamoto H, Kitamura T, Yoshimura A. Mitogen-activated protein kinase plays an essential role in the erythropoietin-dependent proliferation of CTLL-2 cells. J Biol Chem. 2000;275:35857–62.
48. Yamamura Y, Noda M, Ikawa Y. Erythropoietin receptor and interleukin-2 receptor use different downstream signaling pathways for proliferation and apoptosis-block. Leukemia. 1994;8:s107–10.
49. Wakao H, Harada N, Kitamura T, Mui AL, Miyajima A. Interleukin 2 and erythropoietin activate STAT5/MGF via distinct pathways. EMBO J. 1995;14:2527–35.
50. Yamamura Y, Kageyama Y, Matuzaki T, Noda M, Ikawa Y. Distinct downstream signaling mechanism between erythropoietin receptor and interleukin-2 receptor. EMBO J. 1992;11:4909–15.
51. Minamoto S, Treisman J, Hankins WD, Sugamura K, Rosenberg SA. Acquired erythropoietin responsiveness of interleukin-2-dependent T lymphocytes retrovirally transduced with genes encoding chimeric erythropoietin/interleukin-2 receptors. Blood. 1995;86:2281–7.

52. Eschbach JW, Kelly MR, Haley NR, Abels RI, Adamson JW. Treatment of the anemia of progressive renal failure with recombinant human erythropoietin. N Engl J Med. 1989;321:158–63.

53. Guthrie M, Cardenas D, Eschbach JW, et al. Effects of erythropoietin on strength and functional status of patients on hemodialysis. Clin Nephrol. 1993;39:97–102.

54. Locatelli F, Baldamus CA, Villa G, Ganea A, Martin de Francisco AL. Once-weekly compared with three-times-weekly subcutaneous epoetin beta: results from a randomized, multicenter, therapeutic-equivalence study. Am J Kidney Dis. 2002;40:119–25.

55. Macdougall IC. An overview of the efficacy and safety of novel erythropoiesis stimulating protein (NESP). Nephrol Dial Transplant. 2001;16:14–21.

56. Glaspy JA. Hematopoietic management in oncology practice. Part 2: Erythropoietic factors. Oncology (Huntington). 2003;17:1724–30.

57. Singh AK, Szczech L, Tang KL, et al. Correction of anemia with epoetin alfa in chronic kidney disease. N Engl J Med. 2006;355:2085–98.

58. Nowrousian MR, Dunst J, Vaupel P. Erythropoiesis-stimulating agents: favorable safety profile when used as indicated. Strahlenther Onkol. 2008;184:121–36.

59. Rush RS, Derby PL, Smith DM, et al. Microheterogeneity of erythropoietin carbohydrate structure. Anal Chem. 1995;67:1442–52.

60. Sasaki H, Bothner B, Dell A, Fukuda M. Carbohydrate structure of erythropoietin expressed in Chinese hamster ovary cells by a human erythropoietin cDNA. J Biol Chem. 1987;262:12059–76.

61. Takeuchi M, Kobata A. Structures and functional roles of the sugar chains of human erythropoietins. Glycobiology. 1991;1:337–46.

62. Wide L, Bengtsson C. Molecular charge heterogeneity of human serum erythropoietin. Br J Haematol. 1990;76:121–7.

63. Lasne F, Martin L, Crepin N, De Ceaurriz J. Detection of isoelectric profiles of erythropoietin in urine: differentiation of natural and administered recombinant hormones. Anal Biochem. 2002;311:119–26.

64. Takeuchi M, Takasaki S, Miyazaki H, et al. Comparative study of the asparagine-linked sugar chains of human erythropoietins purified from urine and the culture medium of recombinant Chinese hamster ovary cells. J Biol Chem. 1988;263:3657–63.

65. Noguchi A, Mukuria CJ, Suzuki E, Naiki M. Failure of human immunoresponse to *N*-glycolylneuraminic acid epitope contained in recombinant human erythropoietin. Nephron. 1996;72:599–603.

66. Hokke CH, Bergwerff AA, Van Dedem GW, Kamerling JP, Vliegenthart JF. Structural analysis of the sialylated N- and O-linked carbohydrate chains of recombinant human erythropoietin expressed in Chinese hamster ovary cells. Sialylation patterns and branch location of dimeric *N*-acetyllactosamine units. Eur J Biochem. 1995;228:981–1008.

67. Kawasaki N, Haishima Y, Ohta M, et al. Structural analysis of sulfated N-linked oligosaccharides in erythropoietin. Glycobiology. 2001;11:1043–9.

68. Strickland T, Adler B, Aoki K, et al. Occurrence of sulfate on the N-linked oligosaccharides of human erythropoietin. J Cell Biochem. 1992;Suppl 16D:167.

69. Elliott S, Egrie J, Browne J, et al. Control of rHuEPO biological activity: the role of carbohydrate. Exp Hematol. 2004;32:1146–55.

70. Sinclair AM, Elliott S. Glycoengineering: the effect of glycosylation on the properties of therapeutic proteins. J Pharm Sci. 2005;94:1626–35.

71. Bernard BA, Yamada KM, Olden K. Carbohydrates selectively protect a specific domain of fibronectin against proteases. J Biol Chem. 1982;257:8549–54.

72. Runkel L, Meier W, Pepinsky RB, et al. Structural and functional differences between glycosylated and non-glycosylated forms of human interferon-beta (IFN-beta). Pharm Res. 1998;15:641–9.

73. Sola RJ, Griebenow K. Effects of glycosylation on the stability of protein pharmaceuticals. J Pharm Sci. 2009;98:1223–45.

74. Cleland JL, Powell MF, Shire SJ. The development of stable protein formulations: a close look at protein aggregation, deamidation, and oxidation. Crit Rev Ther Drug Carrier Syst. 1993;10:307–77.
75. Covic A, Kuhlmann MK. Biosimilars: recent developments. Int Urol Nephrol. 2007;39: 261–6.
76. Roger SD, Goldsmith D. Biosimilars: it's not as simple as cost alone. J Clin Pharm Ther. 2008;33:459–64.
77. Bouchet JL, Brunet P, Canaud B, et al. Position statements regarding usage of biosimilars of Epoetins. Position paper of the Societe de nephrologie, Societe francophone de dialyse, and Societe de nephrologie pediatrique. Nephrol Ther. 2009;5:61–6.
78. Antonetti F, Finocchiaro O, Mascia M, Terlizzese MG, Jaber A. A comparison of the biologic activity of two recombinant IFN-beta preparations used in the treatment of relapsing–remitting multiple sclerosis. J Interferon Cytokine Res. 2002;22:1181–4.
79. Crommelin DJ, Storm G, Verrijk R, et al. Shifting paradigms: biopharmaceuticals versus low molecular weight drugs. Int J Pharm. 2003;266:3–16.
80. Rosenberg AS. Immunogenicity of biological therapeutics: a hierarchy of concerns. Dev Biol. 2003;112:15–21.
81. Schellekens H. Recombinant human erythropoietins, biosimilars and immunogenicity. J Nephrol. 2008;21:497–502.
82. Smalling R, Foote M, Molineux G, Swanson SJ, Elliott S. Drug-induced and antibody-mediated pure red cell aplasia: a review of literature and current knowledge. Biotechnol Annu Rev. 2004;10:237–49.
83. Casadevall N, Nataf J, Viron B, et al. Pure red-cell aplasia and antierythropoietin antibodies in patients treated with recombinant erythropoietin. N Engl J Med. 2002;346:469–75.
84. Verhelst D, Rossert J, Casadevall N, et al. Treatment of erythropoietin-induced pure red cell aplasia: a retrospective study. Lancet. 2004;363:1768–71.
85. Schellekens H. Bioequivalence and the immunogenicity of biopharmaceuticals. Nat Rev Drug Discov. 2002;1:457–62.
86. Schellekens H. Follow-on biologics: challenges of the 'next generation'. Nephrol Dial Transplant. 2005;20:iv31–36.
87. Park SS, Park J, Ko J, et al. Biochemical assessment of erythropoietin products from Asia versus US Epoetin alfa manufactured by Amgen. J Pharm Sci. 2009;98:1688–99.
88. Keithi-Reddy SR, Kandasamy S, Singh AK. Pure red cell aplasia due to follow-on epoetin. Kidney Int. 2008;74:1617–22.
89. Belalcazar V, Ventura R, Segura J, Pascual JA. Clarification on the detection of epoetin delta and epoetin omega using isoelectric focusing. Am J Hematol. 2008;83:754–5.
90. Elliott S, Lorenzini T, Asher S, et al. Enhancement of therapeutic protein in vivo activities through glycoengineering. Nat Biotechnol. 2003;21:414–21.
91. Egrie JC, Dwyer E, Browne JK, Hitz A, Lykos MA. Darbepoetin alfa has a longer circulating half-life and greater in vivo potency than recombinant human erythropoietin. Exp Hematol. 2003;31:290–9.
92. Macdougall IC, Gray SJ, Elston O, et al. Pharmacokinetics of novel erythropoiesis stimulating protein compared with epoetin alfa in dialysis patients. J Am Soc Nephrol. 1999;10:2392–5.
93. Jarsch M, Brandt M, Lanzendorfer M, Haselbeck A. Comparative erythropoietin receptor binding kinetics of C.E.R.A. and epoetin-beta determined by surface plasmon resonance and competition binding assay. Pharmacology. 2008;81:63–9.
94. Macdougall IC, et al. Pharmacokinetics and pharmacodynamics of intravenous and subcutaneous continuous erythropoietin receptor activator (C.E.R.A.) in patients with chronic kidney disease. Clin J Am Soc Nephrol. 2006;1:1211–15.
95. Fan Q, Leuther KK, Holmes CP, et al. Preclinical evaluation of hematide, a novel erythropoiesis stimulating agent, for the treatment of anemia. Exp Hematol. 2006;34:1303–11.
96. Connolly PJ, Wetter SK, Murray WV, et al. Synthesis and erythropoietin receptor binding affinities of N, N-disubstituted amino acids. Bioorg Med Chem Lett. 2000;10:1995–9.

97. Suzuki N, Obara N, Yamamoto M. Use of gene-manipulated mice in the study of erythropoietin gene expression. Methods Enzymol. 2007;435:157–77.
98. Erslev AJ. Clinical erythrokinetics: a critical review. Blood Rev. 1997;11:160–7.
99. Schuster SJ, Badiavas EV, Costa-Giomi P, et al. Stimulation of erythropoietin gene transcription during hypoxia and cobalt exposure. Blood. 1989;73:13–16.
100. Jiang BH, Rue E, Wang GL, Roe R, Semenza GL. Dimerization, DNA binding, and transactivation properties of hypoxia-inducible factor 1. J Biol Chem. 1996;271:17771–8.
101. Wang GL, Jiang BH, Rue EA, Semenza GL. Hypoxia-inducible factor 1 is a basic-helix-loop-helix-PAS heterodimer regulated by cellular O_2 tension. Proc Natl Acad Sci USA. 1995;92:5510–14.
102. Kaelin WG Jr, Ratcliffe PJ. Oxygen sensing by metazoans: the central role of the HIF hydroxylase pathway. Mol Cell. 2008;30:393–402.
103. Epstein AC, Gleadle JM, McNeill LA, et al. *C. elegans* EGL-9 and mammalian homologs define a family of dioxygenases that regulate HIF by prolyl hydroxylation. Cell. 2001;107:43–54.
104. Masson N, Willam C, Maxwell PH, Pugh CW, Ratcliffe PJ. Independent function of two destruction domains in hypoxia-inducible factor-alpha chains activated by prolyl hydroxylation. EMBO J. 2001;20:5197–206.
105. Bruick RK, McKnight SL. A conserved family of prolyl-4-hydroxylases that modify HIF. Science. 2001;294:1337–40.
106. Ivan M, Kondo K, Yang H, et al. HIFalpha targeted for VHL-mediated destruction by proline hydroxylation: implications for O_2 sensing. Science. 2001;292:464–8.
107. Hon WC, Wilson MI, Harlos K, et al. Structural basis for the recognition of hydroxyproline in HIF-1 alpha by pVHL. Nature. 2002;417:975–8.
108. Maxwell PH, Pugh CW, Ratcliffe PJ. Insights into the role of the von Hippel–Lindau gene product. A key player in hypoxic regulation. Exp Nephrol. 2001;9:235–40.
109. Heatherington AC. Clinical pharmacokinetic properties of rHuEpo: a review. In: Molineux G, Foot MA, Elliott SG, editors. Erythropoietins and erythropoiesis: molecular, cellular, preclinical and clinical biology. Basel: Birkhauser; 2003. pp. 87–112.
110. Eckardt KU, Boutellier U, Kurtz A, et al. Rate of erythropoietin formation in humans in response to acute hypobaric hypoxia. J Appl Physiol. 1989; 66: 1785–8.
111. Cheung WK, Goon BL, Guilfoyle MC, Wacholtz MC. Pharmacokinetics and pharmacodynamics of recombinant human erythropoietin after single and multiple subcutaneous doses to healthy subjects. Clin Pharmacol Ther. 1998;64:412–23.
112. McMahon FG, Vargas R, Ryan M, et al. Pharmacokinetics and effects of recombinant human erythropoietin after intravenous and subcutaneous injections in healthy volunteers. Blood. 1990;76:1718–22.
113. Boxenbaum H. Pharmacokinetics tricks and traps: flip–flop models. J Pharm Pharm Sci. 1998;1:90–1.
114. Padhi D, Ni L, Cooke B, Marino R, Jang G. An extended terminal half-life for darbepoetin alfa: results from a single-dose pharmacokinetic study in patients with chronic kidney disease not receiving dialysis. Clin Pharmacokinet. 2006;45:503–10.
115. Glaspy J, Henry D, Patel R, et al. Effects of chemotherapy on endogenous erythropoietin levels and the pharmacokinetics and erythropoietic response of darbepoetin alfa: a randomised clinical trial of synchronous versus asynchronous dosing of darbepoetin alfa. Eur J Cancer. 2005;41:1140–9.
116. Blumer J, Berg S, Adamson PC, et al. Pharmacokinetic evaluation of darbepoetin alfa for the treatment of pediatric patients with chemotherapy-induced anemia. Pediatr Blood Cancer. 2007;49:687–93.
117. Fukuda MN, Sasaki H, Lopez L, Fukuda M. Survival of recombinant erythropoietin in the circulation: the role of carbohydrates. Blood. 1989;73:84–9.
118. Spivak JL, Hogans BB. The in vivo metabolism of recombinant human erythropoietin in the rat. Blood. 1989;73:90–9.

119. Fu J-S, Lertora JJL, Brookins J, Rice JC, Fisher JW. Pharmacokinetics of erythropoietin in intact and anephric dogs. J Lab Clin Med. 1988;111:669–76.

120. Widness JA, Veng-Pedersen P, Schmidt RL, et al. In vivo 125I-erythropoietin pharmacokinetics are unchanged after anesthesia, nephrectomy and hepatectomy in sheep. J Pharmacol Exp Ther. 1996;279:1205–10.

121. Kindler J, Eckardt KU, Ehmer B, et al. Single-dose pharmacokinetics of recombinant human erythropoietin in patients with various degrees of renal failure. Nephrol Dial Transplant. 1989;4:345–9.

122. Macdougall IC, Roberts DE, Coles GA, Williams JD. Clinical pharmacokinetics of epoetin (recombinant human erythropoietin). Clin Pharmacokinet. 1991;20:99–113.

123. Sawyer ST, Krantz SB, Goldwasser E. Binding and receptor-mediated endocytosis of erythropoietin in Friend virus-infected erythroid cells. J Biol Chem. 1987;262:5554–62.

124. Gross AW, Lodish HF. Cellular trafficking and degradation of erythropoietin and novel erythropoiesis stimulating protein (NESP). J Biol Chem. 2006;281:2024–32.

125. Agoram B, Aoki K, Doshi S, et al. Investigation of the effects of altered receptor binding activity on the clearance of erythropoiesis-stimulating proteins: Nonerythropoietin receptor-mediated pathways may play a major role. J Pharm Sci. 2009;98(6):2198–211.

126. Porter CJ, Charman SA. Lymphatic transport of proteins after subcutaneous administration. J Pharm Sci. 2000;89:297–310.

127. Yoshioka E, Kato K, Shindo H, et al. Pharmacokinetic study of darbepoetin alfa: absorption, distribution, and excretion after a single intravenous and subcutaneous administration to rats. Xenobiotica. 2007;37:74–90.

128. Agoram B, Sutjandra L, Molineux G, Jang G, Elliott S. Tissue distribution and excretion of 125I darbepoetin alfa in Sprague Dawley rats following a single subcutaneous or IV administration [abstract]. Nephrol Dial Transplant. 2006;21:304.

129. Erslev AJ. Erythropoietin titers in health and disease. Semin Hematol. 1991;28:2–7.

130. Eschbach JW, Egrie JC, Downing MR, Browne JK, Adamson JW. Correction of the anemia of end-stage renal disease with recombinant human erythropoietin. Results of a combined phase I and II clinical trial. N Engl J Med. 1987;316:73–8.

131. Egrie JC, Strickland TW, Lane J, et al. Characterization and biological effects of recombinant human erythropoietin. Immunobiology. 1986;172:213–24.

132. Hodges VM, Rainey S, Lappin TR, Maxwell AP. Pathophysiology of anemia and erythrocytosis. Crit Rev Oncol Hematol. 2007;64:139–58.

133. Bokemeyer C, Oechsle K, Hartmann JT. Anaemia in cancer patients: pathophysiology, incidence and treatment. Eur J Clin Invest. 2005;35:26–31.

134. Finch CA, Harker LA, Cook JD. Kinetics of the formed elements of human blood. Blood. 1977;50:699–707.

135. Hillman RS, Finch CA. Erythropoiesis: normal and abnormal. Semin Hematol. 1967;4:327–36.

136. Brines M, Cerami A. Discovering erythropoietin's extra-hematopoietic functions: biology and clinical promise. Kidney Int. 2006;70:246–50.

137. Hardee ME, Arcasoy MO, Blackwell KL, Kirkpatrick JP, Dewhirst MW. Erythropoietin biology in cancer. Clin Cancer Res. 2006;12:332–9.

138. Laugsch M, Metzen E, Svensson T, Depping R, Jelkmann W. Lack of functional erythropoietin receptors of cancer cell lines. Int J Cancer. 2008;122:1005–11.

139. Sinclair AM, Rogers N, Busse L, et al. Erythropoietin receptor transcription is neither elevated nor predictive of surface expression in human tumour cells. Br J Cancer. 2008;98:1059–67.

140. Keller MA, Addya S, Vadigepalli R, et al. Transcriptional regulatory network analysis of developing human erythroid progenitors reveals patterns of coregulation and potential transcriptional regulators. Physiol Genomics. 2006;28:114–28.

141. Jeong JY, Feldman L, Solar P, Szenajch J, Sytkowski AJ. Characterization of erythropoietin receptor and erythropoietin expression and function in human ovarian cancer cells. Int J Cancer. 2008;122:274–80.

142. Brown WM, Maxwell P, Graham AN, et al. Erythropoietin receptor expression in non-small cell lung carcinoma: a question of antibody specificity. Stem Cells. 2007;25:718–22.
143. Della Ragione F, Cucciolla V, Borriello A, Oliva A, Perrotta S. Erythropoietin receptors on cancer cells: a still open question. J Clin Oncol. 2007;25:1812–13.
144. Kirkeby A, van Beek J, Nielsen J, Leist M, Helboe L. Functional and immunochemical characterisation of different antibodies against the erythropoietin receptor. J Neurosci Methods. 2007;164:50–8.
145. Ulich TR, del Castillo J, Yin SM, Egrie JC. The erythropoietic effects of interleukin 6 and erythropoietin in vivo. Exp Hematol. 1991;19:29–34.
146. Grossi A, Vannucchi AM, Rafanelli D, Rossi FP. Recombinant human erythropoietin has little influence on megakaryocytopoiesis in mice. Br J Haematol. 1989;71:463–8.
147. Suzuki N, Ohneda O, Takahashi S, et al. Erythroid-specific expression of the erythropoietin receptor rescued its null mutant mice from lethality. Blood. 2002;100:2279–88.
148. Banks WA, Jumbe NL, Farrell CL, Niehoff ML, Heatherington AC. Passage of erythropoietic agents across the blood–brain barrier: a comparison of human and murine erythropoietin and the analog darbepoetin alfa. Eur J Pharmacol. 2004;505:93–101.
149. Buemi M, Allegra A, Corica F, et al. Intravenous recombinant erythropoietin does not lead to an increase in cerebrospinal fluid erythropoietin concentration. Nephrol Dial Transplant. 2000;15:422–3.
150. Hardee ME, Kirkpatrick JP, Shan S, et al. Human recombinant erythropoietin (rEpo) has no effect on tumour growth or angiogenesis. Br J Cancer. 2005;93:1350–5.
151. Sinclair AM, Todd MD, Forsythe K, et al. Expression and function of erythropoietin receptors in tumors: implications for the use of erythropoiesis-stimulating agents in cancer patients. Cancer. 2007;110:477–88.
152. Katavetin P, Tungsanga K, Eiam-Ong S, Nangaku M. Antioxidative effects of erythropoietin. Kidney Int. 2007;72:S10–S15.
153. Yazihan N, Uzuner K, Salman B, et al. Erythropoietin improves oxidative stress following spinal cord trauma in rats. Injury. 2008;39:1408–13.

Chapter 5
Thrombopoietin Factors

Ping Wei

Abstract Megakaryopoiesis and thrombopoiesis are the central biological processes of platelet generation. Severe thrombocytopenia is a major morbidity and mortality factor in several diseases and represents a significant unmet medical need. Since the discovery of thrombopoietin (TPO) as the primary physiological regulator of megakaryopoiesis, a number of therapeutics have been developed for thrombocytopenia and been tested in preclinical models and human clinical trials. The TPO mimetics romiplostim (Nplate® or AMG531) and eltrombopag (Promacta®) have recently been approved for the treatment of adult chronic idiopathic (immune) thrombocytopenic purpura (ITP) and are successful examples of these endeavors. This chapter will review scientific progress over the last 20 years on various thrombopoietic factors with an emphasis on the biology, physiology, and pharmacology of TPO, its cognate receptor, c-Mpl, and various TPO mimetics.

Introduction

Megakaryopoiesis and thrombopoiesis involve the commitment of hematopoietic stem and progenitor cells to the megakaryocytic lineage, megakaryocyte proliferation, maturation, and differentiation, and ultimately platelet generation and release into the blood stream (Fig. 5.1) [1, 2]. These are highly ordered and specialized processes governed by the interplay between hematopoietic cells, stromal cells, and humoral factors. On average, an adult human produces approximately 1×10^{11} platelets daily and this can be increased by more than tenfold under physiological demand [2, 3]. Platelets play an essential role in hemostasis, ranging from the repair of minute vascular damage to thrombus formation following a large vascular injury. Low platelet counts due to dysregulation of megakaryopoiesis or thrombopoiesis and/or excessive platelet consumption can result in the development of various pathological conditions [2, 4].

P. Wei (✉)
Department of Hematology, Amgen, Inc., Thousand Oaks, CA 91320, USA
e-mail: pwei@amgen.com

G.H. Lyman, D.C. Dale (eds.), *Hematopoietic Growth Factors in Oncology*,
Cancer Treatment and Research 157, DOI 10.1007/978-1-4419-7073-2_5,
© Springer Science+Business Media, LLC 2011

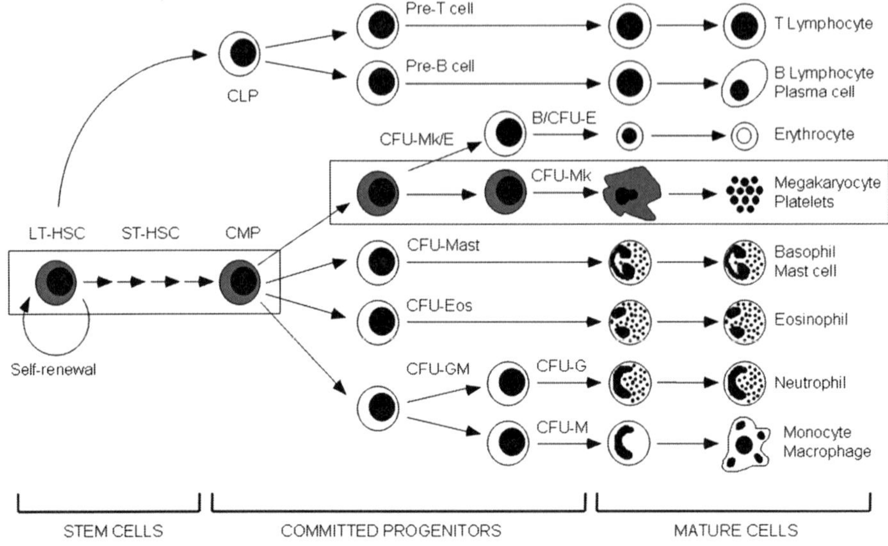

Fig. 5.1 The megakaryopoiesis and thrombopoiesis pathways (*boxed*) of the hematopoietic system. Cells known to express the c-Mpl receptor and to respond to TPO are *shaded* in *gray*. These include long-term (LT) and short-term (ST) hematopoietic stem cells (HSCs), common myeloid progenitors (CMPs), colony-forming units for the megakaryocyte/erythroid (CFU-Mk/E) and megakaryocyte (CFU-Mk) lineages, mature megakaryocytes, and platelets. CLP, common lymphoid progenitor; Mast, basophilic mast cell; Eos, eosinophil; G, neutrophilic granulocyte; M, monocyte/macrophage

Thrombocytopenia, when severe, can lead to serious and life-threatening hemorrhage [4, 5]. It can be seen in a variety of different disease states as either an acute or chronic condition. Chronic thrombocytopenia is a common medical problem found in certain autoimmune diseases such as ITP, bone marrow-related malignancies such as aplastic anemia (AA) and myelodysplastic syndromes (MDS), and virus-induced diseases such as hepatitis C virus (HCV)-mediated chronic liver disease (CLD) and human immunodeficiency virus (HIV)-induced acquired immunodeficiency syndrome (AIDS) [6]. It also includes several rare inherited diseases such as congenital amegakaryocytic thrombocytopenia (CAMT) and X-linked thrombocytopenia [2]. Chemotherapy-induced thrombocytopenia (CIT) is also a major clinical problem in the management of cancer patients receiving high-dose, multi-cycle, and/or multi-agent chemotherapies. Such treatments often kill megakaryocytes and their progenitor cells which are essential for platelet production. Risk of serious bleeding associated with CIT could restrict the usefulness of chemotherapy in these cancer patients [6].

Platelet transfusion is often used to reduce the risk of bleeding in severe thrombocytopenia (platelet counts $<50 \times 10^9$/L). Currently, over 4 million platelet units are transfused in the United States yearly [1]. However, platelet transfusion is associated with many problems including limited blood supply and high cost, alloimmunization and refractoriness, transfusion reactions, and transmission of infectious diseases [6]. In autoimmune-induced ITP patients, the standard initial treatment is corticosteroids and is often followed by intravenous administration of immunoglobulin and/or anti-D immunoglobulin [5]. However, these therapies usually provide only temporary improvement in platelet numbers and long-term use of corticosteroids is associated with serious side effects. Splenectomy is often considered for patients who are refractory to the initial treatments but this invasive procedure carries its own risks, is not appropriate for all patients, and relapse is also common in post-splenectomized patients [5]. Rituximab, an anti-CD20 antibody originally developed for use in lymphoid malignancy, has been used in patients with ITP. However, rituximab is not approved for this indication, and may be associated with severe side effects, based on its relatively non-selective immunosuppressive mode of action. Clearly, better and safer therapies are needed for managing severe thrombocytopenia.

Hematopoietic growth factors have been recognized as important regulators of megakaryopoiesis since they were first discovered and as potential therapeutics for treating thrombocytopenia in different disease states [3, 6, 7]. Recombinant granulocyte–macrophage colony-stimulating factor (GM-CSF), erythropoietin (EPO), interleukin (IL)-3, IL-6, IL-11, leukemia inhibitory factor (LIF), and stem cell factor (SCF), either alone or in combination, have been shown to stimulate megakaryocyte proliferation from $CD34^+$ progenitor cells in vitro [7]. IL 1a and LIF were also shown to enhance megakaryocyte maturation and platelet release [7]. Several of the interleukins, including IL-1a, IL-6, IL-11, and LIF, were studied in early clinical trials and shown to increase platelet counts and accelerate platelet recovery after chemotherapy [6]. However, the effects of these cytokines in humans were modest and often associated with a variety of unacceptable side effects. Double-knockout studies in mice that lack the genes for c-Mpl and one other growth factor have also demonstrated that IL-3, IL-6, IL-11, GM-CSF, and LIF are not physiological mediators of megakaryopoiesis or thrombopoiesis [8–10]. Despite its limited potency and toxic side effects, Oprelvekin (Neumega or recombinant IL-11) was approved for the prevention of severe thrombocytopenia due to chemotherapy and to reduce the need for platelet transfusions in patients with non-myeloid malignancies [11].

The discovery of the most potent thrombopoietic factor, thrombopoietin (TPO), and its primary role in megakaryopoiesis led to significant advancement in both the scientific understanding of megakaryopoiesis and thrombopoiesis and the development of therapeutics for thrombocytopenia. This chapter will review the biology of TPO and its cognate receptor, c-Mpl, and the development of different platelet-stimulating agents including both protein therapeutics and small molecule TPO mimetics.

Discovery of Thrombopoietin (TPO)

The existence of a humoral regulator of megakaryopoiesis was first demonstrated in 1958 when serum from thrombocythemic humans was found to increase platelet counts in recipient mice [12]. However, the identification of the thrombopoietic factor in this complex mixture was hindered over the next few decades by the difficulties in purifying this molecule and the slow development of technologies to measure its activity. The breakthrough came in 1990 when a viral oncogene, *v-mpl*, was identified from the murine myeloproliferative leukemia virus that causes an acute myeloproliferative syndrome in mice [13]. The cloning of its cellular homolog, *c-Mpl*, in 1992 and subsequent analysis of its amino acid sequence together with structural and functional studies revealed that c-Mpl is a new member of the hematopoietic growth factor receptor superfamily and plays a unique role in megakaryopoiesis [14, 15]. These findings led to the purification and cloning of the ligand for c-Mpl and the demonstration that it was the long-sought thrombopoietic factor, TPO, in 1994 [16–20] (TPO is also called megakaryocyte growth and development factor, MGDF, or megapoietin.). Recombinant human TPO (rhTPO) stimulates the growth of megakaryocyte colony-forming units (MK-CFUs) in vitro and megakaryopoiesis and platelet production in vivo [6]. The role of TPO as the primary physiological regulator of thrombopoiesis was established with subsequent gene targeting studies, in which genetic elimination of *TPO* or *c-Mpl* in mice resulted in severe thrombocytopenia with 85–95% reduction in megakaryocytes and platelet numbers [21–23]. The identification of TPO and c-Mpl opened a new era of research on megakaryocyte development and platelet biology and provided the scientific foundation for the subsequent development of therapeutics for thrombocytopenia.

Biology of TPO and c-Mpl

TPO Molecular Structure

Human TPO is a 353-amino acid glycoprotein with an apparent molecular weight (MW) of 85 kDa, which is greater than the predicted 38 kDa due to glycosylation. In addition to a 21-amino acid signal peptide, the 332 residue mature TPO protein is composed of two subdomains: a 153-residue N-terminal receptor-binding domain (RBD) and a 179-residue C-terminal domain that is highly glycosylated and important for TPO secretion and stability [24]. Both domains are well conserved across species with over 90 and 70% homology between human and mouse, respectively [24]. Although the RBD of TPO has <25% primary sequence identity with other prototypic type I cytokines, its 3D structure is strikingly similar to the RBDs of EPO, granulocyte colony-stimulating factor (G-CSF), growth hormone (GH), and prolactin (PL) [25, 26]. When crystallized with a neutralizing antibody fragment, the RBD of TPO folds into a four-helix bundle structure with two small antiparallel β(beta)-pleated sheets in the loop regions, a topology most resembling that of EPO [26–28]. Also similar to EPO, TPO has high- and low-affinity ligand-binding sites (Kd in nM and mM range, respectively) and binds to the receptor with a 1:2 stoichiometry [26, 28].

TPO Expression and Regulation

TPO is produced primarily by liver hepatocytes and kidney proximal tubule cells [29–31]. Liver transplantation studies in both humans and mice suggest that the liver contributes at least 60% of the circulating TPO [32, 33]. The expression from liver and kidney appears to be constitutive with no apparent transcriptional or translational regulation [29, 30]. Although bone marrow stromal cells do not express TPO in normal circumstances, TPO mRNA has been detected in these cells from thrombocytopenic patients with AA, post-chemotherapy marrow aplasia, and ITP, as well as from chemotherapy and/or radiation-induced thrombocytopenic mice [29, 31]. This inducible mode of TPO expression has also been reported in inflammatory conditions and the acute-phase cytokine IL-6 was shown to induce TPO expression both in vitro and in vivo [3, 24, 34]. The physiological significance of this inducible TPO expression is still under investigation.

TPO is cleared from the circulation mainly through receptor-mediated uptake and degradation by megakaryocytes and platelets [30, 35–38]. Decreased megakaryocyte and/or platelet counts lead to reduced TPO binding and clearance. This leads to an increase in circulating TPO concentration that stimulates megakaryopoiesis and platelet production. Conversely, high megakaryocyte and/or platelet numbers lead to increased elimination of TPO from the circulation and consequently attenuated megakaryopoiesis. In normal individuals, the serum TPO level is around 50–150 pg/mL [39]. In many thrombocytopenic conditions, such as AA and myelosuppressive therapy-induced thrombocytopenia, plasma TPO levels are significantly elevated, up to 20-fold above normal levels, in an inverse relationship with platelet counts [35].

c-Mpl Molecular Structure and Signal Transduction

Human c-Mpl, the TPO receptor, is a 635-amino acid transmembrane protein and a member of the hematopoietic growth factor receptor superfamily [25]. Together with the receptors for EPO, G-CSF, growth hormone (GH), and prolactin (PL), c-Mpl belongs to the single-chain, type I cytokine receptor subfamily that activates signal transduction through receptor homodimerization. Unlike the other subfamily members that each contains one cytokine receptor module (CRM) in the extracellular domain, c-Mpl has two. Each CRM is approximately 200 amino acids in length and contains four conserved cysteines in the N-terminal region and a pentapeptide WSXWS motif near the C-terminal end [25]. Biochemical studies suggest that TPO binds to the distal CRM that plays an inhibitory role in c-Mpl signaling as its deletion results in c-Mpl autoactivation [40]. The 122-residue cytoplasmic domain of c-Mpl is composed of two 60-amino acid regions. The membrane-proximal region that includes two conserved sequence motifs, box 1 and box 2, is essential for binding to Janus kinase 2 (JAK2) to initiate signal transduction and for receptor surface expression [41–43]. In contrast to the EPO receptor (EpoR), which depends completely on JAK2 for cell surface expression, c-Mpl exhibits both JAK2-dependent and JAK2-independent surface expressions [43]. The distal 60-amino acid region is not required for megakaryopoiesis or platelet production under normal conditions, however, it appears to be important in acute response to stress as its deletion results in delayed platelet recovery following myelosuppression [41].

TPO binding to c-Mpl is believed to induce receptor homodimerization and subsequent phosphorylation and activation of JAK2 that is prebound to the intracellular domain [3, 24]. Activated JAK2 then phosphorylates tyrosine residues in c-Mpl and associated signaling tyrosine kinases and phosphatases, and triggers multiple signaling pathways. These include the JAK/signal transducers and activators of transcription (STAT) pathway involving mostly JAK2, STAT3, and STAT5, the mitogen-activated kinase (MAPK) pathways involving both the extracellular signal-regulated kinases (ERK) and p38 kinases, and the phosphatidylinositol-3-kinase (PI3K) pathway [3, 24, 44]. Together these culminate in changes in gene expression and the TPO-stimulated biological responses.

c-Mpl Expression and Regulation

Human c-Mpl is primarily expressed in hematopoietic tissues and specifically on the surface of hematopoietic stem and progenitor cells, megakaryocytes, and platelets (Fig. 5.1) [14, 45–47]. Both c-Mpl mRNA and protein have been detected in human pluripotent $CD34^+CD38^-$ cells, cultured human megakaryocytes, and purified platelets but not in committed erythroid, myeloid, or lymphoid cells. On average, human megakaryocytes have $\sim$12,000 surface c-mpl receptors/cell while platelets have 25–200 [37, 38, 48]. RT-PCR analysis failed to detect any c-Mpl mRNA in 38 of 39 human solid tumor cell lines or 20 primary tissue samples of various types [49]. These included brain, breast, colon, lung, ovarian, pancreatic, prostate, skin, and other cancers. In vitro studies have also demonstrated a lack of correlation between c-Mpl mRNA expression and functional receptor and/or cellular responses [50].

The expression of c-Mpl appears to be constitutive in hematopoietic tissues and cell surface levels are modulated by TPO binding and subsequent receptor internalization [3, 37, 38]. Although c-Mpl expression has also been reported on endothelial cells in vitro [14, 51, 52], the physiological significance of this finding is not clear. For example, bone marrow transplantation studies demonstrated that despite a potentially 100-fold higher mass of c-Mpl on the surface of blood vessels than on megakaryocytes and platelets, endothelial c-Mpl has no effect on serum TPO levels [53], arguing against any biological functions of the c-Mpl found on endothelial cells. Another mode of c-Mpl regulation was suggested by the discovery of three different splice variants of c-Mpl [54–56]. While in vitro studies showed that the K form has no apparent function, c-Mpl-tr caused the degradation of the full-length receptor when co-expressed in cell lines [54–56]. More studies are clearly needed to fully understand the distribution and the physiological roles of these different forms of c-Mpl.

Physiological Role of TPO

TPO is the primary and most potent regulator of megakaryopoiesis and functions in almost all stages of megakaryocyte development (Fig. 5.1) [2, 3]. It supports the survival and expansion of hematopoietic stem cells (HSCs) and early progenitor cells with megakaryocytic differentiation potential, promotes the proliferation, maturation, and differentiation of megakaryocytes, and enhances the platelet response upon activation [2, 3]. Interestingly, TPO does not appear to play a direct role in the final stage of platelet formation including proplatelet formation and platelet release [57]. On the other hand, nuclear factor erythroid 2 (NF-E2) has been shown to be essential for this final stage of platelet production [58].

Both genetic and biochemical studies in humans and animals have demonstrated that TPO also plays an important role in HSC expansion and survival. Children with congenital absence of c-Mpl develop CAMT that progresses to pancytopenia and bone marrow failure at early ages, underscoring the non-redundant role of TPO/c-Mpl pathway in HSC physiology [2, 3]. Genetic deletion of TPO or c-Mpl in mice leads to severe thrombocytopenia with accompanying deficiencies in HSC and progenitor cells of all hematopoietic lineages [21, 59, 60]. Enriched stem cell populations from c-Mpl-deficient mice were sevenfold less potent than those from wild-type mice in a competitive repopulation study, and human $CD34^+CD38$ c-Mpl^+ cells were significantly more efficient in engraftment of immunodeficient mice than $CD34^+CD38$-c-Mpl^- cells [46]. Moreover, TPO promoted the growth and survival of HSC in vitro and in vivo with no apparent effect on lineage fate determination [59, 61]. TPO synergizes with IL-3 and/or SCF in vitro to enhance the proliferation of HSC in both human and murine systems [61, 62]. Other cytokines, such as IL-11 and EPO, were also found to synergize with TPO to promote the proliferation of primitive progenitor cells [63].

Development of Recombinant Thrombopoietic Factors

The discovery of TPO and its essential role in megakaryopoiesis and platelet production stimulated the development of rhTPO as a potential therapeutic for thrombocytopenia. Two related molecules, rhTPO and PEG-rHuMGDF, were the first to be generated and evaluated extensively in preclinical and clinical studies [6, 64]. Recombinant hTPO is a glycosylated full-length human TPO produced in Chinese hamster ovary (CHO) cells. It has the same amino acid sequence as native human TPO. PEG-rHuMGDF is a non-glycosylated truncated human TPO containing only the first 163 residues of native TPO. It is produced in *Escherichia coli* and subsequently conjugated to a 20-kDa polyethylene glycol (PEG) moiety. These recombinant proteins represented the first generation of c-Mpl agonistic agents, had similar pharmacologic characteristics, and exhibited comparable preclinical and clinical effects [6, 64]. Administration of either agent significantly elevated platelet counts in normal animals and those rendered thrombocytopenic by chemotherapy and/or radiotherapy [65–68]. In clinical studies of cancer patients with thrombocytopenia caused by non-myeloablative chemotherapy, both agents reduced the severity and duration of thrombocytopenia, accelerated platelet recovery, and reduced the requirement for platelet transfusions [69]. However, in patients with severe thrombocytopenia induced by myeloablative chemotherapy, rhTPO or PEG-rHuMGDF was not effective in improving the platelet count nadir, time to platelet recovery, or the number of platelet transfusions [70–72]. Besides chemotherapy-induced thrombocytopenia, PEG-rHuMGDF also showed promising effects in ameliorating ITP which was refractory to standard therapy. In the majority of patients tested, PEG-rHuMGDF increased platelet counts and reduced bleeding events [73].

Despite these initial promising findings, the clinical development of recombinant TPO was terminated in 1998 after it was discovered that some patients and healthy volunteers who received repeated injections of PEG-rHuMGDF developed antibodies against the protein. These antibodies cross-reacted with and neutralized endogenous TPO and resulted in prolonged treatment-refractory thrombocytopenia [74, 75]. A third recombinant thrombopoietic agent, the chimeric TPO/IL-3 fusion protein promegapoietin, showed potent activity in vitro and in vivo but did not enter clinical trials [76].

Development of TPO Mimetics

The knowledge and experience gained from the first generation of c-Mpl agonistic molecules provided preliminary evidence and paved the road for the development of the second generation of thrombopoiesis-stimulating agents. Efforts were then devoted to the generation of TPO mimetics that have little sequence or structural homology with native TPO to avoid autoantibody production [64]. These agonists include peptide and small molecule mimetics and c-Mpl agonistic antibodies. Although these molecules differ in their biochemical properties and pharmacological characteristics, they shared the ability to bind specifically to and activate the c-Mpl receptor and promote platelet production. At least eight such agents have been developed and progressed through various preclinical and clinical studies (Table 5.1). Among these, romiplostim (AMG531 or Nplate®), a TPO mimetic peptibody, was the first to complete clinical evaluation and gain regulatory approval in the United States, Australia, Canada, and the European Union for the treatment of thrombocytopenia associated with adult ITP.

TPO Peptide Mimetics

Phage display technology was used to screen peptide libraries for sequences that bind specifically to c-Mpl and stimulate the proliferation of TPO-dependent cell lines. One 14-amino acid peptide (Ile-Glu-Gly-Pro-Thr-Leu-Arg-Gln-Trp-Leu-Ala-Ala-Arg-Ala) was identified that shares no primary sequence similarity with native TPO but binds to c-Mpl with high affinity and elicits similar biological effects to

Table 5.1 Status of TPO mimetics in preclinical and clinical development

TPO receptor agonist	Current stage of development				
	Preclinical	Phase 1	Phase 2	Phase 3	Marketed
TPO peptide mimetics					
Fab 59	√				
Peg-TPOmp	√	√			
Romiplostim (Nplate® or AMG531)			√	√	√
			CIT	ITP	ITP
			MDS	Ped. ITP	
TPO non-peptide mimetics					
AKR-501		√	√		
			ITP		
Eltrombopag (Promacta®s or SB-497115)			√	√	√
			CIT	ITP	ITP
			HCV		
NIP-401	√				
c-Mpl agonistic antibodies					
VB22B sc(Fv)2	√				
MA01G4344U	√				

CIT, chemotherapy-induced thrombocytopenia; ITP, immune thrombocytopenic purpura; MDS, myelodysplastic syndromes; Ped. ITP, pediatric ITP; PEG-TPOmp, polyethylene glycol-thrombopoietin mimetic peptide.
Modified with permission from Kuter [100].

the native protein [77]. Dimerization of this TPO peptide mimetic significantly enhanced its potency in stimulating the in vitro proliferation and maturation of megakaryocytes from human bone marrow and ability to increase platelet counts when administered to normal mice. However, the short half-life of the peptide in the circulation limited its therapeutic utility and various strategies were employed to increase its stability in serum. These included the generation of a fusion protein in which the peptide was either fused with a more stable protein component or pegylated to a PEG moiety (see below).

Fab59: Fab59 is a rationally designed fusion protein in which two of the above 14-amino acid TPO peptide mimetics were inserted into different complementary-determining regions (CDRs) of a human Fab, one in the heavy chain CDR3 and the other in the light chain CDR2 [78]. The CDR regions of antibodies are known to be highly variable sequences and insertion of a peptide was therefore not expected to be more immunogenic than the native molecule. Although mice injected repeatedly with human Fab59 did develop antibodies against the fusion protein, these did not cross-react with murine or human TPO. Fab59 showed similar potency to rhTPO in an in vitro reporter assay. However, it was at least 30-fold less potent than rhTPO in stimulating platelet production in normal mice and was difficult to express [79]. No human studies have been reported.

Peg-TPOmp: Peg-TPOmp is a pegylated TPO mimetic peptide with a half-life ranging from 18 to 36 h in humans, demonstrating that the addition of a large PEG moiety protected it from degradation and increased its pharmacokinetic properties in vivo [80]. Peg-TPOmp was potent in stimulating TPO-dependent cell growth in vitro and induced dose-dependent increases in platelet counts in mice, rats, and dogs. A phase 1 study in healthy male volunteers showed that a single administration of Peg-TPOmp produced a dose-dependent increase in platelet counts that ranged from 1.4-fold to 3.2-fold above baseline with peak counts seen on days 10–12. Peg-TPOmp was well tolerated in humans and no reactive antibodies were detected. However, further clinical development of this molecule has not been reported.

Romiplostim (AMG531 or Nplate®): Romiplostim is a 59-kDa non-glycosylated fusion protein produced in *E. coli*. It contains an N-terminal human immunoglobulin (IgG$_1$) Fc fragment linked covalently through polyglycine to two copies of a 14-amino acid TPO peptide mimetic at the C-terminus of each heavy chain (Fig. 5.2). Thus, each romiplostim molecule has a total of four TPO peptide mimetics fused to a human Fc fragment. This class of Fc-peptide fusion proteins are referred to as "peptibodies." Mechanistic studies in knockout mice demonstrated that the neonatal Fc receptor (FcRn) expressed on endothelial cells interacts with the human Fc domain and functions as a salvage receptor for romiplostim, protecting it from degradation and extending its half-life in serum. Romiplostim does not interact with Fc-gamma receptors (FcγR) due to the lack of glycans on the Fc fragment after *E. coli* expression [81].

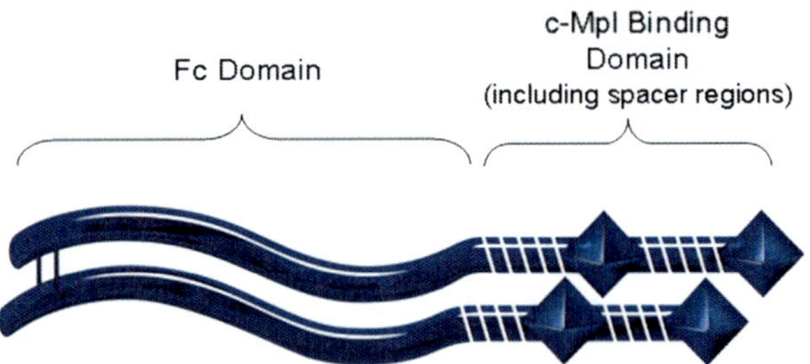

Fig. 5.2 Structure of romiplostim (AMG531 or Nplate®). This peptibody contains two domains: an N-terminal disulfide-bonded Fc domain that prolongs the serum half-life of the whole molecule and a C-terminal c-Mpl receptor interaction domain composed of four 14-amino acid TPO mimetic peptides (*diamond shaped*). Polyglycine linkers, shown as *slashed bars*, covalently link the Fc fragment with the peptides

In vitro studies have shown that romiplostim exhibits similar biological activities and mechanism of action to native TPO [82]. Competition studies with ^{125}I-rhTPO revealed that romiplostim binds to c-Mpl on human, cynomolgus monkey, and rat platelets at sites similar to those that bind rhTPO. Romiplostim binding results in receptor and JAK2 phosphorylation and subsequent signal transduction. Romiplostim stimulates the proliferation of TPO-dependent cell lines as well as the growth and maturation of megakaryocytic progenitor cells from cynomolgus monkeys, baboons, and humans. In in vivo preclinical studies in mice, rats, rhesus and cynomolgus monkeys, and baboons, single or repeated administration of romiplostim was well tolerated and induced dose-dependent increases in platelet counts [83]. Clearance of romiplostim was meditated by the kidney and platelets, but not the spleen. In rodents, romiplostim also ameliorated CIT induced by carboplatin or 5-fluorouracil (5-FU) [84].

In healthy human subjects, romiplostim was well tolerated and induced dose-dependent platelet responses that can be seen as early as 3–5 days after a single intravenous (IV) or subcutaneous (SC) injection, with peak platelet counts occurring on days 12–16, returning to baseline counts by day 28 [85]. Romiplostim has not been found in preclinical or clinical studies to induce the production of neutralizing antibodies that cross-react with endogenous TPO or inhibited TPO's biological activities [4, 83, 86]. Romiplostim was evaluated extensively in multiple phase I–III studies (reviewed in detail in Part IV, "The Thrombopoietic Agents") and found to be effective and safe in ameliorating thrombocytopenia in adult patients with chronic ITP who have had an insufficient response to corticosteroids, immunoglobulins, or splenectomy [4]. In a recently completed long-term safety and efficacy study, romiplostim was found to increase platelet counts in the majority of patients for up to 3 years and have an acceptable safety profile [86]. Romiplostim is currently under clinical investigation in pediatric patients with ITP and adult subjects with MDS or CIT.

TPO Small Molecule Mimetics

Small molecular weight chemical compounds (MW ~500 Da) are not immunogenic and therefore are alternative sources of TPO mimetics. To this end, several groups have screened large chemical libraries in high-throughput, cell-based assays and identified novel small molecule c-Mpl agonists that stimulate cell growth or signaling. At least three different TPO small molecule mimetics have been reported and are in different stages of development (Fig. 5.3). Notably, all of them appear to bind to c-Mpl at sites different from native TPO, are much less potent at equal molar concentrations, and have more restricted species specificity than rhTPO or TPO peptide mimetics.

AKR-501: AKR-501 (formally known as YM477) is an orally active small molecule c-Mpl agonist [87]. Similar to rhTPO, AKR-501 activates the JAK/STAT and MAPK signaling pathways and promotes the growth and maturation of megakaryocytes from human CD34$^+$ cells, although it is 30–1,000-fold less potent than rhTPO in these assays. The exact binding site of AKR-501 on c-Mpl is not known although it did not inhibit ^{125}I-rhTPO binding to human platelets [88], suggesting that AKR-501 binds at a site different from native TPO. In the presence of a supra-physiological concentration (3 nM) of rhTPO, AKR-501 further augmented the growth of human megakaryocytic and non-megakaryocytic progenitor cells, and megakaryocytes in vitro. AKR-501 is highly species specific as it induced STAT5 activation only from platelets from humans and chimpanzees, but not from rodents or other non-human primates tested [87].

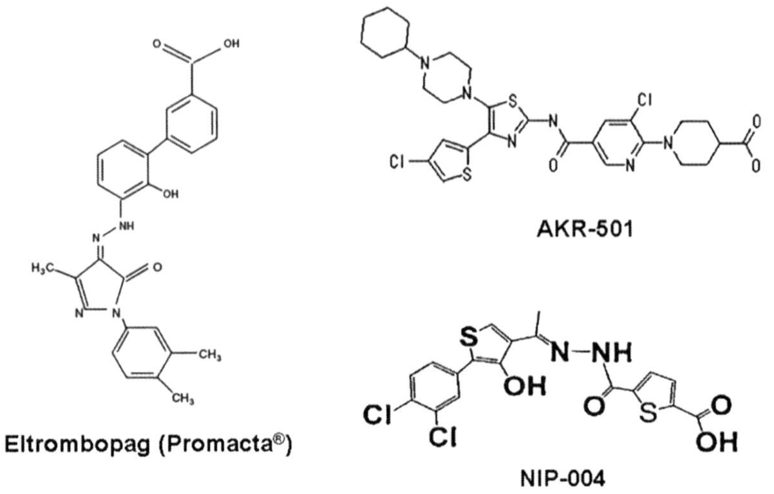

AKR-501

Eltrombopag (Promacta®)

NIP-004

Fig. 5.3 Chemical structures of AKR-501, eltrombopag (Promacta®), and NIP-004

Single-dose and multiple-dose studies were conducted in healthy volunteers. Daily oral administration of AKR-501 at 3, 10, or 20 mg for 14 days induced dose-dependent increases in platelets with peak counts reaching 1.3-fold, 2.25-fold, and 2.8-fold above baseline, respectively. No adverse effects were observed and AKR-501 exhibited a serum half-life of 16 h [89]. A phase II clinical investigation on AKR-501 is underway for chronic ITP.

Eltrombopag (Promacta® or SB-497115): Eltrombopag is a first-in-class, orally active, small molecule (MW 564 Da) c-Mpl agonist [90–92]. In vitro, it exhibits c-Mpl-specific activity, activates the JAK/STAT and MAPK signaling pathways, and stimulates the proliferation and differentiation of human bone marrow $CD34^+$ cells into megakaryocytes. However, on a molar basis it is 1,000–100,000-fold less potent than rhTPO in these assays [92]. Similar to AKR-501, eltrombopag also shows additive effects when combined with rhTPO (>0.1 nM) in promoting the proliferation of a TPO-responsive cell line and exhibited anti-apoptotic effects at concentrations above 30 nM. Since endogenous TPO levels in normal and diseased humans are usually significantly (up to 100-fold) less than 0.1 nM [39], the physiological significance of this additive effect is not clear.

Eltrombopag is highly species specific, binding to and activating c-Mpl only on human and chimpanzee cells but not cells from cynomolgus monkey, cat, mouse, rat, dog, pig, ferret, or tree shrew. Receptor domain swapping, mutagenesis, and NMR structural studies using earlier generations of eltrombopag demonstrated that the extracellular juxtamembrane region (JMR) and the transmembrane domain (TM) of c-Mpl determine the species specificity and are responsible for binding this small molecule agonist [91, 93]. In particular, a 13-amino acid region in the extracellular JMR immediately adjacent to the TM and the His residue at amino acid 499 of the TM are key elements for this interaction and for receptor activation. Sequence analysis further confirmed that His 499 is only present in the TM of human and chimpanzee c-Mpl but not in those of mouse, rat, hamster, guinea pig, rabbit, rhesus macaques, cynomolgus monkey, common marmoset, or squirrel monkey [94].

Although no effect was seen with a single dose of eltrombopag, it stimulated platelet production to 1.5-fold above baseline after repeated daily oral dosing in chimpanzees and in healthy humans [64, 92]. A dose-dependent increase was seen in humans at doses of ≥ 30 mg with a half-life of 9–12 h. Phase I–III studies were completed in adult chronic ITP and eltrombopag became the second molecule to be approved for treating ITP [95] (reviewed in detail in Part IV, "The Thrombopoietic Agents"). It is currently in phase II trials for HCV-induced thrombocytopenia [96].

NIP-004: NIP-004 is another small molecule c-Mpl agonist (MW 455 Da) [94]. It stimulates the proliferation and differentiation of human CD34$^+$ cells but does not act on murine or cynomolgus monkey cells. Similar to eltrombopag, His 499 in the TM of c-Mpl appears to be essential for NIP-004 activity and at least partly determines the species specificity. To study the in vivo efficacy of NIP-004, immunodeficient mice were reconstituted with human umbilical cord blood-derived CD34$^+$ cells. NIP-004 was found to increase the number of human megakaryocytic progenitor cells, megakaryocyte number and ploidy, and functional circulating human platelet levels in these mice. Clinical studies of NIP-004 have not been reported.

c-Mpl Agonistic Antibodies

Antibodies are large molecules with high affinity and specificity to their targets and a long serum half-life. They are also known to have low risk of inducing the development of neutralizing antibodies that cross-react with the therapeutic antibody target. With these properties, c-Mpl agonistic antibodies were also evaluated preclinically as potential therapeutics for thrombocytopenia. Initially, full length anti-c-Mpl monoclonal antibodies were generated by immunizing immunocompromised mice with recombinant human c-Mpl protein or cells engineered to express human c-Mpl. Most isolated anti-c-Mpl-specific antibodies showed no or weak agonist activity in promoting TPO-dependent cell growth, possibly due to steric hindrance and inefficient dimerization of the receptor. However, using powerful tools of antibody engineering, these whole IgGs can be converted into strong c-Mpl agonists. Two such TPO agonist antibodies have been reported and are described below.

VB22B sc(Fv)2: VB22B sc(Fv)2 was generated by cloning two copies of the heavy chain variable region (VH) and the light chain variable region (VL) connected by a short linker sequence into a single-chain (sc) variable fragment (Fv) [97]. With a 55-kDa MW, this molecule is similar in size to an antigen-binding fragment (Fab) of IgG and possesses two antigen-binding sites. It retained the high-affinity binding to c-Mpl (Kd = 10 nM) but exhibited dramatically increased agonistic activity in vitro comparable to that of rhTPO. VB22B sc(Fv)2 induces phosphorylation of JAK2, STAT3, and STAT5, promotes the growth of a TPO-dependent megakaryocytic cell line, and stimulates the differentiation of human CD34$^+$ cells into megakaryocytes. In vivo studies showed that it has an apparent half-life of 8–9 h in cynomolgus monkeys and induced an increase in platelet counts after repeated daily dosing [97]. No clinical development of this molecule has been reported.

MA01G4344U: MA01G4344U was generated through two steps of domain subclass conversion [98]: First, the IgG$_1$ Fc region of an anti-c-Mpl antibody, MA01, was replaced with that of IgG$_4$ to produce MA01G4. This resulted in reduced antibody-dependent cell-mediated cytotoxicity (ADCC) and complement-dependent cytotoxicity (CDC) of target cells compared to MA01. Second, the upper hinge region was changed to one from human IgG$_3$. The end product, MA01G4344U, exhibited tenfold higher agonistic activity than MA01 with no change in receptor affinity. In vitro, MA01G4344U activated the JAK/STAT, MAPK, and PI3K/AKT signaling pathways and stimulated differentiation of human cord blood-derived CD34$^+$ cells into megakaryocytic progenitors. In vivo, a single dose of 3 or 10 mg MA01G4344U stimulated a dose-dependent increase in platelet counts in human c-Mpl-transgenic mice. Platelet levels returned to baseline after 60 and 75 days, respectively [98]. In a xenotransplantation model, weekly administration of MA01G4344U significantly increased the number of human CD41$^+$ cells in the peripheral blood and CD45$^+$/CD34$^+$ cells and myeloid colony-forming cells in the bone marrow [99]. No human studies have been reported.

Conclusions

Over the past 20 years, great progress has been made in understanding the regulation of megakaryopoiesis and thrombopoiesis through the discovery and study of TPO and its receptor, c-Mpl. This period also witnessed the remarkable development of TPO-based pharmaceutics from the first-generation recombinant proteins to the second-generation mimetics that do not stimulate the production of TPO-neutralizing antibodies. Two such agents, romiplostim and eltrombopag, have completed the successful transition from bench to bedside and are currently being used for the treatment of adults with chronic ITP. As we continue to explore their utility in other thrombocytopenia disorders such as CIT, MDS, and HCV-mediated CLD, more will be learned about their efficacy and safety.

References

1. Battinelli EM, Hartwig JH, Italiano JE Jr. Delivering new insight into the biology of megakaryopoiesis and thrombopoiesis. Curr Opin Hematol. 2007;14(5):419–26.
2. Deutsch VR, Tomer A. Megakaryocyte development and platelet production. Br J Haematol. 2006;134(5):453–66.
3. Kaushansky K. The molecular mechanisms that control thrombopoiesis. J Clin Invest. 2005;115(12):3339–47.
4. Kuter DJ, Bussel JB, Lyons RM, et al. Efficacy of romiplostim in patients with chronic immune thrombocytopenic purpura: a double-blind randomised controlled trial. Lancet. 2008;371(9610):395–403.
5. Rodeghiero F. First-line therapies for immune thrombocytopenic purpura: re-evaluating the need to treat. Eur J Haematol Suppl. 2008;(69):19–26.

6. Kuter DJ, Begley CG. Recombinant human thrombopoietin: basic biology and evaluation of clinical studies. Blood. 2002;100(10):3457–69.

7. Gordon MS, Hoffman R. Growth factors affecting human thrombocytopoiesis: potential agents for the treatment of thrombocytopenia. Blood. 1992;80(2):302–7.

8. Gainsford T, Nandurkar H, Metcalf D, Robb L, Begley CG, Alexander WS. The residual megakaryocyte and platelet production in c-mpl-deficient mice is not dependent on the actions of interleukin-6, interleukin-11, or leukemia inhibitory factor. Blood 2000;95(2):528–34.

9. Gainsford T, Roberts AW, Kimura S, et al. Cytokine production and function in c-mpl-deficient mice: no physiologic role for interleukin-3 in residual megakaryocyte and platelet production. Blood. 1998;91(8):2745–52.

10. Scott CL, Robb L, Mansfield R, Alexander WS, Begley CG. Granulocyte–macrophage colony-stimulating factor is not responsible for residual thrombopoiesis in mpl null mice. Exp Hematol. 2000;28(9):1001–7.

11. Kaye JA. FDA licensure of NEUMEGA to prevent severe chemotherapy-induced thrombocytopenia. Stem Cells. 1998;16(Suppl 2):207–23.

12. Kelemen E, Cserhati I, Tanos B. Demonstration and some properties of human thrombopoietin in thrombocythaemic sera. Acta Haematol. 1958;20(6):350–55.

13. Souyri M, Vigon I, Penciolelli JF, Heard JM, Tambourin P, Wendling F. A putative truncated cytokine receptor gene transduced by the myeloproliferative leukemia virus immortalizes hematopoietic progenitors. Cell. 1990;63(6):1137–47.

14. Methia N, Louache F, Vainchenker W, Wendling F. Oligodeoxynucleotides antisense to the proto-oncogene c-mpl specifically inhibit in vitro megakaryocytopoiesis. Blood. 1993;82(5):1395–401.

15. Vigon I, Dreyfus F, Melle J, et al. Expression of the c-mpl proto-oncogene in human hematologic malignancies. Blood. 1993;82(3):877–83.

16. Bartley TD, Bogenberger J, Hunt P, et al. Identification and cloning of a megakaryocyte growth and development factor that is a ligand for the cytokine receptor Mpl. Cell. 1994;77(7):1117–24.

17. de Sauvage FJ, Hass PE, Spencer SD, et al. Stimulation of megakaryocytopoiesis and thrombopoiesis by the c-Mpl ligand. Nature. 1994;369(6481):533–8.

18. Kato T, Ogami K, Shimada Y, et al. Purification and characterization of thrombopoietin. J Biochem. 1995;118(1):229–36.

19. Kuter DJ, Beeler DL, Rosenberg RD. The purification of megapoietin: a physiological regulator of megakaryocyte growth and platelet production. Proc Natl Acad Sci USA. 1994;91(23):11104–8.

20. Lok S, Kaushansky K, Holly RD, et al. Cloning and expression of murine thrombopoietin cDNA and stimulation of platelet production in vivo. Nature 1994;369(6481):565–8.

21. Alexander WS, Roberts AW, Nicola NA, Li R, Metcalf D. Deficiencies in progenitor cells of multiple hematopoietic lineages and defective megakaryocytopoiesis in mice lacking the thrombopoietic receptor c-Mpl. Blood 1996;87(6):2162–70.

22. de Sauvage FJ, Carver-Moore K, Luoh SM, et al. Physiological regulation of early and late stages of megakaryocytopoiesis by thrombopoietin. J Exp Med. 1996;183(2):651–6.

23. Gurney AL, Carver-Moore K, de Sauvage FJ, Moore MW. Thrombocytopenia in c-mpl-deficient mice. Science 1994;265(5177):1445–7.

24. Kaushansky K, Drachman JG. The molecular and cellular biology of thrombopoietin: the primary regulator of platelet production. Oncogene 2002;21(21):3359–67.

25. Boulay JL, O'Shea JJ, Paul WE. Molecular phylogeny within type I cytokines and their cognate receptors. Immunity 2003;19(2):159–63.

26. Feese MD, Tamada T, Kato Y, et al. Structure of the receptor-binding domain of human thrombopoietin determined by complexation with a neutralizing antibody fragment. Proc Natl Acad Sci USA 2004;101(7):1816–21.

27. Cheetham JC, Smith DM, Aoki KH, et al. NMR structure of human erythropoietin and a comparison with its receptor bound conformation. Nat Struct Biol. 1998;5(10):861–6.

28. Syed RS, Reid SW, Li C, et al. Efficiency of signalling through cytokine receptors depends critically on receptor orientation. Nature 1998;395(6701):511–16.
29. McCarty JM, Sprugel KH, Fox NE, Sabath DE, Kaushansky K. Murine thrombopoietin mRNA levels are modulated by platelet count. Blood 1995;86(10):3668–75.
30. Stoffel R, Wiestner A, Skoda RC. Thrombopoietin in thrombocytopenic mice: evidence against regulation at the mRNA level and for a direct regulatory role of platelets. Blood 1996;87(2):567–73.
31. Sungaran R, Markovic B, Chong BH. Localization and regulation of thrombopoietin mRNA expression in human kidney, liver, bone marrow, and spleen using in situ hybridization. Blood 1997;89(1):101–7.
32. Peck-Radosavljevic M, Wichlas M, Zacherl J, et al. Thrombopoietin induces rapid resolution of thrombocytopenia after orthotopic liver transplantation through increased platelet production. Blood 2000;95(3):795–801.
33. Qian S, Fu F, Li W, Chen Q, de Sauvage FJ. Primary role of the liver in thrombopoietin production shown by tissue-specific knockout. Blood 1998;92(6):2189–91.
34. Kaser A, Brandacher G, Steurer W, et al. Interleukin-6 stimulates thrombopoiesis through thrombopoietin: role in inflammatory thrombocytosis. Blood 2001;98(9):2720–5.
35. Emmons RV, Reid DM, Cohen RL, et al. Human thrombopoietin levels are high when thrombocytopenia is due to megakaryocyte deficiency and low when due to increased platelet destruction. Blood 1996;87(10):4068–71.
36. Fielder PJ, Gurney AL, Stefanich E, et al. Regulation of thrombopoietin levels by c-mpl-mediated binding to platelets. Blood 1996;87(6):2154–61.
37. Fielder PJ, Hass P, Nagel M, et al. Human platelets as a model for the binding and degradation of thrombopoietin. Blood 1997;89(8):2782–8.
38. Li J, Xia Y, Kuter DJ. Interaction of thrombopoietin with the platelet c-mpl receptor in plasma: binding, internalization, stability and pharmacokinetics. Br J Haematol. 1999;106(2):345–56.
39. Nichol JL. Endogenous TPO (eTPO) levels in health and disease: possible clues for therapeutic intervention. Stem Cells. 1998;16(Suppl 2):165–75.
40. Sabath DF, Kaushansky K, Broudy VC. Deletion of the extracellular membrane-distal cytokine receptor homology module of Mpl results in constitutive cell growth and loss of thrombopoietin binding. Blood 1999;94(1):365–7.
41. Luoh SM, Stefanich E, Solar G, et al. Role of the distal half of the c-Mpl intracellular domain in control of platelet production by thrombopoietin in vivo. Mol Cell Biol. 2000;20(2):507–15.
42. Morita H, Tahara T, Matsumoto A, Kato T, Miyazaki H, Ohashi H. Functional analysis of the cytoplasmic domain of the human Mpl receptor for tyrosine-phosphorylation of the signaling molecules, proliferation and differentiation. FEBS Lett. 1996;395(2–3):228–34.
43. Tong W, Sulahian R, Gross AW, Hendon N, Lodish HF, Huang LJ. The membrane-proximal region of the thrombopoietin receptor confers its high surface expression by JAK2-dependent and -independent mechanisms. J Biol Chem. 2006;281(50):38930–40.
44. Majka M, Ratajczak J, Villaire G, et al. Thrombopoietin, but not cytokines binding to gp130 protein-coupled receptors, activates MAPKp42/44, AKT, and STAT proteins in normal human CD34$^+$ cells, megakaryocytes, and platelets. Exp Hematol. 2002;30(7):751–60.
45. Graf G, Dehmel U, Drexler HG. Expression of thrombopoietin and thrombopoietin receptor MPL in human leukemia-lymphoma and solid tumor cell lines. Leuk Res. 1996;20(10):831–8.
46. Solar GP, Kerr WG, Zeigler FC, et al. Role of c-mpl in early hematopoiesis. Blood 1998;92(1):4–10.
47. Debili N, Wendling F, Cosman D, et al. The Mpl receptor is expressed in the megakaryocytic lineage from late progenitors to platelets. Blood 1995;85(2):391–401.
48. Sato T, Fuse A, Niimi H, Fielder PJ, Avraham H. Binding and regulation of thrombopoietin to human megakaryocytes. Br J Haematol. 1998;100(4):704–11.

49. Columbyova L, Loda M, Scadden DT. Thrombopoietin receptor expression in human cancer cell lines and primary tissues. Cancer Res. 1995;55(16):3509–12.

50. Drexler HG, Quentmeier H. Thrombopoietin: expression of its receptor MPL and proliferative effects on leukemic cells. Leukemia 1996;10(9):1405–21.

51. Cardier JE, Dempsey J. Thrombopoietin and its receptor, c-mpl, are constitutively expressed by mouse liver endothelial cells: evidence of thrombopoietin as a growth factor for liver endothelial cells. Blood 1998;91(3):923–9.

52. Brizzi MF, Battaglia E, Montrucchio G, et al. Thrombopoietin stimulates endothelial cell motility and neoangiogenesis by a platelet-activating factor-dependent mechanism. Circ Res. 1999;84(7):785–96.

53. Geddis AE, Fox NE, Kaushansky K. The Mpl receptor expressed on endothelial cells does not contribute significantly to the regulation of circulating thrombopoietin levels. Exp Hematol. 2006;34(1):82–6.

54. Coers J, Ranft C, Skoda RC. A truncated isoform of c-Mpl with an essential C-terminal peptide targets the full-length receptor for degradation. J Biol Chem. 2004;279(35):36397–404.

55. Li J, Sabath DF, Kuter DJ. Cloning and functional characterization of a novel c-mpl variant expressed in human CD34 cells and platelets. Cytokine 2000;12(7):835–44.

56. Millot GA, Feger F, Garcon L, Vainchenker W, Dumenil D, Svinarchuk F. MplK, a natural variant of the thrombopoietin receptor with a truncated cytoplasmic domain, binds thrombopoietin but does not interfere with thrombopoietin-mediated cell growth. Exp Hematol. 2002;30(2):166–75.

57. Choi ES, Nichol JL, Hokom MM, Hornkohl AC, Hunt P. Platelets generated in vitro from proplatelet-displaying human megakaryocytes are functional. Blood 1995;85(2):402–13.

58. Lecine P, Villeval JL, Vyas P, Swencki B, Xu Y, Shivdasani RA. Mice lacking transcription factor NF-E2 provide in vivo validation of the proplatelet model of thrombocytopoiesis and show a platelet production defect that is intrinsic to megakaryocytes. Blood 1998;92(5):1608–16.

59. Carver-Moore K, Broxmeyer HE, Luoh SM, et al. Low levels of erythroid and myeloid progenitors in thrombopoietin-and c-mpl-deficient mice. Blood 1996;88(3):803–8.

60. Kimura S, Roberts AW, Metcalf D, Alexander WS. Hematopoietic stem cell deficiencies in mice lacking c-Mpl, the receptor for thrombopoietin. Proc Natl Acad Sci USA. 1998;95(3):1195–200.

61. Sitnicka E, Lin N, Priestley GV, et al. The effect of thrombopoietin on the proliferation and differentiation of murine hematopoietic stem cells. Blood 1996;87(12):4998–5005.

62. Kobayashi M, Laver JH, Kato T, Miyazaki H, Ogawa M. Thrombopoietin supports proliferation of human primitive hematopoietic cells in synergy with steel factor and/or interleukin-3. Blood 1996;88(2):429–36.

63. Broudy VC, Lin NL, Kaushansky K. Thrombopoietin(c-mpl ligand) acts synergistically with erythropoietin, stem cell factor, and interleukin-11 to enhance murine megakaryocyte colony growth and increases megakaryocyte ploidy in vitro. Blood 1995;85(7):1719–26.

64. Kuter DJ. New thrombopoietic growth factors. Blood 2007;109(11):4607–16.

65. Akahori H, Shibuya K, Obuchi M, et al. Effect of recombinant human thrombopoietin in nonhuman primates with chemotherapy-induced thrombocytopenia. Br J Haematol. 1996;94(4):722–8.

66. Harker LA, Marzec UM, Hunt P, et al. Dose–response effects of pegylated human megakaryocyte growth and development factor on platelet production and function in nonhuman primates. Blood 1996;88(2):511–21.

67. Hokom MM, Lacey D, Kinstler OB, et al. Pegylated megakaryocyte growth and development factor abrogates the lethal thrombocytopenia associated with carboplatin and irradiation in mice. Blood 1995;86(12):4486–92.

68. Neelis KJ, Hartong SC, Egeland T, Thomas GR, Eaton DL, Wagemaker G. The efficacy of single-dose administration of thrombopoietin with coadministration of either

granulocyte/macrophage or granulocyte colony-stimulating factor in myelosuppressed rhesus monkeys. Blood 1997;90(7):2565–73.

69. Basser RL, Underhill C, Davis I, et al. Enhancement of platelet recovery after myelosuppressive chemotherapy by recombinant human megakaryocyte growth and development factor in patients with advanced cancer. J Clin Oncol. 2000;18(15):2852–61.

70. Archimbaud E, Ottmann OG, Yin JA, et al. A randomized, double-blind, placebo-controlled study with pegylated recombinant human megakaryocyte growth and development factor (PEG-rHuMGDF) as an adjunct to chemotherapy for adults with de novo acute myeloid leukemia. Blood. 1999;94(11):3694–701.

71. Bolwell B, Vredenburgh J, Overmoyer B, et al. Phase 1 study of pegylated recombinant human megakaryocyte growth and development factor (PEG-rHuMGDF) in breast cancer patients after autologous peripheral blood progenitor cell (PBPC) transplantation. Bone Marrow Transplant. 2000;26(2):141–5.

72. Nash RA, Kurzrock R, DiPersio J, et al. A phase I trial of recombinant human thrombopoietin in patients with delayed platelet recovery after hematopoietic stem cell transplantation. Biol Blood Marrow Transplant. 2000;6(1):25–34.

73. Nomura S, Dan K, Hotta T, Fujimura K, Ikeda Y. Effects of pegylated recombinant human megakaryocyte growth and development factor in patients with idiopathic thrombocytopenic purpura. Blood 2002;100(2):728–30.

74. Basser RL, O'Flaherty E, Green M, et al. Development of pancytopenia with neutralizing antibodies to thrombopoietin after multicycle chemotherapy supported by megakaryocyte growth and development factor. Blood 2002;99(7):2599–602.

75. Li J, Yang C, Xia Y, et al. Thrombocytopenia caused by the development of antibodies to thrombopoietin. Blood 2001;98(12):3241–8.

76. Doshi PD, Giri JG, Abegg AL, et al. Promegapoietin, a family of chimeric growth factors, supports megakaryocyte development through activation of IL-3 and c-Mpl ligand signaling pathways. Exp Hematol. 2001;29(10):1177–84.

77. Cwirla SE, Balasubramanian P, Duffin DJ, et al. Peptide agonist of the thrombopoietin receptor as potent as the natural cytokine. Science 1997;276(5319):1696–9.

78. Frederickson S, Renshaw MW, Lin B, et al. A rationally designed agonist antibody fragment that functionally mimics thrombopoietin. Proc Natl Acad Sci USA 2006;103(39): 14307–12.

79. Lin B, Renshaw MW, Autote K, et al. A step-wise approach significantly enhances protein yield of a rationally-designed agonist antibody fragment in *E. coli*. Protein Expr Purif. 2008;59(1):55–63.

80. Cerneus D, Brown K, Harris R, et al. Stimulation of platelet production in healthy volunteers by a novel pegylated peptide-based thrombopoietin (TPO) receptor agonist. ASH Annu Meet Abstr. 2005;106(11):1249.

81. Jefferis R, Lund J, Pound JD. IgG-Fc-mediated effector functions: molecular definition of interaction sites for effector ligands and the role of glycosylation. Immunol Rev. 1998;163:59–76.

82. Broudy VC, Lin NL. AMG531 stimulates megakaryopoiesis in vitro by binding to Mpl. Cytokine 2004;25(2):52–60.

83. Nichol JL. AMG 531: an investigational thrombopoiesis-stimulating peptibody. Pediatr Blood Cancer 2006;47(5 Suppl):723–5.

84. Hartley C, McElroy T, Molineux G, et al. The novel thrombopoietic agent AMG531 is effective in preclinical models of chemo/radiotherapy induced thrombocytopenia. Proc Am Assoc Cancer Res. 2005;46:1233–8.

85. Wang B, Nichol JL, Sullivan JT. Pharmacodynamics and pharmacokinetics of AMG 531, a novel thrombopoietin receptor ligand. Clin Pharmacol Ther. 2004;76(6):628–38.

86. Bussel JB, Kuter DJ, Pullarkat V, Lyons RM, Guo M, Nichol JL. Safety and efficacy of long-term treatment with romiplostim in thrombocytopenic patients with chronic ITP. Blood 2009;113(10):2161–71.

87. Fukushima-Shintani M, Suzuki K, Iwatsuki Y, et al. AKR-501 (YM477) a novel orally-active thrombopoietin receptor agonist. Eur J Haematol. 2009;82(4):247–54.
88. Fukushima-Shintani M, Suzuki K, Iwatsuki Y, et al. AKR-501 (YM477) in combination with thrombopoietin enhances human megakaryocytopoiesis. Exp Hematol. 2008;36(10): 1337–42.
89. Desjardins RE, Tempel DL, Lucek R, Kuter DJ. Single and multiple oral doses of AKR-501 (YM477) increase the platelet count in healthy volunteers. ASH Annu Meet Abstr. 2006;108(11):477.
90. Duffy KJ, Darcy MG, Delorme E, et al. Hydrazinonaphthalene and azonaphthalene thrombopoietin mimics are nonpeptidyl promoters of megakaryocytopoiesis. J Med Chem. 2001;44(22):3730–45.
91. Erickson-Miller CL, Delorme E, Iskander M, et al. Species specificity and receptor domain interaction of a small molecule TPO receptor agonist. ASH Annu Meet Abstr. 2004;104(11):2909.
92. Erickson-Miller CL, Delorme E, Tian SS, et al. Preclinical activity of eltrombopag (SB-497115), an oral, non-peptide thrombopoietin receptor agonist. Stem Cells 2008;27(2): 424–30.
93. Kim MJ, Park SH, Opella SJ, et al. NMR structural studies of interactions of a small, nonpeptidyl TPO mimic with the thrombopoietin receptor extracellular juxtamembrane and transmembrane domains. J Biol Chem. 2007;282(19):14253–61.
94. Nakamura T, Miyakawa Y, Miyamura A, et al. A novel nonpeptidyl human c-Mpl activator stimulates human megakaryopoiesis and thrombopoiesis. Blood 2006;107(11):4300–7.
95. Bussel JB, Provan D, Shamsi T, et al. Effect of eltrombopag on platelet counts and bleeding during treatment of chronic idiopathic thrombocytopenic purpura: a randomised, double-blind, placebo-controlled trial. Lancet 2009;373(9664):641–8.
96. McHutchison JG, Dusheiko G, Shiffman ML, et al. Eltrombopag for thrombocytopenia in patients with cirrhosis associated with hepatitis C. N Engl J Med. 2007;357(22):2227–36.
97. Orita T, Tsunoda H, Yabuta N, et al. A novel therapeutic approach for thrombocytopenia by minibody agonist of the thrombopoietin receptor. Blood 2005;105(2):562–6.
98. Kai M, Motoki K, Yoshida H, et al. Switching constant domains enhances agonist activities of antibodies to a thrombopoietin receptor. Nat Biotechnol. 2008;26(2):209–11.
99. Kai M, Hagiwara T, Emuta C, et al. In vivo efficacy of anti-MPL agonist antibody in promoting primary human hematopoietic cells. Blood 2009;113(10):2213–16.
100. Kuter DJ. New drugs for familiar therapeutic targets: thrombopoietin receptor agonists and immune thrombocytopenic purpura. Eur J Hematol. 2008;80(Suppl. 69):9–18.

Part II
The Colony-Stimulating Factors

Chapter 6
Cyclic and Chronic Neutropenia

David C. Dale and Karl Welte

Abstract Patients with severe chronic neutropenia have blood neutrophil level <0.5 × 10^9/L, predisposing them to increased susceptibility to life-threatening bacterial infections. This chapter focuses on cyclic and congenital neutropenia, two very interesting and rare hematological conditions causing severe chronic neutropenia. Both disorders respond well to treatment with the myeloid growth factor, granulocyte colony-stimulating factor (G-CSF). This chapter describes the basic features of these diseases and addresses several current clinical issues regarding their diagnosis and management. Cyclic neutropenia is a rare, inherited autosomal dominant disorder due to mutations in the gene for neutrophil elastase (*ELA-2* or *ELANE*). Usually these patients have regular oscillation of blood neutrophil counts with periods of severe neutropenia occurring every 21 days. During these periods, they have painful mouth ulcers, fevers, and bacterial infections. The most severe consequences are gangrene, bacteremia, and septic shock. Cyclic neutropenia patients respond well to treatment with granulocyte colony-stimulating factor (G-CSF) given by subcutaneous injections on a daily or alternate-day basis. Severe congenital neutropenia is also a rare hematological disease, but it is probably more common than cyclic neutropenia. Blood neutrophils are extremely low on a continuing basis; the levels may be <0.2 × 10^9/L, and the risk of severe bacterial infections is even greater than in cyclic neutropenia. The majority of cases are due to autosomal dominant inheritance of mutations in the *ELA-2* or *ELANE* gene. Less commonly, mutations in *HAX-1*, *G6PC3*, and other genes cause this disorder. Treatment with G-CSF is usually effective, but the dose of G-CSF required to normalize blood neutrophils varies greatly. Ten to thirty percent of severe congenital neutropenia patients evolve to develop acute myeloid leukemia, necessitating careful clinical monitoring.

D.C. Dale (✉)
Department of Medicine, University of Washington, Seattle, WA 98195, USA
e-mail: dcdale@u.washington.edu

G.H. Lyman, D.C. Dale (eds.), *Hematopoietic Growth Factors in Oncology*,
Cancer Treatment and Research 157, DOI 10.1007/978-1-4419-7073-2_6,
© Springer Science+Business Media, LLC 2011

Introduction

In healthy individuals, the blood neutrophil count is relatively stable within a range of approximately 2.0–7.0 × 10^9/L. Each person tends to have their own normal level within this range. There are many factors which increase blood neutrophils, including activity, eating, infections, excitement, and despair. Smoking and a few medications cause neutrophilia, including catecholamines, glucocorticosteroids, lithium, and the colony-stimulating factors – granulocyte colony-stimulating factor (G-CSF) and granulocyte–macrophage colony-stimulating factor (GM-CSF) [1].

Neutropenia is usually defined as a reduction in the blood neutrophil count below or 2.0 × 10^9/L. Severe neutropenia is a neutrophil level < 0.5 × 10^9/L and is generally associated with increased susceptibility to infections. In the intermediate range of counts, i.e., from 0.5 to 2.0 × 10^9/L, there may be some enhanced susceptibility, depending upon the event or challenge and the state of the bone marrow, that is, whether or not the patient's marrow can respond to the natural stimuli associated with infections and deliver an increased number of neutrophils into the blood and tissues. In this regard, the blood neutrophil count is a "proxy" for the risk of infections associated with neutropenia. In addition, other host defense factors such as the body's supply of monocytes and lymphocytes and their functions, the integrity of the skin and mucosal membranes, and the functional aspects of the immune system, including the capacity to produce immunoglobulins and complement, are important in determining the consequences of neutropenia [1].

Neutropenia can be either acute (lasting for only a few days to a few weeks) or chronic (lasting for many weeks or even a lifetime). Acute neutropenia is a common occurrence after administration of cancer chemotherapy and following large doses of many immunosuppressive drugs. Many drugs can also suppress neutrophil numbers in the blood and bone marrow as idiosyncratic or allergic reactions [1].

This chapter focuses on two very interesting and rare hematological conditions that cause chronic neutropenia, the diseases are cyclic and congenital neutropenia. Both of these disorders are usually recognized in the first few months or years of life and are associated with enhanced susceptibility to infection secondary to neutropenia and respond well to treatment with the myeloid growth factor, granulocyte colony-stimulating factor (G-CSF). This chapter describes the basic features of these diseases and addresses several current clinical issues regarding their diagnosis and management.

Cyclic Neutropenia

Clinical Characteristics

Cyclic neutropenia is a rare condition affecting perhaps one in a million persons in the general population [2]. It is inherited as an autosomal dominant disorder due to mutations in the gene for neutrophil elastase (*ELA-2*); thus affected patients also often have affected relatives [3]. Sporadic cases occur through new mutations in the

ELA-2 gene. Patients usually present in the first few years of life with recurrent, painful mouth ulcers, fevers, and bacterial infections, most commonly pharyngitis, sinusitis, otitis, and cellulitis. Less frequently, patients get deeper tissue infections, such as pneumonia, peri-anal abscesses, cellulites, and bacteremia. Classically, the patients present with severe neutropenia at the time of fever and infections. They may resolve their clinical symptoms without antibiotics as their neutrophil counts recover. The most severe consequences of cyclic neutropenia are gangrene, bacteremia, and septic shock due to perforating colonic ulcers and infections with *Clostridium septicum* [4, 5]. The occurrence of fever, abdominal pain, and clinical picture of sepsis or a rapidly spreading area of cellulitis are critical and often life-threatening events in these patients.

The hematological features of cyclic neutropenia are classically a regular oscillation of blood neutrophil counts approximately every 21 days. Blood neutrophil levels are usually nearly 0 for 3–5 days, followed by a period of recovering counts to levels near the lower limit of normal [4, 5]. The oscillations and symptoms may be more severe in early childhood, but some patients have the same symptom pattern lasting into their adult years. More commonly, however, symptoms abate, which is probably due to less severe oscillations in blood counts. In families, some affected individuals appear to have more severe disease than others for unknown reasons [6].

Pathophysiology

Cyclic neutropenia is attributable to oscillations in production of neutrophils and other blood cells by the bone marrow. Examining the marrow when neutrophil counts are very low usually shows "maturation arrest" at the promyelocytes or myelocytes stage of development. When counts are higher, the marrow is normal or almost normal [4, 7]. At least 80% of cases of cyclic neutropenia are attributable to mutations in the gene for neutrophil elastase (*ELA-2* mutations) [3, 8]. The effect of these mutations is to shorten the survival of neutrophil progenitors through accelerated apoptosis, making neutrophil production very inefficient. It is not known if any other mutations can cause this disease.

The cause of acquired cyclic neutropenia is also not known. Based upon the mathematical modeling studies of Mackey et al., oscillations in hematopoiesis are a natural consequence of the loss of cells early in the developmental process and the normal feedback system for regulating neutrophil production [9]. The 21-day cycle length in humans is probably attributable to the time for a single cohort of cells to pass through the marrow to their ultimate utilization and removal from the blood or tissues [10].

Diagnosis

The diagnosis of cyclic neutropenia depends upon observing a pattern of regularly recurring neutropenia associated with concomitant fever and inflammatory signs and symptoms. The cycle length is usually approximately 21 days. Regularly recurring mouth ulcers, often deep and painful during neutropenia, are a very common and helpful sign for making this diagnosis. Mutations in the gene for neutrophil elastase in patients with cyclic neutropenia are usually confined to exons four and five and intron four and five of the *ELA-2* gene. Genetic testing for mutations in the gene for neutrophil elastase may be helpful in the diagnosis, but *ELA-2* sequencing is not yet established as a primary way to diagnose this disease because some patients with severe congenital neutropenia will have mutations in the same region of this gene [8].

Treatment

Cyclic neutropenia patients respond well to treatment with granulocyte colony-stimulating factor (G-CSF) [11–13]. Treatment needs to be given by subcutaneous injections on a daily or alternate-day basis and is usually well tolerated by patients of all ages. The response to treatment is to shorten the duration of severe neutropenia, to elevate counts at all other phases of the cycle, and to shorten the cycle length, i.e., the time interval between neutrophil nadirs. G-CSF treatment can usually be titrated to minimize the duration of neutropenia, usually reflected by the elimination or near-elimination of mouth ulcers, fever, and the other inflammatory symptoms which go with the neutropenic periods. Avoidance of very high counts by constant low dose treatment also avoids many of the adverse affects associated with G-CSF therapy. The usual starting dose of G-CSF is 1–2 mg/kg/day and most patients can be managed on less than 3 mg/kg/day.

Current Clinical Issues

Diagnosis

Work is in progress to determine if genetic testing can be a substitute for serial blood counts to make the diagnosis of cyclic neutropenia, since serial blood counts are cumbersome to obtain, particularly for periods of 6 weeks or longer, which is sometimes necessary. Thus finding a mutation in the loci currently associated with cyclic neutropenia supports the diagnosis [14].

How Many Blood Counts to Make the Diagnosis?

Serial blood counts obtained at least 3 days a week for 6 weeks or longer are necessary to make the diagnosis of cyclic neutropenia. It is necessary to do a long series in order to see at least two nadirs, expecting the cycle length to be about 21 days. Counts approximately every other day should show two low counts, i.e., counts below 0.2×10^9/L, during the neutropenic period, concomitant with mouth ulcers and other inflammatory features. For assurance in making the diagnosis it is important to establish both the occurrence of nadirs and the regularity with which they recur.

Is Genetic Diagnosis Possible from Sequencing of the *ELA-2* Gene?

Patients with both cyclic neutropenia and severe congenital neutropenia have mutations in the *ELA-2* gene. The mutations overlap; this is the principal reason that genetic sequencing cannot be used to make the diagnosis of cyclic neutropenia. At present, there are no other genetic mutations known to cause cyclic neutropenia, although careful mathematical analysis may show cyclic oscillations in counts of patients with severe congenital neutropenia, either before or on G-CSF treatment [14].

Do All Patients Need to Be Treated with G-CSF?

Some patients with a history of cyclic neutropenia and typical mutation in the *ELA-2* gene are relatively asymptomatic and do not need G-CSF treatment. The patient's history is the best guide as to whether or not to treat and should always be used in conjunction with blood counts in making this determination.

Are There Alternatives to G-CSF Treatment?

There is no other therapy predictably effective for cyclic neutropenia. GM-CSF has been used in cyclic neutropenia, but usually has more side effects and is less potent for its treatment. No other hematopoietic cytokines are in current use. Corticosteroids are ineffective, as are other therapies such as lithium and androgens.

Is Bone Marrow Transplant an Option for Treatment?

Cyclic neutropenia has been transferred from an affected patient to his/her sibling by bone marrow transplantation, but stem cell transplantation has generally not been used as a treatment for cyclic neutropenia because of the effectiveness of G-CSF.

How Should Clinicians Care for and Follow Patients with Cyclic Neutropenia?

Generally, the most important step is to be sure of the diagnosis based upon serial blood counts, clinical records, and bone marrow examination as necessary to rule out other diagnoses [14]. Once this diagnosis is established, if the patient has recurrent symptoms, treatment with low dose G-CSF is very effective and can be initiated and followed largely with records of the occurrence of mouth ulcers, fever, and other symptoms. Blood counts should be obtained periodically to be sure the patient is not being over-treated or under-treated. Once on a stable dose of G-CSF patients can be followed with blood counts only every few months as a part of their general care. Adverse effects are those generally associated with G-CSF treatment, including bone pain, myalgias and arthralgias, and headaches early in treatment, which generally subside if treatment is maintained at a stable dose.

Does Cyclic Neutropenia Transform to Chronic Neutropenia or Evolve to Leukemia?

Longitudinal records suggest that patients cycle with lesser amplitude as they get older, but this is not a predictable transition, and data are relatively sparse to establish when and how frequently this may occur. Long-term observations of patients with cyclic neutropenia and data from family studies suggest that patients with cyclic neutropenia do not evolve to develop leukemia treated or not treated with G-CSF. If this happens, it must be a very infrequent event, and the risk is substantially less than for patients with severe congenital neutropenia. For this reason, regular bone marrow examinations or other testing for leukemic transformation is not thought to be necessary. Evolution to myelodysplasia is not reported. One case of evolution to chronic myelogenous leukemia, another disease associated with oscillations of blood cell counts, is known to have occurred [15].

Severe Congenital Neutropenia

Dr. Rolf Kostmann, a Swedish pediatrician described a family in northern Sweden with autosomal recessive severe neutropenia in the mid-1950s, early in the era of recognizing congenital immune deficiency disorders [16]. Affected members of this family had very severe neutropenia, recurrent severe infections, and early deaths from infections. Subsequently, similar cases were described with autosomal dominant inheritance [17] and severe neutropenia was observed in association with a number of other hereditable diseases [18]. From a clinical perspective, we now know that severe congenital neutropenia is the consequence of several disorders which affect neutrophil formation from hematopoietic stem cells. All of its forms are quite rare; the combined prevalence is probably only a few cases per million.

Clinical Characteristics

Characteristically, children with severe congenital neutropenia have absolute neutrophil counts of less than 0.5×10^9/L or lower on a continuing basis and patients with the lowest counts, counts less than 0.1×10^9/L often have deep tissue infections with lung abscesses, liver abscesses, and severe skin infections [19]. As a consequence, they are chronically ill from soon after birth with secondary anemia, thrombocytosis, and monocytosis, reflecting the chronicity of their problems with infections. The bone marrow usually shows "promyelocytic maturation arrest" with a paucity of mature cells but many early forms of the myeloid lineage. Other cells in the marrow generally appear normal.

Pathophysiology

Autosomal recessive severe congenital neutropenia is attributable to mutations in the *HAX1* gene, a *BCL2* family-related gene responsible for the production of a mitochondrial protein that is essential for stabilization of mitochondria and to prevent apoptosis of developing cells [20]. The consequence of *HAX1* mutations is accelerated apoptosis of myeloid precursors and the picture of "maturation arrest" of the marrow. Several of families with *HAX1* mutations have now been described, principally in families of Middle Eastern origin in addition to the original family described by Kostmann [20, 21].

A very similar autosomal dominant disorder occurs in patients with *ELA-2* mutations occurring at many loci in exons two through five of the *ELA-2* gene [8]. Pathophysiologically, the expression of the mutant protein from this gene leads to the same consequence, that is, accelerated apoptosis of developing myeloid cells [22]. It is interesting to note that the *ELA-2* gene is expressed only in myeloid tissues and therefore, the clinical phenotype involves only the hematopoietic system. By contrast, the *HAX1* gene, which is expressed in many tissues, leads to other abnormalities, and patients have neurological and neuropsychological abnormalities, at least in some cases [23].

Recently, a similar phenotype with severe neutropenia and maturation arrest of myeloid development was described as an autosomal recessive disorder in patients having mutations of glucose-6-phosphatase (*G6PC3*) [24]. Five of the patients were from two consanguineous pedigrees and seven other isolated cases were also reported. Some of these patients had cardiac and urogenital abnormalities and thrombocytopenia, probably reflecting the wide expression of this gene. Severe neutropenia also occurs rarely with GFI1 and with mutations of the WAS gene [25, 26].

Diagnosis

Severe congenital neutropenia is usually recognized in very young children because of fever and infections and the finding of a very low absolute neutrophil count on the initial blood studies [19]. Characteristically, there may be a very slight neutrophil response to infections, but it is insufficient and chronic infections and fevers usually occur. Milder cases are now being identified based on mutational studies and the full clinical spectrum of severity of illness and consequences for patients with congenital neutropenia is still being discovered. In some cases, serial blood counts and a carefully maintained calendar of clinical events – mouth ulcers, fevers, pharyngitis, otitis, etc. – can be very helpful in ruling in or out the diagnosis of cyclic neutropenia.

Severe congenital neutropenia is relatively easy to diagnosis with standard blood cell counts and a bone marrow aspirate and biopsy. The blood count usually shows severe neutropenia, monocytosis, and may show eosinophilia. The marrow shows maturation arrest and may show increased eosinophils and their progenitors. The marrow is also useful to rule out acute myeloid leukemia. It is particularly important in this regard to observe the characteristics of myeloblasts, since they may appear prominent in patients with severe congenital neutropenia, in part because of the paucity of more mature cells.

Mutations of the *ELA-2* gene are the most common cause for severe congenital neutropenia [18]. Thus for genetic diagnosis, this gene should be sequenced first, unless there is a family history of consanguinity or other clues suggesting an autosomal recessive pattern of inheritance. Similarly, a careful physical examination is helpful in selective genetic testing. *HAX-1* mutations are associated with neurological and behavioral abnormalities, *G6PC3* are associated with cardiac and urogenital abnormalities, and GFI-1 and WAS mutation may be associated with immunological abnormalities.

Treatment

Severe congenital neutropenia, like cyclic neutropenia, responds well to treatment with G-CSF, but usually at higher doses and with some treatment failures [16, 18]. Usually daily treatment with G-CSF in doses of 5–10 mg/kg/day is necessary, starting at a dose of 2–3 μg/kg and gradually increasing the dose to prevent adverse effects. The myeloid growth factor GM-CSF is generally ineffective. Other cytokines have been tried without success. Corticosteroids, androgens, and other treatments are also ineffective. The only significant alternative is hematopoietic transplantation.

Current Clinical Issues

Genetic Testing in the Diagnosis of Severe Congenital Neutropenia

About 60% of cases of severe congenital neutropenia are attributable to mutations in the *ELA-2* gene. For this reason, for genetic diagnosis, this gene should be sequenced first and then consideration given to the other known mutations causing this condition. Mutations of *HAX1*, *G6PC3*, and other genetic mutations are far less common [18].

The Treatment Strategy

It is generally best to start with G-CSF treatment at 2–3 μg/kg/day administered subcutaneously on a daily basis and then to increase the dose gradually, titrating for a response that yields a neutrophil count of 1–2,000. Higher counts can be achieved in responsive patients but this level of stimulation of neutrophil production appears to be unwarranted. Antibiotics and supportive care are important for general management of the patients.

Hematopoietic Transplantation

Patients who are non-responders to G-CSF will benefit from hematopoietic transplantation if they have a good donor. Because donor availability with a perfect or near-perfect match is difficult, often the risk of G-CSF treatment is substantially less than hematopoietic transplantation, except for patients who are poor responders. Individualization of care and consideration of local health resources are always necessary [27, 28].

Risk of Transformation to Myelodysplasia and Leukemia

Patients with severe congenital neutropenia have a 10–30% or perhaps higher risk of evolving to AML in their lifetime [29]. Because of this substantial risk, careful observation is needed to offer the best therapy, since treatment will probably involve chemotherapy and hematopoietic transplantation. Patients with or without *ELA-2* mutations are at approximately equal risk [30]. The requirement for higher does of G-CSF is an indicator or risk, probably because of more severe disease, although a contributing effect of G-CSF to risk cannot be excluded. Studies to determine if certain mutations are more frequently associated with more severe disease or greater likelihood of leukemic transformation are ongoing and no definitive answer to this important question is currently available.

Chemotherapy has been relatively ineffective for patients with AML evolving from severe congenital neutropenia and treatment difficult because of the underlying problem of neutropenia. For this reason, it is recommended that patients have an annual bone marrow examination, blood counts on a regular basis, with observation for changes in the response to G-CSF or for other changes in their hematopoietic state. Any significant change is a signal to consider transplantation.

How to Follow Patients with Severe Congenital Neutropenia

In general, patients who are responsive to G-CSF can be followed on a quarterly basis with regular reporting by the patient or their caregivers about their general health or changes in their general health. Early antibiotics therapy is important for patients who are poor responders or when any of these patients develop signs of a bacterial infection. Although mutations in the G-CSF receptor are associated with leukemic transformation, serial sequencing of this gene is not routinely done to follow patients. Hematopoietic transplantation should be considered for all patients who are poor responders to G-CSF, i.e., requiring more than approximately 20 μg/kg/day or with any significant change in their hematological status or response to G-CSF. It is also prudent to consider patients requiring greater than 8–10 μg/kg/day for transplantation, if there is a well-matched donor, based on the G-CSF dose as a predictor of the risk of leukemic evolution [29].

General Advice

Patients with cyclic neutropenia and congenital neutropenia have a much improved prognosis since the availability of G-CSF as a treatment for this condition. Although this cytokine must be administered subcutaneously, daily or alternate-day therapy is well tolerated and the acute adverse events are generally readily managed. Because of the concern about evolution to acute myeloid leukemia, patients with severe congenital neutropenia should be monitored more closely. The Severe Chronic Neutropenia International Registry is a valuable resource in the care of these patients, a valuable clinical information and information about participation in this registry is available at: http://depts.washington.edu/registry/ and http://www.scner.de/.

References

1. Dale DC. Neutropenia and neutrophilia. In: Williams WJ, et al., editors. Hematology. 7th ed. New York, NY: McGraw-Hill; 2006. pp. 907–19.
2. Dale DC, Bolyard AA, Aprikyan A. Cyclic neutropenia. Semin Hematol. 2002;39:89–94.
3. Horwitz M, Benson KF, Person RE, Aprikyan AG, Dale DC. Mutations in ELA2, encoding neutrophil elastase, define a 21-day biological clock in cyclic haematopoiesis. Nat Genet. 1999;23:433–6.
4. Wright DG, Dale DC, Fauci AS, Wolff SM. Human cyclic neutropenia: clinical review and long-term follow-up of patients. Medicine (Baltimore). 1981;60(1):1–13.
5. Dale DC, Hammond WP IV. Cyclic neutropenia: a clinical review. Blood Rev. 1988;2(3): 178–85.
6. Palmer SE, Dale DC, Livingston RJ, Wijsman EM, Stephens K. Autosomal dominant cyclic hematopoiesis: exclusion of linkage to the major hematopoietic regulatory gene cluster on chromosome 5. Hum Genet. 1994;93:195–7.
7. Guerry D, Dale DC, Omine M, Perry S, Wolff SM. Periodic hematopoiesis in human cyclic neutropenia. J Clin Invest. 1973;52:3220–30.
8. Dale DC, Person RE, Bolyard AA, Aprikyan AG, Bos C, Bonilla MA, Boxer LA, Kannourakis G, Zeidler C, Welte K, Benson KF, Horwitz M. Mutations in the gene encoding neutrophil elastase in congenital and cyclic neutropenia. Blood. 2000;96:2317–22.
9. Haurie C, Dale DC, Mackey MC. Cyclical neutropenia and other periodic hematological disorders: a review of mechanisms and mathematical models. Blood. 1998;92:2629–40.
10. Cartwright GE, Athens JW, Wintrobe MM. The kinetics of granulopoiesis in normal man. Blood. 1964;24:780–803.

11. Hammond WP, Price TH, Souza LM, Dale DC. Treatment of cyclic neutropenia with granulocyte colony stimulating factor. N Engl J Med. 1989;320:1306–11.
12. Dale DC, Bonilla MA, Davis MW, Nakanishi A, Hammond WP, Kurtzberg J, Wang W, Jakubowski A, Winton E, Lalezari P, Robinson W, Glaspy JA, Emerson S, Gabrilove J, Vincent M, Boxer LA. A randomized controlled phase III trial of recombinant human G-CSF for treatment of severe chronic neutropenia. Blood. 1993;81:2496–502.
13. Dale DC, Cottle TE, Fier CJ, Bolyard AA, Bonilla MA, Boxer LA, Cham B, Freedman MH, Kannourakis G, Kinsey SE, Davis R, Scarlata D, Schwinzer B, Zeidler C, Welte K. Severe chronic neutropenia: treatment and follow-up of patients in the Severe Chronic Neutropenia International Registry. Am J Hematol. 2003;72:82–93. PMID: 12555210.
14. Dale DC. ELA2-related neutropenia. In: GeneReviews at GeneTests: medical genetics information resource. Updated Jul 2008. Copyright, University of Washington, Seattle. Available at http://www.genetests.org
15. Dale DC, Bolyard AA, Schwinzer BG, Pracht G, Bonilla MA, Boxer L, Freedman MH, Donadieu J, Kannourakis G, Alter BP, Cham BP, Winkelstein J, Kinsey SE, Fier CJ, Zeidler C, Welte K. The Severe Chronic Neutropenia International Registry: 10-year follow-up report. Support Cancer Ther. 2006;3:220–31.
16. Kostmann R. Infantile genetic agranulocytosis. Acta Paediatr Scand. 1956;45:1–78.
17. Boxer LA, Stein S, Buckley D, Bolyard AA, Dale DC. Strong evidence for autosomal dominant inheritance of severe congenital neutropenia associated with ELA2 mutations. J Pediatr. 2006;148:633–6. PMID: 16737875.
18. Dale DC, Link DC. The many causes of congenital neutropenia. N Engl J Med. 2009;360:3–5.
19. Welte K, Zeidler C, Dale DC. Severe congenital neutropenia. Semin Hematol. 2006;43: 189–95. PMID: 16822461.
20. Klein C, Grudzien M, Appaswamy G, Germeshausen M, Sandrock I, Schäffer AA, Rathinam C, Boztug K, Schwinzer B, Rezaei N, Bohn G, Melin M, Carlsson G, Fadeel B, Dahl N, Palmblad J, Henter JI, Zeidler C, Grimbacher B, Welte K. HAX1 deficiency causes autosomal recessive severe CN (Kostmann disease). Nat Genet. 2007;39:86–92.
21. Carlsson G, Melin M, Dahl N, Ramme KG, Nordenskjöld M, Palmblad J, Henter JI, Fadeel B. Kostmann syndrome or infantile genetic agranulocytosis. Part 2: Understanding the underlying genetic defects in severe congenital neutropenia. Acta Paediatr. 2007;96(6):813–19. Review.
22. Carlsson G, Aprikyan AG, Tehranchi R, Dale DC, Porwit A, Hellstrom-Lindberg E, Palmblad J, Henter JI, Fadeel B. Kostmann syndrome: severe congenital neutropenia associated with defective expression of Bcl-2, constitutive mitochondrial release of cytochrome c, and excessive apoptosis of myeloid progenitor cells. Blood. 2004;103:3355–61. PMID: 14764541.
23. Carlsson G, van't Hooft I, Melin M, Entesarian M, Laurencikas E, Nennesmo I, Trebińska A, Grzybowska E, Palmblad J, Dahl N, Nordenskjöld M, Fadeel B, Henter JI. Central nervous system involvement in severe congenital neutropenia: neurological and neuropsychological abnormalities associated with specific HAX1 mutations. J Intern Med. 2008;264(4):388–400. Epub 2008 May 29.
24. Boztug K, Appaswamy G, Ashikov A, Schäffer AA, Salzer U, Diestelhorst J, Germeshausen M, Brandes G, Lee-Gossler J, Noyan F, Gatzke AK, Minkov M, Greil J, Kratz C, Petropoulou T, Pellier I, Bellanné-Chantelot C, Rezaei N, Mönkemöller K, Irani-Hakimeh N, Bakker H, Gerardy-Schahn R, Zeidler C, Grimbacher B, Welte K, Klein C. A syndrome with congenital neutropenia and mutations in G6PC3. N Engl J Med. 2009;360:32–43.
25. Person RE, Li FQ, Duan Z, Benson KF, Wechsler J, Papadaki HA, Eliopoulos G, Kaufman C, Bertolone SJ, Nakamoto B, Papayannopoulou T, Grimes HL, Horwitz M. Mutations in proto-oncogene GFI1 causes human neutropenia and target ELA2. Nat Genet. 2003;34:208–12.
26. Devriendt K, Kim AS, Mathijs G, Frints SG, Schwartz M, Van Den Oord JJ, Verhoef GE, Boogaerts MA, Fryns JP, You D, Rosen MK, Vandenberghe P. Constitutively activating mutation in WASP causes X-linked severe congenital neutropenia. Nat Genet. 2001;27(3):313–17.

27. Zeidler C, Welte K, Barak Y, Barriga F, Bolyard AA, Boxer L, Cornu G, Cowan MJ, Dale DC, Flood T, Freedman M, Gadner H, Mandel H, O'Reilly RJ, Ramenghi U, Reiter A, Skinner R, Vermylen C, Levine JE. Stem cell transplantation in patients with severe congenital neutropenia without evidence of leukemic transformation. Blood. 2000;95(4):1195–8.
28. Choi SW, Boxer LA, Pulsipher MA, Roulston D, Hutchinson RJ, Yanik GA, Cooke KR, Ferrara JL, Levine JE. Stem cell transplantation in patients with severe congenital neutropenia with evidence of leukemic transformation. Bone Marrow Transplant. 2005;35(5):473–7.
29. Rosenberg PS, Alter BP, Bolyard AA, Bonilla MA, Boxer LA, Cham B, Fier C, Freedman M, Kannourakis G, Kinsey S, Schwinzer B, Zeidler C, Welte K, Dale DC. Severe Chronic Neutropenia International Registry. The incidence of leukemia and mortality from sepsis in patients with severe congenital neutropenia receiving long-term G-CSF therapy. Blood. 2006;107:4628–35.
30. Rosenberg PS, Alter BP, Link DC, Stein S, Rodger E, Bolyard AA, Aprikyan AA, Bonilla MA, Dror Y, Kannourakis G, Newburger PE, Boxer LA, Dale DC. Neutrophil elastase mutations and risk of leukaemia in severe congenital neutropenia. Br J Haematol. 2008;140:210–13.

Chapter 7
The Myeloid Growth Factors

Gary H. Lyman

Introduction

The myeloid growth factors (MGFs) are an important class of biologic agents for the support of cancer patients receiving myelosuppressive chemotherapy by augmenting the production and functional maturation of hematopoietic cells for the purpose of reducing hematologic complications while enabling the safe delivery of effective treatment. This chapter will focus on MGFs with known clinical importance for hematopoiesis in the patient with cancer. Myelosuppression and its sequelae represent the most common dose-limiting complications of cancer chemotherapy and are associated with considerable morbidity, mortality, and costs. In addition to direct chemotherapy-associated complications such as neutropenia, anemia, and thrombocytopenia, myelosuppression often results in chemotherapy dose reductions and delays, reducing delivered chemotherapy dose intensity and potentially compromising disease control and long-term survival in patients with responsive and potentially curable malignancies.

Endogenous production of MGFs occurs in a wide variety of both hematopoietic and nonhematopoietic cells (Table 7.1). Figure 7.1 displays the hematopoietic lineages derived from the myeloid stem cell and modulated by the various MGFs. The concept of the colony-stimulating factors (CSFs) is related to early studies that demonstrated that selected glycoproteins could support the development of colonies of hematopoietic precursors by bone marrow cells in culture [1, 2]. The production of CSFs in various systems using recombinant DNA technology arose from the identification of genes encoding for G-CSF, GM-CSF, and interleukin-3 (IL-3) [3]. The clinically available MGFs are recombinant human (rhu) G-CSF (filgrastim,

G.H. Lyman (✉)
Duke University and the Duke Comprehensive Cancer Center, Durham, NC 27705, USA
e-mail: gary.lyman@duke.edu

G.H. Lyman, D.C. Dale (eds.), *Hematopoietic Growth Factors in Oncology*,
Cancer Treatment and Research 157, DOI 10.1007/978-1-4419-7073-2_7,
© Springer Science+Business Media, LLC 2011

Table 7.1 Characteristics of hematopoietic growth factors

Cytokine	Other names	Generic names	Expression vector	Brand names	No. of amino acids	Human chromosome location	Normal endogenous sources
G-CSF	Granulocyte colony-stimulating factor	Filgrastim Lenograstim	*E. coli* CHO	Neupogen (Amgen) Granocyte (Chugai)	174	17	Monocytes/macrophages, fibroblasts, endothelial cells, keratinocytes
GM-CSF	Granulocyte–macrophage colony-stimulating factor	Sargramostim Molgramostim Regramostim	Yeast *E. coli* CHO	Leukine (Immunex) Leucomax (Schering)	127	5	T lymphocytes, mono-cytes/macrophages, fibroblasts, endothelial cells, osteoblasts, epithelial cells

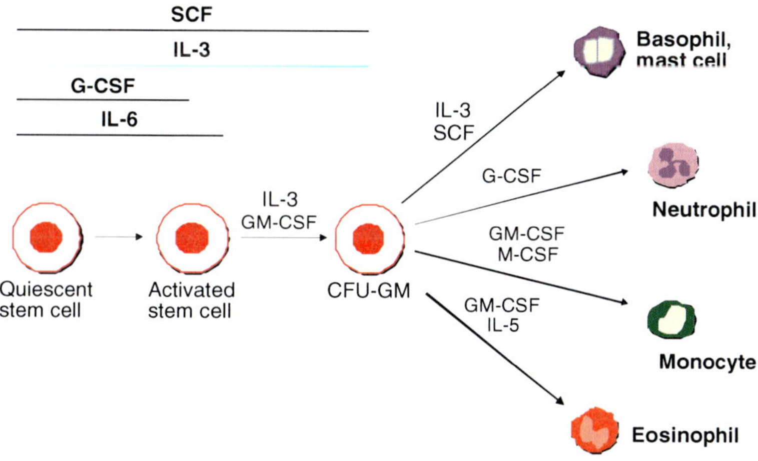

Fig. 7.1 Representation of myeloid hematopoietic differentiation

Table 7.2 Pharmacokinetics of hematopoietic growth factors

CSF	Route	N	Half-life (h)	T_{max} (h)	Cl (mL/min/kg)
G-CSF	SQ	37	2.5–5.8	4–8	19–56
Peg G-CSF	SQ	10	27–47	72–120	0.04–0.68
G-CSF	IV	58	(α 8[a], β 1.8) 1.3–5.1	NA	4–21
GM-CSF	SQ	55	1.6–5.8	2.7–20	249–312
GM-CSF	IV	63	(α 5–20[a], β 1.1–2.5)	NA	9.9–178

Cl, systemic clearance (values are "apparent" for SQ route); CSF, colony-stimulating factor; G-CSF, granulocyte colony-stimulating factor; GM-CSF, granulocyte–macrophage colony-stimulating factor; N, number of patients; NA, not applicable; Peg, pegylated; T_{max}, time of maximal concentration after SQ injection.
Data presented are ranges of mean values in the reviewed studies [96–99].
[a]Values are in minutes.

lenograstim), pegylated rhu G-CSF (pegylated filgrastim), and rhu GM-CSF (sargramostim, molgramostim, regramostim). The pharmacokinetic properties of the CSFs are summarized in Table 7.2.

Granulocyte Colony-Stimulating Factors (G-CSFs)

Filgrastim

A glycoprotein with an ability to induce granulocyte differentiation of a myelomonocytic leukemia cell line subsequently recognized as G-CSF was first identified in 1980 in the serum of mice [4, 5]. Endogenous human G-CSF molecule is an 18.8-kDa glycoprotein with 174 amino acids encoded by a single gene on chromosome 17 and produced by monocytes, macrophages, fibroblasts, endothelial cells, mesenchymal cells, and bone marrow stromal cells. Baseline low G-CSF concentrations are stimulated to high levels by inflammatory cytokines [6, 7]. The receptor for G-CSF, composed of 813 amino acids and encoded by a gene located on chromosome 1, is expressed on the surface of functional neutrophils and neutrophil precursors. While consisting of both cytokine-specific and signal-transducing subunits, the receptor lacks intrinsic kinase activity. Binding of G-CSF to its receptor results in dimerization of signaling proteins linked to the receptor cytoplasmic domains. The biologic action of G-CSF is orchestrated primarily by the Janus kinase–signal transducers and activators of transcription (JAK–STAT) signaling pathway. Once phosphorylated, STAT proteins translocate to the nucleus and result in transcriptional activation. The ras-mitogen-activated protein (MAP) kinases necessary for G-CSF-directed cellular proliferation represent the other important signaling pathways.

G-CSF acts primarily on late myeloid progenitors by increasing cell proliferation and reducing transit time through the bone marrow to the circulation and target tissues. It functions by inducing neutrophil differentiation and functional maturation and increasing chemotaxis, phagocytosis, and antibody-dependent cellular toxicity. Normal neutrophil production as well as any neutrophil response to stress requires the action of G-CSF as demonstrated by the development of chronic neutropenia in G-CSF knockout mice [6, 7]. In neutropenic states, and most dramatically with febrile neutropenia, endogenous G-CSF levels rise. Filgrastim and other unpegylated CSFs are cleared by glomerular filtration and renal excretion. Metabolism is through binding to the G-CSF receptor and internalization, as well as by hepatic enzymes.

The CSFs are the only biological agents used in clinical practice to reduce the risk of neutropenic complications and to maintain chemotherapy dose intensity [8]. Primary prophylaxis with G-CSF starting within 3–5 days of the initial cycle of chemotherapy is based on evidence that the risk of neutropenic complications including febrile neutropenia (FN) is greatest during the first cycle of chemotherapy [9–11]. Multiple randomized controlled trials (RCTs) of primary prophylaxis with G-CSF have been reported in a variety of malignancies and treatment regimens [12]. Filgrastim is approved by the US Food and Drug Administration (FDA) to decrease the incidence of infection, as manifested by FN, in patients with nonmyeloid malignancies receiving myelosuppressive anticancer drugs associated with a significant incidence of severe neutropenia with fever. Lenograstim is a glycosylated G-CSF not available in the United States but with similar biologic, functional, and clinical activity to filgrastim.

Pegylated G-CSF (Pegfilgrastim)

Pegfilgrastim represents recombinant G-CSF covalently bound at the N terminus to a 20-kDa polyethylene glycol molecule which increases the total molecular weight to 39 kDa [13]. The pegfilgrastim molecule retains the biological activity of filgrastim resulting in increased cell division, more rapid transit through the bone marrow, and increased differentiation and end-cell functional activation of neutrophils but is too large for renal clearance resulting in a prolonged half-life of approximately 33 h. Pegfilgrastim has saturable, self-regulating neutrophil-mediated elimination characterized by stimulation of neutrophil production when neutrophil counts are low followed by rapid clearance when neutrophil counts recover and fresh receptors are available for binding. Knockout mice for the G-CSF receptor demonstrate significantly lower clearance, longer half-life as well as greater area under the curve for both filgrastim and pegfilgrastim [14]. In bilateral nephrectomized rats, filgrastim clearance is reduced by 60–70% resulting in similar concentration–time profiles to that of pegfilgrastim [15]. Serum clearance of pegfilgrastim decreases with increasing dose confirming the saturation and neutrophil-mediated clearance while its elimination is prolonged and action sustained during recovery from chemotherapy-induced neutropenia [16] (Fig. 7.2). Pegfilgrastim acts by binding to cell surface G-CSF receptors on neutrophils similar to filgrastim increasing cell division, differentiation, and functional maturation shortening bone marrow transit to the circulation and tissues [17].

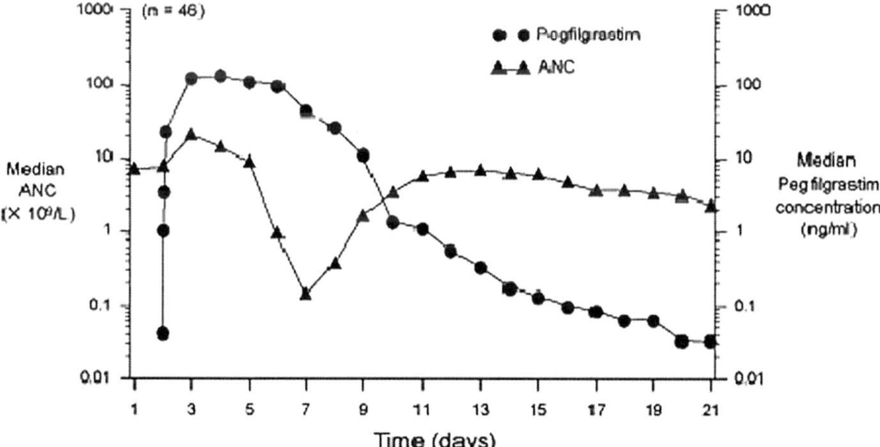

Fig. 7.2 Pegfilgrastim serum concentrations (*circles*) and absolute neutrophil count (ANC) (*triangles*) in patients with breast cancer who received pegfilgrastim as an adjunct to chemotherapy. Adapted from Green et al. [20]

Approval of pegfilgrastim by the FDA was based on two pivotal RCTs comparing pegfilgrastim to filgrastim as an active control in the setting of chemotherapy associated with a risk of febrile neutropenia without MGF support of approximately 40% [18]. Pegfilgrastim was dosed based on weight (100 µg/kg) in one trial and at a fixed dose at 6 mg in the other [19, 20]. As shown in Fig. 7.3, patients in these trials received either a single injection of pegfilgrastim 24 h after chemotherapy followed by placebo or filgrastim at 5 µg/kg daily for up to 14 days. The incidence of FN was lower in patients who received pegfilgrastim with the combined treatment

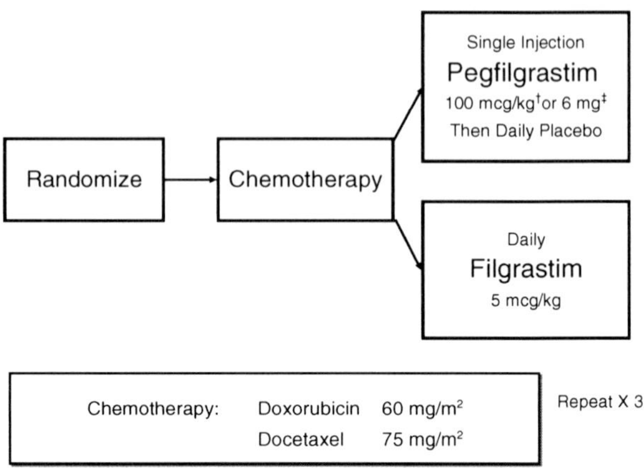

Fig. 7.3 Design of pivotal phase III randomized trials of pegfilgrastim versus filgrastim in patients receiving chemotherapy for stage II–IV breast cancer. †Holmes et al. [19], ‡Green et al. [20]

effect from both studies demonstrating an additional relative risk reduction for FN with pegfilgrastim of 44% ($P = 0.015$) [13]. However, there was no significant difference in the primary outcome in these trials consisting of the duration of severe neutropenia. In a large, double-blind, placebo-controlled RCT, pegfilgrastim was compared to placebo in women with breast cancer receiving docetaxel 100 mg/m² every 3 weeks for four cycles. Patients receiving pegfilgrastim experienced a lower risk of FN (1% vs 17%; $P < 0.001$) and FN hospitalization (1% vs 14%, $P < 0.001$) than control subjects [21]. Pegfilgrastim has been approved to reduce the risk of infection in patients with nonmyeloid malignancies receiving myelosuppressive chemotherapy associated with an incidence of FN of 17% or greater risk. Based on the equivalency in two a pivotal trials, the currently recommended dose of pegfilgrastim is 6 mg single sc injection 24 h after administration of chemotherapy.

Evidence Summary and Clinical Practice Guidelines

A systematic review of RCTs of primary prophylaxis with G-CSF administered according to guideline recommendations has been reported in patients with solid tumors and lymphoma [12]. As shown in Fig. 7.4, the relative risk reduction for febrile neutropenia with G-CSF prophylaxis compared to control was 46% [95%CI 33–57%] ($P < 0.0001$). Importantly, for the first time, the systematic review demonstrated that across eligible RCTs, the relative risk reduction for infection-related and early all-cause mortality with G-CSF was 45% [95%CI 10–67%] ($P = 0.018$) and 40% [95%CI 17–57%] ($P = 0.002$), respectively. Median relative dose intensity (RDI) was 88.5% and 95.5% among control and G-CSF-treated patients, respectively. Improved clinical outcomes have been demonstrated in recent RCTs by increasing the RDI of chemotherapy utilizing abbreviated treatment schedules (dose-dense schedules) with G-CSF support [22–24]. Although no RCTs have

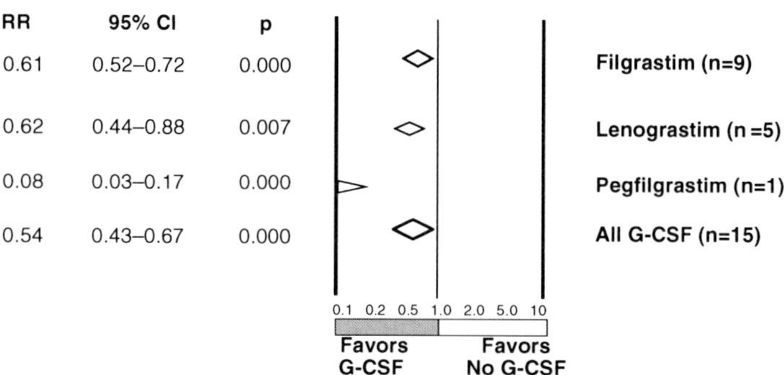

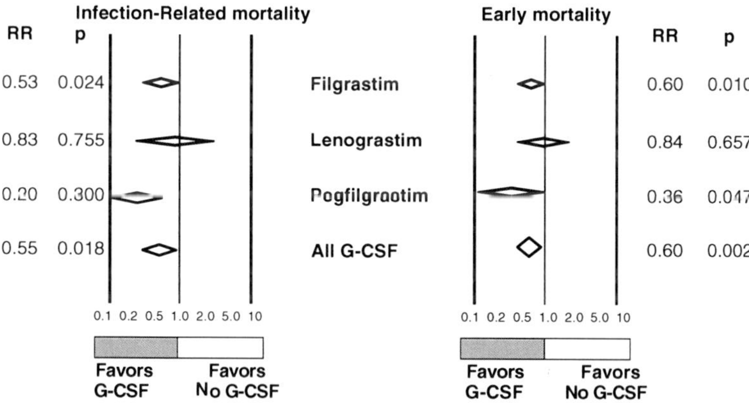

Fig. 7.4 Forest plots of summary results from a meta-analysis of randomized controlled trials of G-CSF prophylaxis in solid tumor and lymphoma patients receiving systemic chemotherapy with or without prophylactic G-CSF including filgrastim, lenograstim, or pegfilgrastim. *Top figure* displays reported rates of febrile neutropenia [12]. *Bottom graphs* reflect results for infection-related and all-cause early mortality reported across trials

directly evaluated the use of the CSFs as secondary prophylaxis following neutropenic complications, primary prophylaxis starting in the first cycle is associated with significantly greater reduction in febrile neutropenia than delayed prophylaxis among RCTs permitting cross-over among control patients after experiencing FN ($P = 0.046$) [12]. Importantly, filgrastim prophylaxis administered after developing neutropenia does not reduce the incidence or duration of neutropenic complications compared to placebo [25]. Finally, CSF treatment utilized along with empiric antibiotics for management of febrile neutropenia is associated with a reduction in the duration of neutropenia and hospitalization and a reduction in infection-related mortality [26].

Several international professional organizations have developed clinical practice guidelines for the use of MGFs in patients receiving cancer chemotherapy [8, 27, 28]. As shown in Table 7.3, recommendations across these guidelines, which include primary prophylaxis with the CSFs when the risk of FN is 20% or greater, are quite consistent despite the differences in methodology. Prophylactic use of myeloid growth factors is also recommended with regimens associated with

Table 7.3 Summary of primary prophylaxis recommendations [8]

ASCO white blood cell growth factor guidelines update summary		
Setting/indication	√ Recommended	✗ Not recommended
General circumstances	FN risk in the range of 20% or higher	
Special circumstances	Clinical factors dictate use	
Secondary prophylaxis	Based on chemotherapy reaction among other factors	
Therapy of afebrile neutropenia		Not to be used routinely
Therapy of febrile neutropenia	If high risk for complications or poor clinical outcomes	Not to be used routinely as adjunctive treatment with antibiotic therapy
Acute myeloid leukemia	Following induction therapy, patients > 55 years old most likely to benefit After the completion of consolidation chemotherapy	Not to be used for priming effects
Myelodysplastic syndrome		Intermittent administration for a subset of patients with severe neutropenia and recurrent infection
Acute lymphocytic leukemia	After the completion of initial chemotherapy or first post-remission course	
Radiotherapy	Consider if receiving radiation therapy alone and prolonged delays are expected	Avoid in patients receiving concomitant chemotherapy and radiation therapy
Older patients	If ≥ 65 years old with diffuse aggressive lymphoma and treated with curative chemotherapy	
Pediatric population	For the primary prophylaxis of pediatric patients with a likelihood of FN and the secondary prophylaxis or therapy for high-risk patients	G-CSF use in children with Acute Lymphocytic Leukemia should be considered carefully

a lower risk of febrile neutropenia in patients with additional individual risk factors for neutropenic complications including older age and major comorbidities. Age represents a consistently reported risk factor with the greatest risk for febrile neutropenia observed in the first cycle of chemotherapy [10, 11]. Risk factors for febrile neutropenia among older cancer patients include prior chemotherapy, anthracycline-based chemotherapy, and hepatic or renal dysfunction [29]. G-CSF reduces the risk of febrile neutropenia in older cancer patients without major medical complications to a similar degree as it does in younger patients [30–33]. Primary prophylaxis with G-CSF in older patients is associated with less febrile neutropenia, hospitalizations for febrile neutropenia, and fewer dose reductions and delays than patients receiving G-CSF only after an initial episode of severe neutropenia [34].

Hematologic Malignancies and Stem Cell Transplantation (SCT)

In patients with acute myeloid leukemia (AML), the MGFs have been used following induction chemotherapy, priming before induction chemotherapy, and after consolidation chemotherapy. Mixed results have been reported in studies of the MGFs administered prior to chemotherapy as priming therapy to increase the number of leukemic blasts in growth phase [35]. MGFs administered after induction or consolidation therapy have been shown to reduce the severity and duration of neutropenia [36, 37]. The CSFs have also been shown to shorten the duration of neutropenia and are recommended after initial induction and post-remission chemotherapy in patients with acute lymphocytic leukemia (ALL) [38–41].

The use of the MGFs had demonstrated efficacy when utilized either to mobilize peripheral blood progenitor cells (PBPCs) for increased stem cell collection or in support of autologous SCT to decrease the duration of neutropenia [42–48]. G-CSF alone or following myelosuppressive chemotherapy is often employed increasing PBPC production for SCT. G-CSF administered for several days prior to SCT appears to increase the numbers of PBPCs for reinfusion [49–51]. Mobilization kinetics with pegfilgrastim are similar to those of filgrastim and associated with earlier recovery and peak concentrations of CD34$^+$ cells and rapid hematopoietic recovery when reinfused [52–56].

G-CSF administered after high-dose chemotherapy with autologous PBPC reinfusion enhances neutrophil recovery and marrow engraftment [43, 57–64]. Both filgrastim and pegfilgrastim treatment are associated with a lower risk and shorter duration of febrile neutropenia when given after SCT [65]. However, conflicting data are available on the use of these agents after allogeneic SCT. While CSF support was associated with more graft versus host disease (GVHD), transplantation-related mortality, and lower survival in a retrospective study of patients with AML undergoing allogeneic SCT, a meta-analysis of RCTs of CSF administration following allogeneic SCT demonstrated more rapid engraftment, shorter hospitalizations, and intravenous antibiotic use and reduced transplant-related mortality [66, 67].

Toxicity and Safety

Approximately, 20–30% of patients receiving G-CSF will experience mild-to-moderate bone pain occurring concurrently with neutrophil recovery following chemotherapy-induced neutropenia [12]. Occasional laboratory abnormalities reported include leukocytosis and elevations of uric acid, alkaline phosphatase, and lactate dehydrogenase. Other reported rare complications of G-CSF treatment when used in the setting of PBSC mobilization have included splenomegaly, splenic rupture, and thrombocytopenia. Pegfilgrastim use has been associated with a very similar safety profile bone pain representing the most common adverse event reported. No significant differences in incidence, severity, or duration of bone pain were reported in retrospective analyses of the pivotal phase III studies of pegfilgrastim versus filgrastim [16, 20]. Pegfilgrastim may also be safely administered in support of dose-dense regimens despite label restrictions to the contrary [19, 68, 69].

Concern has been expressed about a possible increased risk of AML or myelodysplastic syndrome (MDS) in patients receiving G-CSF. Hershman et al. reported an increased risk of AML in elderly women with early-stage breast cancer who previously were treated with adjuvant chemotherapy along with G-CSF or GM-CSF from SEER-Medicare linked data [70]. It is difficult, however, to identify and adjust for all possible confounding factors in such retrospective analyses. Since it is difficult to distinguish any effects of the MGFs from the recognized leukemogenicity of ionizing radiation and many commonly utilized chemotherapeutic agents, the ability of these agents to sustain or increase chemotherapy dose and/or dose intensity further confounds any proposed causal influence on the risk of AML or MDS. A meta-analysis of RCTs of G-CSF-supported chemotherapy with at least 2 years of follow-up has recently reported an increased risk of AML/MDS among G-CSF-treated patients with an absolute risk increase of 4/1,000 [71]. However, a 10% reduction in the relative risk for all-cause mortality with G-CSF support was also observed across trials with an absolute reduction of 3.4%. Therefore, even if some of the observed increased risk of AML/MDS is due to the addition of G-CSF support, the benefit in terms of reduced mortality appears to be some tenfold greater.

Granulocyte–Macrophage Colony-Stimulating Factor (GM-CSF)

GM-CSF is a 14–35-kDa glycoprotein first identified in 1977. It is encoded by a gene located on chromosome 5 and is produced by monocytes, macrophages, fibroblasts, and endothelial cells [6, 7, 72, 73]. In distinction to G-CSF, GM-CSF gene knockout mice demonstrate no impairment in hematopoiesis under steady-state conditions [6, 7]. Receptors for GM-CSF are present on the surface of neutrophils, monocytes, eosinophils, myeloid progenitors, and myeloid leukemia cells. Downstream signaling after binding of GM-CSF to its receptor is primarily through the JAK-STAT pathways [6, 7]. GM-CSF is associated with an increase in phagocytosis and other functional activity of neutrophils, macrophages, monocytes, and eosinophils. GM-CSF enhances the proliferation and survival elements of the granulocytic and macrophage lineages and sustains high concentrations of megakaryocyte progenitors. While GM-CSF stimulates dendritic cells in vitro and in vivo, it has been shown to inhibit neutrophil migration into sterile inflammatory fields [74]. Human GM-CSF was purified in 1984 and recombinant GM-CSF is available as sargramostim derived from yeast and molgramostim derived from *Escherichia coli*. The FDA has approved GM-CSF as an adjunct in the treatment of AML and in the setting of autologous and allogeneic SCT as well as stem cell mobilization.

Hematologic Malignancies and Stem Cell Transplantation

Sargramostim was shown to enhance neutrophil recovery, reduce infection, and improve survival in elderly patients with AML in a large, phase III placebo-controlled RCT [75]. Similarly, reduced time to neutrophil recovery and improved disease-free survival were reported in 240 elderly patients with AML receiving molgramostim during and after induction chemotherapy in a randomized, placebo-controlled study [76].

Several studies have demonstrated the utility of GM-CSF or GM-CSF alone or following chemotherapy in the mobilization of PBPCs for subsequent leukapheresis [50, 77–80]. Improved myeloid and platelet recovery compared to controls has been shown with administration of GM-CSF-primed PBPCs following cytotoxic chemotherapy, with autologous SCT [81]. RCTs of GM-CSF in the setting of high-dose chemotherapy with SCT have demonstrated enhanced neutrophil recovery when bone marrow supported SCT [82–91].

Toxicity and Safety

GM-CSF is most frequently associated with fever, dyspnea, myalgias, bone pain, and fluid retention particularly when made in *E. coli* [92]. GM-CSF induces other endogenous cytokines, which may be responsible for some of the adverse effects reported. Side effects that appear to be unrelated to GM-CSF dose include fever, pleuritis, myalgia, bone pain, pulmonary infiltrates, rash, and thrombophlebitis. Dose-dependent adverse effects include hypotension, capillary leak syndrome, and central vein thrombosis. There have been reports of transient hypoxia and hypotension following the initial but not subsequent doses of GM-CSF [93]. Increased myelosuppression has been reported with the simultaneous administration of GM-CSF and cycle-specific chemotherapy or radiation therapy [94, 95].

References

1. Metcalf D. Studies on colony formation in vitro by mouse bone marrow cells. I. Continuous cluster formation and relation of clusters to colonies. J Cell Physiol. 1969;74:323–32.
2. Metcalf D, Foster R. Bone marrow colony-stimulating activity of serum from mice with viral-induced leukemia. J Natl Cancer Inst. 1967;39:1235–45.
3. Clark SC, Kamen R. The human hematopoietic colony-stimulating factors. Science. 1987;236:1229–37.
4. Burgess AW, Metcalf D. Characterization of a serum factor stimulating the differentiation of myelomonocytic leukemic cells. Int J Cancer. 1980;26:647–54.
5. Moore MA. G-CSF: its relationship to leukemia differentiation-inducing activity and other hemopoietic regulators. J Cell Physiol Suppl. 1982;1:53–64.
6. Bagby G, Heinrich M. Growth factors cytokines, and the control of hematopoiesis. In: Hoffman R, Shattil SJ, editors. Hematology basic principles and practice. Philadelphia, PA: Churchill Livingstone; 2000. pp. 154–202.
7. Moore M. Colony stimulating factors: basic principles and preclinical studies. In: Rosenberg S, editor. Principles and practice of the biologic therapy of cancer. Philadelphia, PA: Lippincott Williams & Wilkins; 2000. pp. 113–40.
8. Smith TJ, Khatcheressian J, Lyman GH, et al. 2006 update of recommendations for the use of white blood cell growth factors: an evidence-based clinical practice guideline. J Clin Oncol. 2006;2006(24):3187–205.
9. Crawford J, Dale DC, Kuderer NM, et al. Risk and timing of neutropenic events in adult cancer patients receiving chemotherapy: the results of a prospective nationwide study of oncology practice. J Natl Compr Canc Netw. 2008;6:109–18.
10. Lyman GH, Delgado DJ. Risk and timing of hospitalization for febrile neutropenia in patients receiving CHOP, CHOP-R, or CNOP chemotherapy for intermediate-grade non-Hodgkin lymphoma. Cancer. 2003;98:2402–9.
11. Lyman GH, Morrison VA, Dale DC, et al. Risk of febrile neutropenia among patients with intermediate-grade non-Hodgkin's lymphoma receiving CHOP chemotherapy. Leuk Lymphoma. 2003;44:2069–76.
12. Kuderer NM, Dale DC, Crawford J, et al. Impact of primary prophylaxis with granulocyte colony-stimulating factor on febrile neutropenia and mortality in adult cancer patients receiving chemotherapy: a systematic review. J Clin Oncol. 2007;25:3158–67.
13. Lyman GH. Pegfilgrastim: a granulocyte colony-stimulating factor with sustained duration of action. Expert Opin Biol Ther. 2005;5:1635–46.
14. Kotto-Kome AC, Fox SE, Lu W, et al. Evidence that the granulocyte colony-stimulating factor (G-CSF) receptor plays a role in the pharmacokinetics of G-CSF and PegG-CSF using a G-CSF-R KO model. Pharmacol Res. 2004;50:55–8.
15. Yang BB, Lum PK, Hayashi MM, et al. Polyethylene glycol modification of filgrastim results in decreased renal clearance of the protein in rats. J Pharm Sci. 2004;93:1367–73.
16. Holmes FA, Jones SE, O'Shaughnessy J, et al. Comparable efficacy and safety profiles of once-per-cycle pegfilgrastim and daily injection filgrastim in chemotherapy-induced neutropenia: a multicenter dose-finding study in women with breast cancer. Ann Oncol. 2002;13:903–9.
17. Molineux G. The design and development of pegfilgrastim (PEG-rmetHuG-CSF, Neulasta). Curr Pharm Des. 2004;10:1235–44.
18. Misset JL, Dieras V, Gruia G, et al. Dose-finding study of docetaxel and doxorubicin in first-line treatment of patients with metastatic breast cancer. Ann Oncol. 1999;10:553–60.
19. Holmes FA, O'Shaughnessy JA, Vukelja S, et al. Blinded, randomized, multicenter study to evaluate single administration pegfilgrastim once per cycle versus daily filgrastim as an adjunct to chemotherapy in patients with high-risk stage II or stage III/IV breast cancer. J Clin Oncol. 2002;20:727–31.

20. Green MD, Koelbl H, Baselga J, et al. A randomized double-blind multicenter phase III study of fixed-dose single-administration pegfilgrastim versus daily filgrastim in patients receiving myelosuppressive chemotherapy. Ann Oncol. 2003;14:29–35.
21. Vogel CL, Wojtukiewicz MZ, Carroll RR, et al. First and subsequent cycle use of pegfilgrastim prevents febrile neutropenia in patients with breast cancer: a multicenter, double-blind, placebo-controlled phase III study. J Clin Oncol. 2005;23:1178–84.
22. Citron ML, Berry DA, Cirrincione C, et al. Randomized trial of dose-dense versus conventionally scheduled and sequential versus concurrent combination chemotherapy as postoperative adjuvant treatment of node-positive primary breast cancer: first report of Intergroup Trial C9741/Cancer and Leukemia Group B Trial 9741. J Clin Oncol. 2003;21:1431–9.
23. Pfreundschuh M, Trumper L, Kloess M, et al. Two-weekly or 3-weekly CHOP chemotherapy with or without etoposide for the treatment of elderly patients with aggressive lymphomas: results of the NHL-B2 trial of the DSHNHL. Blood. 2004;104:634–41.
24. Pfreundschuh M, Trumper L, Kloess M, et al. Two-weekly or 3-weekly CHOP chemotherapy with or without etoposide for the treatment of young patients with good-prognosis (normal LDH) aggressive lymphomas: results of the NHL-B1 trial of the DSHNHL. Blood. 2004;104:626–33.
25. Hartmann LC, Tschetter LK, Habermann TM, et al. Granulocyte colony-stimulating factor in severe chemotherapy-induced afebrile neutropenia. N Engl J Med. 1997;336:1776–80.
26. Clark OA, Lyman GH, Castro AA, et al. Colony-stimulating factors for chemotherapy-induced febrile neutropenia: a meta-analysis of randomized controlled trials. J Clin Oncol. 2005;23:4198–214.
27. Aapro MS, Cameron DA, Pettengell R, et al. EORTC guidelines for the use of granulocyte-colony stimulating factor to reduce the incidence of chemotherapy-induced febrile neutropenia in adult patients with lymphomas and solid tumours. Eur J Cancer. 2006;42:2433–53.
28. Crawford J, Armitage J, Balducci L, et al. Myeloid growth factors. J Natl Compr Canc Netw. 2009;7:64–83.
29. Shayne M, Culakova E, Poniewierski MS, et al. Dose intensity and hematologic toxicity in older cancer patients receiving systemic chemotherapy. Cancer. 2007;110:1611–20.
30. Doorduijn JK, van der Holt B, van Imhoff GW, et al. CHOP compared with CHOP plus granulocyte colony-stimulating factor in elderly patients with aggressive non-Hodgkin's lymphoma. J Clin Oncol. 2003;21:3041–50.
31. Lyman GH, Kuderer N, Agboola O, et al. Evidence-based use of colony-stimulating factors in elderly cancer patients. Cancer Control. 2003;10:487–99.
32. Osby E, Hagberg H, Kvaloy S, et al. CHOP is superior to CNOP in elderly patients with aggressive lymphoma while outcome is unaffected by filgrastim treatment: results of a Nordic Lymphoma Group randomized trial. Blood. 2003;101:3840–8.
33. Zinzani PL, Pavone E, Storti S, et al. Randomized trial with or without granulocyte colony-stimulating factor as adjunct to induction VNCOP-B treatment of elderly high-grade non-Hodgkin's lymphoma. Blood. 1997;89:3974–9.
34. Balducci L, Al-Halawani H, Charu V, et al. Elderly cancer patients receiving chemotherapy benefit from first-cycle pegfilgrastim. Oncologist. 2007;12:1416–24.
35. Lowenberg B, van Putten W, Theobald M, et al. Effect of priming with granulocyte colony-stimulating factor on the outcome of chemotherapy for acute myeloid leukemia. N Engl J Med. 2003;349:743–52.
36. Harousseau JL, Witz B, Lioure B, et al. Granulocyte colony-stimulating factor after intensive consolidation chemotherapy in acute myeloid leukemia: results of a randomized trial of the Groupe Ouest-Est Leucemies Aigues Myeloblastiques. J Clin Oncol. 2000;18:780–7.
37. Heil G, Hoelzer D, Sanz MA, et al. A randomized, double-blind, placebo-controlled, phase III study of filgrastim in remission induction and consolidation therapy for adults with de novo acute myeloid leukemia. The International Acute Myeloid Leukemia Study Group. Blood. 1997;90:4710–18.

38. Larson RA, Dodge RK, Linker CA, et al. A randomized controlled trial of filgrastim during remission induction and consolidation chemotherapy for adults with acute lymphoblastic leukemia: CALGB study 9111. Blood. 1998;92:1556–64.
39. Laver J, Amylon M, Desai S, et al. Randomized trial of r-metHu granulocyte colony-stimulating factor in an intensive treatment for T-cell leukemia and advanced-stage lymphoblastic lymphoma of childhood: a Pediatric Oncology Group pilot study. J Clin Oncol. 1998;16:522–6.
40. Pui CH, Boyett JM, Hughes WT, et al. Human granulocyte colony-stimulating factor after induction chemotherapy in children with acute lymphoblastic leukemia. N Engl J Med. 1997;336:1781–7.
41. Ottmann OG, Hoelzer D, Gracien E, et al. Concomitant granulocyte colony-stimulating factor and induction chemoradiotherapy in adult acute lymphoblastic leukemia: a randomized phase III trial. Blood. 1995;86:444–50.
42. D'Hondt L, Emmons RV, Andre M, et al. The administration of 10 microg/kg granulocyte colony-stimulating factor (G-CSF) alone results in a successful peripheral blood stem cell collection when previous mobilization with chemotherapy and hematopoietic growth factor failed. Leuk Lymphoma. 1999;34:105–9.
43. Klumpp TR, Mangan KF, Goldberg SL, et al. Granulocyte colony-stimulating factor accelerates neutrophil engraftment following peripheral-blood stem-cell transplantation: a prospective, randomized trial. J Clin Oncol. 1995;13:1323–7.
44. Kroger N, Zander AR. Dose and schedule effect of G-GSF for stem cell mobilization in healthy donors for allogeneic transplantation. Leuk Lymphoma. 2002;43:1391–4.
45. Kroger N, Zeller W, Hassan HT, et al. Successful mobilization of peripheral blood stem cells in heavily pretreated myeloma patients with G-CSF alone. Ann Hematol. 1998;76:257–62.
46. Lefrere F, Makke J, Fermand J, et al. Blood stem cell collection using chemotherapy with or without systematic G-CSF: experience in 52 patients with multiple myeloma. Bone Marrow Transplant. 1999;24:463–6.
47. Nemunaitis J, Appelbaum F, Singer J. Effect of GM-CSF on circulating granulocyte–monocyte progenitors in autologous bone marrow transplantation. Lancet. 1989;2:1405–6.
48. Spitzer G, Adkins D, Mathews M, et al. Randomized comparison of G-CSF$^+$ GM-CSF vs G-CSF alone for mobilization of peripheral blood stem cells: effects on hematopoietic recovery after high-dose chemotherapy. Bone Marrow Transplant. 1997;20:921–30.
49. Chao NJ, Schriber JR, Grimes K, et al. Granulocyte colony-stimulating factor "mobilized" peripheral blood progenitor cells accelerate granulocyte and platelet recovery after high-dose chemotherapy. Blood. 1993;81:2031–5.
50. Peters WP, Rosner G, Ross M, et al. Comparative effects of granulocyte–macrophage colony-stimulating factor (GM-CSF) and granulocyte colony-stimulating factor (G-CSF) on priming peripheral blood progenitor cells for use with autologous bone marrow after high-dose chemotherapy. Blood. 1993;81:1709–19.
51. Sheridan WP, Begley CG, Juttner CA, et al. Effect of peripheral-blood progenitor cells mobilised by filgrastim (G-CSF) on platelet recovery after high-dose chemotherapy. Lancet. 1992;339:640–4.
52. Steidl U, Fenk R, Bruns I, et al. Successful transplantation of peripheral blood stem cells mobilized by chemotherapy and a single dose of pegylated G-CSF in patients with multiple myeloma. Bone Marrow Transplant. 2005;35:33–6.
53. Isidori A, Tani M, Bonifazi F, et al. Phase II study of a single pegfilgrastim injection as an adjunct to chemotherapy to mobilize stem cells into the peripheral blood of pretreated lymphoma patients. Haematologica. 2005;90:225–31.
54. Kroschinsky F, Holig K, Poppe-Thiede K, et al. Single-dose pegfilgrastim for the mobilization of allogeneic CD34$^+$ peripheral blood progenitor cells in healthy family and unrelated donors. Haematologica. 2005;90:1665–71.
55. Noga S, Oroszlan M, Hetherington J. Use of pegfilgrastim for autologous peripheral blood stem cell mobilization: comparison to a daily filgrastim regimen. Bone Marrow Transplant. 2003;31:S18.

56. Noga SJ, Oroszlan M, Zhang YL. Single dose pegfilgrastim successfully mobilizes optimal numbers of autologous CD34$^+$ cells for peripheral blood stem cell collection. Blood. 2002;100:826a. Abstract 3262.

57. Asano S, Masaoka T, Takaku F. Beneficial effect of recombinant human glycosylated granulocyte colony-stimulating factor in marrow-transplanted patients: results of multicenter phase II–III studies. Transplant Proc. 1991;23:1701–3.

58. Bishop MR, Tarantolo SR, Geller RB, et al. A randomized, double-blind trial of filgrastim (granulocyte colony-stimulating factor) versus placebo following allogeneic blood stem cell transplantation. Blood. 2000;96:80–5.

59. Schmitz N, Dreger P, Zander AR, et al. Results of a randomised, controlled, multicentre study of recombinant human granulocyte colony-stimulating factor (filgrastim) in patients with Hodgkin's disease and non-Hodgkin's lymphoma undergoing autologous bone marrow transplantation. Bone Marrow Transplant. 1995;15:261–6.

60. Stahel RA, Jost LM, Cerny T, et al. Randomized study of recombinant human granulocyte colony-stimulating factor after high-dose chemotherapy and autologous bone marrow transplantation for high-risk lymphoid malignancies. J Clin Oncol. 1994;12:1931–8.

61. Kawano Y, Takaue Y, Mimaya J, et al. Marginal benefit/disadvantage of granulocyte colony-stimulating factor therapy after autologous blood stem cell transplantation in children: results of a prospective randomized trial. The Japanese Cooperative Study Group of PBSCT. Blood. 1998;92:4040–6.

62. Lee SM, Radford JA, Dobson L, et al. Recombinant human granulocyte colony-stimulating factor (filgrastim) following high-dose chemotherapy and peripheral blood progenitor cell rescue in high-grade non-Hodgkin's lymphoma: clinical benefits at no extra cost. Br J Cancer. 1998;77:1294–9.

63. McQuaker IG, Hunter AE, Pacey S, et al. Low-dose filgrastim significantly enhances neutrophil recovery following autologous peripheral-blood stem-cell transplantation in patients with lymphoproliferative disorders: evidence for clinical and economic benefit. J Clin Oncol. 1997;15:451–7.

64. Shimazaki C, Oku N, Uchiyama H, et al. Effect of granulocyte colony-stimulating factor on hematopoietic recovery after peripheral blood progenitor cell transplantation. Bone Marrow Transplant. 1994;13:271–5.

65. Staber PB, Holub R, Linkesch W, et al. Fixed-dose single administration of pegfilgrastim vs daily filgrastim in patients with haematological malignancies undergoing autologous peripheral blood stem cell transplantation. Bone Marrow Transplant. 2005;35:889–93.

66. Ringden O, Labopin M, Gorin NC, et al. Treatment with granulocyte colony-stimulating factor after allogeneic bone marrow transplantation for acute leukemia increases the risk of graft-versus-host disease and death: a study from the Acute Leukemia Working Party of the European Group for Blood and Marrow Transplantation. J Clin Oncol. 2004;22: 416–23.

67. Komrokji RS, Lyman GH. The colony-stimulating factors: use to prevent and treat neutropenia and its complications. Expert Opin Biol Ther. 2004;4:1897–910.

68. Younes A, Fayad L, Romaguera J, et al. Safety and efficacy of once-per-cycle pegfilgrastim in support of ABVD chemotherapy in patients with Hodgkin lymphoma. Eur J Cancer. 2006;42:2976–81.

69. Lopez A, Fernandez de Sevilla A, Castaigne S. Pegfilgrastim supports delivery of CHOP-R chemotherapy administered every 14 days: a randomised phase II study. Blood. 2004;104:904a–5a. Abstract 3311.

70. Hershman D, Neugut AI, Jacobson JS, et al. Acute myeloid leukemia or myelodysplastic syndrome following use of granulocyte colony-stimulating factors during breast cancer adjuvant chemotherapy. J Natl Cancer Inst. 2007;99:196–205.

71. Lyman GH, Dale DC, Wolff DA, et al. Acute myeloid leukemia or myelodysplastic syndrome in randomized controlled clinical trials of cancer chemotherapy with granulocyte colony-stimulating factor: a systematic review. J Clin Oncol. 2010;28(17):2914–24.

72. Burgess AW, Camakaris J, Metcalf D. Purification and properties of colony-stimulating factor from mouse lung-conditioned medium. J Biol Chem. 1977;252:1998–2003.
73. Gough NM, Gough J, Metcalf D, et al. Molecular cloning of cDNA encoding a murine haematopoietic growth regulator, granulocyte–macrophage colony stimulating factor. Nature. 1984;309:763–7.
74. Peters WP, Stuart A, Affronti ML, et al. Neutrophil migration is defective during recombinant human granulocyte–macrophage colony-stimulating factor infusion after autologous bone marrow transplantation in humans. Blood. 1988;72:1310–15.
75. Rowe JM, Andersen JW, Mazza JJ, et al. A randomized placebo-controlled phase III study of granulocyte–macrophage colony-stimulating factor in adult patients (> 55–70 years of age) with acute myelogenous leukemia: a study of the Eastern Cooperative Oncology Group (E1490). Blood. 1995;86:457–62.
76. Witz F, Sadoun A, Perrin MC, et al. A placebo-controlled study of recombinant human granulocyte–macrophage colony-stimulating factor administered during and after induction treatment for de novo acute myelogenous leukemia in elderly patients. Groupe Ouest Est Leucemies Aigues Myeloblastiques (GOELAM). Blood. 1998;91:2722–30.
77. Boiron JM, Marit G, Faberes C, et al. Collection of peripheral blood stem cells in multiple myeloma following single high-dose cyclophosphamide with and without recombinant human granulocyte–macrophage colony-stimulating factor (rhGM-CSF). Bone Marrow Transplant. 1993;12:49–55.
78. Elias AD, Ayash L, Anderson KC, et al. Mobilization of peripheral blood progenitor cells by chemotherapy and granulocyte–macrophage colony-stimulating factor for hematologic support after high-dose intensification for breast cancer. Blood. 1992;79:3036–44.
79. Huan SD, Hester J, Spitzer G, et al. Influence of mobilized peripheral blood cells on the hematopoietic recovery by autologous marrow and recombinant human granulocyte–macrophage colony-stimulating factor after high-dose cyclophosphamide, etoposide, and cisplatin. Blood. 1992;79:3388–93.
80. Legros M, Fleury J, Bay JO, et al. rhGM-CSF vs placebo following rhGM-CSF-mobilized PBPC transplantation: a phase III double-blind randomized trial. Bone Marrow Transplant. 1997;19:209–13.
81. Kritz A, Crown JP, Motzer RJ, et al. Beneficial impact of peripheral blood progenitor cells in patients with metastatic breast cancer treated with high-dose chemotherapy plus granulocyte–macrophage colony-stimulating factor. A randomized trial. Cancer. 1993;71:2515–21.
82. Advani R, Chao NJ, Horning SJ, et al. Granulocyte–macrophage colony-stimulating factor (GM-CSF) as an adjunct to autologous hemopoietic stem cell transplantation for lymphoma. Ann Intern Med. 1992;116:183–9.
83. De Witte T, Gratwohl A, Van Der Lely N, et al. Recombinant human granulocyte–macrophage colony-stimulating factor accelerates neutrophil and monocyte recovery after allogeneic T-cell-depleted bone marrow transplantation. Blood. 1992;79:1359–65.
84. Gorin NC, Coiffier B, Hayat M, et al. Recombinant human granulocyte–macrophage colony-stimulating factor after high-dose chemotherapy and autologous bone marrow transplantation with unpurged and purged marrow in non-Hodgkin's lymphoma: a double-blind placebo-controlled trial. Blood. 1992;80:1149–57.
85. Gulati SC, Bennett CL. Granulocyte–macrophage colony-stimulating factor (GM-CSF) as adjunct therapy in relapsed Hodgkin disease. Ann Intern Med. 1992;116:177–82.
86. Hiraoka A, Masaoka T, Mizoguchi H, et al. Recombinant human non-glycosylated granulocyte–macrophage colony-stimulating factor in allogeneic bone marrow transplantation: double-blind placebo-controlled phase III clinical trial. Jpn J Clin Oncol. 1994;24:205–11.
87. Khwaja A, Linch DC, Goldstone AH, et al. Recombinant human granulocyte–macrophage colony-stimulating factor after autologous bone marrow transplantation for malignant lymphoma: a British National Lymphoma Investigation double-blind, placebo-controlled trial. Br J Haematol. 1992;82:317–23.

88. Link H, Boogaerts MA, Carella AM, et al. A controlled trial of recombinant human granulocyte–macrophage colony-stimulating factor after total body irradiation, high-dose chemotherapy, and autologous bone marrow transplantation for acute lymphoblastic leukemia or malignant lymphoma. Blood. 1992;80:2188–95.
89. Nemunaitis J, Rabinowe SN, Singer JW, et al. Recombinant granulocyte–macrophage colony-stimulating factor after autologous bone marrow transplantation for lymphoid cancer. N Engl J Med. 1991;324:1773–8.
90. Nemunaitis J, Rosenfeld CS, Ash R, et al. Phase III randomized, double-blind placebo-controlled trial of rhGM-CSF following allogeneic bone marrow transplantation. Bone Marrow Transplant. 1995;15:949–54.
91. Powles R, Smith C, Milan S, et al. Human recombinant GM-CSF in allogeneic bone-marrow transplantation for leukaemia: double-blind, placebo-controlled trial. Lancet. 1990;336: 1417–20.
92. Dorr RT. Clinical properties of yeast-derived versus *Escherichia coli*-derived granulocyte–macrophage colony-stimulating factor. Clin Ther. 1993;15:19–29, discussion 18.
93. Lieschke GJ, Cebon J, Morstyn G. Characterization of the clinical effects after the first dose of bacterially synthesized recombinant human granulocyte–macrophage colony-stimulating factor. Blood. 1989;74:2634–43.
94. Bunn PA Jr, Crowley J, Kelly K, et al. Chemoradiotherapy with or without granulocyte–macrophage colony-stimulating factor in the treatment of limited-stage small-cell lung cancer: a prospective phase III randomized study of the Southwest Oncology Group. J Clin Oncol. 1995;13:1632–41.
95. Shaffer DW, Smith LS, Burris HA, et al. A randomized phase I trial of chronic oral etoposide with or without granulocyte–macrophage colony-stimulating factor in patients with advanced malignancies. Cancer Res. 1993;53:5929–33.
96. Hovgaard D, Mortensen BT, Schifter S, et al. Comparative pharmacokinetics of single-dose administration of mammalian and bacterially-derived recombinant human granulocyte–macrophage colony-stimulating factor. Eur J Haematol. 1993;50:32–6.
97. Petros WP, Rabinowitz J, Stuart AR, et al. Disposition of recombinant human granulocyte–macrophage colony-stimulating factor in patients receiving high-dose chemotherapy and autologous bone marrow support. Blood. 1992;80:1135–40.
98. Petros WP, Rabinowitz J, Stuart A, et al. Clinical pharmacology of filgrastim following high-dose chemotherapy and autologous bone marrow transplantation. Clin Cancer Res. 1997;3:705–11.
99. Jenkins JM, Williams D, Deng Y, et al. Phase 1 clinical study of eltrombopag, an oral, nonpeptide thrombopoietin receptor agonist. Blood. 2007;109:4739–41.

Chapter 8
Meta-Analysis of Randomized Controlled Trials of Granulocyte Colony-Stimulating Factor Prophylaxis in Adult Cancer Patients Receiving Chemotherapy

Nicole M. Kuderer

Introduction

Granulocyte colony-stimulating factor (G-CSF) reduces the severity and duration of neutropenia associated with cancer chemotherapy [1–5]. In the pivotal phase III trial in patients with small cell lung cancer, patients were randomized to either G-CSF or placebo following combination chemotherapy in a double-blind fashion [3]. A significant difference in the cumulative risk of febrile neutropenia (FN) between the control (77%) and the G-CSF (40%) groups was observed despite the allowed use of secondary G-CSF prophylaxis after an initial occurrence of FN in the control group ($P < 0.001$). Several additional clinical trials of prophylactic G-CSF in patients with various malignancies receiving different treatment regimens have been reported [6–11]. The effectiveness of prophylactic G-CSF varies across disease groups and treatment regimens with the majority of reported trials employing relatively small sample size. There is, therefore, a need for a comprehensive systematic review of all relevant randomized controlled trials (RCTs) of primary prophylaxis with G-CSF in solid tumor and malignant lymphoma patients. In addition to providing more precise estimates of the clinical efficacy and toxicity, such an overview should permit an evaluation of the impact of G-CSF on other clinical outcomes including infection-related and all-cause treatment-related mortality.

Despite major improvements in supportive care, myelosuppression and its complications continue to represent the major dose-limiting toxicity of cancer chemotherapy. FN remains a medical emergency associated with substantial morbidity, mortality, and cost [12–15]. FN mortality in hospitalized cancer patients ranges from 5% to 11% and may be as high as 50% or greater among patients with major comorbidities [12–20].

N.M. Kuderer (✉)
Duke University School of Medicine, Durham, NC 27705, USA
e-mail: nicole.kuderer@duke.edu

G.H. Lyman, D.C. Dale (eds.), *Hematopoietic Growth Factors in Oncology*,
Cancer Treatment and Research 157, DOI 10.1007/978-1-4419-7073-2_8,
© Springer Science+Business Media, LLC 2011

Systematic Review

A systematic literature review of RCTs of primary G-CSF prophylaxis versus control in adult cancer patients receiving conventional chemotherapy for solid tumor or lymphoma was performed utilizing Medline, EMBASE, Cancerlit, Cochrane Database of Systematic Reviews, Cochrane Central Register of Controlled Trials (CENTRAL), and Database of Abstracts of Reviews of Effect (DARE) without language restrictions. References from included articles and reviewers were also hand searched. Keywords used in the search process included the following: (1) G-CSF: granulocyte colony-stimulating factor, colony-stimulating factors (CSFs), recombinant G-CSF, lenograstim, filgrastim, pegfilgrastim, and pegylated filgrastim; (2) randomized controlled trials: the standard search strategy recommended by the Cochrane Collaboration was utilized and modified for different databases [21, 22].

Primary G-CSF prophylaxis was defined as use in cycle 1 of chemotherapy prior to onset of neutropenia while secondary prophylaxis represented use in the chemotherapy cycle following an FN event. Studies allowing control patients to receive subsequent G-CSF prophylaxis after FN in the first cycle were included. Prophylactic antibiotic use was allowed if it was administered the same in both arms. Except for pegfilgrastim, G-CSF was to be administered daily until neutrophil recovery. RCTs were eligible if G-CSF was administered 1–3 days after the completion of myelosuppressive chemotherapy in each cycle as recommended in current guidelines [23–32].

Excluded studies encompassed those with granulocyte–macrophage colony-stimulating factor (GM-CSF), RCTs in children, leukemia or multiple myeloma patients, bone marrow or peripheral blood stem cell transplantation, and studies of established neutropenia or FN. RCTs were excluded if patients on G-CSF received different drugs, doses, or schedules of chemotherapy including dose-dense or dose-escalated regimens.

The primary outcome for meta-analysis was the percentage of patients experiencing FN. Secondary outcomes included infection-related mortality, all-early mortality during chemotherapy, bone pain or musculoskeletal pain, and relative dose intensity. Data on study design, patient characteristics, study outcomes, and measures of study quality were extracted by two independent reviewers with discrepancies resolved by consensus. Study quality was evaluated by the scoring system of Jadad [33].

Methodology

Heterogeneity was evaluated based on Cochran's Q statistic and the inconsistency index (I^2) of Higgins [34–36]. Fixed effects models were used to estimate relative risk ±95% confidence limits for infection-related and all-cause early mortality since no significant heterogeneity was observed and the I^2 was zero. Random effects models were employed for analyses of FN and bone pain due to the significant heterogeneity found. Sensitivity analyses were performed for a priori defined subgroups including type of G-CSF, cancer type, patient age, use of prophylactic antibiotics, permitted use of secondary G-CSF in control patients, placebo versus other trials, and single versus multicenter studies. Significance of summary effect estimates was based on the z-statistic [37]. Formal tests for interaction compared treatment group and a priori specified subgroups for the primary and secondary outcomes comparing the ratio of the difference in the natural logarithm of the relative risks and the standard error of the difference in log relative risks to the standard normal distribution [38, 39]. The standardized mean difference in relative dose intensity was estimated [40].

Evidence Synthesis

Figure 8.1 presents the reasons for exclusion of other studies based on a Quorom Statement Diagram [33]. Seventeen eligible RCTs ($N = 3,493$ patients) of primary G-CSF prophylaxis were identified (Table 8.1) [3, 4, 6–10, 41–48]. Filgrastim was studied in ten trials (59%) [3, 4, 6, 8, 10, 44–47], lenograstim in six (35%) [7, 9, 41–43], and pegfilgrastim in one (6%) [48]. Eleven trials (65%) involved patients with solid tumors [3, 4, 7, 10, 41–43, 46–48], and six (35%) were in patients with lymphoma including four (24%) limited to elderly subjects [6, 8, 9, 44, 45]. Eight studies utilized placebo control [3, 4, 7, 9, 42, 43, 48]. Three RCTs permitted secondary G-CSF in control patients [3, 7, 48], two explicitly prohibited its use [4, 45], and the remaining studies did not specify if it was permitted. Five RCTs prohibited the use of prophylactic antibiotics [7, 9, 44, 45, 48], three utilized antibiotic prophylaxis [6, 8, 46], while the remaining studies did not specify.

Febrile neutropenia: The risk of FN among control subjects across studies ranged from 17% to 78%. FN was reported in 15 trials ($N = 3,182$ patients) occurring one or more times in 22.4% of G-CSF patients and 39.5% of controls [RR = 95% CI: 0.54; 0.43–0.67; $P < 0.0001$] (Figs. 8.2 and 8.5). The study of pegfilgrastim reported greater efficacy than filgrastim and lenograstim [RR = 0.08; 95% CI: 0.03–0.18; $Z_{interaction} < 0.0001$]. Greater risk reduction was observed in studies with lower control risk of FN ($P = 0.05$).

Infection-related mortality: Infection-related mortality was reported in 12 RCTs and reported in 2.8% of control and 1.5% of G-CSF-supported patients [RR = 0.55; 95% CI: 0.34–0.90; $P = 0.018$] (Fig. 8.3). Filgrastim was associated with a significant reduction in infection-related mortality [RR = 0.53; 0.30–0.92; $P = 0.024$]. While lenograstim and pegfilgrastim were not associated with significant reductions in infection-related mortality, power for this outcome was low with only nine and two events, respectively, reported in these subgroups.

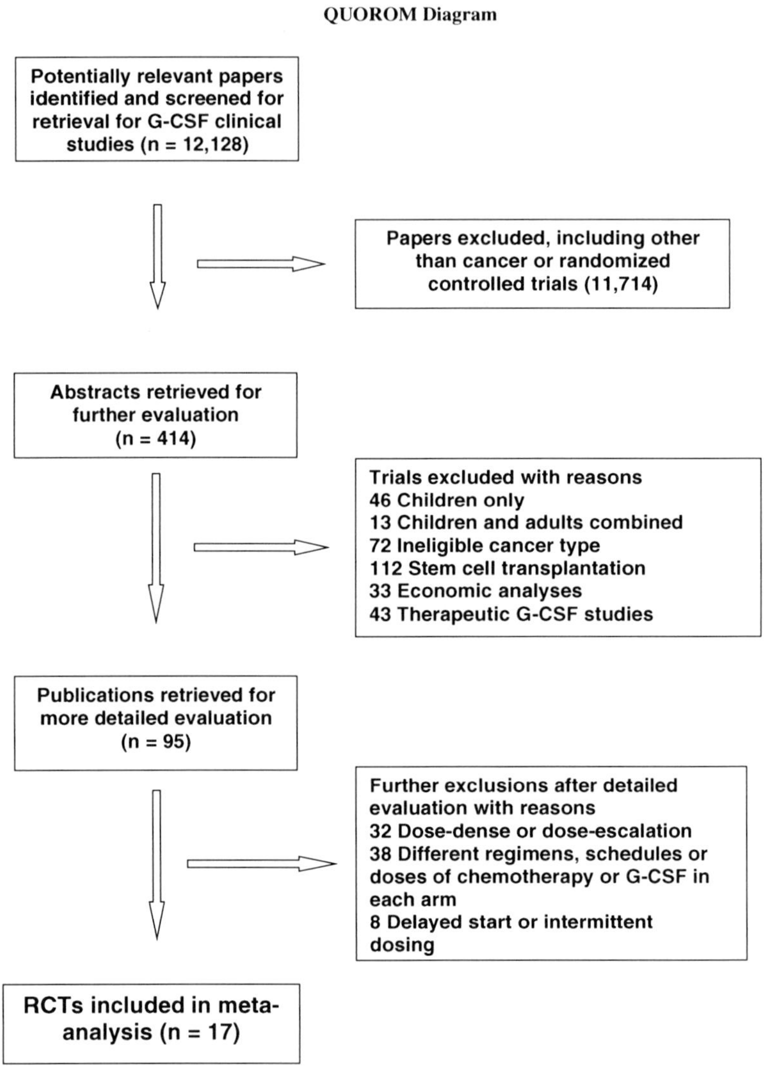

QUOROM Diagram

Potentially relevant papers identified and screened for retrieval for G-CSF clinical studies (n = 12,128)

Papers excluded, including other than cancer or randomized controlled trials (11,714)

Abstracts retrieved for further evaluation (n = 414)

Trials excluded with reasons
46 Children only
13 Children and adults combined
72 Ineligible cancer type
112 Stem cell transplantation
33 Economic analyses
43 Therapeutic G-CSF studies

Publications retrieved for more detailed evaluation (n = 95)

Further exclusions after detailed evaluation with reasons
32 Dose-dense or dose-escalation
38 Different regimens, schedules or doses of chemotherapy or G-CSF in each arm
8 Delayed start or intermittent dosing

RCTs included in meta-analysis (n = 17)

Fig. 8.1 Quorom diagram. Flow chart demonstrating the number of trials included and excluded along with the reasons for study exclusion

Early mortality: Early all-cause mortality was reported in 13 RCTs and described in 5.7% of control and 3.4% of G-CSF-supported patients [RR = 0.60; 95% CI: 0.43–0.83; $P = 0.002$] (Fig. 8.4). Filgrastim [RR = 0.60; 95% CI: 0.41–0.89; $P = 0.010$] and pegfilgrastim [RR = 0.36; 95% CI: 0.13–0.99;

Table 8.1 Summary of randomized controlled trials of primary prophylactic G-CSF in adult patients receiving conventional chemotherapy

References	No. of Pts	Tumor category	Age range	G-CSF type and dosing[a]	Start day[b] (cycle day)[c]	Length of G-CSF therapy (early stop criteria)[d]	Prophylactic antibiotics[f]	Secondary G-CSF prophylaxis in controls[e]
Crawford et al. [3]	199	Solid tumor	31–80	Filgrastim 230 μg/m^2 QD	1 (4)	9–14 days (after 9 d if ANC >10 × 10^9/L)	Unknown	Yes
Pettengell et al. [6]	80	Lymphoma	16–71	Filgrastim 230 μg/m^2 QD	1 (2)	5 or 12 days (1 day prior to next chemo)	Yes	Unknown
Trillet-Lenoir et al. [4]	129	Solid tumor	Unknown	Filgrastim 230 μg/m^2 QD	1 (4)	9–14 days (after 9 d if ANC >10 × 10^9/L)	Unknown	No
Gebbia et al. [42]	86	Solid tumor	38–66	Lenograstim 5 μg/kg QD	1 (unknown)	7–10 days (none)	Unknown	Unknown
Gebbia et al. [43]	51	Solid tumor	40–75	Lenograstim 5 μg/kg QD	2 (unknown)	≥7 days (none)	Unknown	Unknown
Chevallier [74]	120	Solid tumor	23–65	Lenograstim 5 μg/kg QD	2 (6)	10 days (none)	No	Unknown
Bui et al. [7]	48	Solid tumor	21–69	Lenograstim 5 μg/kg QD	1 (4)	10–14 days (sooner if ANC > 30 × 10^9/L)	Unknown	Yes
Muhonen et al. [47]	31	Solid tumor	34–65	Filgrastim 5 μg/kg QD	2 or 3 (3 or 4)	14 days (none)	Unknown	Unknown

Table 8.1 (continued)

References	No. of Pts	Tumor category	Age range	G-CSF type and dosing[a]	Start day[b] (cycle day)[c]	Length of G-CSF therapy (early stop criteria)[d]	Prophylactic antibiotics[f]	Secondary G-CSF prophylaxis in controls[e]
Zinzani et al.[g] [8]	149	Lymphoma	60–82	Filgrastim[g] 5 μg/kg QD	2 (3)	5 days (none)	Yes	Unknown
Gisselbrecht et al. [9]	162	Lymphoma	15–55	Lenograstim 5 μg/kg QD	1 (6)	8 days (none)	No	Unknown
Fossa et al. [10]	259	Solid tumor	15–65	Filgrastim 5 μg/kg QD	1 (3 or 6)	7 or 14 days (depends on chemo)	Unknown	Unknown
Gatzemeier et al. [41]	280	Solid tumor	39–75	Lenograstim 150 μg/m^2 QD	1 (4)	10 days (none)	Unknown	Unknown
Doorduijn et al.[h] [44]	389	Lymphoma	65–90	Filgrastim[h] 300 μg QD	1 (2)	10 days (none)	No	Unknown
Ösby et al. CHOP [45]	205	Lymphoma	60–86	Filgrastim 5 μg/kg QD	1 (2)	10–14 days (after 10 d if ANC > 10 × 10^9/L)	No	No
Ösby et al. CNOP [45]	203	Lymphoma	60–86	Filgrastim 5 μg/kg QD	1 (2)	10–14 days (after 10 d if ANC > 10 × 10^9/L)	No	No

Table 8.1 (continued)

References	No. of Pts	Tumor category	Age range	G-CSF type and dosing[a]	Start day[b] (cycle day)[c]	Length of G-CSF therapy (early stop criteria)[d]	Prophylactic antibiotics[f]	Secondary G-CSF prophylaxis in controls[e]
Timmer-Bonte et al. [46]	174	Solid tumor	36–81	Filgrastim 300/450 µg QD	1 (4)	10 days (none)		Unknown
Vogel et al. [48]	928	Solid tumor	21–88	Pegfilgrastim 6 mg once per cycle	1 (2)	1 day (none)	No	Yes

Abbreviations: G-CSF, granulocyte colony-stimulating factor; No, number; Pts, patients; d, days; Chemo, chemotherapy; QD, daily; Proph, prophylactic; ANC, absolute neutrophil count; L, liter

[a]G-CSF was given subcutaneously in all the studies.

[b]Number indicates the number of days after the completion of chemotherapy administration when G-CSF treatment was started.

[c]Number in brackets indicates the actual day of the chemotherapy cycle, on which G-CSF was started.

[d]Stopping criteria reported for G-CSF treatment by length of therapy or absolute neutrophil count.

[e]Secondary G-CSF Proph. in controls: Studies allowing secondary prophylaxis in control group with same type of G-CSF after the first chemotherapy cycle (G-CSF prophylaxis started in chemotherapy cycle following first episode of FN).

[f]Proph. Antibiotics: Studies investigating G-CSF plus prophylactic antibiotics compared to prophylactic antibiotics alone.

[g]The type of G-CSF was not specified in this publication, however, lenograstim was not commercially available at the study site during the study period.

[h]Study administered G-CSF based on a fixed-dose compared to weight-based dosing in all other studies of lenograstim or filgrastim.

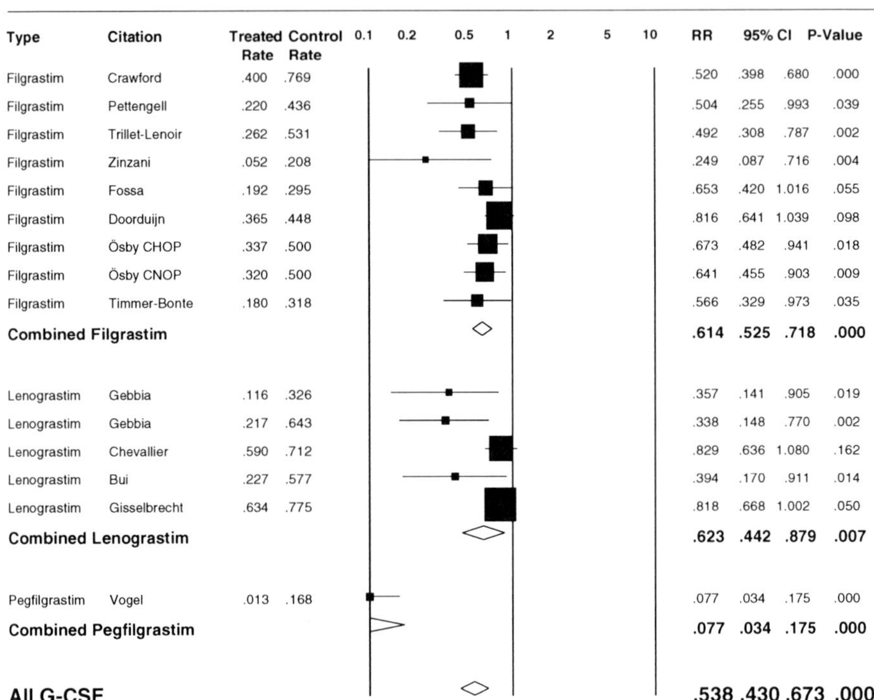

Febrile Neutropenia

Type	Citation	Treated Rate	Control Rate		RR	95% CI		P-Value
Filgrastim	Crawford	.400	.769		.520	.398	.680	.000
Filgrastim	Pettengell	.220	.436		.504	.255	.993	.039
Filgrastim	Trillet-Lenoir	.262	.531		.492	.308	.787	.002
Filgrastim	Zinzani	.052	.208		.249	.087	.716	.004
Filgrastim	Fossa	.192	.295		.653	.420	1.016	.055
Filgrastim	Doorduijn	.365	.448		.816	.641	1.039	.098
Filgrastim	Ösby CHOP	.337	.500		.673	.482	.941	.018
Filgrastim	Ösby CNOP	.320	.500		.641	.455	.903	.009
Filgrastim	Timmer-Bonte	.180	.318		.566	.329	.973	.035
Combined Filgrastim					**.614**	**.525**	**.718**	**.000**
Lenograstim	Gebbia	.116	.326		.357	.141	.905	.019
Lenograstim	Gebbia	.217	.643		.338	.148	.770	.002
Lenograstim	Chevallier	.590	.712		.829	.636	1.080	.162
Lenograstim	Bui	.227	.577		.394	.170	.911	.014
Lenograstim	Gisselbrecht	.634	.775		.818	.668	1.002	.050
Combined Lenograstim					**.623**	**.442**	**.879**	**.007**
Pegfilgrastim	Vogel	.013	.168		.077	.034	.175	.000
Combined Pegfilgrastim					**.077**	**.034**	**.175**	**.000**
All G-CSF					**.538**	**.430**	**.673**	**.000**

Fig. 8.2 Febrile neutropenia. Forest plot of the relative risk (RR) of FN comparing G-CSF and control study arms for each study with a weighted summary relative risk estimate by type of G-CSF

$P = 0.047$] but not lenograstim [RR $= 0.84$; 0.38–1.83; $P = 0.657$] were associated with significant reductions in early mortality.

Bone and musculoskeletal pain: Fourteen trials reported bone or musculoskeletal pain in 19.6% in G-CSF-treated patients compared to 10.4% of controls [RR $= 4.023$; 1.56–7.52; $P < 0.0001$] (Fig. 8.6).

Relative dose intensity: Relative dose intensity was reported in ten RCTs with mean and median values of 86.7% and 88.5%, respectively, among control patients (range 71%–95%) compared to 95.1% and 95.5%, respectively, among G-CSF-treated patients (range 91%–99%). Differences in relative dose intensity averaged 8.4% ($P = 0.001$) between study arms ranging from 2.8% to 20.0%. Six of ten control arms (60%) reported average relative dose intensities less than 90% while none of the G-CSF-supported study arms experienced relative dose intensities less than 90%.

Additional analyses: Patients with both lymphoma [RR $= 0.71$; 0.59–0.85; $P < 0.001$] and solid tumors [RR $= 0.44$; 0.30–0.65; $P < 0.001$] experienced

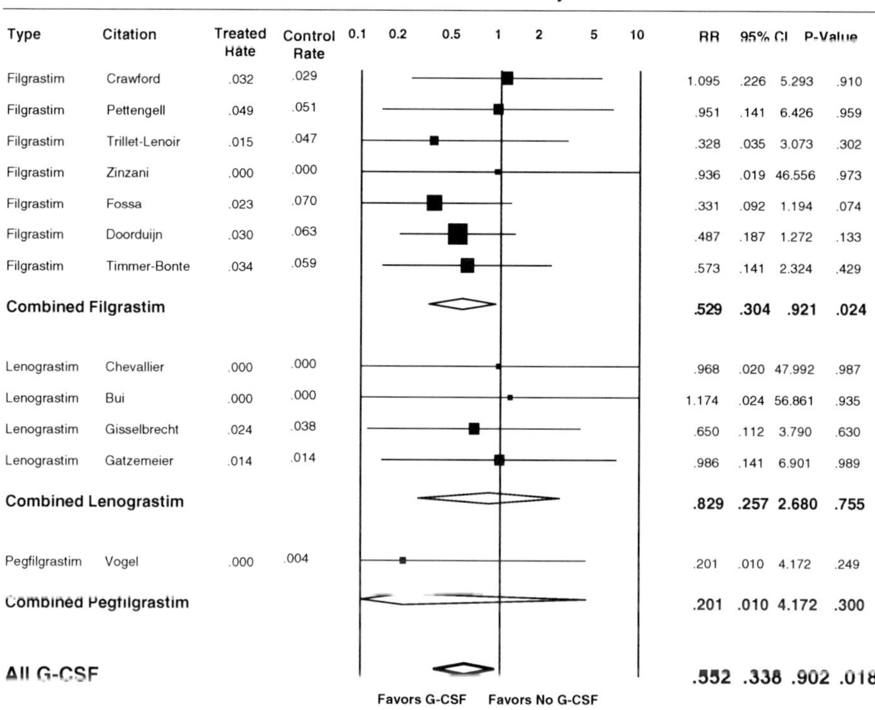

Fig. 8.3 Infection-related mortality. Forest plot of the relative risk (RR) of infection-related mortality comparing G-CSF and control study arms for each study with a weighted summary relative risk estimate by type of G-CSF

significant reductions in risk of FN. Similarly, studies with concurrent prophylactic antibiotics [RR = 0.49; 0.33–0.72; $P < 0.001$] as well as those without prophylactic antibiotics [RR = 0.55; 0.43–0.71; $P < 0.001$] experienced significant reductions in FN among those randomized to receive G-CSF. Finally, significant treatment effects with G-CSF for FN were seen in all age groups, with and without blinded randomization and with and without the use of secondary G-CSF prophylaxis in control patients. No significant differences were found between these subgroups (Table 8.2).

Reductions in infection-related and early mortality with G-CSF were seen in patients with solid tumors but not among those with lymphoma. Although, similar trends in relative risk were observed and the power was low to demonstrate statistical significance in the lymphoma subgroup.

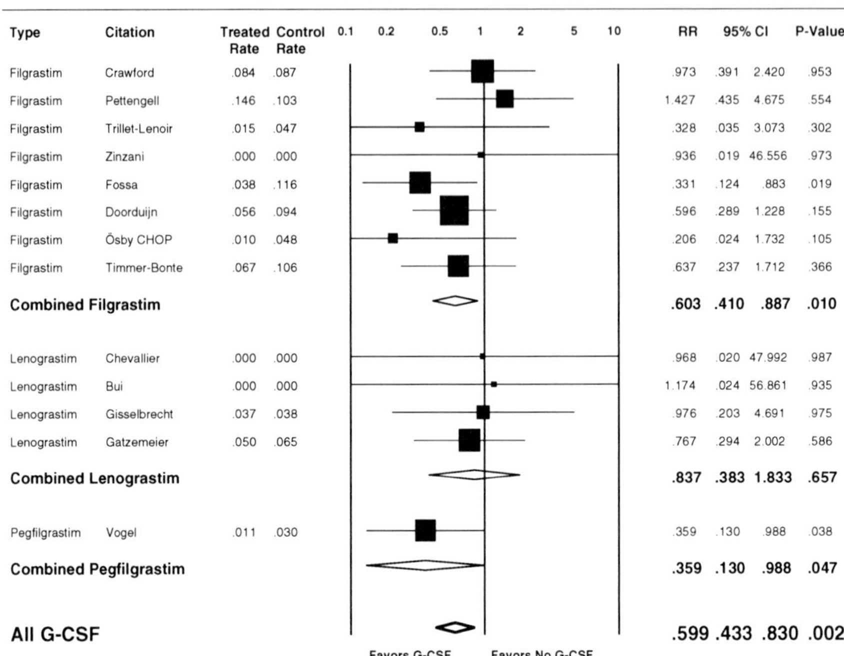

Fig. 8.4 Early all-cause mortality. Forest plot of the relative risk (RR) of early mortality during the course of chemotherapy comparing G-CSF and control study arms for each study with a weighted summary relative risk estimate by type of G-CSF

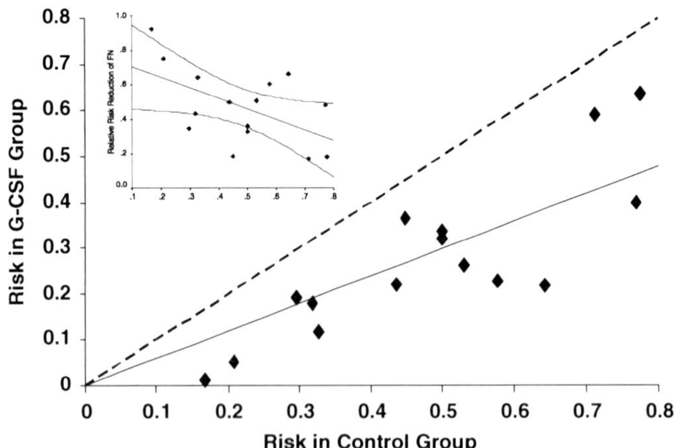

Fig. 8.5 Risk of FN among controls (*x*-axis) and G-CSF-treated patients (*y*-axis) for each study. Studies below the *dashed line* representing the null hypothesis reflect a reduced risk of FN in the G-CSF arms compared to control group. A *solid fitted linear regression line* is shown through the reported data. The *inset* represents a linear regression line and 95% confidence limits of the correlation between the relative risk reduction for FN with G-CSF (*y*-axis) and the risk of FN among control patients (*x*-axis) across trials

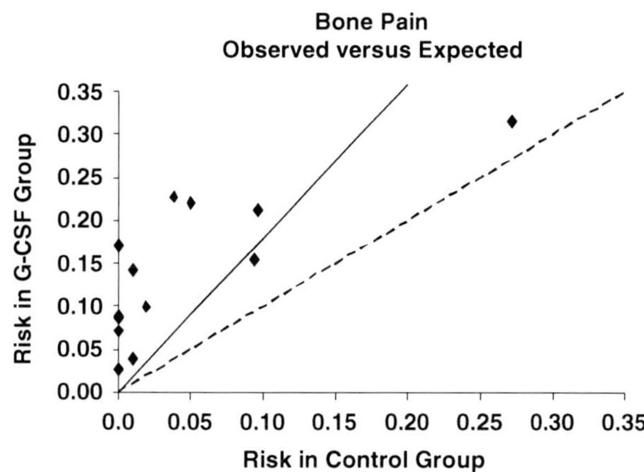

Fig. 8.6 Musculoskeletal symptoms (bone pain) reported among controls (*x*-axis) and G-CSF-treated patients (*y*-axis) for each study. The *dashed line* represents the null hypothesis while the *solid fitted linear regression line* is shown through the reported data

Table 8.2 Summary measures for a priori defined study subgroups: relative risk (RR) and 95% confidence intervals [95% CI] for febrile neutropenia, early mortality, and infection-related mortality

Study categories/subgroups	Outcomes, RR [95% CI]		
	Febrile neutropenia	Early mortality	Infection-related mortality
Tumor type			
Lymphoma	0.71 [0.59–0.85]	0.69 [0.40–1.17]	0.58 [0.28–1.23]
Solid tumors	0.44 [0.30–0.65]	0.55 [0.37–0.84]	0.53 [0.28–1.02]
Age group			
Elderly only[a]	0.68 [0.53–0.87]	0.52 [0.27–1.02]	0.51 [0.20–1.28]
Younger ages included	0.48 [0.35–0.67]	0.63 [0.43–0.91]	0.57 [0.32–1.02]
Prophylactic antibiotics[b]			
No[c]	0.55 [0.43–0.71]	0.55 [0.38–0.79]	0.52 [0.30–0.90]
Yes	0.49 [0.33–0.72]	0.88 [0.42–1.84]	0.70 [0.24–2.05]
Secondary G-CSF prophylaxis in controls[d]			
No[e]	0.66 [0.56–0.77]	0.60 [0.41–0.87]	0.53 [0.31–0.90]
Yes	0.26 [0.07–0.97]	0.60 [0.32–1.16]	0.72 [0.21–2.49]

[a]Studies with patients' age ≥ 60 in aggressive non-Hodgkin's lymphoma patients.
[b]G-CSF plus prophylactic antibiotics compared to prophylactic antibiotics alone.
[c]Studies not providing any information on antibiotic prophylaxis.
[d]Secondary prophylaxis permitted in control group after the first chemotherapy cycle.
[e]Studies not providing information on secondary G-CSF prophylaxis in control groups.

Summary

This systematic review and meta-analysis confirm that primary prophylaxis with G-CSF significantly reduces the risk of FN in patients receiving conventional chemotherapy across a broad range of baseline risk in eligible trials ranging from

17% to 78% among control patients. The reduction in risk of FN and its complications with G-CSF occurred despite improvement in delivered relative dose intensity. The major toxicity across trials was an increase in reported bone or musculoskeletal pain. Perhaps the most important and previously unreported observation emerging from this overview is the observed reduction in infection-related and all-cause early mortality in patients randomized to receive primary prophylaxis with G-CSF. While the majority of trials demonstrated a reduction in the relative risk of infection-related and early mortality, the mortality rates among often highly selected patients were generally low and failed to reach statistical significance in the individual trials. However, when systematically pooled, the average reduction in risk observed with G-CSF support was highly significant. It is important to note that the relative reduction in FN correlated with the relative risk reduction in both infection-related and early mortality.

In a meta-analysis by Clark et al. [49], therapeutic growth factor administered along with empiric antibiotic treatment for established FN resulted in a significant reduction in infection-related but not overall mortality [49].

Randomized controlled trials of select patient populations not only underreport the occurrence of neutropenic events but also underestimate the risk of mortality and cost associated with FN [13–15, 50–56]. Studies of hospitalization for FN in the general cancer population have reported mortality rates of 5%–11% [12]. Mortality rates ranging from 24% to 82% have been reported in patients with major comorbidities including pulmonary, liver, renal, cardiac, or cerebrovascular disorders, pulmonary embolism, invasive fungal infections, bacteremia, hypotension, or septic shock [12–20].

A significant reduction in the risk of FN with G-CSF support was observed in all subgroups based on age, type of G-CSF, concurrent prophylactic antibiotics, and use of secondary G-CSF prophylaxis in the control group. The results presented here also suggest that greater relative risk reduction for FN is seen with G-CSF in settings with a lower baseline risk of FN. In addition to the reduction in neutropenic complications, the relative dose intensity was significantly greater for the G-CSF treatment arms in eligible studies than among controls where 60% averaged below 90%. The results reported here in selected patients eligible for these RCTs very likely underestimate the potential impact on delivered dose intensity among the general population of cancer patients receiving systemic chemotherapy where increased age, poor performance status, and one or more major comorbidities are frequently encountered [50, 56]. These findings are also consistent with those from dose-dense trials where G-CSF support enables intensification of chemotherapy dosing that could not otherwise be tolerated [57–62]. In addition, many of the trials did not consider dose reductions, delays, and missed chemotherapy cycles in patients prematurely discontinuing their treatment and considered only those patients who completed all cycles of chemotherapy in estimating relative dose intensity.

In the interpretation of the results presented here, it is important to summarize the limitations of this overview. Dose-dense and dose-escalation trials with and without G-CSF support were excluded from this meta-analysis since the risk of neutropenic complications including FN and delivered relative dose intensity were not considered otherwise comparable [32, 57–61, 63–67]. In addition, only RCTs evaluating the impact of primary prophylaxis with G-CSF administered according to current guideline recommendations were included. Previous studies have shown that myeloid growth factors administered on the same day as chemotherapy, delayed more than 4 days following chemotherapy, delayed until the onset of neutropenia, or administered using a discontinuous schedule are significantly less effective [23–31, 68, 69]. Since such deviations from current product label and guideline recommendations often occur in clinical practice, the results presented here may not be generalized to all settings [23, 24]. While evidence summaries based on individual patient data represent an ideal, this meta-analysis was based on aggregate patient data derived from peer-review publications, similar to some 95% of all meta-analyses in oncology [70]. Meta-analyses utilizing such aggregate data have been found to result in estimates very similar to those based on individual patient data [71–73]. It also must be noted that comparison of subgroups, even when defined a priori as in this study, should be interpreted cautiously and considered exploratory in nature. Nevertheless, exploration of the sources of heterogeneity represents one of the most interesting and productive aspects of any meta-analysis. Since none of the randomized clinical trials included in this analysis had sufficient numbers of patients to evaluate the effect of G-CSF on secondary outcomes such as infection-related mortality, early mortality, or relative dose intensity with confidence, the lack of significant treatment effects in some subgroups could be either due to the absence of a true treatment effect or inadequate power to demonstrate such an effect.

Appropriately administered primary G-CSF prophylaxis in patients receiving conventional cancer chemotherapy consistently reduces the risk of FN across a broad range of risk while sustaining or enhancing chemotherapy dose delivery. For the first time, it is also clear based on pooled estimates that G-CSF prophylaxis is also associated with significant reductions in infection-related and early all-cause mortality in such patients. Nevertheless, the availability of validated febrile neutropenia prediction tools and updated economic analyses are also needed to guide clinicians and policymakers in the most effective and cost-effective application of G-CSF prophylaxis.

References

1. Gabrilove JL, Jakubowski A, Scher H, et al. Effect of granulocyte colony-stimulating factor on neutropenia and associated morbidity due to chemotherapy for transitional-cell carcinoma of the urothelium. N Engl J Med. 1988;318:1414–22.
2. Morstyn G, Campbell L, Lieschke G, et al. Treatment of chemotherapy-induced neutropenia by subcutaneously administered granulocyte colony-stimulating factor with optimization of dose and duration of therapy. J Clin Oncol. 1989;7:1554–62.
3. Crawford J, Ozer H, Stoller R, et al. Reduction by granulocyte colony-stimulating factor of fever and neutropenia induced by chemotherapy in patients with small-cell lung cancer. N Engl J Med. 1991;325:164–70.

4. Trillet-Lenoir V, Green J, Manegold C, et al. Recombinant granulocyte colony stimulating factor reduces the infectious complications of cytotoxic chemotherapy. Eur J Cancer. 1993;29A:319–24.
5. Welte K, Gabrilove J, Bronchud MH, et al. Filgrastim (r-metHuG-CSF): the first 10 years. Blood. 1996;88:1907–29.
6. Pettengell R, Gurney H, Radford JA, et al. Granulocyte colony-stimulating factor to prevent dose-limiting neutropenia in non-Hodgkin's lymphoma: a randomized controlled trial. Blood. 1992;80:1430–6.
7. Bui BN, Chevallier B, Chevreau C, et al. Efficacy of lenograstim on hematologic tolerance to MAID chemotherapy in patients with advanced soft tissue sarcoma and consequences on treatment dose-intensity. J Clin Oncol. 1995;13:2629–36.
8. Zinzani PL, Pavone E, Storti S, et al. Randomized trial with or without granulocyte colony-stimulating factor as adjunct to induction VNCOP-B treatment of elderly high-grade non-Hodgkin's lymphoma. Blood. 1997;89:3974–9.
9. Gisselbrecht C, Haioun C, Lepage E, et al. Placebo-controlled phase III study of lenograstim (glycosylated recombinant human granulocyte colony-stimulating factor) in aggressive non-Hodgkin's lymphoma: factors influencing chemotherapy administration. Groupe d'Etude des Lymphomes de l'Adulte. Leuk Lymphoma. 1997;25:289–300.
10. Fossa SD, Kaye SB, Mead GM, et al. Filgrastim during combination chemotherapy of patients with poor-prognosis metastatic germ cell malignancy. European Organization for Research and Treatment of Cancer, Genito-Urinary Group, and the Medical Research Council Testicular Cancer Working Party, Cambridge, United Kingdom. J Clin Oncol. 1998;16:716–24.
11. Lyman GH, Kuderer NM, Djulbegovic B. Prophylactic granulocyte colony-stimulating factor in patients receiving dose-intensive cancer chemotherapy: a meta-analysis. Am J Med. 2002;112:406–11.
12. Kuderer NM, Dale DC, Crawford J, et al. Mortality, morbidity, and cost associated with febrile neutropenia in adult cancer patients. Cancer. 2006;106:2258–66.
13. Talcott JA, Siegel RD, Finberg R, et al. Risk assessment in cancer patients with fever and neutropenia: a prospective, two-center validation of a prediction rule. J Clin Oncol. 1992;10:316–22.
14. Klastersky J, Paesmans M, Rubenstein EB, et al. The multinational association for supportive care in cancer risk index: a multinational scoring system for identifying low-risk febrile neutropenic cancer patients. J Clin Oncol. 2000;18:3038–51.
15. Gonzalez-Barca E, Fernandez-Sevilla A, Carratala J, et al. Prognostic factors influencing mortality in cancer patients with neutropenia and bacteremia. Eur J Clin Microbiol Infect Dis. 1999;18:539–44.
16. Malik I, Hussain M, Yousuf H. Clinical characteristics and therapeutic outcome of patients with febrile neutropenia who present in shock: need for better strategies. J Infect. 2001;42:120–5.
17. Darmon M, Azoulay E, Alberti C, et al. Impact of neutropenia duration on short-term mortality in neutropenic critically ill cancer patients. Intensive Care Med. 2002;28:1775–80.
18. Elting LS, Rubenstein EB, Rolston KV, et al. Outcomes of bacteremia in patients with cancer and neutropenia: observations from two decades of epidemiological and clinical trials. Clin Infect Dis. 1997;25:247–59.
19. Carratala J, Roson B, Fernandez-Sevilla A, et al. Bacteremic pneumonia in neutropenic patients with cancer: causes, empirical antibiotic therapy, and outcome. Arch Intern Med. 1998;158:868–72.
20. Rossini F. Prognosis of infections in elderly patients with haematological diseases. Support Care Cancer. 1996;4:46–50.
21. Dickersin K, Scherer R, Lefebvre C. Identifying relevant studies for systematic reviews. BMJ. 1994;309:1286–91.
22. Higgins JPT, Green S, editors. Cochrane handbook for systematic reviews of interventions 4.2.5 [updated May 2005].

23. Burton C, Linch D, Hoskin P, et al. A phase III trial comparing CHOP to PMitCEBO with or without G-CSF in patients aged 60 plus with aggressive non-Hodgkin's lymphoma. Br J Cancer. 2006;94:806–13.
24. Aapro MS, Cameron DA, Pettengell R, et al. EORTC guidelines for the use of granulocyte-colony stimulating factor to reduce the incidence of chemotherapy-induced febrile neutropenia in adult patients with lymphomas and solid tumours. Eur J Cancer. 2006;42:2433–53.
25. Crawford J, Althaus B, Armitage J, et al. Myeloid growth factors clinical practice guidelines in oncology. J Natl Compr Canc Netw. 2005;3:540–55.
26. Hartmann LC, Tschetter LK, Habermann TM, et al. Granulocyte colony-stimulating factor in severe chemotherapy-induced afebrile neutropenia. N Engl J Med. 1997;336:1776–80.
27. Dunlop DJ, Eatock MM, Paul J, et al. Randomized multicentre trial of filgrastim as an adjunct to combination chemotherapy for Hodgkin's disease. West of Scotland Lymphoma Group. Clin Oncol (R Coll Radiol). 1998;10:107–14.
28. Bassan R, Lerede T, Di Bona E, et al. Granulocyte colony-stimulating factor (G-CSF, filgrastim) after or during an intensive remission induction therapy for adult acute lymphoblastic leukaemia: effects, role of patient pretreatment characteristics, and costs. Leuk Lymphoma. 1997;26:153–61.
29. Crawford J, Kreisman H, Garewal H, et al. The impact of filgrastim schedule variation on hematopoietic recovery post-chemotherapy. Ann Oncol. 1997;8:1117–24.
30. Lokich JJ. Same day pegfilgrastim and CHOP chemotherapy for non-Hodgkin lymphoma. Am J Clin Oncol. 2006;29:361–3.
31. Kaufman PA, Paroly W, Rinaldi D, et al. Randomized double-blind phase 2 study evaluating same-day vs next-day administration of pegfilgrastim with docetaxel, doxorubicin, and cyclophosphamide (TAC) in women with early stage and advanced breast cancer. Breast Cancer Res Treat. 2004;88(1):S59.
32. Bohlius J, Reiser M, Schwarzer G, et al. Impact of granulocyte colony-stimulating factor (CSF) and granulocyte–macrophage CSF in patients with malignant lymphoma: a systematic review. Br J Haematol. 2003;122:413–23.
33. Moher D, Jadad AR, Nichol G, et al. Assessing the quality of randomized controlled trials: an annotated bibliography of scales and checklists. Control Clin Trials. 1995;16:62–73.
34. Cochran WG. The combination of estimates from different experiments. Biometrics. 1954;10:101–29.
35. Higgins JP, Thompson SG. Quantifying heterogeneity in a meta-analysis. Stat Med. 2002;21:1539–58.
36. Higgins JP, Thompson SG, Deeks JJ, et al. Measuring inconsistency in meta-analyses. BMJ. 2003;327:557–60.
37. Fleiss JL. The statistical basis of meta-analysis. Stat Methods Med Res. 1993;2:121–45.
38. Yusuf S, Wittes J, Probstfield J, et al. Analysis and interpretation of treatment effects in subgroups of patients in randomized clinical trials. JAMA. 1991;266:93–98.
39. Altman DG, Bland JM. Interaction revisited: the difference between two estimates. BMJ. 2003;326:219.
40. Cohen J. Statistical power analysis for the behavioral sciences. 2nd ed. Hillsdale: Lawrence Earlbaum Associates; 1988.
41. Gatzemeier U, Kleisbauer JP, Drings P, et al. Lenograstim as support for ACE chemotherapy of small-cell lung cancer: a phase III, multicenter, randomized study. Am J Clin Oncol. 2000;23:393–400.
42. Gebbia V, Testa A, Valenza R, et al. A prospective evaluation of the activity of human granulocyte-colony stimulating factor on the prevention of chemotherapy-related neutropenia in patients with advanced carcinoma. J Chemother. 1993;5:186–90.
43. Gebbia V, Valenza R, Testa A, et al. A prospective randomized trial of thymopentin versus granulocyte – colony stimulating factor with or without thymopentin in the prevention of febrile episodes in cancer patients undergoing highly cytotoxic chemotherapy. Anticancer Res. 1994;14:731–4.

44. Doorduijn JK, van der Holt B, van Imhoff GW, et al. CHOP compared with CHOP plus granulocyte colony-stimulating factor in elderly patients with aggressive non-Hodgkin's lymphoma. J Clin Oncol. 2003;21:3041–50.
45. Ösby E, Hagberg H, Kvaloy S, et al. CHOP is superior to CNOP in elderly patients with aggressive lymphoma while outcome is unaffected by filgrastim treatment: results of a Nordic Lymphoma Group randomized trial. Blood. 2003;101:3840–8.
46. Timmer-Bonte JN, de Boo TM, Smit HJ, et al. Prevention of chemotherapy-induced febrile neutropenia by prophylactic antibiotics plus or minus granulocyte colony-stimulating factor in small-cell lung cancer: a Dutch randomized phase III study. J Clin Oncol. 2005;23:7974–84.
47. Muhonen T, Jantunen I, Pertovaara H, et al. Prophylactic filgrastim (G-CSF) during mitomycin-C, mitoxantrone, and methotrexate (MMM) treatment for metastatic breast cancer. A randomized study. Am J Clin Oncol. 1996;19:232–4.
48. Vogel CL, Wojtukiewicz MZ, Carroll RR, et al. First and subsequent cycle use of pegfilgrastim prevents febrile neutropenia in patients with breast cancer: a multicenter, double-blind, placebo-controlled phase III study. J Clin Oncol. 2005;23:1178–84.
49. Clark OA, Lyman GH, Castro AA, et al. Colony-stimulating factors for chemotherapy-induced febrile neutropenia: a meta-analysis of randomized controlled trials. J Clin Oncol. 2005;23:4198–214.
50. Dale DC, McCarter GC, Crawford J, et al. Myelotoxicity and dose intensity of chemotherapy: reporting practices from randomized clinical trials. J Natl Comp Cancer Net. 2003;1:440–54.
51. Hassett MJ, O'Malley AJ, Pakes JR, et al. Frequency and cost of chemotherapy-related serious adverse effects in a population sample of women with breast cancer. J Natl Cancer Inst. 2006;98:1108–17.
52. Russo A, Autelitano M, Re BL. Frequency and cost of chemotherapy-related serious adverse effects in a population sample of women with breast cancer. J Natl Cancer Inst. 2006;98:1826–7.
53. Timmer-Bonte JN, Adang EM, Smit HJ, et al. Cost-effectiveness of adding granulocyte colony-stimulating factor to primary prophylaxis with antibiotics in small-cell lung cancer. J Clin Oncol. 2006;24:2991–7.
54. Lyman GH, Kuderer N, Greene J, et al. The economics of febrile neutropenia: implications for the use of colony-stimulating factors. Eur J Cancer. 1998;34:1857–64.
55. Calhoun EA, Schumock GT, McKoy JM, et al. Granulocyte colony-stimulating factor for chemotherapy-induced neutropenia in patients with small cell lung cancer: the 40% rule revisited. Pharmacoeconomics. 2005;23:767–75.
56. Cosler LE, Calhoun EA, Agboola O, et al. Effects of indirect and additional direct costs on the risk threshold for prophylaxis with colony-stimulating factors in patients at risk for severe neutropenia from cancer chemotherapy. Pharmacotherapy. 2004;24:488–94.
57. Citron ML, Berry DA, Cirrincione C, et al. Randomized trial of dose-dense versus conventionally scheduled and sequential versus concurrent combination chemotherapy as postoperative adjuvant treatment of node-positive primary breast cancer: first report of Intergroup Trial C9741/Cancer and Leukemia Group B Trial 9741. J Clin Oncol. 2003;21:1431–9.
58. Pfreundschuh M, Trumper L, Kloess M, et al. Two-weekly or 3-weekly CHOP chemotherapy with or without etoposide for the treatment of elderly patients with aggressive lymphomas: results of the NHL-B2 trial of the DSHNHL. Blood. 2004;104:634–41.
59. Pfreundschuh M, Trumper L, Kloess M, et al. Two-weekly or 3-weekly CHOP chemotherapy with or without etoposide for the treatment of young patients with good-prognosis (normal LDH) aggressive lymphomas: results of the NHL-B1 trial of the DSHNHL. Blood. 2004;104:626–33.
60. Wunderlich A, Kloess M, Reiser M, et al. Practicability and acute haematological toxicity of 2- and 3-weekly CHOP and CHOEP chemotherapy for aggressive non-Hodgkin's lymphoma: results from the NHL-B trial of the German High-Grade Non-Hodgkin's Lymphoma Study Group (DSHNHL). Ann Oncol. 2003;14:881–93.

61. Burstein HJ, Parker LM, Keshaviah A, et al. Efficacy of pegfilgrastim and darbepoetin alfa as hematopoietic support for dose-dense every-2-week adjuvant breast cancer chemotherapy. J Clin Oncol. 2005;23:8340–47.

62. Kummel S, Krocker J, Kohls A, et al. Randomised trial: survival benefit and safety of adjuvant dose-dense chemotherapy for node-positive breast cancer. Br J Cancer. 2006;94:1237–44.

63. Diehl V, Franklin J, Pfreundschuh M, et al. Standard and increased-dose BEACOPP chemotherapy compared with COPP-ABVD for advanced Hodgkin's disease. N Engl J Med. 2003;348:2386–95.

64. Woll PJ, Hodgetts J, Lomax L, et al. Can cytotoxic dose-intensity be increased by using granulocyte colony-stimulating factor? A randomized controlled trial of lenograstim in small-cell lung cancer. J Clin Oncol. 1995;13:652–9.

65. Hidalgo M, Mendiola C, Lopez-Vega JM, et al. A multicenter randomized phase II trial of granulocyte-colony stimulating factor-supported, platinum-based chemotherapy with flexible midcycle cisplatin administration in patients with advanced ovarian carcinoma. PSAMOMA Cooperative Group, Spain. Cancer. 1998;83:719–25.

66. Fukuoka M, Masuda N, Negoro S, et al. CODE chemotherapy with and without granulocyte colony-stimulating factor in small-cell lung cancer. Br J Cancer. 1997;75:306–9.

67. Sternberg CN, de Mulder PH, Schornagel JH, et al. Randomized phase III trial of high-dose-intensity methotrexate, vinblastine, doxorubicin, and cisplatin (MVAC) chemotherapy and recombinant human granulocyte colony-stimulating factor versus classic MVAC in advanced urothelial tract tumors: European Organization for Research and Treatment of Cancer Protocol No. 30924. J Clin Oncol. 2001;19:2638–46.

68. American Society of Clinical Oncology. Recommendations for the use of hematopoietic colony-stimulating factors: evidence-based, clinical practice guidelines. J Clin Oncol. 1994;12:2471–508.

69. Gerhartz HH, Engelhard M, Brittinger G, et al. Recombinant human granulocyte–macrophage colony-stimulating factor as adjunct to chemotherapy in aggressive non-Hodgkin's lymphomas. Semin Oncol. 1994;21:25–28.

70. Lyman GH, Kuderer NM. The strengths and limitations of meta-analyses based on aggregate data. BMC Med Res Methodol. 2005;5:14.

71. Olkin I, Sampson A. Comparison of meta-analysis versus analysis of variance of individual patient data. Biometrics. 1998;54:317–22.

72. Mathew T, Nordstrom K. On the equivalence of meta-analysis using literature and using individual patient data. Biometrics. 1999;55:1221–3.

73. Angelillo IF, Villari P. Meta-analysis of published studies or meta-analysis of individual data? Caesarean section in HIV-positive women as a study case. Public Health. 2003;117:323–8.

74. Chevallier B, Chollet P, Merrouche Y, et al. Lenograstim prevents morbidity from intensive induction chemotherapy in the treatment of inflammatory breast cancer. J Clin Oncol. 1995;13:1564–1771.

Chapter 9
Summary and Comparison of Myeloid Growth Factor Guidelines in Patients Receiving Cancer Chemotherapy

Gary H. Lyman and Jessica Malone Kleiner

Abstract Chemotherapy-induced neutropenia and its complications are major dose-limiting toxicities of cancer chemotherapy. The myeloid growth factors have been shown to reduce the risk of neutropenic events across malignancies, regimens, and associated risk categories often enabling the delivery of greater chemotherapy dose intensity. Three different practice guidelines for the myeloid growth factors have recently been published by major professional organizations. A comprehensive review and comparison of the guidelines using a priori structured content criteria and a previously validated quality appraisal tool are reported. Consistency in the final recommendations from these guidelines is observed for primary prophylaxis with the colony-stimulating factors (CSFs) when the risk of febrile neutropenia is in the range of 20% or greater. There is also consistency in the recommendation that patients receiving regimens associated with lower risk should have CSF use guided by individual risk assessment. Critical quality appraisal indicates that the scope and purpose, stakeholder involvement, and applicability of the guidelines differ little. There is more emphasis on comprehensive literature reviews in the ASCO and EORTC guidelines while the NCCN guidelines are more current based on systematic annual updates. The clarity of presentation also favors the NCCN guidelines with recommendations generally presented as both text and algorithmic diagram. All three new or updated guidelines recommend prophylactic use of the myeloid growth factors in patients at greater than a 20% risk of febrile neutropenia and in those with important factors increasing individual risk of neutropenic complications.

G.H. Lyman (✉)
Duke University and the Duke Comprehensive Cancer Center, Durham, NC 27705, USA
e-mail: gary.lyman@duke.edu

This chapter is reproduced from *J Natl Compr Canc Netw*. 2007 Feb;5(2):217–28. With kind permission of Cold Spring Publishing

G.H. Lyman, D.C. Dale (eds.), *Hematopoietic Growth Factors in Oncology*,
Cancer Treatment and Research 157, DOI 10.1007/978-1-4419-7073-2_9,
© Springer Science+Business Media, LLC 2011

Introduction

Chemotherapy-induced neutropenia, including febrile neutropenia (FN), is a major dose-limiting toxicity of many common systemic chemotherapy regimens. Although the reported risk of hematologic toxicity including FN has been consistently under-reported in randomized controlled trials (RCTs), it clearly varies across treatment regimens and patient populations [1]. The risk of the initial FN event for many regimens appears to be greatest during the early cycles of chemotherapy [2]. However, when a prophylactic colony-stimulating factor (CSF) is not employed and dose intensity of the same regimen is maintained, the rates of severe or FN are nearly constant across cycles with approximately one-third experiencing two or more events [3]. Most patients with FN require hospitalization for prompt clinical evaluation and the administration of empiric, broad-spectrum antibiotics to reduce the mortality associated with delayed treatment of serious infections in the neutropenic patient. Whatever the risk of occurrence, FN and its consequences are associated with substantial morbidity, mortality, and cost [4].

Neutropenic complications are frequently associated with dose reductions and treatment delays resulting in reduced delivered chemotherapy dose intensity potentially compromising disease control and long-term survival in patients treated with curative intent [5, 6]. Both retrospective studies and prospective RCTs of adjuvant chemotherapy in early-stage breast cancer (ESBC) with patients randomized to different dose intensities have demonstrated a significant relationship between the chemotherapy dose intensity and both disease-free and overall survival [7–10]. In addition, dose-dense regimens based on shortened treatment intervals with CSF support permitting upward of 50% increase in relative dose intensity (RDI) have been shown to improve survival over standard regimens in ESBC and non-Hodgkin lymphoma (NHL) [11, 12]. Nevertheless, a large proportion of patients receiving chemotherapy for potentially curable malignancies are undertreated in the United States [5, 6]. In a study of nearly 20,000 women with ESBC treated in 1,200 oncology practices, more than half received less than 85% of standard dose intensity for their regimen often following an episode of severe or FN [5]. Undertreatment was more prevalent among elderly patients, those receiving certain regimens and over-weight or obese patients [13]. Many authors have concluded that such reductions in dose intensity represent a major reason for subsequent treatment failure in patients with responsive malignancies [14].

The myeloid growth factors have been shown to reduce the incidence, duration, and severity of neutropenic events across a broad range of malignancies and regimens often enabling the delivery of full chemotherapy dose intensity [15, 16]. A number of additional RCTs confirming the impact of the myeloid growth factors on reducing the risk of FN have been published over the past few years [17–20]. An updated meta-analysis of RCTs of primary prophylactic G-CSF administered within 3 days of completing myelosuppressive chemotherapy in adult cancer patients has recently been presented [21]. Significant reductions in the risk of FN were observed in both NHL and solid tumor studies, in studies limited to elderly patients as well as all adult age groups and with all forms of G-CSF. In addition to confirming a reduction in the relative risk of FN, this analysis has demonstrated a significant reduction in infection-related mortality.

The decision to use primary CSF prophylaxis in support of patients receiving cancer chemotherapy is generally based on clinical judgment including (1) the estimated risk of neutropenic complications expected based on the treatment regimen; (2) patient-specific characteristics, including age, functional status, and comorbidities; and (3) the treatment intention, balancing the anticipated *benefit* of chemotherapy with the *risk* of serious and life-threatening complications [22]. Treatment intention determines the relevance or potential harm associated with alternative options to the addition of CSF support, such as dose reduction, treatment delay, use of an alternative chemotherapy regimen, or withholding treatment altogether. When there are no compelling clinical indications for the use of myeloid growth factors based on reducing the risk of FN or infection-related mortality, the decision to use these agents may be based on economic considerations [23–25].

Older age is consistently identified as a predictor of neutropenic complications, including dose reductions and delays. Other predictors include poor performance status, the presence of comorbid conditions, and baseline laboratory abnormalities. A risk model for time to initial FN in aggressive non-Hodgkin's lymphoma patients receiving CHOP was derived from a retrospective series of 577 patients and included 6 independent risk factors: age, baseline hemoglobin, heart disease, renal disease, planned dose intensity, and no CSF prophylaxis [2]. A risk model for first-cycle severe or FN based on a prospective registry of nearly 4,500 patients treated with a new chemotherapy regimen at 117 randomly selected practices in the United States is under development [26]. Independent risk factors in multivariate analysis included the type of cancer, treatment regimen, age, certain comorbidities (liver disease, renal disease, diabetes) and concomitant medications, baseline blood counts, the intention to provide full-dose chemotherapy, and no prophylactic CSF support. Once fully validated, such a risk model may guide clinicians and patients on the most efficacious and cost-effective use of myeloid growth factors.

Clinical practice guidelines statements are generally based on a systematic review of a topic in order to guide practitioners and patients in making informed decisions about appropriate health care. This chapter summarizes and contrasts recently developed or updated guidelines for the use of the myeloid growth factors. The results of recently conducted RCTs and meta-analyses of these trials were reviewed by the respective guidelines panels. The similarities and differences between the guidelines content and process are summarized and contrasted.

Methods

Three sets of clinical practice guidelines for the use of the myeloid growth factors have recently been developed or updated by major professional oncology organizations. These include guidelines updates by The American Society of Clinical Oncology (ASCO) and the National Comprehensive Cancer Network (NCCN) along with newly developed guidelines by the European Organization for Research and Treatment of Cancer (EORTC). ASCO published their initial clinical practice guideline for the use of the hematopoietic CSFs in 1994 [27]. These guidelines were subsequently updated in 1996, 1997, and 2000, only recently completing the most recent update in 2006 with the most extensive revision provided since the original report [28, 29]. In 2005, the NCCN presented and published their initial guidelines on the use of the myeloid growth factors which were updated in 2006 as a part of a systematic annual update [30, 31]. In 2006, the EORTC published guidelines for the use of the CSFs in adults with lymphoma and solid tumors [32]. The EORTC guidelines were intended to complement previously published guidelines on the use of the CSFs in the elderly [33].

The authors undertook a comprehensive review and comparison of the three guidelines using a priori structured content criteria and previously validated quality appraisal tools. Content areas extracted for each guideline included recommendations related to: primary prophylaxis; secondary prophylaxis; therapeutic use; afebrile neutropenia; sustaining dose intensity; progenitor cell transplant; acute leukemia and myelodysplasia; older patients; pediatric patients; schedule and dose; G-CSF versus GM-CSF; and radiation injury. In addition, risk factors associated with disease, treatment, and patient-specific factors such as age, gender, ethnicity, performance status, the presence of comorbidities, and laboratory abnormalities. Guideline content was also contrasted for the major chemotherapy regimens and assumed rates of FN associated with each regimen.

The quality of the recently updated or developed guidelines was then critically appraised using the Appraisal of Guidelines Research and Evaluation (AGREE) Instrument which provides a framework for assessing the quality of clinical practice guidelines based on the potential for bias in guideline development as well as the internal and external validity and feasibility for practice [34]. The AGREE instrument was developed using a sequential process including item generation, selection, scaling, field evaluation, and finalization. An initial list of 82 items was extracted from existing tools and relevant literature addressing these domains [35]. A draft was field tested on the 100 guidelines by 194 appraisers and after further refinement, a final instrument underwent further validation The internal consistency of the final instrument was acceptable with Cronbach's alpha ranging from 0.64 to 0.88 and intraclass correlation coefficients ranging from 0.57 to 0.91 with different appraisers [36]. The use of the AGREE instrument involves taking into account the benefits, harms, and costs of the recommendations, as well as their practical use. Therefore, the assessment includes judgments about the methods used for developing the guidelines, the content of the final recommendations, and the factors linked to their application. The AGREE Instrument assesses both the quality of the recommendations as well as reporting. The tool consists of 23 key items organized in 6 domains, each intended to capture a separate dimension of quality. Items 1–3 assess the scope and purpose of guideline, the clinical questions being asked, and the target population. Items 4–7 reflect the stakeholder involvement or the extent to which the guideline represents the views of its users. Items 8–14 assess the rigor of guideline development or the process used to gather and synthesize the evidence, the methods of developing the recommendations as well as to update them. Items

15–18 evaluate the clarity and presentation of the guidelines in terms of language and format. Items 19–21 assess the applicability of the guidelines including the impact on behavior and costs. Items 22–23 evaluate the editorial independence of the recommendations and any conflicts of interest. As recommended by the developers, the guidelines were assessed by two independent appraisers (GHL, JMK). Each scale item was rated from 4 "Strongly Agree" to 1 "Strongly Disagree", with 3 "Agree" and 2 "Disagree." Domain scores were calculated by summing up all the scores of the individual scale items in a domain. The total score was standardized by presenting the score as a percentage of the maximum possible score for each domain. The developers recommend that the domain scores not be aggregated into a single score and that they be presented and compared independently.

Results

Myeloid growth factor guidelines from the NCCN were initially put forward in 2005 and then updated in 2006. As summarized in Fig. 9.1, these guidelines recommend a stepwise process of starting with an initial evaluation based on the type of cancer, chemotherapy regimen, patient-specific risk factors, and treatment intention. This is to be followed by a formal risk assessment, then a recommendation on the use of

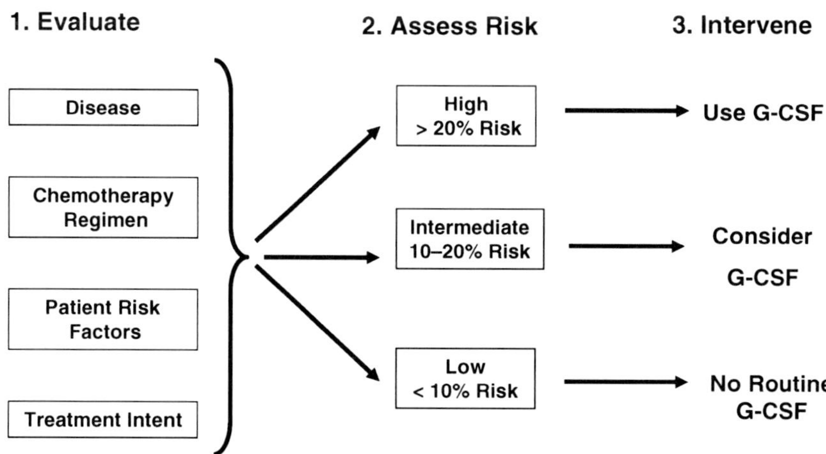

Fig. 9.1 Schematic diagram of the decision process for the use of the myeloid growth factors based on the NCCN Guidelines [3]. After an initial evaluation based on disease, regimen, patient risk factors, and the intention of treatment, the risk of febrile neutropenia should be formally assessed with each patient classified as high (>20%), intermediate (10–20%), or low (<10%) risk. The use of prophylactic CSFs can then be based on the individual patient's assessed risk

the myeloid growth factors based on the level of risk. Unlike the ASCO guidelines in effect at the time, the NCCN guidelines recommended use of G-CSF prophylaxis when patients are thought to be at 20% or greater risk. Patients at intermediate risk, 10–20%, may be considered for prophylactic G-CSF if there are additional considerations that either may place the patient at greater risk for FN or for serious consequences of FN such as prolonged hospitalization or death. Routine prophylaxis with G-CSF should not be employed in patients thought to have a low risk of FN (under 10%). The 2006 ASCO White Blood Cell Growth Factor Guidelines Update Committee agreed unanimously that reduction in FN was an important clinical outcome that justified use of the CSFs when the risk of FN was about 20% and no other equally effective regimen that did not require CSF was available. This was a distinct change from the threshold recommended in previous ASCO guidelines for some 12 years. An additional change with the 2006 guidelines was the introduction of several derivative products including executive and patient summaries, a PowerPoint slide set, and a work sheet or flow sheet to assist practitioners in the application of the guidelines as well as monitoring for guidelines compliance when appropriate. As shown in Fig. 9.2, along with other information, this flow sheet assessed the justification for use of the CSFs and the treatment plan including dose, schedule, route, and duration of use of the white blood cell growth factors. The EORTC also issued guidelines for the use of G-CSF in 2006. As shown in Fig. 9.3, the overall recommendation for prophylactic use of G-CSF is remarkably similar to that of the NCCN and revised ASCO guidelines with routine use in those receiving a regimen with a 20% or greater risk, none when the risk is less than 10%, and then an individual risk assessment in those receiving a regimen associated with a risk of 10–20%. If the individual patient risk for FN after such assessment is deemed to be 20% or greater, primary prophylaxis with G-CSF is recommended.

Table 9.1 summarizes and compares recommendations of the three myeloid growth factor guidelines for the major topics considered as discussed in the methods section. Clearly, not every topic was discussed or equally considered across all guidelines. However, remarkable similarity in the final recommendations is observed for the three guidelines for primary prophylaxis, secondary prophylaxis, sustaining dose intensity, and management of the elderly. There is consistency across the guidelines in the recommendation to consider prophylactic use of the CSFs when the risk of FN is in the range of 20% or greater (Table 9.2). Likewise, there is consistency in the recommendations that patients at lower levels of risk should have their individual risk assessed by the clinician and CSF use considered if there are sufficient risk factors such as advanced age to indicate a greater level of individual patient risk than the RCTs for a given regimen might otherwise   indicate.

Table 9.3 summarizes and contrasts the disease-related, treatment-related, and patient-related factors considered to increase the risk of FN and its complications in each of the guidelines. While some differences in emphasis exist, there is consistency across guidelines in recognizing the importance of assessing patient-specific risk factors such as advanced disease, previous episodes of FN, prior extensive chemotherapy, age $\geq$ 65, poor performance or nutritional status, serious

White Blood Cell Growth Factors (CSF) Orders and Flow Sheet

Patient Name: ____ Date:______________ Weight: _________

Diagnosis: _________________________________ Most recent chemotherapy date: ______________ Regimen: ___________

Insurance: _________________________________ Approved by: ______________________ Date Approved: ___________

JUSTIFICATION FOR USE:

Primary Administration (Preventive)

☐ Chemotherapy regimen with the risk of febrile neutropenia (FN) at 20% or higher

☐ "Dose dense" chemotherapy regimen

☐ Patient is ≥ 65 years old, has diffuse aggressive lymphoma and receives curative chemotherapy

☐ Pediatric patient with likelihood of developing FN

☐ Patient is at higher risk for chemotherapy-induced infectious complications including, but not limited to:

○ >65 years old   ○ Previous episodes of FN   ○ Extensive prior tx (large radiation ports, prior chemotherapy)
○ Poor performance status   ○ Administration of combined chemoradiotherapy   ○ Cytopenias due to bone marrow involvement by tumor
○ Poor nutritional status   ○ Presence of open wounds/active infections   ○ Advanced cancer
○ Other serious comorbidities: ____

Secondary Administration (Preventive)

☐ Patient had a neutropenic complication from prior chemotherapy (primary prophylaxis not received) and dose reduction or delay may compromise survival or treatment outcome

☐ Pediatric patient is high-risk

Therapeutic Use

☐ Patient has FN and is at high-risk for infection-associated complications

☐ Pediatric patient is high-risk

☐ Patient has prognostic factors that predict a poor clinical outcome:

○ Expected prolonged (>10days) and profound (<0.1 x 109/L) neutropenia   ○ Uncontrolled primary disease
○ Patient age >65 years (esp. with poor performance status, consider additional risk factors)   ○ Pneumonia
○ Hypotension and multi-organ dysfunction (sepsis syndrome)   ○ Invasive fungal infection
○ Patient gets radiotherapy-only (if prolonged delays secondary to neutropenia are expected)   ○ Hospitalization at time of fever development

Other Clinical Circumstance

☐ Patient has AML and tx follows completion of consolidation chemotherapy or patient is >55 years old and tx follows initial induction therapy

☐ Patient has ALL and tx follows the completion of the initial days of chemotherapy of the initial induction or first post-remission course

☐ Patient has MDS and severe neutropenia with recurrent infection(s)

☐ To mobilize PBPC (esp. in conjunction with chemotherapy and their administration after autologous, but not allogeneic, PBPC transplant)

☐ Patient exposed to lethal doses of total body radiotherapy (prompt administration of CSF or pegylated G-CSF)

☐ Other: ____

PLAN:

Growth Factor	Setting	Dose/basis	Dose	Route	Schedule
G-CSF (filgrastim)	Myelotoxic chemotherapy	Adults: 5 ug/kg/d		Sub Q	Continue until ANC at least 2-3 x 10^9/L— 24-72 hours after administration of myelotoxic chemotherapy
	High-dose therapy and autologous stem cell rescue	Adults: 5 ug/kg/d		Sub Q	Continue until ANC at least 2-3 x 10^9/L — 24-120 hours after administration of high-dose therapy
	PBPC mobilization	Adults: 10 ug/kh/d		Sub Q	Continue until last leukapheresis — Start at least 4 days before first leukapheresis
Pegylated G-CSF (pegfilgrastim)	Myelotoxic chemotherapy	6mg (6mg=0.6mL)		Sub Q	Once in each chemotherapy cycle — 24 hours after completion of chemotherapy
GM-CSF (sargramostim)	Bone marrow transplant or AML	Adults: 250 ug/m^2/d		Sub Q IV Infusion	Continue until ANC >1.5 x 10^9/L for 3 consecutive days — Day of bone marrow infusion and not less than 24 hours from the last chemotherapy and 12 hours from most recent radiotherapy

Write dose to be given in appropriate box. After it is administered, write in site and your initials.

Cycle #	Day of cycle	Date to be given	Dose to be given	MD Initials	Dose given	Site	RN Initials

Reviewed by________________on ____

Insurance: _________________________________ Approved by: ______________________ Date: ______________

Fig. 9.2 Flow sheet developed by ASCO to accompany the updated 2006 White Blood Cell Growth Factor Guidelines [29]. The flow sheet assesses the justification for use of a white blood cell growth factor for primary or secondary prevention, therapeutic use, or other reasons and then provides a framework for documenting the dose, schedule, and actual administration of such support. The flow sheet is available on the website of the *Journal of Oncology Practice*. http://www.jopasco.org/jopasco/Main/

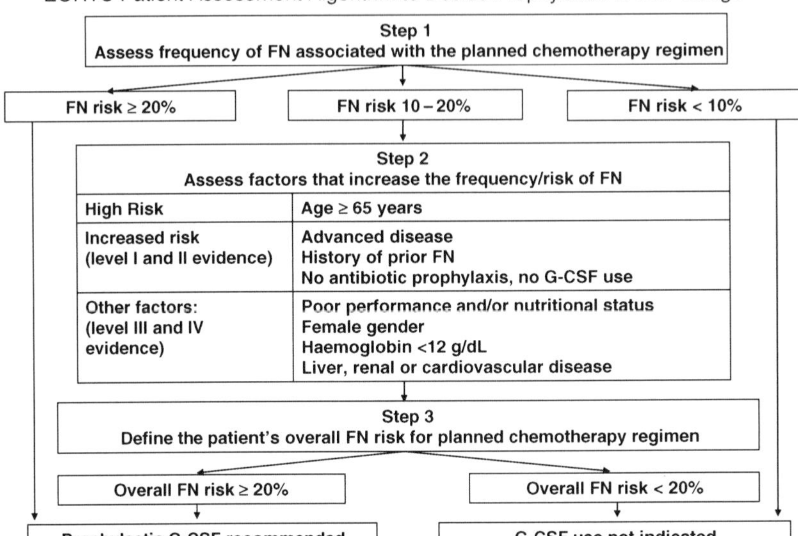

Fig. 9.3 Schematic of the clinical decision pathway for the use of prophylactic G-CSF from the recently published EORTC CSF Guidelines [32]. Primary prophylaxis is recommended routinely for a risk of FN ≥ 20% and not for patients at a <10% risk. Patients with a risk of FN of 10–20% should be further assessed for their individual risk based on age and other disease-specific, treatment-specific, and patient-specific risk factors. Patients should be considered for primary G-CSF prophylaxis if their individual risk is thought to be ≥20%

comorbidities, and low baseline blood counts or bone marrow involvement. The issues related to the use of the CSFs for treating FN, afebrile neutropenia, progenitor cell transplantation, acute leukemia and myelodysplastic syndrome (MDS), pediatric patients, and the recommended dose and schedule are not addressed by all of the guidelines (Table 9.1).

Each of the guidelines lists common regimens associated with varying levels of risk for FN. Table 9.4 summarizes and compares the regimens that were considered representative of those used in the treatment of common cancers and the assumed level of risk for FN associated with these regimens. Given the differences in process and the inherent variation in oncology practice between Europe and the United States, differences in the regimens mentioned are not a surprise. The EORTC guidelines present considerably more regimens including many that are not mentioned in the ASCO and NCCN guidelines probably reflecting differences in oncology practice in Europe. Although the presumed risk of FN associated with regimens presented across guidelines is relatively comparable, there are some differences evident in the interpretation of clinical trial data on the risk of FN with common regimens presented in these guidelines including doxorubicin and cyclophosphamide (AC) and AC–Docetaxel in breast cancer and cisplatin and paclitaxel (DP) in lung cancer.

Table 9.1 Comparison of guidelines recommendations

Topic	ASCO	EORTC	NCCN
Primary prophylaxis			
CSFs indicated	Risk of FN associated with chemotherapy is approximately 20% or greater[a] Prior FN[b]	Risk of FN > 20% when individual patient risk factors for FN are considered[a] Prior FN[b]	Risk of FN > 20% when individual patient risk factors for FN are considered Prior FN[b]
Consider use of CSFs	If risk of FN < 20%, consider individual risk factors that may increase risk of neutropenic complications[a]	If risk of FN = 10–20%, consider individual risk factors that may increase risk of FN	If risk of FN = 10–20%[c]
No indication for CSFs	Risk of FN < 20% and patient low risk for neutropenic complications	Risk of FN associated with chemotherapy is <10%	Risk of FN <10% and patient low risk for neutropenic complications
Secondary prophylaxis	Patients with previous FN in which dose reduction/delay would compromise outcome	Consider with previous FN when dose reduction/delay would compromise care	Patients with previous FN in which dose reduction/delay would compromise outcome
Therapeutic use for febrile neutropenia	Should not use routinely but consider in patients at high risk for infectious complications	Should not use routinely; consider when unresponsive to antibiotics or with life-threatening complications	Not addressed
Afebrile neutropenia	Not indicated	Not addressed	Not addressed
Sustain dose intensity	Indicated when there is a survival benefit for dose-dense schedules or dose reduction/delay would compromise care	Indicated when there is a survival benefit for dose-dense schedules or dose reduction/delay would compromise care	Indicated when there is a survival benefit for dose-dense schedules or dose reduction/delay would compromise care
Progenitor cell transplant	*Autologous*: indicated for stem cell mobilization and after transplantation *Allogeneic*: indicated for stem cell mobilization only	Not addressed	Not addressed

Table 9.1 (continued)

Topic	ASCO	EORTC	NCCN
Acute leukemia and MDS	*AML*: indicated after induction and consolidation *MDS*: indicated with severe neutropenia and recurrent infection *ALL*: indicated after initial induction and first post-remission chemotherapy	Not addressed	GM-CSF indicated in older adults with AML following induction chemotherapy
Older patients	Indicated in patients $\geq$ 65 years with aggressive lymphoma receiving curative chemotherapy	Indicated in elderly patients to sustain doses and schedule and reduce risk of neutropenic complications[d]	Use in all patients $\geq$ 65 years receive chemotherapy equivalent to CHOP[d]
Pediatric patients	*See adult guidelines*: use in ALL with caution	Not addressed	Not addressed
Schedule	Initiate 24–72 h after chemotherapy or 24–120 h after high-dose chemotherapy. Continue until ANC 2–3 $\times 10^9$/L	Not addressed	Initiated 1–3 days after completion of chemotherapy and continued until post-nadir ANC recovery

Table 9.1 (continued)

Topic	ASCO	EORTC	NCCN
Dose	G-CSF 5 μg/kg/d GM-CSF 250 μg/m^2/d; pegylated G-CSF 6 mg 24 h after completion of chemotherapy	Not addressed	G-CSF 5 μg/kg/d[e] GM-CSF 250 μg/m^2/d; pegylated G-CSF 6 mg 24 h after completion of chemotherapy[e]
G-CSF vs GM-CSF	No recommendations can be made regarding the equivalency of G-CSF and GM-CSF. Further trials are needed to compare activity, toxicity, and cost-effectiveness	Filgrastim, lenograstim, and pegfilgrastim are all recommended to prevent FN or FN-related complications	Level 1 evidence to support filgrastim or pegfilgrastim for the prevention of FN. Insufficient evidence to recommend GM-CSF for the prevention of FN. GM-CSF is indicated in older adults with AML
Radiation injury	Prompt administration indicated immediately following lethal doses of total body irradiation	Not addressed	Not addressed

FN, febrile neutropenia; CSF, colony-stimulating factor.

[a]When no equally efficacious regimen available with less risk of FN.

[b]Patients who have had a neutropenic complication during previous cycle and in which dose reduction/delay would compromise cure/care.

[c]Physician–patient discussion indicated. If indication for treatment is palliation, consider an alternative CTR.

[d]Separate Guidelines for CSF use in the elderly:

    EORTC, Repetto et al. [33]

    NCCN Senior Adult Oncology Guidelines, NCCN, v.1.2005.

[e]Insufficient data available to support pegylated G-CSF in chemotherapy schedules less than 2 weeks.

Table 9.2 Summary of primary prophylaxis recommendations

Neutropenic event risk	ASCO 2006	EORTC 2006	NCCN 2006
Moderate to high	Use CSF $\geq$ 20%	Use CSF > 20%	Use CSF > 20%
Intermediate	Recommend <20% (with risk factors)	Consider CSF (10–20% with risk factors)	Consider CSF (10–20% with risk factors)
Low	Not further specified	CSF is not recommended <10%	CSF is not recommended for most patients <10%

Table 9.3 Risk factors for febrile neutropenia and its complications

Category	ASCO	EORTC	NCCN
Disease-related	Advanced stage disease	Advanced disease/metastasis	Advanced stage disease; bone marrow involvement; elevated LDH (lymphoma); leukemia; lung cancer
Treatment-related	Previous episode of FN; extensive prior chemotherapy Concurrent XRT or large prior radiation ports	Previous episode of FN; no antibiotic prophylaxis[a]; no G-CSF use; planned dose intensity > 80%	Prior history of severe neutropenia; planned dose intensity > 80% Extensive prior chemotherapy Concurrent/prior radiation
Patient-related			
–Age	Age $\geq$ 65	Age $\geq$ 65	Age $\geq$ 65
–Gender		Female	Female
–Ethnicity		Asian origin	
–Performance status	Poor performance status	Poor performance status	Poor performance status (ECOG $\geq$ 2)
–Comorbidities	Poor nutritional status; open or infected wounds; serious comorbidities	Poor nutritional status; cardiovascular, renal disease; $\geq$1 comorbidity Body surface area <2.0 m^2	Poor nutritional, immune status; open or infected wounds; COPD; cardiovascular disease; diabetes mellitus
–Laboratory	Cytopenia secondary to bone marrow involvement	Abnormal liver transaminases Hb < 12 g/dL; serum albumin $\leq$ 3.5 g/dL; pre-treatment ANC < 1,500	Elevated bilirubin or alkaline phosphatase Low hg; pre-existing ANC <1,000 or lymphocytopenia

[a]Indiscriminant use of antibiotic prophylaxis is not recommended.

Table 9.4 Incidence of febrile neutropenia for selected chemotherapy regimens: reported rates across guidelines

Cancer type	Regimen	Myeloid growth factor guideline (%FN)		
		ASCO	EORTC	NCCN
Breast	AC	10	10–20	10–20
	AC–Doc	3–6	5–25	>20
	A–T–C	3	3	
	CEF	8–9	14	
	TAC	24–34	21–24	>20
	APac		21–32	>20
	ADoc	33	33–48	
	FEC120		9–14	
	FEC100		0–2	
	FAC		5	
	CMFiv		0–3	
	CMFpo		1	
	Doc	21	16–17	10–20
	DocCapec		13	10–20
SCLC	Carbo/VP-16			10–20
	TopC			10–20
	CAE		24–57	>20
	Topotecan		28	>20
	TopT		>20	>20
	ICE		24	
	VICE		70	
NSCLC	VIG		25	>20
	DP	3.7	26	>20
	Cis/Pac	16	16	10–20
	Cis/Gem	4	1–7	
	Cis/Doc	11	5–11	
	Carbo/Pac	4	0–9	
	VP-16/Cis		54	
	Vinor/Cis		1–10	
NHL	ESHAP	30	30–64	>20
	ACOD		11	10–20
	FM		11	10–20
	CHOP		17–50	
	RCHOP	18	19	10–20
	DHAP	48	48	
Colorectal	5-FU/LV		1–15	
	FOLFIRI		3–14	
	FOLFOX		0–8	
	IFL		3–7	
	Irinotecan		2–7	
Germ cell	VIP			>20
	EC		10	10–20
	BEP → EP		13	
	BOP → VIP-B		46	
Ovary	Top	18	10–18	>20, 10–20
	Pac		22	>20

Table 9.4 (continued)

		Myeloid growth factor guideline (%FN)		
Cancer type	Regimen	ASCO	EORTC	NCCN
	Doc		33	>20
	Cis/Pac	Rare		
	Carbo/Pac		3–8	
	Gem/Cis		9	
Sarcoma	MAID		58	>20
	Doxorubicin			>20
	Dox/Ifos			>20

AC, doxorubicin/cyclophosphamide; AC–Doc, doxorubicin/cyclophosphamide/docetaxel; A–T–C, doxorubicin/paclitaxel/cyclophosphamide; CEF, cyclophosphamide/epirubicin/fluorouracil; TAC, docetaxel/doxorubicin/cyclophosphamide; APac, doxorubicin/paclitaxel; ADoc, doxorubicin/docetaxel; FEC120, cyclophosphamide/epirubicin/fluorouracil; FEC100, cyclophosphamide/epirubicin/fluorouracil; FAC, fluorouracil/doxorubicin/cyclophosphamide; CMFiv, cyclophosphamide/methotrexate/fluorouracil-intravenous; CMFpo, cyclophosphamide/methotrexate/fluorouracil-oral; Doc, docetaxel; DocCapec, docetaxel/capecitabine; Carbo/VP-16, carboplatin/etoposide; TopC, topotecan/cisplatin; CAE, cyclophosphamide/doxorubicin/etoposide; TopT, topotecan/paclitaxel; ICE, ifosfamide/carboplatin/etoposide; VICE, vincristine/ifosfamide/carboplatin/etoposide; VIG, gemcitabine/ifosfamide/dacarbazine; DP, docetaxel/carboplatin; Cis/Pac, cisplatin/paclitaxel; Cis/Gem, cisplatin/gemcitabine; Cis/Doc, cisplatin/docetaxel; Carbo/Pac, carboplatin/paclitaxel; VP-16/Cis, etoposide/cisplatin; Vinor/Cis, vinorelbine/cisplatin; ESHAP, etoposide/methylprednisolone/cisplatin/cytarabine; ACOD, doxorubicin/cyclophosphamide/vincristine/prednisone; FM, fludarabine/mitoxantrone; CHOP, cyclophosphamide/doxorubicin/vincristine/prednisone; RCHOP, cyclophosphamide/doxorubicin/vincristine/prednisone/rituximab; DHAP, cisplatin/cytarabine/dexamethasone; 5-FU/LV, 5-FU/leucovorin; FOLFIRI, 5-FU/leucovorin/irinotecan; FOLFOX, 5-FU/leucovorin/oxaliplatin; IFL, irinotecan/fluorouracil/leucovorin; VIP, vinblastine/ifosfamide/cisplatin; EC, etoposide/cisplatin; BEP → EP, bleomycin/etoposide/cisplatin → etoposide/cisplatin; BOP → VIP-B, bleomycin/vincristine/cisplatin → cisplatin/ifosfamide/etoposide/bleomycin; Top, topotecan; Pac, paclitaxel; MAID, mesna/adriamycin/ifosfamide/dacarbazine; Dox/Ifos, doxorubicin/ifosfamide.

Finally, each guideline was critically appraised by the authors independently using the previously validated AGREE measurement tool and discrepancies resolved as discussed in the methods section. Table 9.5 summarizes and contrasts the results of this critical appraisal by domain of focus of the scale. For issues related to the scope and purpose, stakeholder involvement, and applicability of the guidelines, little or no differences in appraisal were found. The NCCN guideline was appraised as less rigorous in its development largely related to the recognized consensus process employed compared to a more rigorous evidence-based approach used by ASCO and EORTC. While a literature review was undertaken by each of the Panels, the review process was found to be more systematic and comprehensive in the ASCO and EORTC guidelines than in the NCCN guidelines in which no criteria for the search and selection of relevant literature are presented. Differences are also noted in the review process with an explicit process for independent and external review of the ASCO and EORTC guidelines. Similarly, there appears to

Table 9.5 Critical appraisal of myeloid growth factor guidelines

	ASCO 2006	EORTC	NCCN
Scope and purpose			
1. The overall objectives of the guideline are specifically described	4 To update the 2000 ASCO guideline on the use of CSFs	4 To develop European focused guidelines to assist in the use of CSF in patients at risk for FN	4 To develop guidelines to assist clinicians in the appropriate prophylactic use of CSFs
2. Clinical questions covered by the guideline are specifically described	4 Clinical questions are clearly described	4 Clinical questions are clearly described	4 Clinical questions are clearly described
3. Patients to whom the guideline is meant to apply are specifically described	4 Population is clear within each specific clinical area. Much broader populations than other guidelines	4 Adult cancer patients at risk for chemotherapy-induced FN	4 Adult patients with solid tumors and non-myeloic malignancies
Domain score	100%	100%	100%
Stakeholder involvement			
4. Guideline development group includes individuals from all the relevant professional groups	3 A full list of committee members are provided, but their areas of specialty/interest are not indicated	4 The development group members are representative of relevant professional groups	3 The development group members are representative of NCCN member institutions with some external consultation
5. Patients' views and preferences have been sought	2 Literature review addressing QOL completed. Direct patient interviews were not conducted. No patient representative	2 Literature review addressing QOL completed. No indication that direct patient interviews were conducted	2 Literature review addressing QOL completed. No indication that direct patient interviews were conducted
6. Target users of the guidelines are clearly defined	3 Specific user of the guideline is never stated directly, although it is strongly implied	3 Specific user of the guideline is never stated directly, although it is strongly implied	3 Specific user of the guideline is never stated directly, although it is strongly implied
7. Guideline has been piloted among target users	1 No indication that the guideline had been tested prior to its publication	1 No indication that the guideline had been tested prior to its publication	1 No indication that the guideline had been tested prior to its publication
Domain score	42%	50%	42%

Table 9.5 (continued)

	ASCO 2006	EORTC	NCCN
Rigor of development			
8. Systematic methods were used to search for evidence	4 Systematic method used for searching the literature was clearly delineated	4 Systematic method used for searching the literature was clearly delineated	2 No systematic literature search. Updated literature is reviewed, guidelines consensus based
9. Criteria for selecting the evidence clearly described	4 Criteria for evidence selection was clearly delineated	4 Criteria for evidence selection was clearly delineated	1 No indication of the criteria used for selecting relevant evidence
10. Methods used for formulating the recommendations are clearly described	4 Clear description of the methods used to formulate the guideline recommendations provided	4 Clear description of the methods used to formulate the guideline recommendations provided	2 Guidelines are consensus based. Specifics of how the consensus was obtained are not provided
11. Health benefits, side effects and risks considered in formulating the recommendations	3 Benefits of CSFs are clearly stated. Some side effects and risks of growth factors are not addressed at all	2 Benefits of CSFs are clearly stated. Side effects and risks of growth factors are not addressed at all	2 Benefits of CSFs are clearly stated. Side effects and risks of growth factors are not addressed at all
12. Explicit link between recommendations and supporting evidence	4 Each point in the guideline is backed with a reference	4 Each point in the guideline is backed with a reference	4 Each point in the guideline is backed with a reference
13. Guideline has been externally reviewed by experts prior to publication	3 Reviewed by ASCO Health Service Committee and Board of Directors. No description of the reviewers' areas of expertise. No indication of review outside of ASCO	4 External review by experts in several fields was performed	1 Guideline drafts are reviewed by experts at each center. No indication that external review occurred

Table 9.5 (continued)

	ASCO 2006	EORTC	NCCN
14. Procedure for updating the guideline is provided	1 No clear statement of when the next ASCO update will occur available in the guidelines	1 No clear procedure for updating the guideline is indicated	4 Guidelines updated annually and based on evaluation of scientific data integrated with expert judgment by multidisciplinary panels of experts from NCCN institutions
Domain score	76%	76%	48%
Clarity and presentation			
15. Recommendations are specific and unambiguous	4 Recommendations are specific and unambiguous	4 Recommendations are specific and unambiguous	4 Recommendations are specific and unambiguous
16. Different options for management are clearly presented	4 Patient management options are discussed	4 Patient management options are discussed	4 Patient management options are discussed
17. Key recommendations are easily identifiable	3 Key recommendations are easy to identify in guideline manuscript and guideline summary, but are wordy	4 Key recommendations are italicized in the manuscript	4 Key recommendations are available in manuscript text and as user-friendly diagrams and tables
18. The guideline is supported with tools for application	4 Guideline summary available as an appendix to the manuscript. Derivative slide set and flow sheet available	2 User-friendly diagram provided in the manuscript directing CSF use. No other application tools are provided	4 User-friendly tables and diagrams are provided online with convenient links between relevant treatment decision points
Domain score	92%	83%	100%

Table 9.5 (continued)

	ASCO 2006	EORTC	NCCN
Applicability			
19. Potential organizational barriers in applying recommendations discussed	1 Guideline did not contain discussion of potential organizational barriers to applying the guidelines	1 Guideline did not contain discussion of potential organizational barriers to applying the guidelines	1 Guideline did not contain discussion of potential organizational barriers to applying the guidelines
20. Cost implications of applying recommendations considered	4 Clear discussion of cost benefit analysis was provided	4 Clear discussion of cost benefit analysis was provided	4 Clear discussion of cost benefit analysis was provided
21. Guideline presents key review criteria for monitoring or audit purposes	4 Separate worksheet developed for review and audits	4 Flow chart presented that outlines details criteria to meet recommendations	4 Flow chart presented that outlines criteria to meet recommendations
Domain score	67%	67%	67%
Editorial independence			
22. Guideline is editorially independent from the funding body	2 Guideline approved by ASCO Panel, Health Services Committee and Board of Directors. Process has industry input but is editorially independent	2 Guideline approved by EORTC Panel, Infectious Disease Group and Governing Board. Process has industry input but is editorially independent	2 Guideline approved by NCCN Panel and Institutions. Process has industry input and receives industry support for distribution of the guideline library on CD-ROM but is editorially independent
23. Conflicts of interest of guideline development members have been recorded	4 Conflicts of interest of guideline committee members are clearly stated	4 Conflicts of interest of guideline committee members are clearly stated	2 Conflicts of interest statement made for entire panel is available
Domain score	67%	67%	33%

CSFs, colony-stimulating factors; QOL, quality of life.

be no indication of individual conflicts of interest for Panel members of the NCCN Panel as there are for the ASCO and EORTC guidelines. In contrast, the NCCN guidelines are updated on an annual basis while no explicit process for update of the ASCO and EORTC guidelines are stated. In addition, the clarity of presentation favors the NCCN guidelines with the recommendations generally presented in both text and algorithmic diagrams for ease of access and use. While no meaningful overall summary measure can be derived from the critical appraisal, the differences observed are largely accountable by the differences in process employed by the different professional groups involved. All guidelines in the end recommend further clinical investigation of a number of areas that remain unclear.

Discussion

Chemotherapy-induced neutropenia and its complications are major dose-limiting toxicities of cancer chemotherapy. The myeloid growth factors have been shown to reduce the risk of FN and its related complications. Three different practice guidelines for the myeloid growth factors have recently been published by major professional organizations. A comprehensive review and comparison of the guidelines demonstrates remarkable consistency in the final recommendations from these guidelines for the use of CSF primary prophylaxis in patients at approximately a 20% risk of FN or greater. All guidelines also recommend CSF use be considered when individual risk assessment by the clinician concludes a patient is at increased risk.

The quality of clinical practice guidelines has recently been brought into question [37]. Overall, the quality of the myeloid growth factor guidelines was rated as good with little or no difference between guidelines in the stated scope and purpose, stakeholder involvement, and applicability of the guidelines. There is clearly more emphasis on systematic and comprehensive literature reviews in the ASCO and EORTC guidelines, while the NCCN guidelines are updated on an annual basis and appear to offer better clarity of presentation.

References

1. Dale DC, McCarter GC, Crawford J, et al. Myelotoxicity and dose intensity of chemotherapy: reporting practices from randomized clinical trials. J Natl Compr Canc Netw. 2003;1:440–54.
2. Lyman GH, Morrison VA, Dale DC, Crawford J, et al. Risk of febrile neutropenia among patients with intermediate-grade non-Hodgkin's lymphoma receiving CHOP chemotherapy. Leuk Lymphoma. 2003;44:2069–76.
3. Lyman GH. Guidelines of the National Comprehensive Cancer Network on the use of the myeloid growth factors with cancer chemotherapy: a review of the evidence. J Natl Compr Canc Netw. 2005;3:557–71.
4. Kuderer NM, Dale D, Crawford J, Cosler L, Lyman GH. The morbidity, mortality and cost of febrile neutropenia in cancer patients. Cancer. 2006;106:2258–66.

5. Lyman GH, Dale D, Crawford J. Incidence, practice patterns and predictors of low dose intensity in adjuvant breast cancer chemotherapy: results of a nationwide study of community practices. J Clin Oncol. 2003;21:4524–31.

6. Lyman GH, Dale D, Friedberg J, Crawford J, Fisher RI. Incidence and predictors of low chemotherapy dose intensity in aggressive non-Hodgkin's lymphoma: a nationwide study. J Clin Oncol. 2004;22:4302–11.

7. Bonadonna G, Valagussa P, Moliterni A, et al. Adjuvant cyclophosphamide, methotrexate, and fluorouracil in node-positive breast cancer: the results of 20 years of follow-up. N Engl J Med. 1995;332:901–6.

8. Early Breast Cancer Trialists' Collaborative Group. Effects of chemotherapy and hormonal therapy for early breast cancer on recurrence and 15-year survival: an overview of the randomized trials. Lancet 2005;365:1687–1717.

9. Budman DR, Berry DA, Cirrincione CT, et al. Dose and dose intensity as determinants of outcome in the adjuvant treatment of breast cancer. The Cancer and Leukemia Group B. J Natl Cancer Inst. 1998;90:1205–11.

10. Bonneterre J, Roche H, Kerbrat P, et al. Epirubicin increases long-term survival in adjuvant chemotherapy of patients with poor-prognosis, node-positive, early breast cancer: 10-year follow-up results of the French Adjuvant Study Group 05 randomized trial. J Clin Oncol. 2005;23:2686–93.

11. Citron ML, Berry DA, Cirrincione C, et al. Randomized trial of dose-dense versus conventionally scheduled and sequential versus concurrent combination chemotherapy as postoperative adjuvant treatment of node-positive primary breast cancer: first report of Intergroup Trial C9741/Cancer and Leukemia Group B Trial 9741. J Clin Oncol. 2003;21:1431–9.

12. Pfreundschuh M, Trümper L, Kloess M, et al. 2-weekly or 3-weekly CHOP chemotherapy with or without etoposide for the treatment of elderly patients with aggressive lymphomas: results of the NHL-B2 trial of the DSHNHL. Blood. 2004;104:634–41.

13. Griggs JJ, Sorbero MES, Lyman GH. Undertreatment of obese women receiving breast cancer chemotherapy. Int Arch Med. 2005;165:1267–73.

14. Chu E, DeVita V. Principles of medical oncology. In: DeVita VT, Rosenberg SA, editors. Cancer: principles and practice of oncology. 7th ed. Philadelphia, PA: Lippincott; 2006. pp. 295–306.

15. Crawford J, Ozer H, Stoller R, et al. Reduction by granulocyte colony-stimulating factor of fever and neutropenia induced by chemotherapy in patients with small-cell lung cancer. N Engl J Med. 1991;325:164–70.

16. Lyman GH, Kuderer NM, Djulbegovic B. Prophylactic granulocyte colony-stimulating factor in patients receiving dose-intensive cancer chemotherapy: a meta-analysis. Am J Med. 2002;112:406–11.

17. Osby E, Hagberg H, Kvaloy S, et al. CHOP is superior to CNOP in elderly patients with aggressive lymphoma while outcome is unaffected by filgrastim treatment: results of a Nordic Lymphoma Group randomized trial. Blood. 2003;101:3840–8.

18. Doorduijn JK, van der HB, van Imhoff GW, et al. CHOP compared with CHOP plus granulocyte colony-stimulating factor in elderly patients with aggressive non-Hodgkin's lymphoma. J Clin Oncol. 2003;21:3041–50.

19. Timmer-Bonte JN, de Boo TM, Smit HJ, et al. Prevention of chemotherapy-induced febrile neutropenia by prophylactic antibiotics plus or minus granulocyte colony-stimulating factor in small-cell lung cancer: a Dutch randomized phase III study. J Clin Oncol. 2005;23:7974–84.

20. Vogel C, Wojtukiewicz MZ, Caroll RR, et al. First and subsequent cycle use of pegfilgrastim prevents febrile neutropenia in patients with breast cancer: a multicenter, double-blind, placebo-controlled phase III study. J Clin Oncol. 2005;23:1178–84.

21. Kuderer NM, Crawford J, Dale DC, Lyman GH. Meta-analysis of prophylactic granulocyte colony-stimulating factor (G-CSF) in cancer patients receiving chemotherapy. J Clin Oncol. 2005;23:758 s. Abstract 8117.

22. Lyman GH, Lyman CH, Agboola O. Risk models for predicting chemotherapy-induced neutropenia. Oncologist. 2005;10:427–37.
23. Lyman GH, Lyman CG, Sanderson RA, Balducci L. Decision analysis of hematopoietic growth factor use in patients receiving cancer chemotherapy. J Natl Cancer Inst. 1993;85: 488–93.
24. Lyman GH, Kuderer N, Greene J, Balducci L. The economics of febrile neutropenia: implications for the use of colony-stimulating factors. Eur J Cancer. 1998;34:1857–64.
25. Lyman GH, Kuderer NM. Economics of hematopoietic growth factors. In: Morstyn G, Foote M, Lieschke GJ, editors. Cancer drug discovery and development. Hematopoietic growth factors in oncology: basic science and clinical therapeutics. Totowa, NJ: Humana Press Inc; 2004. pp. 409–443.
26. Lyman GH, Kuderer NM, Crawford J, et al. Prospective validation of a risk model for first cycle neutropenic complications in patients receiving cancer chemotherapy. J Clin Oncol. 2006;24:483 s. Abstract 8561.
27. American Society of Clinical Oncology. Recommendations for the use of hematopoietic colony-stimulating factors: evidence-based, clinical practice guidelines. J Clin Oncol. 1994;12(11):2471–508.
28. Ozer H, Armitage JO, Bennett CL, et al. Update of recommendations for the use of hematopoietic colony-stimulating factors: evidence-based, clinical practice guidelines. American Society of Clinical Oncology Growth Factors Expert Panel. J Clin Oncol. 2000;2000(18):3558–85.
29. Smith TJ, Khatcheressian J, Lyman GH, et al. Update of recommendations for the use of white blood cell growth factors: an evidence-based clinical practice guideline. J. Clin Oncol. 2006;24:3187–205.
30. Crawford J, Althaus B, Armitage J, et al. Myeloid growth factors. J Natl Compr Canc Netw. 2005;3:540–55.
31. Crawford J, Althaus B, Armitage J, Blayney DW, Cataland S, Dale DC, Demetri GD, Foran J, Heaney ML, Htoy S, Kloth DD, Lyman GH, Michaud L, Motl S, Vadham-Raj S, Wong MK. Myeloid growth factors. 2006. http://www.nccn.org/professionals/physician_gls/PDF/myeloid_growth.pdf.
32. Aapro MS, Cameron DA, Pettengell R, et al. European Organisation for Research and Treatment of Cancer (EORTC) Granulocyte Colony-Stimulating Factor (G-CSF) Guidelines Taskforce. EORTC guidelines for the use of granulocyte colony-stimulating factor in adult patients with chemotherapy-induced febrile neutropenia. Eur J Cancer 2006;42: 2433–53.
33. Repetto L, Biganzoli L, Koehne CH, et al. EORTC cancer in the elderly task force guidelines for the use of colony-stimulating factors in elderly patients with cancer. Eur J Cancer. 2003;39(16):2264–72.
34. The AGREE Collaboration. Appraisal of the Guidelines for Research and Evaluation (AGREE) Instrument. http://www.agreecollaboraiton.org.
35. AGREE Collaboration. Development and validation of an international appraisal instrument for assessing the quality of clinical practice guidelines: the AGREE project. Qula Saf Health Care. 2003;12:18–23.
36. Burgers JS, Fervers B, Haugh M, et al. International assessment of the quality of clinical practice guidelines in oncology using the appraisal of guidelines and research and evaluation instrument. J Clin Oncol. 2004;22:2000–7.
37. Shanaeyfelt TM, Mayo-Snith MF, Rothwangl J. Are guidelines following guidelines? The methodological quality of clinical practice guidelines in the peer-reviewed medical literature. JAMA. 2006;281:1900–5.

Chapter 10
Granulocyte Colony-Stimulating Factors and Risk of Acute Myeloid Leukemia and Myelodysplastic Syndrome

Gary H. Lyman and Nicole M. Kuderer

Introduction

Granulocyte colony-stimulating factors (G-CSFs) in patients receiving cancer chemotherapy have been shown to reduce the severity and duration of neutropenia as well as the risk of febrile neutropenia, documented infection, and infection-related mortality while enabling an increase in delivered chemotherapy dose intensity [1, 2]. Meta-analyses of randomized controlled trials (RCTs) of the myeloid growth factors have been reported for both adults and children consistently demonstrating the impact of these agents on neutropenia and its complications [3–5]. Clinical practice guidelines have been put forward by the American Society of Clinical Oncology and other professional organizations for the use of these agents [6–8].

Systemic cancer chemotherapy and radiation therapy have been associated with an increased risk of secondary acute myeloid leukemia (AML) in a number of previous studies [9, 10]. Multiple studies of cancer survivors have confirmed an association of treatment with myelosuppresive chemotherapy across a range of malignancies and chemotherapeutic programs [11–14]. Recent retrospective studies have suggested a possible increased risk of AML and myelodysplastic syndrome (MDS) in patients receiving chemotherapy with myeloid growth factor support [15, 16]. Interpretation of those studies has been difficult due to their post hoc design and to the limited ability to adjust for relevant confounding factors since the G-CSF was not randomly assigned and pre-existing hematologic disorders, chemotherapy and radiation therapy, low baseline blood counts as well as unrecognized inherited or acquired childhood, occupational, and other environmental exposures could not be adjusted for. None of the reported RCTs of the myeloid growth factors were adequately powered to address any possible risk for second malignancies including AML or MDS associated with the colony-stimulating factors. Previous meta-analyses of RCTs searched for studies where the chemotherapy was the same

G.H. Lyman (✉)
Duke University and the Duke Comprehensive Cancer Center, Durham, NC 27705, USA
e-mail: gary.lyman@duke.edu

G.H. Lyman, D.C. Dale (eds.), *Hematopoietic Growth Factors in Oncology*,
Cancer Treatment and Research 157, DOI 10.1007/978-1-4419-7073-2_10,
© Springer Science+Business Media, LLC 2011

in both arms and the primary outcome was a reduction in neutropenic complications [5, 17, 18].

Perhaps the greatest challenge in understanding the potential risk of G-CSF for the occurrence of AML and MDS is the acknowledged leukemogenicity of many of the commonly employed cancer chemotherapeutic agents given in conjunction with these agents. In addition to ionizing radiation, several chemotherapeutic agents are considered to be leukemogenic in both animals and humans [11–13, 19–21]. Since G-CSF is frequently utilized to minimize chemotherapy dose reductions and delays and to enable the delivery of dose-intense and dose-escalating chemotherapy regimens, the use of these agents is often accompanied by greater chemotherapy dose intensity or greater cumulative exposure to chemotherapy.

Systematic Review of Randomized Controlled Trials

A systematic review was undertaken to assess any association between G-CSF support and the risk of second malignancies, including AML or MDS and overall mortality in patients receiving cancer chemotherapy. RCTs of adult cancer patients receiving systemic chemotherapy with or without primary G-CSF support between January 1, 1990 and October 1, 2008 were identified by searching Medline, EMBASE, the Cochrane Library, clinical practice guidelines from the National Guideline Clearinghouse, and conference proceedings from the American Society of Clinical Oncology and the American Society of Hematology. References of eligible articles were also searched for relevant citations (Fig. 10.1). Abstracts were selected for further evaluation if they represented randomized clinical trials of G-CSF with concurrent placebo or non-placebo controls in cancer patients receiving systemic chemotherapy. The initial search identified 3,794 articles that were further reviewed (Fig. 10.1).

Eligible studies included cancer patients receiving conventional chemotherapy for lymphoma or solid tumors randomized to G-CSF or a control group without initial G-CSF. Eligible studies were required to have at least 24 months of follow-up and report the incidence of AML and/or MDS or all secondary malignancies as well as overall survival. Studies of patients with leukemia or undergoing stem cell or bone marrow transplant were excluded. Data extraction was performed by two independent reviewers with a third reviewer resolving all conflicts. Occurrence of AML or MDS and all-cause mortality represented the primary outcomes for analysis. Relative risk (RR) or absolute risk (AR) difference in G-CSF versus control patient outcomes was estimated as the weighted sum of the individual estimates where the weights are the reciprocal of the variance [22]. Exploratory analyses planned a priori included subgroup comparisons based on the type of cancer, the type of chemotherapy regimen, and chemotherapy relative dose intensity (RDI) defined as the ratio of the dose intensity in the G-CSF-supported arm to that in the control arm. Planned and actual chemotherapy dose intensity with G-CSF support relative to that in control patients was regressed on the natural logarithm of the relative risk for mortality.

QUORUM Diagram

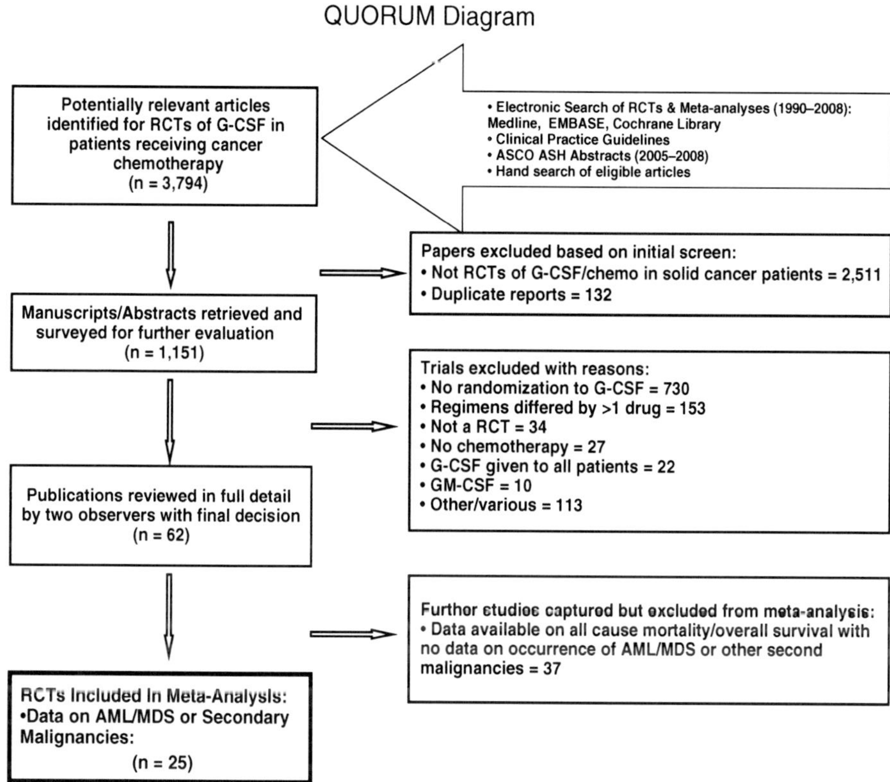

Fig. 10.1 Quorum diagram of the systematic review reported here summarizing results of search and exclusion criteria resulting in the final 25 studies for full analysis

Heterogeneity was based on Cochran's Q statistic and the inconsistency index (I^2) representing the proportion of variation across studies due to heterogeneity rather than chance. Statistical analysis was based on the z-statistic for individual studies as well as the overall effect estimate [23].

As shown in Fig. 10.1, subsequent review of the 3,794 articles identified with the initial search culminated in 25 eligible RCTs [24–52]. Overall, 12,804 patients were included in these trials (6,058 randomized to G-CSF and 6,746 controls) with mean and median follow-up of 60 and 53 months, respectively. Deaths totaled 3,944 including 1,845 in those randomized to G-CSF and 2,099 in control patients. RDI was reported in 16 studies with mean and median of 110.9 and 98.1% in G-CSF patients and 91.6 and 93.5% among controls, respectively. Among the 16 RCTs where the RDI in each study arm was provided, the median RDIs with G-CSF support and controls were 98.1 and 93.5%, respectively. The excess RDI of chemotherapy with G-CSF support compared to control was 18% when the intended dose intensity was the same in each study arm compared to 46 and 23% in dose-dense and dose-escalation studies, respectively.

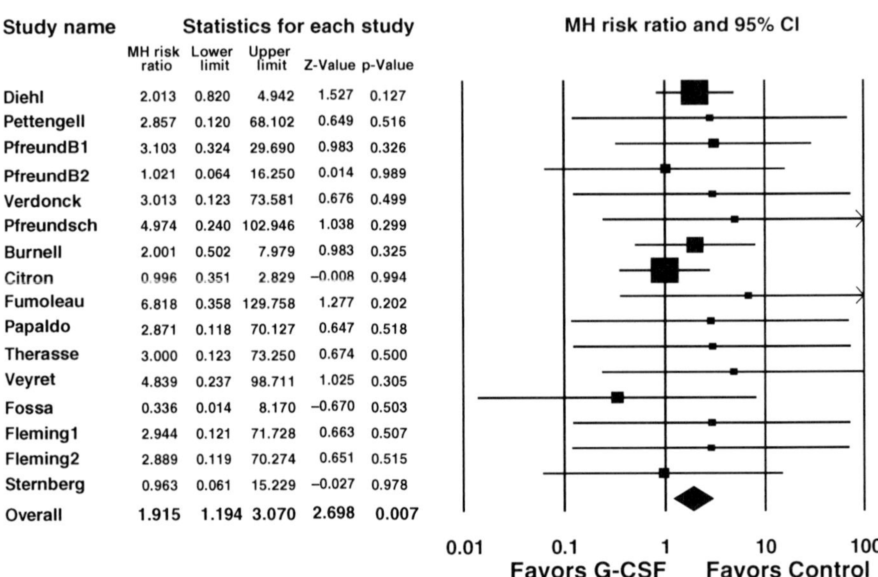

Fig. 10.2 Forest plot of the estimated RR [±95% CI] for AML or MDS comparing G-CSF-supported chemotherapy to control for each study (*squares*) with weighted summary RR (*diamond*) based on the method of Mantel and Haenszel

AML or MDS was reported in 23 eligible studies with study populations of 5,474 in the G-CSF arms and 6,157 in the control arms. AML or MDS occurred in 22 (0.36%) control and 43 (0.79%) G-CSF-supported patients receiving chemotherapy. RR for AML/MDS in those receiving chemotherapy compared to controls was 1.92 [$P = 0.007$] (Fig. 10.2). The AR increase of AML/MDS in patients receiving G-CSF was at 4/1,000 [0.41%; $P = 0.009$]. As also shown in Table 10.1, the AR increase for AML/MDS was least in those receiving dose-dense schedules and greatest in studies with dose or drug escalation. The risk of AML/MDS was greater where G-CSF support was associated with greater total dose of chemotherapy [RR = 2.334; AR = 0.76%; $P = 0.009$]. No significant association between RDI and the RR for AML/MDS with G-CSF support was observed. The number of all second malignancies was reported in 11 eligible studies including two that did not report AML or MDS separately and occurred in 115 (3.28%) patients receiving chemotherapy with G-CSF support and 114 (3.25%) controls [RR = 1.01; $P = 0.941$]. No differences for secondary malignancies between treatment groups for any subgroup were analyzed. In the 25 eligible studies, 2,099 (31.1%) control patients and 1,845 (30.5%) patients receiving G-CSF-supported chemotherapy died over the period of follow-up.

Table 10.1 Absolute and relative risk for AML/MDS and all-cause mortality: by cancer type and regimen category

Group	Subgroup		AML/MDS					All-cause mortality			
					Absolute risk difference					Absolute risk difference	
		N	Relative risk [95% CLs]		(%) [95% CLs]		N	Relative risk [95% CLs]		(%) [95% CLs]	
Overall	–	23	1.915*	1.195, 3.070	0.41*	0.11, 0.73	24	0.897***	0.857, 0.938	−3.40***	−4.80, −2.01
Cancer type	Breast	7	1.811	0.897, 3.656	0.30	−0.06, 0.67	7	0.902**	0.815, 0.998	−1.89**	−3.72, −0.06
	Endometrial	2	2.916	0.305, 27.872	0.68	−0.66, 2.02	2	0.945	0.874, 1.021	−4.64	−10.89, 1.61
	Germ cell	1	0.336	0.014, 8.170	−0.77	−2.90, 1.36	1	0.849	0.568, 1.269	−4.42	−15.23, 6.38
	Hodgkin	1	2.013	0.820, 4.942	0.1.51	−0.39, 3.41	1	0.660**	0.452, 0.963	−4.42**	−8.39, −0.46
	Non-Hodgkin	8	2.732	0.804, 9.280	0.45	−0.13, 1.03	9	0.895*	0.832, 0.963	−4.66*	−7.57, −1.75
	Lung	3	0.956	0.101, 9.072	0.00	−1.66, 1.66	3	0.945	0.875, 1.021	−4.88	−11.46, 1.71
	Urothelial	1	0.963	0.061, 15.229	−0.03	−2.13, 2.07	1	0.868**	0.772, 0.977	−11.45**	−20.79, −2.11
Regimen category	Same drugs, dose and schedule	9	1.947	0.487, 7.779	0.35	−0.51, 1.21	10	0.942	0.881, 1.009	−2.90	−6.22, 0.42
	Dose-dense schedule	6	1.288	0.577, 2.875	0.11	−0.25, 0.48	6	0.841***	0.776, 0.912	−4.79***	−7.01, −2.57
	Dose escalation	3	2.211	0.940, 5.203	1.34	−0.09, 2.78	3	0.785	0.589, 1.045	−2.97	−6.46, 0.52
	Added or substituted agent	5	2.827**	1.013, 7.885	0.56**	0.01, 1.12	5	0.945	0.868, 1.029	−1.65	−4.08, 0.78

N = Number of trials.

AML = acute myeloid leukemia; MDS = myelodysplastic syndrome; CLs = confidence limits.

*$P < 0.01$; **$P < 0.05$; ***$P < 0.001$.

All-Cause Mortality

Study name	MH risk ratio	Z-Value	Lower limit	Upper limit	p-Value
Burton	0.936	−0.978	0.821	1.068	0.328
Diehl	0.660	−2.157	0.452	0.963	0.031
Doorduijn	0.975	−0.333	0.838	1.134	0.739
Pan	1.385	0.397	0.277	6.913	0.692
Pettengell	0.951	−0.274	0.665	1.360	0.784
PfreundB1	0.717	−2.026	0.520	0.989	0.043
PfreundB2	0.845	−2.300	0.732	0.975	0.021
Verdonck	0.862	−1.277	0.687	1.083	0.202
Zinzani	0.970	−0.144	0.637	1.476	0.886
Pfreundschuh	0.995	−0.022	0.625	1.584	0.983
Gisselbrecht	0.813	−1.085	0.559	1.182	0.278
Burnell	0.818	−1.204	0.590	1.134	0.228
Citron	0.828	−1.999	0.689	0.996	0.046
Fumoleau	1.049	0.218	0.684	1.607	0.828
Papaldo	0.938	−0.358	0.659	1.334	0.720
Therasse	1.009	0.095	0.834	1.222	0.925
Venturini	0.890	−0.957	0.701	1.130	0.339
Veyret	1.171	0.630	0.717	1.913	0.529
Fossa	0.849	−0.800	0.568	1.269	0.424
Fleming1	1.027	0.532	0.932	1.131	0.595
Fleming2	0.849	−2.532	0.748	0.964	0.011
Sternberg	0.868	−2.352	0.772	0.977	0.019
Fukuoka	0.969	−0.565	0.868	1.082	0.572
Gatzemeier	0.970	−0.651	0.884	1.064	0.515
Woll	0.807	−1.510	0.610	1.066	0.131
Overall	0.897	−4.765	0.857	0.938	0.000

Fig. 10.3 Forest plot of the estimated RR [±95% CI] for all-cause mortality comparing G-CSF-supported chemotherapy to control for each study (*squares*) with weighted summary RR (*diamond*) based on the method of Mantel and Haenszel

The RR and AR decreases in all-cause mortality in patients receiving chemotherapy with G-CSF support compared to controls were 0.897 [$P < 0.001$] and 3.40% [$P < 0.001$], respectively (Fig. 10.3). The relative risk and AR decrease in all-cause mortality with and without G-CSF support varied by tumor type and chemotherapy regimen category (Table 10.1). The RR for mortality when G-CSF was utilized to support dose-dense chemotherapy regimens was 0.841 [$P < 0.001$] and for chemotherapy dose escalation was 0.785 [$P = 0.097$] compared to when the dose and schedule were the same [RR = 0.942; $P = 0.088$]. A significant inverse association was observed between planned RDI with G-CSF support compared to controls and the RR for all-cause mortality [$P = 0.0159$] (Fig. 10.4). Likewise, a significant inverse association was observed between the RR for mortality and both the RDI with G-CSF support compared to control [$P = 0.0148$] (Fig. 10.5).

No association between the source of funding and the primary outcomes was reported in eligible RCTs in this overview. The RR for AML/MDS was 2.568 in studies funded by industry compared to 1.463 and 1.773 in studies funded by government sources and other independent sources, respectively. Some suggestion of an underrepresentation of smaller negative studies was observed for AML/MDS in this analysis based on Egger's regression intercept method for funnel plot asymmetry [$P = 0.0775$].

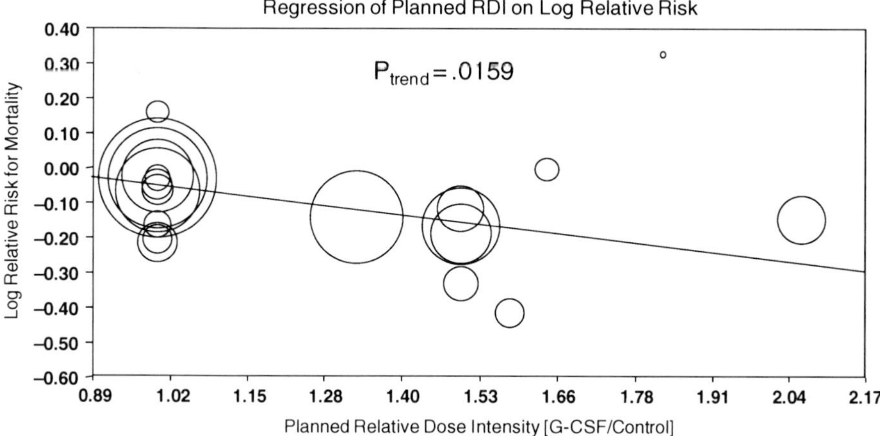

Fig. 10.4 Graphic display of meta-regression of planned RDI on the natural logarithm of the RR for mortality in G-CSF-supported chemotherapy compared to control. Each study is represented by a *circle*, the area of which is proportional to the weight provided by each study to overall estimate

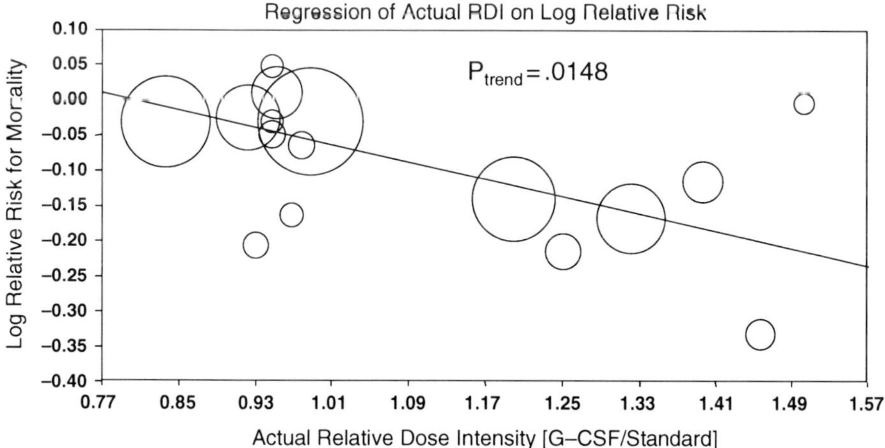

Fig. 10.5 Graphic display of meta-regression of actual delivered RDI compared to standard on the natural logarithm of the RR for mortality in G-CSF-supported chemotherapy. Each study is represented by a *circle*, the area of which is proportional to the weight provided by each study to overall estimate

Summary

Among the 25 RCTs of patients receiving cancer chemotherapy and randomized to initial G-CSF support or not identified in this systematic review, AML/MDS was reported in 23, second malignancies in 11, and survival or mortality data in all 25 while only 12 reported RDI by study treatment assignment. The RR and AR increases for AML/MDS with G-CSF-supported chemotherapy were 1.92 and 0.4%, respectively, at a median follow-up of 54 months. At the same time, the RR and AR decreases in mortality with G-CSF-supported chemotherapy compared to control were 0.897 and 3.4%, respectively. A significant inverse association between delivered RDI and reduced mortality was observed. The results presented here cannot distinguish any effects on the risk of AML/MDS due to the growth factor and those due to greater chemotherapy exposure due to less reduction in dosing or actual dose escalation. Importantly, systemic chemotherapy with G-CSF support was associated with greater reduction in all-cause mortality. The 3–4% reduction in all-cause mortality is some tenfold greater than the 3 to 4/1000 in estimated excess risk of AML and MDS in these trials. Significant reductions in infection-related and all-cause early mortality were observed in a previous meta-analysis of G-CSF primary prophylaxis [4]. Although significant reductions in all-cause mortality were not observed, none of the studies in that review were powered for overall mortality. Likewise, a meta-analysis of myeloid growth factors as additional treatment for febrile neutropenia in addition to antibiotics observed a decrease in infection-related mortality [3]. Again, although no reduction in overall mortality was observed, this did not represent the primary outcome of any of the included trials. Therefore, the most likely explanation for the observed reduction in overall mortality is that of reduced disease recurrence resulting from sustained or enhanced chemotherapy dose and schedule with G-CSF support. Dose-dense regimens were accompanied by greater reductions in mortality while being associated with low risk of AML/MDS. Whether this relates to the delivery of equal total doses of chemotherapy with such regimens or other differences will require further investigation.

In a previous meta-analysis of 7,110 patients with early-stage breast cancer in 19 RCTs of epirubicin-containing regimens, a cumulative risk of AML/MDS of 0.55% at 8 years of follow-up (95% CI, 0.33–0.78%) [13] was observed. Although the intended individual dose and cumulative dose of epirubicin were directly associated with an increased risk of AML/MDS, most also received cyclophosphamide. Cumulative doses of epirubicin and cyclophosphamide were found to be independent risk factors for AML/MDS in multivariate analysis while G-CSF was not a significant risk factor.

An underrepresentation of smaller negative studies for AML/MDS cannot be excluded. However, limitation of this review to larger RCTs with substantial follow-up suggests that few such studies would go unreported or unrecognized. In addition, the observed risk of AML or MDS reported in these trials was actually greater among studies supported by industry than those funded by other sources. Although publication bias must also be considered, there was no evidence of such bias for overall mortality reported across these RCTs.

Many patients randomized to the control arms of identified studies in this systematic review went on to receive G-CSF at a future time representing either a permitted cross-over by trial design or subsequent use of G-CSF off study while receiving future cancer treatment regimens. Likewise, there are insufficient data on G-CSF dosing and duration in the RCTs in this review to permit evaluation of any dose–response relationship for G-CSF with risk of AML/MDS.

In RCTs where patients were planned to receive the same drugs, dose, schedule, duration, and dose intensity of chemotherapy, greater RDI and/or total doses of chemotherapy were actually received due to fewer dose reductions and delays. As a result, an unplanned imbalance in chemotherapy drug exposure occurred along with planned imbalances in studies where G-CSF support permitted dose escalation. These differences in chemotherapy total dose and dose intensity make it difficult if not impossible to separate the effects of known carcinogenic agents such as the alkylating agents and the anthracyclines from any possible risk due to G-CSF [11–13, 19–21].

The reported rates of AML and MDS are likely underestimates due to limited follow-up in some studies and a median follow-up of only 5 years. In addition, the occurrence of AML and MDS was not a primary outcome planned in any of the RCTs included. Nevertheless, leukemia is the earliest malignancy to be identified after exposure to leukemogenic agents including ionizing radiation. In addition, the design of the RCTs included in this review offers a balanced follow-up of patients in the study arms for whatever duration of follow-up is reported. In fact, longer survival in patients receiving G-CSF-supported chemotherapy may result in greater person-years at risk for AML/MDS.

In conclusion, it is difficult if not impossible to distinguish any risk of AML or MDS associated with G-CSF from the recognized dose-dependent leukemogenic effects of many myelosuppressive chemotherapeutic agents. The greater planned or delivered chemotherapy of known leukemogenic potential in patients supported by G-CSF in these studies may represent a major causal source of exposure for the greater risk of AML/MDS observed. While an enhancement of the leukemogenic effect of chemotherapy drugs by G-CSF cannot be ruled out with the data presented here, the observed excess risk of AML associated with chemotherapy dose intensity sustained or escalated with G-CSF support is less than 1% across identified RCTs. The rates of AML reported in this overview are, in fact, similar to those reported in patients receiving myelosuppressive chemotherapy without G-CSF support [11, 13, 14, 19, 53]. At the same time, the reduction in overall mortality in patients receiving chemotherapy with G-CSF support was considerably greater than any associated risk of second malignancies and was consistent with the enhanced chemotherapy dose and schedule received.

References

1. Crawford J, Ozer H, Stoller R, et al. Reduction by granulocyte colony-stimulating factor of fever and neutropenia induced by chemotherapy in patients with small-cell lung cancer. N Engl J Med. 1991;325:164–70.
2. Trillet-Lenoir V, Green J, Manegold C, et al. Recombinant granulocyte colony stimulating factor reduces the infectious complications of cytotoxic chemotherapy. Eur J Cancer. 1993;29A:319–24.
3. Clark OA, Lyman GH, Castro AA, et al. Colony-stimulating factors for chemotherapy-induced febrile neutropenia: a meta-analysis of randomized controlled trials. J Clin Oncol. 2005;23:4198–214.

4. Kuderer NM, Dale DC, Crawford J, et al. Impact of primary prophylaxis with granulocyte colony-stimulating factor on febrile neutropenia and mortality in adult cancer patients receiving chemotherapy: a systematic review. J Clin Oncol. 2007;25:3158–67.

5. Wittman B, Horan J, Lyman GH. Prophylactic colony-stimulating factors in children receiving myelosuppressive chemotherapy: a meta-analysis of randomized controlled trials. Cancer Treat Rev. 2006;32:289–303.

6. Aapro MS, Cameron DA, Pettengell R, et al. EORTC guidelines for the use of granulocyte-colony stimulating factor to reduce the incidence of chemotherapy-induced febrile neutropenia in adult patients with lymphomas and solid tumours. Eur J Cancer. 2006;42:2433–53.

7. Crawford J, Armitage J, Balducci L, et al. Myeloid growth factors. J Natl Compr Canc Netw. 2009;7:64–83.

8. Smith TJ, Khatcheressian J, Lyman GH, et al. 2006 update of recommendations for the use of white blood cell growth factors: an evidence-based clinical practice guideline. J Clin Oncol. 2006;24:3187–205.

9. Castro GA, Church A, Pechet L, et al. Leukemia after chemotherapy of Hodgkin's disease. N Engl J Med. 1973;289:103–4.

10. Preisler HD, Lyman GH. Acute myelogenous leukemia subsequent to therapy for a different neoplasm: clinical features and response to therapy. Am J Hematol. 1977;3:209–18.

11. Leone G, Pagano L, Ben-Yehuda D, et al. Therapy-related leukemia and myelodysplasia: susceptibility and incidence. Haematologica. 2007;92:1389–98.

12. Le Deley MC, Suzan F, Cutuli B, et al. Anthracyclines, mitoxantrone, radiotherapy, and granulocyte colony-stimulating factor: risk factors for leukemia and myelodysplastic syndrome after breast cancer. J Clin Oncol. 2007;25:292–300.

13. Praga C, Bergh J, Bliss J, et al. Risk of acute myeloid leukemia and myelodysplastic syndrome in trials of adjuvant epirubicin for early breast cancer: correlation with doses of epirubicin and cyclophosphamide. J Clin Oncol. 2005;23:4179–91.

14. Smith RE, Bryant J, DeCillis A, et al. Acute myeloid leukemia and myelodysplastic syndrome after doxorubicin–cyclophosphamide adjuvant therapy for operable breast cancer: the National Surgical Adjuvant Breast and Bowel Project Experience. J Clin Oncol. 2003;21:1195–204.

15. Hershman D, Neugut AI, Jacobson JS, et al. Acute myeloid leukemia or myelodysplastic syndrome following use of granulocyte colony-stimulating factors during breast cancer adjuvant chemotherapy. J Natl Cancer Inst. 2007;99:196–205.

16. Relling MV, Boyett JM, Blanco JG, et al. Granulocyte colony-stimulating factor and the risk of secondary myeloid malignancy after etoposide treatment. Blood. 2003;101:3862–7.

17. Lyman GH, Shayne M. Granulocyte colony-stimulating factors: finding the right indication. Curr Opin Oncol. 2007;19:299–307.

18. Sung L, Nathan PC, Alibhai SM, et al. Meta-analysis: effect of prophylactic hematopoietic colony-stimulating factors on mortality and outcomes of infection. Ann Intern Med. 2007;147:400–11.

19. Crump M, Tu D, Shepherd L, et al. Risk of acute leukemia following epirubicin-based adjuvant chemotherapy: a report from the National Cancer Institute of Canada Clinical Trials Group. J Clin Oncol. 2003;21:3066–71.

20. Kalaycio M, Rybicki L, Pohlman B, et al. Risk factors before autologous stem-cell transplantation for lymphoma predict for secondary myelodysplasia and acute myelogenous leukemia. J Clin Oncol. 2006;24:3604–10.

21. Patt DA, Duan Z, Fang S, et al. Acute myeloid leukemia after adjuvant breast cancer therapy in older women: understanding risk. J Clin Oncol. 2007;25:3871–6.

22. Mantel N, Haenszel W:. Statistical aspects of the analysis of data from retrospective studies of disease. J Natl Cancer Inst. 1959;22:719–48.

23. Cochran WG. The combination of estimates from different experiments. Biometrics. 1954;10:101–29.

24. Burnell MJI, Levine MN, Chapman JA, et al. A phase III adjuvant trial of sequenced EC + filgrastim + epoetin-alpha followed by paclitaxel compared to sequenced AC followed by paclitaxel compared to CEF in women with node-positive or high-risk node-negative breast cancer (NCIC CTG MA.21). J Clin Oncol. (ASCO 2007 Meeting Abstract). 2007;25:550.

25. Burton C, Linch D, Hoskin P, et al. A phase III trial comparing CHOP to PMitCEBO with or without G-CSF in patients aged 60 plus with aggressive non-Hodgkin's lymphoma. Br J Cancer. 2006;94:806–13.

26. Chevallier B, Chollet P, Merrouche Y, et al. Lenograstim prevents morbidity from intensive induction chemotherapy in the treatment of inflammatory breast cancer. J Clin Oncol. 1995;13:1564–71.

27. Citron ML, Berry DA, Cirrincione C, et al. Randomized trial of dose-dense versus conventionally scheduled and sequential versus concurrent combination chemotherapy as postoperative adjuvant treatment of node-positive primary breast cancer: first report of Intergroup Trial C9741/Cancer and Leukemia Group B Trial 9741. J Clin Oncol. 2003;21: 1431–9.

28. Clamp AR, Ryder WD, Bhattacharya S, et al. Patterns of mortality after prolonged follow-up of a randomised controlled trial using granulocyte colony-stimulating factor to maintain chemotherapy dose intensity in non-Hodgkin's lymphoma. Br J Cancer. 2008;99: 253–8.

29. Engert A, Diehl V, Franklin J et al. Escalated-Dose BEACOPP in the Treatment of Patients With Advanced-Stage Hodgkin's Lymphoma: 10 Years of Follow-Up of the GHSG HD9 Study. J Clin Oncol 2009;27:4548–54.

30. Diehl V, Franklin J, Pfreundschuh M, et al. Standard and increased-dose BEACOPP chemotherapy compared with COPP-ABVD for advanced Hodgkin's disease. N Engl J Med 2003;348:2386–95.

31. Doorduijn JK, van der Holt B, van Imhoff GW, et al. CHOP compared with CHOP plus granulocyte colony-stimulating factor in elderly patients with aggressive non-Hodgkin's lymphoma. J Clin Oncol. 2003;21:3041–50.

32. Fleming GF, Brunetto VL, Cella D, et al. Phase III trial of doxorubicin plus cisplatin with or without paclitaxel plus filgrastim in advanced endometrial carcinoma: a Gynecologic Oncology Group Study. J Clin Oncol. 2004;22:2159–66.

33. Fleming GF, Filiaci VL, Bentley RC, et al. Phase III randomized trial of doxorubicin + cisplatin versus doxorubicin + 24-h paclitaxel + filgrastim in endometrial carcinoma: a Gynecologic Oncology Group study. Ann Oncol. 2004;15:1173–8.

34. Fossa SD, Kaye SB, Mead GM, et al. Filgrastim during combination chemotherapy of patients with poor-prognosis metastatic germ cell malignancy. European Organization for Research and Treatment of Cancer, Genito-Urinary Group, and the Medical Research Council Testicular Cancer Working Party, Cambridge, United Kingdom. J Clin Oncol. 1998;16:716–24.

35. Fukuoka M, Masuda N, Negoro S, et al. CODE chemotherapy with and without granulocyte colony-stimulating factor in small-cell lung cancer. Br J Cancer. 1997;75:306–9.

36. Fumoleau P, Chauvin F, Namer M, et al. Intensification of adjuvant chemotherapy: 5-year results of a randomized trial comparing conventional doxorubicin and cyclophosphamide with high-dose mitoxantrone and cyclophosphamide with filgrastim in operable breast cancer with 10 or more involved axillary nodes. J Clin Oncol. 2001;19:612–20.

37. Gatzemeier U, Kleisbauer JP, Drings P, et al. Lenograstim as support for ACE chemotherapy of small-cell lung cancer: a phase III, multicenter, randomized study. Am J Clin Oncol. 2000;23:393–400.

38. Gisselbrecht C, Haioun C, Lepage E, et al. Placebo-controlled phase III study of lenograstim (glycosylated recombinant human granulocyte colony-stimulating factor) in aggressive non-Hodgkin's lymphoma: factors influencing chemotherapy administration. Groupe d'Etude des Lymphomes de l'Adulte. Leuk Lymphoma. 1997;25:289–300.

39. Pan D, Qin J, Farber C, et al. CHOP with high dose cyclophosphamide consolidation versus CHOP alone as initial therapy for advanced stage, indolent non-Hodgkin's lymphomas. Leuk Lymphoma. 2003;44:967–71.
40. Papaldo P, Lopez M, Cortesi E, et al. Addition of either lonidamine or granulocyte colony-stimulating factor does not improve survival in early breast cancer patients treated with high-dose epirubicin and cyclophosphamide. J Clin Oncol. 2003;21:3462–8.
41. Pettengell R, Gurney H, Radford JA, et al. Granulocyte colony-stimulating factor to prevent dose-limiting neutropenia in non-Hodgkin's lymphoma: a randomized controlled trial. Blood. 1992;80:1430–6.
42. Pfreundschuh M, Trumper L, Kloess M, et al. Two-weekly or 3-weekly CHOP chemotherapy with or without etoposide for the treatment of elderly patients with aggressive lymphomas: results of the NHL-B2 trial of the DSHNHL. Blood. 2004;104:634–41.
43. Pfreundschuh M, Trumper L, Kloess M, et al. Two-weekly or 3-weekly CHOP chemotherapy with or without etoposide for the treatment of young patients with good-prognosis (normal LDH) aggressive lymphomas: results of the NHL-B1 trial of the DSHNHL. Blood. 2004;104:626–33.
44. Pfreundschuh M, Zwick C, Zeynalova S, et al. Dose-escalated CHOEP for the treatment of young patients with aggressive non-Hodgkin's lymphoma: II. Results of the randomized high-CHOEP trial of the German High-Grade Non-Hodgkin's Lymphoma Study Group (DSHNHL). Ann Oncol. 2008;19:545–52.
45. Sternberg CN, de Mulder P, Schornagel JH, et al. Seven year update of an EORTC phase III trial of high-dose intensity M-VAC chemotherapy and G-CSF versus classic M-VAC in advanced urothelial tract tumours. Eur J Cancer. 2006;42:50–4.
46. Sternberg CN, de Mulder PH, Schornagel JH, et al. Randomized phase III trial of high-dose-intensity methotrexate, vinblastine, doxorubicin, and cisplatin (MVAC) chemotherapy and recombinant human granulocyte colony-stimulating factor versus classic MVAC in advanced urothelial tract tumors: European Organization for Research and Treatment of Cancer Protocol No. 30924. J Clin Oncol. 2001;19:2638–46.
47. Therasse P, Mauriac L, Welnicka-Jaskiewicz M, et al. Final results of a randomized phase III trial comparing cyclophosphamide, epirubicin, and fluorouracil with a dose-intensified epirubicin and cyclophosphamide + filgrastim as neoadjuvant treatment in locally advanced breast cancer: an EORTC–NCIC–SAKK multicenter study. J Clin Oncol. 2003;21:843–50.
48. Venturini M, Del Mastro L, Aitini E, et al. Dose-dense adjuvant chemotherapy in early breast cancer patients: results from a randomized trial.[see comment]. J Natl Cancer Inst. 2005;97:1724–33.
49. Verdonck LF, Notenboom A, de Jong DD, et al. Intensified 12-week CHOP (I-CHOP) plus G-CSF compared with standard 24-week CHOP (CHOP-21) for patients with intermediate-risk aggressive non-Hodgkin lymphoma: a phase 3 trial of the Dutch–Belgian Hemato-Oncology Cooperative Group (HOVON). Blood. 2007;109:2759–66.
50. Veyret C, Levy C, Chollet P, et al. Inflammatory breast cancer outcome with epirubicin-based induction and maintenance chemotherapy: ten-year results from the French Adjuvant Study Group GETIS 02 Trial. Cancer. 2006;107:2535–44.
51. Woll PJ, Hodgetts J, Lomax L, et al. Can cytotoxic dose-intensity be increased by using granulocyte colony-stimulating factor? A randomized controlled trial of lenograstim in small-cell lung cancer. J Clin Oncol. 1995;13:652–9.
52. Zinzani PL, Pavone E, Storti S, et al. Randomized trial with or without granulocyte colony-stimulating factor as adjunct to induction VNCOP-B treatment of elderly high-grade non-Hodgkin's lymphoma. Blood. 1997;89:3974–9.
53. Josting A, Wiedenmann S, Franklin J, et al. Secondary myeloid leukemia and myelodysplastic syndromes in patients treated for Hodgkin's disease: a report from the German Hodgkin's Lymphoma Study Group. J Clin Oncol. 2003;21:3440–6.

Part III
The Erythroid-Stimulating Agents

Chapter 11
Do Erythropoietic-Stimulating Agents Relieve Fatigue? A Review of Reviews

David T. Eton and David Cella

Abstract Interest in the efficacy and potential deleterious consequences of treatment with erythropoietic-stimulating agents (ESAs) is very high. Recently, the ESAs have come under intense scrutiny as several clinical trials have shown their use to be associated with an increased risk of thrombosis, and a concern for increased mortality risk in oncology. In this context, attention to the effect of ESAs upon fatigue and other aspects of quality of life has tended to be lost. To aid inclusion of this endpoint in the important consideration of risks and benefits of ESA therapy, we summarize the many reviews that have been conducted on this topic. The ten selected reviews were all conducted systematically or were otherwise comprehensive. While these reviews acknowledge an overall positive fatigue or quality-of-life effect, some were equivocal about the meaningfulness or magnitude of the benefit. The overall evidence from these reviews supports a fatigue and overall quality-of-life benefit from treatment with ESAs that is unlikely to be due to chance. This information should be included in the risk/benefit consideration of these controversial agents.

Interest in the efficacy and potential deleterious consequences of treatment with erythropoietic-stimulating agents (ESAs) is at a peak. First synthesized in 1985 and approved for use in patients with chronic renal failure, the ESAs were introduced into the oncology setting in the early 1990s as a treatment for chemotherapy-induced anemia (CIA). Since this time a number of oncology clinical trials have shown that the ESAs (including epoetin alfa, epoetin beta, and darbepoetin alfa) are effective at alleviating CIA, decreasing the need for red blood cell transfusion, and decreasing fatigue while improving quality of life. The positive findings of these studies led to an explosion in ESA use with cancer patients, especially in those patients receiving treatments associated with anemia, such as chemotherapy.

D. Cella (✉)
Department of Medical Social Sciences, Prevention and Control, Robert H. Lurie Comprehensive Cancer Center, Northwestern University, Chicago, IL 60611, USA
e-mail: d-cella@northwestern.edu

G.H. Lyman, D.C. Dale (eds.), *Hematopoietic Growth Factors in Oncology*, Cancer Treatment and Research 157, DOI 10.1007/978-1-4419-7073-2_11, © Springer Science+Business Media, LLC 2011

However, more recently the ESAs have come under intense scrutiny as several clinical trials have shown their use to be associated with an increased risk of thrombosis. These concerns as well as the possibility that their use in oncology could pose a mortality risk led the US Food and Drug Administration (FDA) in early 2007 to issue a "black box" warning against using higher than necessary dosages of these drugs. Specifically, this warning cautioned physicians to use the lowest dose needed to gradually raise hemoglobin to *only* the level needed to avoid blood transfusion. Furthermore, the FDA emphasized that target hemoglobin concentrations should not exceed 12 g/dL. These cautions are reflected in the recent update of clinical practice guidelines of the American Society of Clinical Oncology and American Society of Hematology (ASCO/ASH) [1].

In March of 2008, the FDA reconvened its Oncology Drug Advisory Committee to further review safety issues and offer direction for the future. The result of this meeting and subsequent FDA action was to stipulate even greater restriction on package labeling such that ESAs *not be given* to patients who are potentially "curable" and *not be given* to patients with hemoglobin concentrations of 10 g/dL or more. Similarly, the European Medicines Agency (EMEA) has recently recommended that "blood transfusions be preferred in cancer patients with a reasonably long life expectancy." Given that "curable" and "reasonably long life expectancy" are subjective and that blood transfusion typically commences at a hemoglobin level of 8 g/dL, under these new regulatory mandates, clinical usage of the ESAs has been and will continue to be substantially curtailed.

Concern over the safe use of these drugs in the oncology setting is warranted. However, it is important to note that many of the trials demonstrating a higher-mortality risk were published after 2002. Compared with trials published through 2001, those published after 2001 enrolled patients with higher baseline hemoglobin levels, included patients who used higher dosages of ESA, and targeted hemoglobin levels higher than 13 g/dL to prevent anemia recurrence [2]. Thus, in these later trials the ESAs were being used outside of their approved indication – to alleviate mild-to-moderate anemia. While restriction on prophylactic usages would appear to be in order, *over-restriction* of an efficacious drug is ultimately *not* in the best interests of the patient. In the context of today's highly charged debate about safety, it is tempting to revise what is known about efficacy, by highlighting certain findings while simultaneously downplaying or ignoring others. Indeed, many studies of ESA efficacy have shown a symptom or quality-of-life benefit. Given this, a brief review of the evidence to date could be highly illustrative.

Reviewing the Reviews

Sorting through the vast literature on ESAs in oncology requires more focus on patient values and preferences, because it is the patient who must make each individual informed decision about ESA use today. The clinical trials literature on the efficacy of ESAs in cancer patients has been reviewed many times, and several of those reviews have considered the patient perspective, with varying levels of detailed scrutiny. Within the past 5 years alone several high-quality reviews have become available [3–12]. While synthesizing the results of recent clinical trials of ESAs is critical, there is little to be gained by conducting yet another systematic review. A more revealing exercise would be to summarize the findings and evidence outlined in the most recently conducted, high-quality reviews of the ESA literature. Hence, our objective in this chapter is to briefly review the findings of ten systematic reviews of clinical trials in the 5-year period spanning 2004–2008. Half of these reviews were of sufficient quality to serve as the primary evidence base for the 2007 ASCO/ASH practice guideline update (one of which updated a previously conducted report) [4–6, 8–10] and two were used as additional supportive evidence in the guideline update [3, 7]. Two others, including one sponsored by the Cochrane Collaboration, were published after the 2008 publication of the guideline update [11, 12].

Though we summarize findings of salient clinical outcomes such as transfusion rate, hematologic response, survival, and thrombosis risk, we will particularly focus on what these reviews have concluded about patient-reported symptoms and quality-of-life outcomes such as fatigue and self-perception of functioning. We chose to emphasize these outcomes because they are an often neglected component of the complex risk-to-benefit equation in the use of ESAs. There has also been a tendency for some regulatory and systematic reviewers to dismiss these outcomes altogether. As evidence of this neglect, the FDA has stated firmly that fatigue is *not* a benefit of ESA therapy and the pharmaceutical industry has become singly focused on the safety side of the equation. Lack of regard for the quality-of-life outcomes associated with ESA therapy renders the practitioner of evidence-based medicine unable to accurately portray or even define the full range of benefits, harms, and costs of these controversial agents.

Review Summary

Table 11.1 presents the characteristics of the ten systematic reviews. As shown in the table, most of the reviews (seven of ten) provide coverage of studies from 1985, the year that human recombinant erythropoietin was first synthesized. Seven reviews provide coverage of studies up to or through 2005, with one providing coverage through March 2007. Three reviews were supported by the Cochrane Collaboration. Seven of the reviews focused exclusively on randomized trials, while the other three summarize findings from a mix of randomized and un-randomized studies. There were two reviews [3, 12] that focused exclusively on the impact of ESAs on patient quality-of-life (QOL) or self-reported symptoms (i.e., fatigue). The other eight reviews summarize data for a host of clinical outcomes including transfusion rate, hematologic response, survival, and safety (most notably, thrombosis risk) as well as QOL. However, it should be noted that in many of these reviews a smaller subset of the total included studies actually provide QOL data.

Table 11.1 Characteristics and quality-of-life findings of ESA reviews (2004–2008)

References	Coverage years	No. and type of studies[a]	Symptoms/QOL findings[b]
Jones et al. [3]	1985–2002	Twenty-three studies (11,459 patients) RCTs (placebo or supportive care) and single-arm (open-label) studies of epoetin alfa in cancer patients ($\geq$20 patients per treatment arm required)	QOL results from three validated, common-use scales were meta-analyzed (LASA, FACT, and SF-36) Mean changes in LASA scores (energy level, activity, overall QOL) from baseline were positive and substantial in epoetin-treated cohorts. Improvements of 20–25%. Control cohorts remained unchanged or worsened Mean changes in FACT scores from baseline were positive and substantial in epoetin-treated cohorts. Largest improvements observed for the FACT-F (17%) and FACT-Anemia (12%) subscales. Control cohorts remained unchanged or worsened Mean changes on four SF-36 subscales (physical, role-physical, vitality, and social function) from baseline were significant and positive in the epoetin-treated cohorts. Control cohorts worsened on most of these subscales Notably, improvements in LASA scores were significant in epoetin-treated patients in double-blind AND open-label studies; however, the largest improvements were seen in the latter. QOL results remained consistent even when possible placebo effects were controlled
Bohlius et al. [4] (Cochrane review)	1985–2001	Twenty-seven studies (3,287 patients) RCTs of epoetin alfa or epoetin beta vs transfusion Fifteen – epoetin alfa Eight – epoetin beta Three – unspecified One – epoetin alfa or beta (14 placebo-controlled; 13 standard of care control)	QOL data incl. in 14 studies; 2,113 patients. Method and reporting inconsistencies precluded meta-analysis. "Vote counting" used to summarize results. Eight of the 14 studies showed improvement in at least one QOL domain for patients in an epoetin arm Results deemed too inconsistent to conclude that epoetin improves QOL or fatigue

Table 11.1 (continued)

References	Coverage years	No. and type of studies[a]	Symptoms/QOL findings[b]
Bohlius et al. [5] (Cochrane review: update of Bohlius et al. [4])	1985–April, 2005	Fifty-seven studies – incl. 27 from Bohlius et al. [4] review (9,353 patients) RCTs of epoetin (alfa and beta) or darbepoetin vs observation + transfusion Forty – epoetin alfa Eight – epoetin beta Three – unspecified Five – darbepoetin alfa One – epoetin alfa or beta (31 placebo-controlled; 26 standard of care control)	QOL data incl. in 16 studies; 3,670 patients. Method inconsistencies in quantifying and reporting QOL and fatigue data precluded meta-analysis. "Vote counting" used to summarize results Nine studies (incl. five placebo-controlled) used the FACT (general, anemia, and/or fatigue scales). Impact determined by counting the number of stat. significant results favoring epoetin/darbepoetin vs the number of stat. significant results favoring controls: –FACT-G: two epoetin/darbepoetin vs zero control –Anemia subscale: one epoetin/darbepoetin vs zero control –Fatigue subscale: five epoetin/darbepoetin vs zero control Ten studies (incl. five placebo-controlled) used LASA scales (energy, activity level, and overall QOL). Impact determined by counting the number of stat. significant results favoring epoetin/darbepoetin vs the number of stat. significant results favoring controls: –Energy: three epoetin/darbepoetin vs zero control –Activity level: three epoetin/darbepoetin vs zero control –Overall QOL: five epoetin/darbepoetin vs zero control Too few studies use other "generic" measures to draw any conclusions Actual size of QOL effects could not be quantified Evidence is deemed "suggestive" that epoetin and darbepoetin may improve QOL
Seidenfeld et al. [6]	1999–March, 2005	Fifty-nine studies (11,757 patients) Randomized trials: Seven – comparisons of darbepoetin and epoetin Forty-eight – RCTs of epoetin vs control Four – RCTs of darbepoetin vs control	QOL data incl. in 15 studies; 3,610 patients. Method and reporting inconsistencies precluded meta-analysis. "Vote counting" used to summarize results Overall, QOL measures tended to favor treatment with epoetin or darbepoetin compared to control; however, the degree of change varied widely across studies. Eight of 15 studies favored treatment using the FACT-Fatigue subscale. No evidence provided on the clinical significance of results

Table 11.1 (continued)

References	Coverage years	No. and type of studies[a]	Symptoms/QOL findings[b]
Ross et al. [7]	1980–July, 2005	Forty studies (21,378 patients) Randomized and non-randomized (but controlled) trials of patients treated with epoetin or darbepoetin for chemotherapy-induced anemia (CIA: Hgb < 11 g/dL) and prospective, uncontrolled studies enrolling ≥300 CIA patients	Five controlled trials used FACT-Fatigue subscale; four controlled trials used LASA scales for overall fatigue. Results meta-analyzed – effect size (ES) of mean difference in change between epoetin/darbepoetin and control arms Small, but significant improvement in fatigue for epoetin/darbepoetin patients compared to controls: FACT-Fatigue ES = 0.23 (95% CI, 0.10–0.36) and LASA ES = 0.36 (95% CI, 0.14–0.57). No differences on FACT-Fatigue between epoetin and darbepoetin groups (two studies): ES = −0.06 (95% CI, −0.17 to 0.04).
Wilson et al. [8]	1996– September, 2004	Forty-six studies – incl. 27 from Bohlius et al. [4] review (7,304 patients) RCTs comparing epoetin or darbepoetin vs control (placebo or standard of care)	QOL data incl. in 20 studies; 3,185 patients. "Vote counting" and qualitative assessment used to summarize the symptom/QOL data. Studies were classified as having a "positive," "negative," or "neutral" effect (no accounting for effect sizes). Lack of detailed reporting of QOL outcomes made it unfeasible to use meta-analysis Twenty-nine "positive" QOL effects (in favor of epoetin/darbepoetin group); 19 of these effects were statistically significant Eight "neutral" QOL effects (no difference between epoetin/darbepoetin and control groups) One "negative" QOL effect (in favor of control group) Overall, a positive effect of epoetin/darbepoetin on QOL was observed. Notably, less than half of the trials (eight) were placebo-controlled with patients blinded to treatment

Table 11.1 (continued)

References	Coverage years	No. and type of studies[a]	Symptoms/QOL findings[b]
Quirt et al. [9]	1966–March, 2005	Forty-eight studies – 34 in previous guideline + 14 in most recent update (12,048 patients) Thirty-four RCTs: Twenty-three – epoetin vs standard of care Eleven – epoetin vs placebo Two randomized trials comparing darbepoetin to epoetin; two randomized trials comparing two doses of epoetin Ten non-controlled epoetin studies of QOL *Note*: All trials involved cancer patients with non-hematologic malignancies receiving chemotherapy	QOL data incl. in 24 studies (14 randomized, 10 non-controlled); 9,252 patients. "Vote counting" and qualitative assessment used to summarize the symptom/QOL data from common-use instruments (i.e., LASA, FACT, SF-36, NHP, EORTC QLQ-C30) Six RCTs showed significant improvements in QOL (one or more domains of LASA) for epoetin groups compared with controls Among RCTs using other QOL measures, five reported significant increases in QOL for epoetin groups compared with controls; three reported no significant differences between epoetin and control groups Over all measures, only three RCTs showed no significant difference in QOL between epoetin and control groups Among the ten non-controlled (mostly single-arm) studies, four showed significant improvements from baseline on three LASA scales (energy, activity level and overall QOL) and three showed significant improvements from baseline on the FACT-Anemia subscale. All ten studies showed some improvement in QOL for epoetin-treated cohorts (*p*-values not reported in two studies)

Table 11.1 (continued)

References	Coverage years	No. and type of studies[a]	Symptoms/QOL findings[b]
Shehata et al. [10]	1985–2005	Fifteen studies (2,454 patients) Fourteen RCTs: Five – epoetin alfa vs placebo (four double-blind) Four – epoetin alfa vs standard of care Two – darbepoetin vs placebo (both double-blind) Two – epoetin beta vs standard of care One – epoetin beta vs placebo (double-blind) One randomized trial comparing two doses of epoetin beta *Note*: All trials involved cancer patients with hematologic malignancies receiving chemotherapy	QOL data incl. in seven RCTs; 1,699 patients. "Vote counting" and qualitative assessment used to summarize the symptom/QOL data from common-use instruments (i.e., LASA, FACT, SF-36, NHP). Due to method limitations QOL data were not pooled. Across all seven studies, six reported improvement in at least one QOL domain for epoetin/darbepoetin compared with control groups. Four studies used the FACT (general, anemia, and/or fatigue scales). All four reported significant improvement in QOL for epoetin/darbepoetin groups compared with controls. Two studies used LASA scales (energy, activity level, and overall QOL). One study reported significant improvement on all three LASA scales for epoetin group compared with the control group; the other study reported no significant difference between epoetin and control groups on any LASA scale. One study using the NHP reported no differences in improvement of QOL between epoetin and placebo groups
Kimel et al. [11]	1993–September, 2005	Nine cancer studies (1,949 patients) RCTs comparing epoetin alfa vs placebo ($n = 6$) or standard of care ($n = 3$)	All studies used at least one measure from the FACT-Anemia scale and seven studies used LASA scales for energy, daily activities, and overall QOL. Results were not meta-analyzed. Differences in QOL change scores between epoetin and control groups were qualitatively summarized. Absolute differences in FACT-Fatigue change scores ranged from 1.8 to 7.9 with change scores favoring epoetin arms in all but one comparison (70% of these differences were clinically significant, i.e., ≥ 3.0). Absolute differences in LASA-energy change scores ranged from 0.8 to 19.8 mm with change scores favoring epoetin arms in all but one comparison (86% of these differences were clinically significant, i.e., ≥ 8.0)

Table 11.1 (continued)

References	Coverage years	No. and type of studies[a]	Symptoms/QOL findings[b]
Minton et al. [12] (Cochrane review)	1966–March, 2007	Twenty-seven studies in full analysis; 14 epoetin or darbepoetin studies (5,385 patients) RCTs comparing epoetin/darbepoetin vs placebo or standard of care; ten epoetin trials (five open-label; five placebo-controlled) and four darbepoetin trials (all placebo-controlled)	Results of patient-reported fatigue (i.e., FACT-F) were meta-analyzed Overall combined effect size from ten epoetin studies: Z score $= 8.32$ ($p < 0.001$); standardized mean difference (SMD) $= -0.30$ (95% CI -0.46 to -0.29), indicating a fatigue effect of epoetin over control (standard care or placebo) Overall combined effect size from four darbepoetin studies: Z score $= 1.45$ ($p = 0.05$); standardized mean difference (SMD) $= -0.13$ (95% CI -0.27 to 0.00), indicating a small but significant fatigue effect of darbepoetin over placebo control Weighted mean differences (WMDs) were generated for studies using the FACT-F subscale. The WMD for epoetin studies was 4.33, a difference above the threshold for clinical significance. The WMD for darbepoetin studies was -1.96, a difference below the threshold for clinical significance. The WMD for epoetin + darbepoetin studies combined was 3.75, a difference above the threshold for clinical significance

[a]RCT: Randomized Controlled Trial. Hgb: Hemoglobin; g/dL: grams per deciliter; QOL: Quality Of Life.

[b]LASA: Linear Analog Self-Assessment; FACT: Functional Assessment of Cancer Therapy; SF-36: Short Form-36; FACT-F: Functional Assessment of Cancer Therapy-Fatigue scale; FACT-G: Functional Assessment of Cancer Therapy-General scale; NHP: Nottingham Health Profile. EORTC QLQ-C30: European Organization for Research and Treatment of Cancer Quality of Life Questionnaire-Core 30.

Clinical Outcomes

Table 11.2 briefly summarizes the results for clinical outcomes *other than* symptoms and QOL (i.e., transfusion rate, hematologic response, survival, and thrombosis risk). As the table shows, there is extensive support for the efficacy of ESAs when compared to treatment with placebo- or standard of care-control. Among all of the reviews in which it was reported, there were fewer blood transfusions and better hematologic responses among patients treated with ESA versus controls. The results for survival and thrombosis risk (the primary adverse event of interest in studies of ESAs) were mixed. Three reviews reported no differences in survival between patients treated with ESA versus controls, whereas four reviews deemed evidence to be insufficient to draw any conclusion about survival (three reviews did not report survival data). With respect to thrombosis, two reviews found a higher risk in ESA-treated patients versus controls, two reviews found no difference in risk between ESA-treated patients versus controls, and three reviews deemed the evidence insufficient to draw any conclusions about thrombosis risk (three reviews did not report data on thrombosis risk). Overall, the evidence from these reviews would appear to support the conclusion that ESA therapy does reduce the need for blood transfusion and may lead to a clinically significant rise in hemoglobin in anemic cancer patients. Furthermore, while the evidence from these reviews seems to support that there may be an elevated risk of thrombo-embolic complications in patients treated with an ESA, the available evidence is currently insufficient to determine whether the ESAs are associated with decreased survival.

Patient-Reported Symptoms and Quality of Life

Given the somewhat mixed profile of the findings for clinical outcomes, the findings for patient-reported symptoms (i.e., fatigue) and QOL should take on added significance. It is conceivable that such findings could be used to "tip the balance" either for ESA use or against it. If the symptom and QOL data do not consistently favor ESA therapy then treatment with these agents would simply not be worth the risks *under any circumstances*. However, if the symptom and QOL data do consistently favor ESA therapy then continued use of these agents might be warranted and clinical interest should be focused on mitigating any possible risks, that is, *determining those circumstances* when the ESAs can be used safely.

The last column of Table 11.1 presents the findings for patient-reported symptoms and QOL. Symptom and QOL results were synthesized via statistical meta-analysis [3, 7, 12], "vote counting" (counting the number of statistically significant results favoring ESA vs control arms) [4–6, 8–10] or qualitative summary [11]. All ten reviews provide at least some data showing a symptom and/or QOL benefit of ESA therapy. However, not all reviewers draw the same conclusions from these findings. Seidenfeld et al. [6] and Shehata et al. [10] deemed the evidence "insufficient" to draw any definitive conclusions about the effects of ESAs on symptoms and

Table 11.2 Clinical findings of ESA reviews (2004–2008)

References	Transfusion	Hematologic response	Survival	Thrombosis risk
Jones et al. [3]	NR	NR	NR	NR
Bohlius et al. [4]	+	+	IE	IE
Bohlius et al. [5]	+	+	IE	−
Seidenfeld et al. [6]	+	+	IE	−
Ross et al. [7]	+	NR	0	0
Wilson et al. [8]	+	+	0	IE
Quirt et al. [9]	+	NR	NR	IE
Shehata et al. [10]	+	NR[a]	IE	0
Kimel et al. [11]	+	NR[a]	0	NR
Minton et al. [12]	NR	NR	NR	NR

Note: +, results favor ESA over control; −, results favor control over ESA; 0, no difference between ESA and control; IE, insufficient evidence to draw a conclusion; NR, not reported. Hematologic response defined as a rise in hemoglobin $\geq$ 2 g/dL.
[a]On balance, most studies from this review report an increase in hemoglobin concentration that favors ESA over control; however, a 2 g/dL rise was not specified.

QOL. In their first Cochrane review, Bohlius and colleagues [4] claimed that the evidence was "too inconsistent" to conclude that ESAs improve fatigue and/or QOL. In an updated Cochrane review that included data from an additional 30 studies published since 2002, Bohlius and colleagues [5] stated that the evidence was now "suggestive" that ESAs may improve fatigue and/or QOL. In their meta-analysis, Ross and colleagues [7] documented a small, but significant benefit in self-reported fatigue favoring ESA-treated patients versus controls, though there were no fatigue differences between epoetin-treated and darbepoetin-treated patients.

Five other reviews (including two meta-analyses) concluded that ESA therapy does improve symptoms and/or QOL in cancer patients [3, 8, 9, 11, 12]. In the Jones et al. meta-analysis, the QOL benefit of epoetin alfa was maintained even after placebo effects were statistically controlled. Among 20 studies containing QOL data, Wilson et al. counted 29 "positive" QOL effects (favoring ESA-treated patients) and only one "negative" QOL effect (favoring control patients). However, there was no accounting for the size of these effects. In two of the most recent reviews, both Kimel et al. [11] and Minton et al. [12] draw attention to the clinical significance of the QOL effects. Kimel et al. observed that 70% of the differences in

FACT-Fatigue change scores favoring ESA versus control arms were clinically significant (≥ 3 points). Further, 86% of the differences in LASA-energy change scores favoring ESA versus control arms were clinically significant (≥ 8 mm). Finally, in their meta-analysis conducted for the Cochrane Collaboration, Minton et al. generated weighted mean differences (WMDs) for ESA trials that used the FACT-Fatigue subscale. The WMD weights and standardizes change score differences between ESA and control arms. The WMD for epoetin + darbepoetin studies combined was 3.75, a difference above the threshold for clinical significance and indicative of a fatigue benefit for ESA-treated compared with placebo-treated or standard care-treated patients.

When interpreting the findings of these syntheses, several methodological limitations of the reviewed studies must be kept in mind [4–6]. First, not all of the reviewed studies are placebo-controlled or double-blinded. Single-arm, non-randomized, and open-label studies could be subject to placebo effects, an especially salient threat to validity when the outcome is self-reported by patients. Second, many studies failed to report the metrics needed to allow for a more formal statistical meta-analysis of symptom and QOL outcomes (i.e., means and appropriate measures of dispersion). Third, there were substantial losses of symptom and QOL data at follow-up in many studies, plus a number of studies failed to adequately document how the missing follow-up data were handled. In those that did, a last observation carried forward approach was often used to impute the data – an approach that can bias results. Finally, many studies did not provide details of the timing and circumstances under which the symptom and QOL measures were administered. These limitations notwithstanding, the overall evidence from these reviews would seem to support a symptom and QOL benefit from treatment with ESAs that is unlikely to be due to chance.

Conclusions

Our intent in reviewing recent reviews is not to overemphasize symptom and QOL data, while ignoring data on safety. Indeed, we suggest that simultaneous consideration of all the benefits and harms of these agents should be weighed together. Concerns for safety should be considered in the context of efficacy and cost and in the context of survival they become paramount. However, restricting the use of drugs that may be safe and effective *when used appropriately* can be a disservice to patients. Perhaps we are approaching an important crossroads with respect to the ESAs. On the one hand, oncologists could abandon the use of these drugs altogether, on the other, clinical and biological science can probe further into the mechanisms of action and work toward understanding when and how they can be used safely. While there are no guarantees that the latter will be accomplished, premature abandonment of these drugs may leave patients and clinicians with few viable therapeutic alternatives.

So what are the next steps? We feel that specifying the conditions for the safe use of ESA therapy should be the next area of focus. This should include assessments of when and for whom benefits and harms will be expected to occur. Stated more empirically this could involve simultaneous calculations of the number needed to treat and the number needed to harm. It could also include elucidation of whether the benefits and harms of ESA therapy depend on baseline anemia status, and whether this could change based on patient demographic, clinical, or genetic factors. Can an *empirically-derived* cutoff be specified above which ESA therapy is contraindicated? Furthermore, a better understanding of what an appropriate target hemoglobin level is could allay clinician confusion about when ESA therapy should be terminated. While ongoing and future clinical trials will undoubtedly help, many of these issues could also be addressed through detailed analysis of secondary data sources such as the current efforts of the Cochrane Collaborative to meta-analyze individual patient-level data from archival trial data.

Finally, we might also allow the lessons of the past to educate us about the directions for the future. Overenthusiasm for the ESAs laid the foundation for expansive use, often outside of its approved indication. Today, as the momentum shifts from efficacy toward safety, the risk is greater that *appropriate* ESA use will be discouraged if not disallowed. One critical stakeholder in weighing the potential benefits and harms of ESA therapy is the patient. Tools to educate patients about the probabilities of benefit and harm can help guide us toward appropriate ESA use. Patient-reported outcome data, part of the ESA benefit–harm ratio, are the source of the information patients need to understand how their lives are likely to be affected by use (or lack of use) of ESA therapy.

References

1. Rizzo JD, Somerfeld MR, Hagerty KL, Seidenfeld J, Bohlius J, Bennett CL, et al. Use of epoetin and darbepoetin in patients with cancer: 2007 American Society of Clinical Oncology/American Society of Hematology clinical practice guideline update. J Clin Oncol. 2008;26:132–49.
2. Bohlius J, Wilson J, Seidenfeld J, Piper M, Schwarzer G, Sandercock J, et al. Recombinant human erythropoietins and cancer patients: updated meta-analysis of 57 studies including 9353 patients. J Natl Cancer Inst. 2006;98:708–14.
3. Jones M, Schenkel B, Just J, Fallowfield L. Epoetin alfa improves quality of life in patients with cancer: results of a meta-analysis. Cancer. 2004;101:1720–32.
4. Bohlius J, Langensiepen S, Schwarzer G, Seidenfeld J, Piper M, Bennet C, et al. Erythropoietin for patients with malignant disease (review). Cochrane Database Syst Rev. 2005;4:1–153.
5. Bohlius J, Wilson J, Seidenfeld J, Piper M, Schwarzer G, Sandercock J, et al. Erythropoietin or darbepoetin for patients with cancer. Cochrane Database Syst Rev. 2006;3:1–228.
6. Seidenfeld J, Piper M, Bohlius J, Weingart O, Trelle S, Engert A, et al. Comparative effectiveness of epoetin and darbepoetin for managing anemia in patients undergoing cancer treatment. Comparative effectiveness review no. 3. Agency for Healthcare Research & Quality, May 2006.
7. Ross SD, Allen E, Henry DH, Seaman C, Sercus B, Goodnough LT. Clinical benefits and risks associated with epoetin and darbepoetin in patients with chemotherapy-induced anemia: a systematic review of the literature. Clin Ther. 2006;28:1–31.

8. Wilson J, Yao GL, Raftery J, Bohlius J, Brunskill S, Sandercock J, et al. A systematic review and economic evaluation of epoetin alfa, epoetin beta and darbepoetin alfa in anaemia associated with cancer, especially that attributable to cancer treatment. Health Technol Assess. 2007;11:1–220.
9. Quirt I, Bramwell V, Charette M, Oliver T. The role of erythropoietin in the management of cancer patients with non-hematologic malignancies receiving chemotherapy. Practice guideline report #12-1. Toronto, ON: Cancer Care Ontario, 2007.
10. Shehata N, Walker I, Meyer R, Haynes AE, Imrie K. Treatment for anemia with erythropoietic agents in patients with non-myeloid hematological malignancies. A clinical practice guideline. Toronto, ON: Cancer Care Ontario, 2007.
11. Kimel M, Leidy NK, Mannix S, Dixon J. Does epoetin alfa improve health-related quality of life in chronically ill patients with anemia? Summary of trials of cancer, HIV/AIDS, and chronic kidney disease. Value Health. 2008;11:57–75.
12. Minton O, Stone P, Richardson A, Sharpe M, Hotopf M. Drug therapy for the management of cancer-related fatigue. Cochrane Database Syst Rev. 2008;1:1–43.

Chapter 12
Randomized Controlled Trials of the Erythroid-Stimulating Agents in Cancer Patients

John A. Glaspy

Cytopenias, including leukopenia, anemia, and thrombocytopenia, have been commonly encountered in cancer patients since the advent of myelosuppressive chemotherapy and have presented difficult challenges to the management of these patients. Anemia is particularly common [1] and is usually multifactorial, with the major contributing factors including the disturbances in iron metabolism associated with chronic inflammatory illness [2–5] and the myelosuppressive effects of cytotoxic chemotherapy (Fig. 12.1). In addition, these patients may have absolute iron deficiency, related to prior bleeding, surgery, malnutrition or repeated phlebotomy, active bleeding, marrow replacement with tumor, renal insufficiency, or hemolysis contributing to the observed anemia. The cloning and clinical development of the glycoproteins involved in the regulation of hematopoiesis was a watershed event in the practice of oncology, opening new approaches to the cytopenias observed in cancer patients.

The normal physiologic response to anemia is an increase in circulating erythropoietin levels resulting in a compensatory increase in erythropoietic stimulus to the marrow. Early on, it was demonstrated that cancer patients with the anemia of chronic illness – usually referred to in the literature as anemia of cancer (AOC) – often have a blunted erythropoietin response to anemia: a relative erythropoietin deficiency [6]. This important observation formed the initial rationale for clinical trials of the cloned preparations of human erythropoietin in anemic cancer patients. Because the other disturbances in erythropoiesis in AOC, namely, reduced access to storage iron, the suppressive effects of inflammatory cytokines, and the effects of cytotoxic chemotherapy, might act to reduce the erythropoietic response to a given level of circulating erythropoietin, a second rationale for the administration of exogenous erythropoietins was that the level of erythropoietin requisite to maximally support erythropoiesis in this setting might be even higher than that achieved in the normal response to anemia [7]. Hence, in dose-finding clinical trials,

J.A. Glaspy (✉)
Division of Hematology and Oncology, Department of Medicine, David Geffen School of Medicine – UCLA, Los Angeles, CA 90095, USA
e-mail: jglaspy@mednet.ucla.edu

G.H. Lyman, D.C. Dale (eds.), *Hematopoietic Growth Factors in Oncology*,
Cancer Treatment and Research 157, DOI 10.1007/978-1-4419-7073-2_12,
© Springer Science+Business Media, LLC 2011

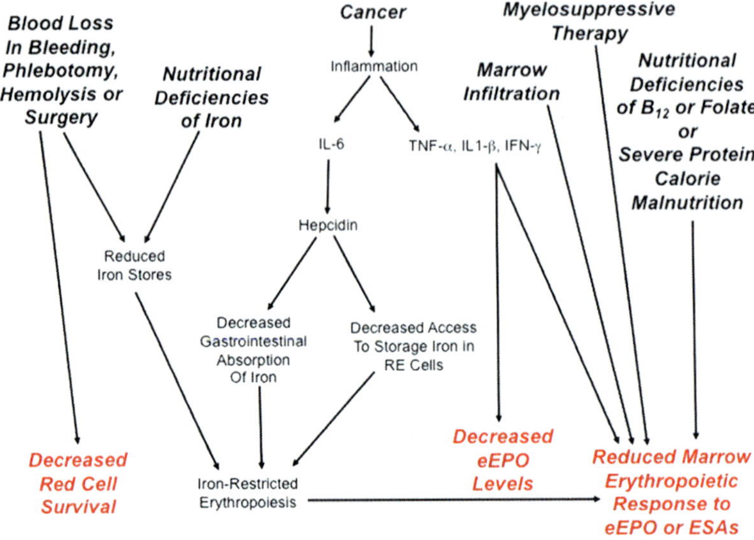

Fig. 12.1 The pathogenesis of anemia in cancer patients. Multiple factors result in three mechanisms of anemia: a reduced response of the erythron to EPO, a relative deficiency of eEPO, and a decrease in red cell survival. Iron-restricted erythropoiesis, due either to reduced iron stores or a diminished access to storage pools mediated by hepcidin, is frequently present in cancer patients. (RE = reticuloendothelial, TNF-α = tumor necrosis factor-alpha, IL1-β = interleukin beta, IFN-γ = interferon gamma, and IL-6 = interleukin 6.)

the endpoint chosen was evidence of increased erythropoiesis and reduction in anemia, not merely correction of the relative erythropoietin deficiency. It was found that the doses of these agents necessary to induce a significant increase in hemoglobin level were significantly higher than that usually required to correct anemia in clinical conditions, such as renal failure, wherein the major erythropoietic challenge is a reduction in erythropoietin levels [8]. Cancer patients are not only relatively erythropoietin deficient, but they are also relatively erythropoietin resistant, especially when they are receiving cytotoxic chemotherapy and this biology has important consequences for the therapeutic use of erythropoietic agents in oncology.

There are now several preparations of cloned human erythropoietin available worldwide [9]. The vast majority of the useful clinical data relevant to cancer patients have been generated using three preparations: recombinant human erythropoietin alfa, recombinant human erythropoietin beta (available only outside the United States), and recombinant darbepoetin alfa. Because the efficacy and safety data appear similar for all three preparations and the few randomized trials that have compared these agents have not identified differences in overall efficacy or safety [10], this chapter will treat them as a group, using the term erythropoiesis-stimulating agents (ESAs). In patients with anemia during cancer chemotherapy – usually referred to in the literature as chemotherapy-induced anemia (CIA) – treatment with ESAs has been clearly and consistently shown to result in an increase in mean hemoglobin levels and a reduction in the incidence of red cell transfusion.

There are also data indicating that responding patients with CIA experience a reduction in fatigue and/or an improvement in functional status, although this has not been as consistent an observation. More recently, safety concerns have arisen regarding ESAs and their use in cancer patients, which will be discussed below following a review of efficacy data in various settings in oncology.

Efficacy in Treatment of Chemotherapy-Induced Anemia

Randomized clinical trials have demonstrated that, when ESAs are utilized to treat chemotherapy-induced anemia, therapy is associated with an increase in mean hemoglobin levels and a reduction in the incidence of red blood cell transfusions. The relative risk of red cell transfusion for ESA-treated compared to control patients reported in summaries of all randomized clinical trials including more than 6,000 patients has been approximately 0.65 and highly statistically significant [11–14]. This finding has been consistent across trials and over time and there is widespread agreement that this is an established benefit of ESAs used to treat patients with CIA. Several studies have also suggested that ESA therapy is associated with a decrease in fatigue and increase in functional capacity [15, 16], although not all studies have identified this effect [17]. Both the multifactorial nature of fatigue in cancer patients and questions regarding the best instruments to measure these patient-reported outcomes have prevented this benefit from being recognized by regulatory authorities such as the Food and Drug Administration.

Efficacy in the Treatment of Anemia of Cancer

Randomized clinical trials of ESAs for the treatment of AOC have generally observed an increase in mean hemoglobin concentrations in treated patients, but have failed to demonstrate a statistically significant reduction in red cell transfusion rates [18, 19]. This failure to translate an observed erythropoietic effect into a demonstrable reduction in transfusion benefit may be due to: (1) some trials having utilized lower ESA doses and/or durations of therapy than the CIA trials and (2) transfusion rates being lower in patients with AOC, reducing the statistical power of trials of a given size to demonstrate an effect. In one sufficiently large randomized trial [19], the majority of patients were enrolled at centers outside the United States, some of which failed to transfuse patients who met criteria for red cell transfusion due to insufficient blood bank resources. Had these patients had access to transfusion services and received the indicated transfusions, the data from this trial indicate that a reduction in transfusions would have been demonstrated. Nevertheless, in randomized trials to date, there has not been a clear demonstration of a reduction of transfusions with ESA therapy for patients with AOC and these agents have accordingly not been labeled by the Food and Drug Administration for this indication. Moreover, in the largest randomized trial of ESAs for AOC, a decreased survival was observed in the ESA-treated patients [19]. This safety concern, coupled with the failure of randomized trials to demonstrate a clinical benefit, clearly supports a conclusion that ESAs should not be utilized to treat anemia in this setting.

Efficacy in the Prevention of Anemia and Tumor Cell Hypoxia

Anemia has been consistently identified as a negative prognostic factor across all cancer histologies, and although it remains entirely possible that anemia is simply a marker for extensive disease or serious co-morbidities, it has been suspected that anemia may play more direct role in the pathophysiology of cancer progression [20, 21]. Owing to both growth kinetics and a disorganized vasculature cells comprising solid tumors are particularly prone to become hypoxic [22] and the effects of anemia on cancer biology are most often attributed to the association of even mild or moderate degrees of anemia with hypoxia in the tumor microenvironment [23]. Hypoxia is associated with a cellular response that includes a rapid increase in levels of the transcription factor, hypoxia-inducible factor (HIF), that leads to an increased activity of several hypoxia response genes, including vascular endothelial growth factor (VEGF), glucose transporters, and erythropoietin [24]. In cancers, this adaptive response to hypoxia will have the effect of increasing angiogenesis and promoting metabolic changes that enhance tumor cell survival [25].

Tumor cell hypoxia has been linked to increased mutation rates and the development of aggressive phenotypes in cancer cells [26–28] and with resistance to radiotherapy [29–33] and cytotoxic chemotherapy [34, 35]. These considerations, coupled with preclinical evidence that treating anemia with ESAs might improve tumor outcomes [36] or reverse hypoxia-induced resistance to radiation [37] and chemotherapy [38], led to an interest in the use of ESAs to prevent anemia and/or to increase hemoglobin concentrations to supra-normal levels, with the goal of enhancing response to radiotherapy or chemotherapy and improve tumor outcomes [39]. However, there are only very limited data on the relationship of hemoglobin concentration to tumor cell oxygenation at supra-normal hemoglobin levels in humans and the available data suggest that increasing hemoglobin levels above 13 g/dL may result in increased tumor cell hypoxia [40], presumably due to the rheology of blood in the tortuous tumor vasculature. In randomized trials of ESAs to enhance tumor oxygenation, hemoglobin levels substantially above 13 g/dL have frequently been achieved in ESA-treated patients, making interpretation of efficacy results complex and leaving the tumor cell hypoxia hypothesis with respect to ESAs essentially unanswered. With this caveat regarding the shortcomings of the available randomized trials, to date, no randomized trials of ESAs to enhance response to radiotherapy or chemotherapy have demonstrated any benefit to ESA therapy in terms of tumor response or survival. Moreover, as delineated below, in some of these oxygenation trials, a reduced survival was observed in ESA-treated patients. There are no clinical data supporting the use of ESAs to prevent anemia or enhance tumor response in cancer patients and there is some indication that increasing hemoglobin concentrations to levels of 13 g/dL or greater may be harmful to cancer patients. There is currently no support for the use of ESAs to prevent anemia and enhance therapeutic outcomes in clinical practice.

Safety Considerations

General Safety Issues with ESAs

Therapy with ESAs has been associated with hypertension and an increased risk of thrombosis in clinical settings outside oncology. Initially, it was believed that this might be due to an expansion of red blood cell mass in patients with renal failure who were unable to appropriately adjust plasma volume. However, these effects have now been well documented in patients, including cancer patients, with normal renal function. This has been taken as indirect evidence that there may be functional erythropoietin receptors (EPO-R) on normal vascular endothelial cells. However, more direct attempts to demonstrate the presence of these receptors have yielded conflicting results and the existence of vascular EPO-R remains controversial and an area of active investigation.

One toxicity unique to cloned human proteins is the potential for the exogenous material to be immunogenic and to induce the production of antibodies that cross-react with and clear the endogenous protein resulting in a sustained deficiency. Several years ago, an increase in the expected incidence of pure red cell aplasia (PRCA) was noted in dialysis patients outside the United States treated with a new recombinant erythropoietin preparation [41]. This was traced to the development of anti-erythropoietin antibodies following therapy with the new preparation; the production issues were addressed and PRCA rates returned to the expected low levels [42]. Although the induction of auto-antibody production is a potential risk of cloned protein therapy, PRCA has been rare with the current preparations and has not been reported to be increased in patients with cancer receiving ESAs. Nevertheless, the stability and immunogenicity of newer ESAs will be a concern relevant to all ESA-treated patients as generic preparations appear in Europe and the United States.

ESA Therapy and Thrombosis in Cancer Patients

Although most randomized trials of ESAs in cancer patients have not observed a statistically significant increase in observed thrombotic events in ESA-treated patients, these trials were not powered with thrombosis as a primary endpoint and in many there were trends suggesting a higher rate of observed thrombosis in the ESA arm. Meta-analyses of the randomized trials of ESAs in cancer patients have consistently found a significantly higher rate of thrombosis in ESA-treated patients, with a relative risk in the range of 1.67 (95% CI 1.35–2.06) [13]. This increase in thrombosis appears to be limited to venous events and have been observed most frequently in patients undergoing radiotherapy and/or patients with gynecological malignancies [43, 44]. There is little evidence linking the risk of thrombosis to the rate of rise in hemoglobin level or peak level of hemoglobin achieved in an individual patient and the mechanism of the increase in thrombosis remains unclear. Possibilities that have been proposed include the following: activation of vascular endothelium [45], interaction with thrombopoietin in priming platelets [46], activation of platelets through their interaction with reticulocytes [47], and increases in blood viscosity associated with a changing hemoglobin level.

Effects of ESAs on Tumor Progression or Survival in Cancer Patients

The major safety issue for ESAs in oncology in recent years has been their potential effects on tumor progression and survival [48, 49]. These concerns have arisen as a result of the publication or presentation of several randomized trials of ESAs in cancer patients in which increased loco-regional progression and/or decreased survival was observed in patients randomized to receive ESAs compared to controls (Fig. 12.2). Overall, the available data are conflicting; in most cases the negative effect on tumor outcomes has not been observed in other, similar randomized trials. The available data are also complex; with randomized trials of ESAs for CIA, AOC, and tumor oxygenation/anemia prevention in a variety of malignancies with therapy initiated at a variety of different hemoglobin levels aiming therapy at various hemoglobin targets.

In the majority of the trials of concern, the objective has been to reduce tumor cell hypoxia by preventing anemia or driving hemoglobin concentrations to supra-normal levels in the ESA-treated arm to improve tumor outcomes. In these trials,

Study	N	Tumor	Indication/Rx	Entry HB	PFS	OS
Leyland-Jones	939	Breast	hypoxia-reduction/ chemotherapy	13 g/dL	neutral	reduced
Henke	351	Head+Neck	hypoxia-reduction/ radiotherapy	12 g/dL F 13 g/dL M	reduced	reduced
Overgaard	484	Head+Neck	hypoxia-reduction/ radiotherapy	12-13 g/dL	reduced	neutral
PREPARE	735	Breast	hypoxia-reduction/ chemotherapy	13 g/dL	trend	trend
GOG 191	109	Cervical	hypoxia-reduction/ chemotherapy+ radiotherapy	12 g/dL	trend	trend
Wright	70	Lung	AOC	<12 g/dL	-	reduced
Smith	985	Multiple	AOC	<11 g/dL	-	reduced
Hedenus	344	B Cell	CIA/chemotherapy	< 11 g/dL	-	reduced

Fig. 12.2 Studies in which ESA therapy has been associated with reduced progression-free or overall survival (OS). (Rx = anticancer therapy.)

patients initiated ESA therapy at hemoglobin concentrations above 12 g/dL and hence their relevance to the use of ESAs for the treatment of CIA, where ESAs have not been administered if the hemoglobin is 12 g/dL or greater, is unclear. In the ENHANCE trial, patients with head and neck cancer scheduled to receive primary radiotherapy (without concomitant chemotherapy) were randomized to receive either ESAs initiated while the hemoglobin concentration was relatively high (12 g/dL in females or 13 g/dL in males) or to undergo radiotherapy without ESA support [50]. A reduced progression-free and overall survival were observed in the ESA arm. Interpretation of this trial is made more difficult because of a relatively high rate of protocol non-compliance and baseline imbalances between the two arms in terms of known prognostic factors for this patient population. In a similar study, the DAHANCA-10 trial, patients with squamous cell head and neck cancer undergoing radiotherapy were randomized to receive or not receive ESAs initiated at hemoglobin levels of 12–13 g/dL, to study the effect of increasing hemoglobin levels during radiation on the efficacy of this therapy [51]. A reduction in progression-free but not in overall survival was observed in the ESA-treated arm and the trial was closed based upon a determination of futility for the prespecified efficacy endpoint. This trial was both larger (484 vs 351 randomized subjects) and executed with fewer protocol violations than the ENHANCE trial. In a third, smaller ($N = 148$) randomized trial, RTOG 99-03, patients with squamous cell cancers of the head and neck undergoing chemoradiotherapy were randomized to receive or not receive ESAs initiated at hemoglobin levels between 9 and 12 g/dL [52]. No differences in progression-free or overall survival were observed between ESA and control patients, but, like the ENHANCE and DAHANCA-10 studies, this trial was not specifically designed to detect a negative survival outcome. Finally, in a larger ($N = 301$) randomized trial of ESAs during radiotherapy for squamous cell cancer of the head and neck, no differences in progression-free or overall survival observed in ESA patients compared to controls [53].

In the GOG 131 trial, 109 patients with cervical cancer undergoing radiotherapy were randomized to receive or not receive ESAs initiated at a hemoglobin level of 12 g/dL. In this trial, trends toward reductions in progression-free and overall survival and a significant increase in thromboses were observed in the ESA arm [54]. In contrast, in a similar ($N = 120$) randomized trial in patients undergoing chemoradiotherapy for cervical cancer, no increase in thrombosis or adverse effects on tumor progression or survival was observed [55]. A much smaller ($N = 74$) trial reported neutral similarly neutral findings [56].

Several trials have explored the use of ESAs for anemia/hypoxia prevention in cancer patients undergoing chemotherapy. In the BEST trial, 939 patients with metastatic breast cancer who were supposed to be initiating first-line chemotherapy were randomized to receive either ESA, initiated at a hemoglobin level of 13 g/dL, or no erythropoietic support in conjunction with that chemotherapy [57]. Although no differences were observed in progression-free survival, in the initial analysis, a reduced overall survival was observed in the ESA arm. The difference in mortality was observed very early, within 4 months of initiating ESA therapy. Interestingly, on later follow-up analyses of the data from this trial, there is no difference in overall survival between the two arms, a finding that has been very difficult to understand. In a second study which has not been published, the PREPARE trial, 735 patients with early breast cancer were randomized to be at risk to receive ESA if their hemoglobin levels fell to 13 g/dL during preoperative adjuvant chemotherapy or to not receive ESA during their chemotherapy. For some patients randomized to ESAs, anemia did not develop and they were therefore never exposed to ESA therapy. No differences in tumor response were observed in the ESA versus the control arm. With a median follow-up of 3 years, an interim analysis has shown that the survival rate was lower (86% vs 90%, HR 1.42) and PFS rate was lower (73% vs 79%, HR 1.33) in patients randomized to receive ESA if and when hemoglobin fell [58]. These trends toward differences in tumor outcomes between the ESA and control arms are substantially reduced when the analysis is confined, as safety analyses traditionally are, to patients who actually became anemic and were exposed to ESA. It is difficult to explain why being randomized to be at risk for ESA and then not requiring it would impart a risk of relapse relative to patients randomized to be observed. In contrast to the BEST trial, these trends did not become apparent until relatively late in the follow-up period, more than 2 years after the discontinuation of ESA therapy. In two additional randomized trials of ESAs for patients undergoing chemotherapy for breast cancer, no differences in progression-free or overall survival have been observed in the ESA arms [59, 60].

In one of the few randomized trials in cancer patients receiving chemotherapy in which survival was a primary endpoint and sample size was sufficient ($N = 600$) to meaningfully examine the effects on overall survival, patients with small cell lung cancer were stratified and randomized to receive ESA or placebo initiating at a hemoglobin level of during the first cycle of chemotherapy, with doses held if the hemoglobin level exceeded 14 g/dL [61]. No significant difference in overall survival was observed (hazard ratio = 0.93; 95% confidence intervals: 0.78–1.11; $p = 0.43$). In this study of ESAs in patients receiving chemotherapy, no adverse effects on tumor outcomes were observed, despite the relatively high hemoglobin target for ESA therapy.

In the 35 randomized trials of ESAs to treat anemia in cancer patients receiving chemotherapy (CIA) in which tumor outcome data are available, inferior tumor outcomes have been reported in the ESA arm in 2 studies. In a trial involving 344 anemic (hemoglobin less than 11 g/dL) patients with B cell neoplasms carried out with red cell transfusion rate as the primary endpoint, a reduced overall survival was reported in the ESA-treated arm [62]. Because survival was not a primary endpoint, no attempt was made to balance prognostic factors at study entry between the two groups. In other randomized trials of ESAs in patients with B cell neoplasms, differences in tumor progression or survival have not been reported between treatment groups, however like the Hedenus trial, these studies were not designed or powered to examine survival as a primary endpoint [63–65].

In a small trial involving 70 anemic (hemoglobin concentration < 12 g/dL) patients with non-small cell lung cancer (NSCLC), patients who were not receiving chemotherapy or who were receiving late-line chemotherapy were randomized to receive or not receive ESAs with the goal being an examination of quality-of-life effects of an increased hemoglobin level in a patient population where palliation is the main goal of therapy [66]. At the time of an interim analysis done to examine the effects of ESA on thrombosis in this trial, a reduced overall survival was noted in ESA-treated patients and the trial was closed. In a much larger ($N = 320$) randomized trial of ESA to treat CIA in lung cancer patients, no differences in progression-free or overall survival were observed between ESA and placebo-treated patients [67]. An additional trial (EPO-GER-022) in non-small cell lung cancer that has not been published has been reported to show no negative effect of ESA on survival [58].

In the largest randomized trial to date with an observed inferior survival outcome in the ESA-treated arm, 985 patients with a variety of non-myeloid malignancies with AOC (hemoglobin concentration < 11 g/dL) who were not receiving any anti-cancer therapy were randomized to receive ESA or placebo [19]. The primary endpoint was red cell transfusion and no attempt was made to balance baseline prognostic factors for survival between the two treatment groups in this very heterogeneous population of patients with a variety of tumor types and stages. Monitoring for tumor progression was not specified in this study. A decrease in overall survival was observed in the intent-to-treat analysis for patients randomized to receive ESA (hazard ratio 1.22, 95% confidence intervals 1.03–1.45, $p = 0.02$). At study entry, there was an imbalance in prognostic factors favoring a better survival outcome in the placebo arm; when the survival analysis is adjusted for these imbalances in stratification factors and covariates, the observed difference between arms is reduced, but still trends in favor of the placebo arm (hazard ratio 1.15, 95% confidence intervals 0.97–1.37, $p = 0.12$). On subset analysis, the survival disadvantage with ESAs was observed in men but not in women, and in patients with B cell malignancy but not with breast or lung cancers. In this trial, achieving a hemoglobin level of 12 g/dL, regardless of treatment group to which a patient was assigned, was associated with a favorable survival outcome and a rapid rise in hemoglobin had a neutral survival effect. Red cell transfusion, whether the patient was assigned to ESA or placebo, was associated with a significantly lower survival. A rise in hemoglobin was associated with improved survival, whether or not a patient was receiving ESA; a deterioration in hemoglobin level sufficient to require red cell transfusion was a substantial negative prognostic factor in both treatment arms.

In the final analysis, the central problem is that there are no published randomized trials specifically studying the tumor progression and survival effects of ESAs used to treat CIA. To be definitive, a trial should focus on a single cancer, employ identical chemotherapy treatments in both treatment arms, stratify to balance baseline prognostic factors in the two arms, follow patients until death, and be sufficiently large to deal with dropouts and have the power to detect or exclude even modest effects on tumor outcomes. The initiation and target hemoglobin levels should model the clinical practice that will result in the lowest transfusion risk. Trials meeting these standards have now been initiated in breast and lung cancers and are accruing patients. They promise to provide more reliable and conclusive answers regarding the safety of ESAs in the CIA setting in which they have demonstrated benefits in terms of red cell transfusion reduction.

Until the results of definitive survival trials are available, we are left to deal with the conflicting data from available randomized trials, which are all suboptimal for studying effects on tumor progression or survival. One approach has been the performance of meta-analyses of available trials to attempt to discern the overall effect of ESAs on tumor outcomes. This too has proven to be a difficult endeavor; the results of study-level meta-analyses have varied, depending upon whether they focus more upon trials for treatment of CIA, where a neutral or even favorable impact on overall survival has been suggested [12] or include as well more recent trials of ESA in AOC or to establish high hemoglobin/tumor oxygenation, where a negative overall effect on survival has been discerned [14]. More recently, meta-analyses have utilized patient-level data from the databases for randomized trials of ESAs in cancer to attempt to increase the power to detect any effects of ESAs on survival. However, even here results have varied depending upon whether the analysis focuses on "on-study" mortality, where the BEST trial, as the single trial with a significant number of on-study deaths in either treatment arm, is a major driver of the result and an overall negative effect (reflective of the BEST's data) is discerned [68, 69], or whether overall survival in the treatment of CIA is the focus, where a neutral effect on tumor progression and survival has been reported [70].

If ESAs Negatively Impact Survival, What Mechanism(s)

If ESAs have the capacity to negatively impact tumor progression or overall survival in cancer patients, it will be extremely important to understand the mechanism(s) through which this effect is mediated if we are to develop an optimized approach to the significant problem of anemia in cancer patients [71]. Because the ESAs that have been utilized to date are cloned erythropoietin proteins, it is very likely that all of their effects are mediated through interaction with cognate, functional erythropoietin receptors (EPO-R) in the tissues. In humans, the only tissue in which functional EPO-R have been incontrovertibly demonstrated is the hematopoietic progenitor cells in the bone marrow, where erythropoietins acting on EPO-R on committed erythroid progenitors enhance survival of these cells and leads to an increase in the production of red cells. More recently, some data have implied that there may be EPO-R on vascular endothelial cells [72–75] although this has not been clearly demonstrated and there are data refuting their existence. If they do exist, these vascular receptors might be important in the increased incidence of hypertension and thrombosis that have been observed in ESA-treated humans. Most recently, several investigators have postulated the existence of functional EPO-R on human cancer cells and suggested that ESAs may enhance survival or induce proliferation of some human cancers [76–83].

Marrow EPO-R

Clearly, ESAs increase hemoglobin levels in humans. Although there has been abundant data for many years linking anemia to tumor cell hypoxia, aggressive tumor behavior and resistance to radiation and chemotherapy, there has been surprisingly little work done on the effects of high hemoglobin levels on tumor oxygenation. Tumor vasculature is unlike that in normal tissues; it is tortuous and characterized by variations in vessel diameter and therefore flow rates. The tumor oxygenation/anemia prevention trials of ESAs in cancer patients carried out to date have been designed with the implicit assumption that the relationship between hemoglobin concentration and tissue oxygenation in human tumors is much the same as in normal tissues, with oxygen delivery increasing as hemoglobin rises until very high hemoglobin levels (>16 g/dL) are reached. What little data exist suggest that the rheology of blood is much different in tumor tissues, with tumor oxygenation increasing with increasing hemoglobin concentration only until hemoglobin levels in the range of 13 g/dL are reached; as hemoglobin levels increase high, oxygenation falls and tumor cell hypoxia increases rather than decreases [40]. It is possible that the adverse impact on tumor progression or survival reported in the tumor oxygenation trials summarized above were due to increases in hemoglobin levels in ESA-treated patients above 13 g/dL, with the result that tumors became more phenotypically aggressive or resistant to radiation or chemotherapy. Paradoxically, trials aimed at demonstrating the benefit of reduced tumor cell hypoxia through ESA-induced increases in hemoglobin may have inadvertently observed the deleterious effects of increased tumor cell hypoxia associated with well intended but ill conceived trial designs that resulted in hemoglobin levels in the ESA arms too high for optimal oxygenation (Fig. 12.3).

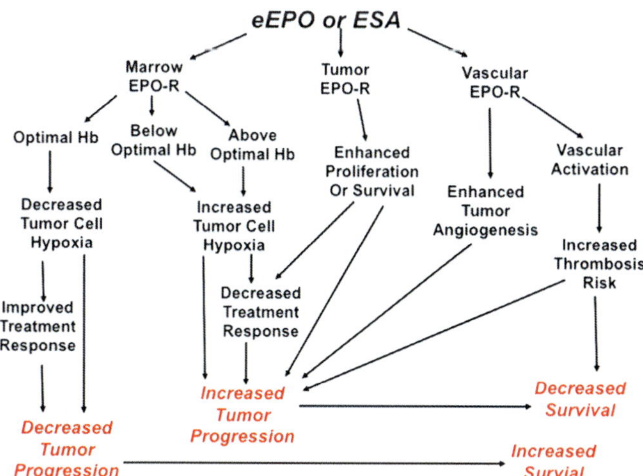

Fig. 12.3 Theoretical framework for the multiple postulated effects of ESA therapy on tumor progression or survival in cancer patients. Although this serves to illustrate the complexity of potential factors involved, it is important to note that none of the hypothesized mechanisms have been demonstrated to occur in ESA-treated cancer patients

Vascular EPO-R, Thrombosis

Although the existence of functional EPO-R on vascular endothelium remains controversial, if they do exist it is possible that they are involved in the increased thromboses that have been observed with ESA treatment. It would also be possible that ESAs acting on vascular EPO-R may have an effect on tumor angiogenesis mediating a deleterious effect on tumor progression or survival [84]. Regardless of whether or not functional vascular EPO-R exist, it is clear that ESA therapy is associated with an increased incidence of venous thrombosis in cancer patients. Although venous thrombosis can result in embolism and death, it is extremely unlikely that excess deaths in the numbers that have been implied in the randomized ESA trials of concern could be due to unsuspected pulmonary embolism. Recently, there has been a renewed interest in the role of local thrombosis in tumors in cancer progression and metastasis. Several clinical trials have examined the effects of anticoagulation on tumor outcomes in patients with cancer who do not have clinical evidence of deep venous thromboses with variable results. A recent systematic meta-analysis of these studies has concluded that there is an overall reduction in mortality associated with parenteral anticoagulation of cancer patients even in the absence of clinical thrombosis [85]. If anticoagulation improves tumor outcomes, it is logical to wonder whether agents that enhance thrombosis, whether or not it is due to vascular activation, might decrease survival. It should be noted, however, that the most significant improvement in survival associated with parenteral anticoagulation has been observed in patients with small cell lung cancer; the one setting in which we have a large and well-designed survival trial of ESAs, a trial that demonstrated identical survival outcomes for ESA and placebo-treated patients [61]. If the literature regarding anticoagulation and tumor outcomes is informative regarding the effects of thrombosis on tumor biology, small cell lung cancer is the setting in which a deleterious effect would have been expected.

Tumor Cell EPO-R

Several investigators have reported detection of EPO-R on human cancer cells [86]. In most instances, these studies have utilized commercially available antibody reagents presumed to be specific for EPO-R. However, the specificity of these reagents has been called into question and it now appears that the available reagents also bind to other cancer-associated entities, including important heat shock proteins [87–90]. Increases in EPO-R transcript levels have not been found in malignant tissue compared to normal tissue counterparts [88]. The presence of tumor cell EPO-R has remained quite controversial [91–94]. This important technical issue may have recently been solved through the development of more specific antibodies to EPO-R [95] and we expect further studies using this reagent to be forthcoming. It has been even more difficult to demonstrate that any EPO-R that may or may not be present on human tumors are functional and therefore relevant to the safety of ESAs. In most reported in vivo and in vitro studies, no effects of ESAs on the proliferation or survival of human cancer cells have been observed, with the predictable exception of erythroleukemia cell lines [96–98]. However in some studies, effects of ESAs on cancer cell biology have been reported [81, 84, 99, 100]. Some data suggest that EPO-R may be expressed on human ovarian cancer cells [82, 101] and that exposure to ESAs may cause these cells to develop resistance to paclitaxel [102]. There are conflicting data indicating that ESAs may enhance the effects of chemotherapy on ovarian cancer [103]. There are limited data regarding the effects of ESAs on tumor progression or survival in patients with ovarian cancer. In the large AOC trial discussed above, no negative effect of ESA therapy on survival was observed in patients with ovarian cancer [19].

In summary, efforts to demonstrate EPO-R on human tumor cells have been hampered by a lack of specific reagents for immunohistochemistry. Studies of the effects of ESAs on the proliferation or survival of human cancer cells have yielded conflicting results, even when efforts are confined to a single, well-defined tumor type such as ovarian cancer. Ultimately, it is likely that this issue will remain controversial until the results of the ongoing survival studies of ESAs in cancer patients are available and provide a practical answer. Parenthetically, it is interesting to note that if ESAs interact with EPO-R on tumor vasculature on tumor cells and promote tumor progression and mortality to the extent suggested by some there should be concern that endogenous erythropoietin is active in the cancer progression process and some consideration of EPO and EPO-R as targets for anticancer therapy.

Future Directions: Iron, Inflammation, and Insight

ESAs have never been approved by the Food and Drug Administration for the treatment of AOC or to increase hemoglobin concentration to supra-normal levels to improve tumor oxygenation and response to therapy. They have been approved for the treatment of CIA with the goal being a reduction in transfusion requirements. To date, there has not been a demonstration that ESAs increase the rate of tumor progression or decrease survival in cancer patients when they are used to treat CIA, with therapy initiated at hemoglobin levels less than 12 g/dL and therapy withheld for hemoglobin levels of 12 g/dL or greater. However, the results of several randomized trials of ESAs used at higher hemoglobin levels and/or without chemotherapy have raised concerns that ESAs may increase the rate of tumor progression or decrease survival in cancer patients, and these data have raised concerns regarding the safety of ESAs in the setting of CIA. Unfortunately, we do not have high-quality randomized trials to definitively establish the safety of ESAs in terms of tumor progression and survival for several common malignancies and the data from settings other than CIA have raised safety concerns in the CIA setting as well. This has resulted in the need to inform patients of the data available to date and in the recommendation that ESA therapy not be initiated for patients with CIA until the hemoglobin level is less than 10 g/dL. While this policy will decrease the total exposure of cancer patients to ESAs, it is likely that it will also result in an increase in the proportion of cancer patients receiving transfusions and in the number of transfusions that individual patients receive [104–106]. Occasionally, a debilitated cancer patient with cardiopulmonary co-morbidities who is undergoing chemotherapy will require transfusion support before the hemoglobin level falls below 10 g/dL and these patients may never have access to ESAs if use is restricted to lower hemoglobin levels. Clearly, we need better insight into the safest approach to anemia in cancer patients and this insight can only come through additional randomized trials.

When ESAs were being developed for the treatment of anemia in cancer, the biology of anemia of chronic illness was poorly understood. The discovery of the iron regulatory peptide hepcidin [2, 4] and its role in the development of anemia in the setting of inflammatory illnesses including cancer has been a very important subsequent event. In the setting of inflammatory illness, hepcidin levels increase and hepcidin acts to decrease iron transport in cells in gastrointestinal tract and in macrophages containing body iron stores. The result is a decrease in iron absorption and its accessibility of storage pool iron [107]. This limitation on access to storage pool iron can lead to functional iron deficiency, in which there is iron-restricted erythropoiesis despite what should be adequate body iron stores. Functional iron deficiency is even more likely to occur with the administration of ESAs, which increase the quantity of iron required for erythropoiesis. This advance in our understanding of the pathophysiology of the anemia of chronic illness provides some explanation for the relative erythropoietin resistance observed in anemic cancer patients; the dose of ESAs required in CIA is approximately threefold higher than that required in patients with renal failure and even with this higher dose, response rates are significantly lower. Because the mechanism(s) of adverse effects of ESAs in cancer patients are not well understood, it is difficult to speculate on whether these higher doses of ESAs in cancer patients are responsible for the observed instances of hypertension or thrombosis or for the effects, if any, on tumor progression or survival. Clearly, these higher and less effective doses of ESAs significantly reduced the cost effectiveness of ESAs used in the oncology setting and led to additional reservations regarding their use [8].

The above considerations raised interest in the use of iron supplementation, particularly parenteral preparations to bypass the reduced gastrointestinal absorption, during ESA therapy for CIA. There have now been several randomized trials of parenteral iron in this setting [108–112]. These trials have indicated that parenteral iron increases the efficacy of ESAs in CIA patients, an effect that can be exploited to either improve the response rate or decrease the ESA dose in this setting. They have also shown that parenteral iron is more effective than oral iron for this purpose; oral iron not been shown to be superior to no iron supplementation [108, 109]. Had this been known when ESAs were being developed in cancer patients, it is likely that parenteral iron would have been integrated into treatment algorithms.

Traditionally, physicians have been concerned about the potential for anaphylaxis associated with the use of parenteral iron due to early experience with the high molecular weight dextran preparations. More recently, lower molecular weight dextran preparations have introduced and the extensive experience in dialysis patients suggests that these preparations are safer than the earlier preparations [113–115]. There are also iron salt preparations available with a reduced risk of adverse events. The interested reader is referred to a recent review of practical aspects of parenteral iron administration [116].

Therapy with ESAs has been shown to provide a clinical benefit to patients with CIA. Used in this setting, with dosing held for hemoglobin levels of 12 g/dL or greater, ESA therapy is associated with an increase in hemoglobin levels and a decrease in transfusion requirements; adverse events include an increased risk of thrombosis and of hypertension. In general, impacts on tumor progression or survival have not been observed with this use of ESAs in oncology. Therapies with ESAs have not been proven to provide clinical benefit to patients with AOC and have never been shown in any randomized trial to improve response to radiotherapy or chemotherapy. In these settings, tumor progression and/or decreased survival have been observed in the ESA-treated cohorts. Given the lack of efficacy and these potential safety concerns, use of ESAs for these indications in clinical practice cannot be supported. Controversy continues to surround the questions of whether ESA therapy alters the behavior of cancers in patients and what, if any, mechanisms may be at work. Controversy has also surrounded the extent to which these observations in AOC and hyperoxygenation trials should change clinical practice in the management of CIA. For the immediate future, guidelines that will decrease exposure of CIA patients to ESAs will likely continue, but these will also likely result in an increase in red cell transfusion rates in cancer patients.

References

1. Groopman JE, Itri LM. Chemotherapy-induced anemia in adults: incidence and treatment. J Natl Cancer Inst. 1999;91:1616–34.
2. Ganz T. Hepcidin, a key regulator of iron metabolism and mediator of anemia of inflammation. Blood. 2003;102:783–8.
3. Nemeth E, Valore EV, Territo M, Schiller G, Lichtenstein A, Ganz T. Hepcidin, a putative mediator of anemia of inflammation, is a type II acute-phase protein. Blood. 2003;101: 2461–3.
4. Andrews NC. Anemia of inflammation: the cytokine–hepcidin link. J Clin Invest. 2004;113:1251–3.
5. Roy CN, Andrews NC. Anemia of inflammation: the hepcidin link. Curr Opin Hematol. 2005;12:107–11.
6. Miller CB, Jones RJ, Piantadosi S, Abeloff MD, Spivak JL. Decreased erythropoietin response in patients with the anemia of cancer. N Engl J Med. 1990;322:1689–92.
7. Glaspy JA. Hematopoietic management in oncology practice. Part 2. Erythropoietic factors. Oncology (Williston Park). 2003;17:1724–30, discussion 31–2, 35, 39.
8. Glaspy JA. The development of erythropoietic agents in oncology. Expert Opin Emerg Drugs. 2005;10:553–67.
9. Greenberg PL, Sun Z, Miller KB, et al. Treatment of myelodysplastic syndrome patients with erythropoietin with or without granulocyte colony-stimulating factor: results of a prospective randomized phase 3 trial by the Eastern Cooperative Oncology Group (E1996). Blood. 2009;114:2393–400.

10. Glaspy J, Vadhan-Raj S, Patel R, et al. Randomized comparison of every-2-week darbepo-etin alfa and weekly epoetin alfa for the treatment of chemotherapy-induced anemia: the 20030125 Study Group Trial. J Clin Oncol. 2006;24:2290–7.

11. Bohlius J, Langensiepen S, Schwarzer G, et al. Erythropoietin for patients with malignant disease. Cochrane Database Syst Rev. 2004(3):CD003189.

12. Bohlius J, Langensiepen S, Schwarzer G, et al. Recombinant human erythropoietin and over-all survival in cancer patients: results of a comprehensive meta-analysis. J Natl Cancer Inst. 2005;97:489–98.

13. Bohlius J, Wilson J, Seidenfeld J, et al. Erythropoietin or darbepoetin for patients with cancer. Cochrane Database Syst Rev. 2006;3:CD003407.

14. Bohlius J, Wilson J, Seidenfeld J, et al. Recombinant human erythropoietins and cancer patients: updated meta-analysis of 57 studies including 9353 patients. J Natl Cancer Inst. 2006;98:708–14.

15. Cella D, Zagari MJ, Vandoros C, Gagnon DD, Hurtz HJ, Nortier JW. Epoetin alfa treatment results in clinically significant improvements in quality of life in anemic cancer patients when referenced to the general population. J Clin Oncol. 2003;21:366–73.

16. Berndt E, Kallich J, McDermott A, Xu X, Lee H, Glaspy J. Reductions in anaemia and fatigue are associated with improvements in productivity in cancer patients receiving chemotherapy. Pharmacoeconomics. 2005;23:505–14.

17. Christodoulou C, Dafni U, Aravantinos G, et al. Effects of epoetin-alpha on quality of life of cancer patients with solid tumors receiving chemotherapy. Anticancer Res. 2009;29: 693–702.

18. Henry DH, Abels RI. Recombinant human erythropoietin in the treatment of cancer and chemotherapy-induced anemia: results of double-blind and open-label follow-up studies. Semin Oncol. 1994;21:21–8.

19. Smith RE, Aapro MS, Ludwig H, et al. Darbepoetin alpha for the treatment of anemia in patients with active cancer not receiving chemotherapy or radiotherapy: results of a phase III, multicenter, randomized, double-blind, placebo-controlled study. J Clin Oncol. 2008;26:1040–50.

20. Caro JJ, Salas M, Ward A, Goss G. Anemia as an independent prognostic factor for survival in patients with cancer: a systemic, quantitative review. Cancer. 2001;91:2214–21.

21. Knight K, Wade S, Balducci L. Prevalence and outcomes of anemia in cancer: a systematic review of the literature. Am J Med. 2004;5:11S–26S.

22. Kallinowski F, Zander R, Hoeckel M, Vaupel P. Tumor tissue oxygenation as evaluated by computerized-pO_2-histography. Int J Radiat Oncol Biol Phys. 1990;19:953–61.

23. Vaupel P, Briest S, Hockel M. Hypoxia in breast cancer: pathogenesis, characterization and biological/therapeutic implications. Wien Med Wochenschr. 2002;152:334–42.

24. Semenza GL. Expression of hypoxia-inducible factor 1: mechanisms and consequences. Biochem Pharmacol. 2000;59:47–53.

25. Semenza GL. Involvement of hypoxia-inducible factor 1 in human cancer. Intern Med. 2002;41:79–83.

26. Graeber TG, Osmanian C, Jacks T, et al. Hypoxia-mediated selection of cells with diminished apoptotic potential in solid tumours. Nature. 1996;379:88–91.

27. Hockel M, Vaupel P. Tumor hypoxia: definitions and current clinical, biologic, and molecular aspects. J Natl Cancer Inst. 2001;93:266–76.

28. Semenza GL. Hypoxia, clonal selection, and the role of HIF-1 in tumor progression. Crit Rev Biochem Mol Biol. 2000;35:71–103.

29. Fyles AW, Milosevic M, Wong R, et al. Oxygenation predicts radiation response and survival in patients with cervix cancer. Radiother Oncol. 1998;48:149–56.

30. Semenza GL. Intratumoral hypoxia, radiation resistance, and HIF-1. Cancer Cell. 2004;5:405–6.

31. Fyles A, Milosevic M, Pintilie M, et al. Long-term performance of interstitial fluid pressure and hypoxia as prognostic factors in cervix cancer. Radiother Oncol. 2006;80:132–7.

32. Dunst J, Kuhnt T, Strauss HG, et al. Anemia in cervical cancers: impact on survival, patterns of relapse, and association with hypoxia and angiogenesis. Int J Radiat Oncol Biol Phys. 2003;56:778–87.

33. Nordsmark M, Bentzen SM, Rudat V, et al. Prognostic value of tumor oxygenation in 397 head and neck tumors after primary radiation therapy. An international multi-center study. Radiother Oncol. 2005;77:18–24.

34. Teicher BA, Holden SA, Al-Achi A, Herman TS. Classification of antineoplastic treatments by their differential toxicity toward putative oxygenated and hypoxic tumor subpopulations in vivo in the FSaIIC murine fibrosarcoma. Cancer Res. 1990;50:3339–44.

35. Van Belle SJ, Cocquyt V. Impact of haemoglobin levels on the outcome of cancers treated with chemotherapy. Crit Rev Oncol Hematol. 2003;47:1–11.

36. Mittelman M, Neumann D, Peled A, Kanter P, Haran-Ghera N. Erythropoietin induces tumor regression and antitumor immune responses in murine myeloma models. Proc Natl Acad Sci USA. 2001;98:5181–6.

37. Thews O, Koenig R, Kelleher DK, Kutzner J, Vaupel P. Enhanced radiosensitivity in experimental tumours following erythropoietin treatment of chemotherapy-induced anaemia. Br J Cancer. 1998;78:752–6.

38. Thews O, Kelleher DK, Vaupel P. Erythropoietin restores the anemia-induced reduction in cyclophosphamide cytotoxicity in rat tumors. Cancer Res. 2001;61:1358–61.

39. Glaspy J, Dunst J. Can erythropoietin therapy improve survival? Oncology. 2004;1:5–11.

40. Vaupel P, Thews O, Mayer A, Hockel S, Hockel M. Oxygenation status of gynecologic tumors: what is the optimal hemoglobin level? Strahlenther Onkol. 2002;178:727–31.

41. Casadevall N, Nataf J, Viron B, et al. Pure red cell aplasia and anticrythropoietin antibodies in patients treated with recombinant erythropoietin. N Engl J Med. 2002;346:469–75.

42. Bennett CL, Luminari S, Nissenson AR, et al. Pure red-cell aplasia and epoetin therapy. N Engl J Med. 2004;351:1403–8.

43. Wun T, Law L, Harvey D, Sieracki B, Scudder SA, Ryu JK. Increased incidence of symptomatic venous thrombosis in patients with cervical carcinoma treated with concurrent chemotherapy, radiation, and erythropoietin. Cancer. 2003;98:1514–20.

44. Lavey RS, Liu PY, Greer BE, et al. Recombinant human erythropoietin as an adjunct to radiation therapy and cisplatin for stage IIB–IVA carcinoma of the cervix: a Southwest Oncology Group Study. Gynecol Oncol. 2004;95:145–51.

45. Stohlawetz PJ, Dzirlo L, Hergovich N, et al. Effects of erythropoietin on platelet reactivity and thrombopoiesis in humans. Blood. 2000;95:2983–9.

46. Wun T, Paglieroni T, Hammond WP, Kaushansky K, Foster DC. Thrombopoietin is synergistic with other hematopoietic growth factors and physiologic platelet agonists for platelet activation in vitro. Am J Hematol. 1997;54:225–32.

47. Valles J, Santos MT, Aznar J, et al. Platelet–erythrocyte interactions enhance alpha(IIb)beta(3) integrin receptor activation and P-selectin expression during platelet recruitment: down-regulation by aspirin ex vivo. Blood. 2002;99:3978–84.

48. Glaspy JA. Cancer patient survival and erythropoietin. J Natl Compr Canc Netw. 2005;3:796–804.

49. Glaspy JA. Erythropoiesis stimulating agents in oncology. J Natl Compr Canc Netw. 2008; 6:565–575.

50. Henke M, Laszig R, Rube C, et al. Erythropoietin to treat head and neck cancer patients with anaemia undergoing radiotherapy: randomised, double-blind, placebo-controlled trial. Lancet. 2003;362:1255–60.

51. Overgaard J, Hoff C, Sand Hansen H, et al. Randomized study of the importance of Novel Erythropoiesis Stimulating Protein (Aranesp®) for the effect of radiotherapy in patients with primary squamous cell carcinoma of the head and neck (HNSCC) – the Danish Head and Neck Cancer Group DAHANCA 10 rand. Eur J Cancer. 2007;5:7. Abstract 6LB.

52. Machtay M, Pajak TF, Suntharalingam M, et al. Radiotherapy with or without erythropoietin for anemic patients with head and neck cancer: a randomized trial of the Radiation Therapy Oncology Group (RTOG 99-03). Int J Radiat Oncol Biol Phys. 2007;69:1008–17.

53. Hoskin PJ, Robinson M, Slevin N, Morgan D, Harrington K, Gaffney C. Effect of epoetin alfa on survival and cancer treatment-related anemia and fatigue in patients receiving radical radiotherapy with curative intent for head and neck cancer. J Clin Oncol. 2009;27: 5751–6.
54. Thomas G, Ali S, Hoebers FJ, et al. Phase III trial to evaluate the efficacy of maintaining hemoglobin levels above 12 g/dL with erythropoietin vs above 10 g/dL without erythropoietin in anemic patients receiving concurrent radiation and cisplatin for cervical cancer. Gynecol Oncol. 2008;108:317–25.
55. Gupta S, Singh PK, Bisth SS, et al. Role of recombinant human erythropoietin in patients of advanced cervical cancer treated "by chemoradiotherapy". Cancer Biol Ther. 2009;8:13–17.
56. Strauss HG, Haensgen G, Dunst J, et al. Effects of anemia correction with epoetin beta in patients receiving radiochemotherapy for advanced cervical cancer. Int J Gynecol Cancer. 2008;18:515–24.
57. Leyland-Jones B, Semiglazov V, Pawlicki M, et al. Maintaining normal hemoglobin levels with epoetin alfa in mainly nonanemic patients with metastatic breast cancer receiving first-line chemotherapy: a survival study. J Clin Oncol. 2005;23:5960–72.
58. Amgen. March 2008 Briefing document. http://wwwfdagov/ohrms/dockets/ac/08/briefing/2008-4345b2-05-AMGENpdf
59. Aapro M, Leonard RC, Barnadas A, et al. Effect of once-weekly epoetin beta on survival in patients with metastatic breast cancer receiving anthracycline- and/or taxane-based chemotherapy: results of the Breast Cancer–Anemia and the Value of Erythropoietin (BRAVE) Study. J Clin Oncol. 2008;26:592–8.
60. Chang J, Couture F, Young S, McWatters KL, Lau CY. Weekly epoetin alfa maintains hemoglobin, improves quality of life, and reduces transfusion in breast cancer patients receiving chemotherapy. J Clin Oncol. 2005;23:2597–605.
61. Pirker R, Ramlau RA, Schuette W, et al. Safety and efficacy of darbepoetin alpha in previously untreated extensive-stage small-cell lung cancer treated with platinum plus etoposide. J Clin Oncol. 2008;26:2342–9.
62. Hedenus M, Hansen S, Taylor K, et al. Randomized, dose-finding study of darbepoetin alfa in anaemic patients with lymphoproliferative malignancies. Br J Haematol. 2002;119: 79–86.
63. Cazzola M, Messinger D, Battistel V, et al. Recombinant human erythropoietin in the anemia associated with multiple myeloma or non-Hodgkin's lymphoma: dose finding and identification of predictors of response. Blood. 1995;86:4446–53.
64. Osterborg A, Boogaerts MA, Cimino R, et al. Recombinant human erythropoietin in transfusion-dependent anemic patients with multiple myeloma and non-Hodgkin's lymphoma – a randomized multicenter study. The European Study Group of Erythropoietin (Epoetin Beta) Treatment in Multiple Myeloma and Non-Hodgkin's Lymphoma. Blood. 1996;87:2675–82.
65. Osterborg A, Brandberg Y, Hedenus M. Impact of epoetin-beta on survival of patients with lymphoproliferative malignancies: long-term follow up of a large randomized study. Br J Haematol. 2005;129:206–9.
66. Wright JR, Ung YC, Julian JA, et al. Randomized, double-blind, placebo-controlled trial of erythropoietin in non-small-cell lung cancer with disease-related anemia. J Clin Oncol. 2007;25:1027–32.
67. Vansteenkiste J, Pirker R, Massuti B, et al. Double-blind, placebo-controlled, randomized phase III trial of darbepoetin alfa in lung cancer patients receiving chemotherapy. J Natl Cancer Inst. 2002;94:1211–20.
68. Bohlius J, Schmidlin K, Brillant C, et al. Recombinant human erythropoiesis-stimulating agents and mortality in patients with cancer: a meta-analysis of randomised trials. Lancet. 2009;373:1532–42.
69. Glaspy J. ESAs to treat anemia – balancing risks and benefits. Nat Rev Clin Oncol. 2009;6:500–2.

70. Ludwig H, Crawford J, Osterborg A, et al. Pooled analysis of individual patient-level data from all randomized, double-blind, placebo-controlled trials of darbepoetin alfa in the treatment of patients with chemotherapy-induced anemia. J Clin Oncol. 2009;27:2838–47.
71. Glaspy J. Erythropoietin in cancer patients. Annu Rev Med. 2009;60:35.1–35.12.
72. Anagnostou A, Lee ES, Kessimian N, Levinson R, Steiner M. Erythropoietin has a mitogenic and positive chemotactic effect on endothelial cells. Proc Natl Acad Sci USA. 1990;87:5978–82.
73. Anagnostou A, Liu Z, Steiner M, et al. Erythropoietin receptor mRNA expression in human endothelial cells. Proc Natl Acad Sci USA. 1994;91:3974–8.
74. Beleslin-Cokic BB, Cokic VP, Yu X, Weksler BB, Schechter AN, Noguchi CT. Erythropoietin and hypoxia stimulate erythropoietin receptor and nitric oxide production by endothelial cells. Blood. 2004;104:2073–80.
75. Zwezdaryk KJ, Coffelt SB, Figueroa YG, et al. Erythropoietin, a hypoxia-regulated factor, elicits a pro-angiogenic program in human mesenchymal stem cells. Exp Hematol. 2007;35:640–52.
76. Acs G, Acs P, Beckwith SM, et al. Erythropoietin and erythropoietin receptor expression in human cancer. Cancer Res. 2001;61:3561–5.
77. Arcasoy MO, Amin K, Chou SC, Haroon ZA, Varia M, Raleigh JA. Erythropoietin and erythropoietin receptor expression in head and neck cancer: relationship to tumor hypoxia. Clin Cancer Res. 2005;11:20–7.
78. Batra S, Perelman N, Luck LR, Shimada H, Malik P. Pediatric tumor cells express erythropoietin and a functional erythropoietin receptor that promotes angiogenesis and tumor cell survival. Lab Invest. 2003;83:1477–87.
79. Feldman L, Wang Y, Rhim JS, Bhattacharya N, Loda M, Sytkowski AJ. Erythropoietin stimulates growth and STAT5 phosphorylation in human prostate epithelial and prostate cancer cells. Prostate. 2006;66:135–45.
80. Lai SY, Childs EE, Xi S, et al. Erythropoietin-mediated activation of JAK–STAT signaling contributes to cellular invasion in head and neck squamous cell carcinoma. Oncogene. 2005;24:4442–9.
81. Lester RD, Jo M, Campana WM, Gonias SL. Erythropoietin promotes MCF-7 breast cancer cell migration by an ERK/mitogen-activated protein kinase-dependent pathway and is primarily responsible for the increase in migration observed in hypoxia. J Biol Chem. 2005;280:39273–7.
82. McBroom JW, Acs G, Rose GS, Krivak TC, Mohyeldin A, Verma A. Erythropoietin receptor function and expression in epithelial ovarian carcinoma. Gynecol Oncol. 2005;99:571–7.
83. Leo C, Horn LC, Rauscher C, et al. Expression of erythropoietin and erythropoietin receptor in cervical cancer and relationship to survival, hypoxia, and apoptosis. Clin Cancer Res. 2006;12:6894–900.
84. Hardee ME, Cao Y, Fu P, et al. Erythropoietin blockade inhibits the induction of tumor angiogenesis and progression. PLoS ONE. 2007;2:e549.
85. Akl EA, van Doormaal FF, Barba M, et al. Parenteral anticoagulation for prolonging survival in patients with cancer who have no other indication for anticoagulation. Cochrane Database Syst Rev. 2007;CD00652.
86. Hardee ME, Arcasoy MO, Blackwell KL, Kirkpatrick JP, Dewhirst MW. Erythropoietin biology in cancer. Clin Cancer Res. 2006;12:332–9.
87. Sinclair AM, Todd MD, Forsythe K, Knox SJ, Elliott S, Begley CG. Expression and function of erythropoietin receptors in tumors: implications for the use of erythropoiesis-stimulating agents in cancer patients. Cancer. 2007;110:477–88.
88. Sinclair AM, Rogers N, Busse L, et al. Erythropoietin receptor transcription is neither elevated nor predictive of surface expression in human tumour cells. Br J Cancer. 2008;98:1059–67.
89. Brown WM, Maxwell P, Graham AN, et al. Erythropoietin receptor expression in non-small cell lung carcinoma: a question of antibody specificity. Stem Cells. 2007;25:718–22.

90. Elliott S, Busse L, Bass MB, et al. Anti-Epo receptor antibodies do not predict Epo receptor expression. Blood. 2006;107:1892–5.
91. Longmore GD. Do cancer cells express functional erythropoietin receptors? N Engl J Med. 2007;356:2447.
92. Della Ragione F, Cucciolla V, Borriello A, Oliva A, Perrotta S. Erythropoietin receptors on cancer cells: a still open question. J Clin Oncol. 2007;25:1812–13. Author reply 5.
93. Jelkmann W, Laugsch M. Problems in identifying functional erythropoietin receptors in cancer tissue. J Clin Oncol. 2007;25:1627–8. Author reply 8.
94. Osterborg A, Aapro M, Cornes P, Haselbeck A, Hayward CR, Jelkmann W. Preclinical studies of erythropoietin receptor expression in tumour cells: impact on clinical use of erythropoietic proteins to correct cancer-related anaemia. Eur J Cancer. 2007;43: 510–19.
95. Elliott S, Busse L, McCaffery I, et al. Identification of a sensitive anti-erythropoietin receptor monoclonal antibody allows detection of low levels of EpoR in cells. J Immunol Methods. 2010;352:126–39.
96. LaMontagne KR, Butler J, Marshall DJ, et al. Recombinant epoetins do not stimulate tumor growth in erythropoietin receptor-positive breast carcinoma models. Mol Cancer Ther. 2006;5:347–55.
97. Belda-Iniesta C, Perona R, Carpeno J de C, et al. Human recombinant erythropoietin does not promote cancer growth in presence of functional receptors expressed in cancer cells. Cancer Biol Ther. 2007;6:1600–5.
98. Laugsch M, Metzen E, Svensson T, Depping R, Jelkmann W. Lack of functional erythropoietin receptors of cancer cell lines. Int J Cancer. 2008;122:1005–11.
99. Hamadmad SN, Hohl RJ. Erythropoietin stimulates cancer cell migration and activates RhoA protein through a mitogen-activated protein kinase/extracellular signal-regulated kinase-dependent mechanism. J Pharmacol Exp Ther. 2008;324:1227–33.
100. Hardee ME, Rabbani ZN, Arcasoy MO, et al. Erythropoietin inhibits apoptosis in breast cancer cells via an Akt-dependent pathway without modulating in vivo chemosensitivity. Mol Cancer Ther. 2006;5:356–61.
101. Yasuda Y, Musha T, Tanaka H, et al. Inhibition of erythropoietin signalling destroys xenografts of ovarian and uterine cancers in nude mice. Br J Cancer. 2001;84:836–43.
102. Solar P, Feldman L, Jeong JY, Busingye JR, Sytkowski AJ. Erythropoietin treatment of human ovarian cancer cells results in enhanced signaling and a paclitaxel-resistant phenotype. Int J Cancer. 2008;122:281–8.
103. Silver DF, Piver MS. Effects of recombinant human erythropoietin on the antitumor effect of cisplatin in SCID mice bearing human ovarian cancer: a possible oxygen effect. Gynecol Oncol. 1999;73:280–4.
104. Crawford J, Robert F, Perry MC, Belani C, Williams D. A randomized trial comparing immediate versus delayed treatment of anemia with once-weekly epoetin alfa in patients with non-small cell lung cancer scheduled to receive first-line chemotherapy. J Thorac Oncol. 2007;2:210–20.
105. Lyman GH, Glaspy J. Are there clinical benefits with early erythropoietic intervention for chemotherapy-induced anemia? A systematic review. Cancer. 2006;106:223–33.
106. Vansteenkiste J, Hedenus M, Gascon P, et al. Darbepoetin alfa for treating chemotherapy-induced anemia in patients with a baseline hemoglobin level < 10 g/dL versus ≥ 10 g/dL: an exploratory analysis from a randomized, double-blind, active-controlled trial. BMC Cancer. 2009;9:311.
107. Rivera S, Liu L, Nemeth E, Gabayan V, Sorensen OE, Ganz T. Hepcidin excess induces the sequestration of iron and exacerbates tumor-associated anemia. Blood. 2005;105:1797–802.
108. Auerbach M, Ballard H, Trout JR, et al. Intravenous iron optimizes the response to recombinant human erythropoietin in cancer patients with chemotherapy-related anemia: a multicenter, open-label, randomized trial. J Clin Oncol. 2004;22:1301–7.

109. Henry DH, Dahl NV, Auerbach M, Tchekmedyian S, Laufman LR. Intravenous ferric gluconate significantly improves response to epoetin alfa versus oral iron or no iron in anemic patients with cancer receiving chemotherapy. Oncologist. 2007;12:231–42.
110. Hedenus M, Birgegard G, Nasman P, et al. Addition of intravenous iron to epoetin beta increases hemoglobin response and decreases epoetin dose requirement in anemic patients with lymphoproliferative malignancies: a randomized multicenter study. Leukemia. 2007;21:627–32.
111. Bastit L, Vandebroek A, Altintas S, et al. Randomized, multicenter, controlled trial comparing the efficacy and safety of darbepoetin alpha administered every 3 weeks with or without intravenous iron in patients with chemotherapy-induced anemia. J Clin Oncol. 2008;26:1611–18.
112. Pedrazzoli P, Farris A, Del Prete S, et al. Randomized trial of intravenous iron supplementation in patients with chemotherapy-related anemia without iron deficiency treated with darbepoetin alpha. J Clin Oncol. 2008;26:1619–25.
113. Fletes R, Lazarus JM, Gage J, Chertow GM. Suspected iron dextran-related adverse drug events in hemodialysis patients. Am J Kidney Dis. 2001;37:743–9.
114. Chertow GM, Mason PD, Vaage-Nilsen O, Ahlmen J. On the relative safety of parenteral iron formulations. Nephrol Dial Transplant. 2004;19:1571–5.
115. Chertow GM, Mason PD, Vaage-Nilsen O, Ahlmen J. Update on adverse drug events associated with parenteral iron. Nephrol Dial Transplant. 2006;21:378–82.
116. Auerbach M, Ballard H, Glaspy J. Clinical update: intravenous iron for anaemia. Lancet. 2007;369:1502–4.

Chapter 13
Ten Years of Meta-analyses on Erythropoiesis-Stimulating Agents in Cancer Patients

Thomy Tonia and Julia Bohlius

Abstract Background: Since erythropoiesis-stimulating agents (ESAs) were licensed in 1993, more than 70 randomized controlled trials and more than 20 meta-analyses and systematic reviews on their effectiveness were conducted. Here, we present a systematic review on the meta-analyses of trials evaluating ESAs in cancer patients. Methods: We included all published meta-analyses of at least five randomized controlled trials that evaluated the effects of ESAs versus control in patients with any type of cancer or myelodysplastic syndrome. Results: We included a total of 23 systematic reviews and meta-analyses (16 literature based and 7 based on individual patient data (IPD)) that assessed several outcomes. All 12 meta-analyses reporting on transfusion risks demonstrated that ESAs significantly reduce the risk of transfusions. Eleven meta-analyses (nine based on published data and two on IPD) evaluated thrombovascular events. An increased risk of thrombovascular events was observed in all but two meta-analyses (relative risks (RRs) ranging from 1.57 to 1.69). However, potential reporting and publication bias as well as detection bias call for a cautious interpretation of these results. Survival and mortality were evaluated in 18 meta-analyses, with the observed effect changing over time. While meta-analyses on studies conducted before 2002 showed beneficial effects of ESAs on survival, contrary results, i.e. worsened survival, was seen in meta-analyses including more recent studies. Discussion: The results from several meta-analyses show that ESAs in cancer patients reduce the risk for red blood cell transfusions and increase the risk for thrombovascular events and mortality. The effect of ESAs on mortality risk in patients receiving chemotherapy remains unclear. In clinical practice, the benefits and risks of ESAs should be carefully considered and decisions should be made based on each patient's situation and preferences.

Since erythropoiesis-stimulating agents (ESAs) were licensed for the treatment of anaemia in cancer patients in 1993 more than 70 randomized controlled trials were

J. Bohlius (✉)
Institute of Social and Preventive Medicine, University of Bern, Bern, Switzerland
e-mail: jbohlius@ispm.unibe.ch

G.H. Lyman, D.C. Dale (eds.), *Hematopoietic Growth Factors in Oncology*,
Cancer Treatment and Research 157, DOI 10.1007/978-1-4419-7073-2_13,
© Springer Science+Business Media, LLC 2011

conducted. In order to systematically organize these studies several meta-analyses were done. The first meta-analysis was published in 1999. Ever since, more than 20 meta-analyses and systematic reviews on the effects of ESAs in cancer patients were published.

We here present a systematic review on these meta-analyses of trials evaluating ESAs in cancer patients and provide an overview of the different methods used, the results achieved, and the main limitations.

Methods

Inclusion Criteria

We included all fully published meta-analyses based on at least five randomized controlled trials evaluating the effects of ESAs versus control in patients with cancer or myelodysplastic syndrome (MDS). Systematic reviews that did not contain a meta-analysis were excluded. Abstract publications of meta-analyses were also excluded. In addition, meta-analyses examining the effects of pre- and perioperative administration of ESAs were excluded.

Search Strategy

We conducted a literature search in Medline and selected Internet pages to identify meta-analyses of primarily randomized controlled trials on ESAs in cancer patients (date of search: May 3, 2009). The following search terms were used in Medline (1985–2009):

#1	"Neoplasms"[Mesh]
#2	Cancer
#3	Cancer*
#4	Darbepoetin alfa
#5	Darbepo*
#6	Epoetin
#7	Epoetin*
#8	("Epoetin Alfa" [Mesh] OR "epoetin beta" [Substance Name] OR "epoetin zeta" [Substance Name] OR "epoetin omega" [Substance Name] OR "epoetin delta" [Substance Name])
#9	Meta-analysis
#10	Meta-analys*
#11	"Meta-analysis" [Publication Type]
#12	(#1 OR #2 OR #3) AND (#4 OR #5 OR #6 OR #7 OR #8) AND (#9 OR #10 OR #11)

We identified 50 references in Medline. Conference proceedings were not searched.

We removed duplicates, reviews not fulfilling the inclusion criteria, i.e. unsystematic reviews or studies not including patients with malignant diseases or MDS, not including randomized controlled trials, or not evaluating the effectiveness of ESAs versus control. Finally, 23 systematic reviews and meta-analyses were included in the present review.

Characteristics of Included Meta-analyses

Of the 23 systematic reviews and meta-analyses included [1–23], 16 were literature based and 7 meta-analyses were based on individual patient data [14–19, 22]. Several meta-analyses were not independent studies but updates of previous meta-analyses or collaborative projects updating previous studies. The meta-analyses are listed in Table 13.1 in ascending order of the last year of literature search or study included. All presented meta-analyses included randomized controlled trials; however, some reviews also included non-randomized controlled studies or uncontrolled studies. All analyses included cancer patients, some reviews excluded patients with MDS, and others were restricted to patients with MDS. There was a range of concomitant interventions. While most reviews included studies with chemotherapy and/or radiotherapy and also studies without anticancer therapy, others were restricted to patients on chemotherapy or patients assumed to be treated within the license indication of the respective ESA. The literature-based meta-analyses mainly included data as published in the literature, few made additional attempts to evaluate FDA documents or contact authors for unreported data.

Results

A wide range of outcomes were assessed in the various meta-analyses, including the risk of receiving a red blood cell transfusion, haematological (Hb) response, Hb change, number of red blood cell units transfused, Quality of Life (QoL), thrombovascular events, hypertension, and other adverse events and survival, for a specification of outcomes assessed per review see Table 13.1. Three of the meta-analyses were restricted to QoL [3, 11, 14]. The outcomes of red blood cell transfusions, thrombovascular events, and survival will be explored in the following section.

Red Blood Cell Transfusions

Transfusion risks have been reported in 12 meta-analyses, see Table 13.2. The first meta-analysis was conducted and published by Quirt et al. [21]. Seidenfeld et al

Table 13.1 Study characteristics

Meta-Analysis	Literature based meta-analyses						
	Quirt 1997	Marsh 1999	Seidenfeld 2001	Clark 2002	Jones 2004	Bohlius 2005	Wilson 2007
Literature search: period covered	1985-1995	up to 1996	1985-1998	up to 2001, no comphrehensive literature search	1985-2002	1985-2001	1996-2004
Types of studies							
Randomised controlled studies	Yes	Yes	Yes	Yes	Yes	Yes	Yes
Otherwise controlled studies	No	Yes	Yes	No	Yes	No	No
Uncontrolled trials	No	No	No	No	Yes	No	No
Minimum study size	NR	>= 10 total study population	>= 10 participants per study arm	NR	20 participants per study arm	> 10 participants per study arm	10 participants per study arm
Types of participants							
Age groups	Adults and children	Adults	Children and adults	Children and adults	Adults	Adults	Children and adults
Cancer	Yes	Yes	Yes	Yes	Yes	Yes	Yes
MDS	No	Yes	No	No	No	Yes	Yes
Co-interventions							
Chemotherapy	Yes	Yes	Yes	Yes	Yes	Yes	Yes
Radiotherapy/radiochemotherapy	No	Yes	Yes	Yes	No	Yes	Yes
No anticancer treatment	No	Yes	No	Yes	No	Yes	Yes
Surgery	No	No	No	No	No	No	No
Stem cell transplant	No	No	No	No	No	No	No
Other inclusion criteria	Excluded trials with haematologic cancer origination in the bone marrow	cancer and renal disease, patients with documented anemia	NR	NR	patients receiving chemotherapy	NR	NR
Source of data							
Full text	Yes	Yes	Yes	Yes	Yes	Yes	Yes
Abstracts	Yes	Yes	Yes	Yes	Yes	Yes	Yes
FDA documents	No	No	No	No	No	Yes	Yes
Unpublished data	No	Yes	No	No	Yes	Yes	Yes
Individual patient data	No	No	No	No	No	For some studies	Yes
Endpoints covered							
Mortality / survival	No	No	No	No	No	Yes	Yes
Transfusion	Yes	No	Yes	Yes	No	Yes	Yes
Hb response	No	Yes	No	No	No	Yes	Yes
Hb change	No	No	No	No	No	Yes	Yes
Number of RBC units	No	No	No	No	No	Yes	Yes
Tumor control	No	No	No	No	No	Yes	Yes
Thromboembolic events	No	No	No	No	No	Yes	Yes
Hypertension/cardiovascular	No	No	No	No	No	Yes	Yes
Other adverse events	No	No	No	No	No	Yes	Yes
Quality of Life	Yes	No	Yes	No	Yes	Yes	Yes

Table 13.1 (continued)

Meta-Analysis	Literature based meta-analyses								
	Bohlius 2006	Seidenfeld 2006	Ross 2006	Ross 2007	Bennett 2008	Minton 2008	Mundle 2009	Tonelli 2009	Lambin 2009
Literature search: period covered	1985-2005	1999-2005	1980-2005	1980-2005	up to 2008, no comprehensive literature	1966-2007	1990-2007	1950-2007	up to 2009
Types of studies									
Randomised controlled studies	Yes	Yes	Yes	Yes	Yes	Yes	Yes	Yes	Yes
Otherwise controlled studies	No	No	Yes	Yes	No	No	Unclear	No	No
Uncontrolled trials	No	No	Yes, not reported here	Yes, not reported here	No	No	Unclear	No	No
Minimum study size	> 10 participants per study arm	10 participants per study arm	10 participants per study arm	10 participants per study arm	NR	NR	NR	30 participants per study arm	NR
Types of participants									
Age groups	Children and adults	Children and adults	Children and adults	Adults	Children and adults	Adults	Adults	Adults	Adults
Cancer	Yes	Yes	Yes	No	Yes	Yes	No	Yes	Yes
MDS	Yes	No	No	Yes	No	No	Yes	Yes	No
Co-interventions									
Chemotherapy	Yes	Yes	Yes	Yes	Yes	Yes	NR	Yes	No
Radiotherapy/radiochemotherapy	Yes	Yes	No	NA	Yes	No	NA	Yes	Radiochemotherapy
No anticancer treatment	Yes	No	Yes	Yes	Yes	Yes	NR	Yes	No
Surgery	No	No	No	NA	No	No	NA	Yes	No
Stem cell transplant	No	No	No	No	No	No	NR	No	No
Other inclusion criteria	NR	NR	treatment of chemotherapy induced anemia in cancer patients with anemia	Only MDS	NR	NR	Only MDS	cancer related anemia	head and neck cancer
Source of data									
Full text	Yes	Yes	Yes	Yes	Yes	Yes	Yes	Yes	Yes
Abstracts	Yes	Yes	Yes	Yes	Yes	Yes	Yes	Yes	Yes
FDA documents	Yes	Yes	No	No	Yes	No	No	No	No
Unpublished data	No	No	No	No	No	No	No	Yes	No
Individual patient data	No	No	No	No	No	No	No	No	No
Endpoints covered									
Mortality / survival	Yes	Yes	Yes	Yes	Yes	No	No	Yes	Yes
Transfusion	Yes	Yes	Yes	Yes	No	No	Yes	Yes	No
Hb response	Yes	Yes	No	Yes	No	No	Yes	No	No
Hb change	Yes	No	No	Yes	No	No	No	No	No
Number of RBC units	Yes	No	No	No	No	No	Yes	No	No
Tumor control	Yes	Yes	No	No	No	No	No	Yes	Yes
Thromboembolic events	Yes	Yes	Yes	Yes	Yes	No	No	Yes	No
Hypertension/cardiovascular	Yes	Yes	No	Yes	No	No	No	Yes	No
Other adverse events	Yes	Yes	No	Yes	No	No	No	Yes	Yes
Quality of Life	Yes	Yes	Yes	Yes	No	Yes	No	Yes	No

Table 13.1 (continued)

Meta-Analysis	Individual patient data meta-analyses						
	Cella 2004	Hedenus 2005	Couture 2005	Aapro 2006	Aapro 2008	Ludwig 2009	Bohlius 2009
Literature search: period covered	No literature search conducted	No literature search conducted	Not stated	No literature search conducted	No literature search conducted	No literature search conducted	1985-2008
Types of studies							
Randomised controlled studies	Yes	Yes	Yes	Yes	Yes	Yes	Yes
Otherwise controlled studies	No	No	No	No	No	No	No
Uncontrolled trials	No	No	No	No	No	No	No
Minimum study size	NR	NR	NR	NR	NR	No	50 evaluated participants per
Types of participants							
Age groups	Adults	Adults	Adults	Adults	Adults	Adults	Children and adults
Cancer	Yes	Yes	Yes	Yes	Yes	Yes	Yes
MDS	No	No	No	NA	NA	No	No
Co-interventions							
Chemotherapy	Yes	Yes	Yes	Yes	Yes	Yes	Yes
Radiotherapy/radiochemotherapy	No	No	No	No	Yes	No	Yes
No anticancer treatment	Yes	No	No	NA	NA	No	Yes
Surgery	No	No	No	Yes	Yes	No	No
Stem cell transplant	No	No	No	NA	NA	No	No
Other inclusion criteria	RCTs conducted by Amgen	RCTs conducted by Amgen	NR	all RCTs by Roche or Boehringer	all RCTs by Roche or Boehringer	only double-blind, placebo-controlled RCTs, darbepoetin, chemotherapy	Individual patient data available
Source of data							
Full text	NA	NA	N/A	NA	NA	NA	NA
Abstracts	NA	NA	N/A	NA	NA	NA	NA
FDA documents	NA	NA	N/A	NA	NA	NA	NA
Unpublished data	Yes	Yes	Yes	Yes	Yes	Yes	Yes
Individual patient data	Yes	Yes	Yes	Yes	Yes	Yes	Yes
Endpoints covered							
Mortality / survival	No	Yes	No	Yes	Yes	Yes	Yes
Transfusion	No	No	Yes	No	No	Yes	No
Hb response	No	No	No	No	No	No	No
Hb change	No	No	No	No	No	No	No
Number of RBC units	No	No	No	No	No	No	No
Tumor control	No	Yes	No	Yes	Yes	Yes	No
Thromboembolic events	No	No	No	Yes	Yes	Yes	No
Hypertension/cardiovascular	No	No	No	No	No	Yes	No
Other adverse events	No	No	No	No	No	Yes	No
Quality of Life	Yes	No	No	No	No	No	No

NR: not reported
NA: not appicable

Table 13.2 Red blood cell transfusions

Meta-analysis	Period covered	Inclusion criteria	Drugs	Data source	Studies included	Patients included	Effect estimate ESA versus control (fixed effects if not reported otherwise)
Seicenfeld et al. [2]	1985–1998	Cancer, MDS, chemotherapy, radiotherapy	Epoetin alpha, epoetin beta	Published data only	12	1,390	OR 0.38 (95% CI 0.28–0.51)[a]
Clark et al. [23]	up to 2001	Cancer, chemotherapy, no therapy	Epoetin alpha, epoetin beta	Published data only	19	1,896	RR 0.61 (95% CI 0.54–0.68)
Bohlius et al. [4]	1985–2001	Cancer, MDS, chemotherapy, radiotherapy, no therapy	Epoetin alpha, epoetin beta	Published and unpublished data	25	3,069	RR 0.67 (95% CI 0.62–0.73)
Wilson et al. [5]	1985–2004	Cancer, MDS, chemotherapy, radiotherapy, no therapy	Epoetin alpha, epoetin beta, darbepoetin	Published data only	35	4,613	RR 0.63 (95% CI 0.58–0.67)
Bohlius et al. [6]	1985–2005	Cancer, MDS, chemotherapy, radiotherapy, no therapy	Epoetin alpha, epoetin beta, darbepoetin	Published data only	42	6,510	RR 0.64 (95% CI 0.60–0.68)
Seicenfeld et al. [7] (Epoetin)	1985–2005	Cancer, MDS, chemotherapy, radiotherapy, no therapy	Epoetin alpha, epoetin beta	Published data only	34	5,210	RR 0.63 (95% CI 0.59–0.67)
Seicenfeld et al. [7] (Darbepoetin)	1985–2005	Cancer, MDS, chemotherapy, radiotherapy, no therapy	Darbepoetin	Published data only	4	950	RR 0.61 (95% CI 0.52–0.72)

Table 13.2 (continued)

Meta-analysis	Period covered	Inclusion criteria	Drugs	Data source	Studies included	Patients included	Effect estimate ESA versus control (fixed effects if not reported otherwise)
Ross et al. [9]	1980–2005	MDS, chemotherapy, no therapy	Epoetin alpha, epoetin beta, darbepoetin	Published data only	1	66	OR 0.3 (95% CI 0.1–1.6)
Tonelli et al. [13]	1950–2007	Cancer, MDS, chemotherapy, radiotherapy, no therapy, surgery	Epoetin alpha, epoetin beta, darbepoetin	Published data only	24	5,321	RR 0.64 (95% CI 0.56–0.73)
Chemotherapy studies							
Quirt et al. [21]	1985–1995	Cancer, chemotherapy	Epoetin alpha, epoetin beta	Published data only	8	813	RR 0.64 (95% CI 0.53–0.78)
Couture et al. [22]	Not stated	Cancer, chemotherapy	Epoetin alpha	Individual patient data	5	934	RR 0.58 (95% CI 0.49–0.69)
Ross et al. [8]	1980–2005	Only studies within license indication, chemotherapy induced anemia	Epoetin alpha, epoetin beta	Published data only	18	2,520	OR 0.45 (95% CI 0.38–0.53)[b]
Ludwig et al. [18]	Not conducted	Only double-blind, placebo-controlled RCTs, darbepoetin, chemotherapy	Darbepoetin	Individual patient data	6	2,004	HR 0.46 (0.39, 0.55)

[a]Note: random effects, Bayesian method used
[b]Only data for studies reporting week 1 onwards included

published another meta-analysis in 2001 [2]. This analysis was updated in a collaborative effort by Bohlius et al. [4]. In 2004/2005 these analyses were updated together with investigators from the University of Birmingham [5] and the agency for healthcare research and quality (AHRQ) [7]. Apart from this collaboration, several independent meta-analyses published results for red blood cell transfusions [5, 8, 9, 13, 21–23].

All but one [9] meta-analyses demonstrated that ESAs reduce the risk for transfusions in a statistically and clinically meaningful way. The effect estimates obtained range from 0.38 (Odds Ratio, OR) [2] to 0.67 (relative risk) [4]. The most conservative result was reported by Bohlius et al. [4]. This was the only meta-analysis that had included unreported data from the investigators. The largest effect (OR 0.38) was reported by Seidenfeld et al. [2], in this meta-analysis both poor and high-quality randomized controlled trials (RCTs) were included. When the analysis was restricted to high-quality RCTs the effect of ESAs on blood transfusions was OR of 0.45 (95% CI 0.33–0.62) [2].

Number Needed to Treat

When applying the results generated by the Bohlius et al. [6] meta-analysis (RR 0.64 (95% CI 0.60–0.68)) to a range of hypothetical populations, the following numbers needed to treat (NNT) emerge, see Table 13.3. In a cancer population with low risk (i.e. 10%) to receive red blood cell transfusion for every 28 (95% CI 25–31.3) patients treated with ESAs, 1 additional patient might be spared from red blood cell transfusions; in a population with an underlying risk to receive red blood cell transfusions of 50%, the NNT is 5.6 (95% CI 5.0–6.3) thus, for every six patients treated with ESAs one additional patient might be spared from red blood cell transfusions.

Table 13.3   Number needed to treat to spare one additional patient from red blood cell transfusions

Underlying risk to receive red blood cell transfusions (%)	RR for red blood cell transfusions, ESA vs control	NNT (95% CI)
10	RR 0.64 (95% CI	28 (95% CI 25–31.3)
30	0.60–0.68)	9.3 (95% CI 8.3–10.4)
50		5.6 (95% CI 5.0–6.3)
70		4.0 (95% CI 3.6–4.5)
90		3.1 (95% CI 2.8–3.5)

Abbreviation: RR, relative risk; NNT, number needed to treat; CI, confidence interval.

In conclusion, various meta-analyses have fairly consistently shown that the use of ESAs effectively reduce the risk for red blood cell transfusions.

Thrombovascular Events

Thrombovascular events were evaluated in 11 meta-analyses [4, 6–8, 10, 13, 16–18], see Table 13.4. Two of these were restricted to studies in which patients were

Table 13.4 Thrombovascular events

Meta-analysis	Period covered	Inclusion criteria	Drugs	Data source	Studies included	Patients included	Effect estimate ESA vs control (fixed effects if not reported otherwise)
Bohlius et al. [19]	1985–2001	Cancer, MDS, chemotherapy, radiotherapy, no therapy	Epoetin alpha, epoetin beta	Published and unpublished data	12	1,738	RR 1.58 (95% CI 0.94–2.66)
Bohlius et al. [6]	1985–2005	Cancer, MDS, chemotherapy, radiotherapy, no therapy	Epoetin alpha, epoetin beta, darbepoetin	Published data only	35	6,769	RR 1.67 (95% CI 1.35–2.06)
Seidenfeld et al. [7] (Epoetin)	1985–2005	Cancer, chemotherapy, radiotherapy	Epoetin alpha, epoetin beta	Published data only	30	6,092	RR 1.69 (95% CI 1.36–2.10)
Seidenfeld et al. [7] (Darbepoetin)	1985–2005	Cancer, chemotherapy, radiotherapy	Darbepoetin	Published data only	1	314	RR 1.44 (95% CI 0.47–4.43)
Ross et al. [8]	1980–2005	Studies with and without chemotherapy-induced anaemia	Epoetin alpha, epoetin beta, darbepoetin	Published data only	11	2,029	OR 1.41 (95% CI 0.92–2.18)
Bennett et al. [10]	Up to 2008	Cancer, chemotherapy, radiotherapy, no therapy	Epoetin alpha, epoetin beta, darbepoetin	Published data only	38	8,172	RR 1.57 (95% CI 1.31–1.87)
Tonelli et al. [13]	1950–2007	Cancer, MDS, chemotherapy, radiotherapy, no therapy, surgery	Epoetin alpha, epoetin beta, darbepoetin	Published data only	13	3,420	RR 1.69 (95% CI 1.27–2.24)

Table 13.4 (continued)

Meta-analysis	Period covered	Inclusion criteria	Drugs	Data source	Studies included	Patients included	Effect estimate ESA vs control (fixed effects if not reported otherwise)
Aapro et al. [17]	No literature search	Studies conducted by Roche or Boehringer	Epoetin beta	Individual patient data	12	2,297	HR 1.62 (95% CI 1.13–2.31)
Ross et al. [9]	1980–2005	MDS	Epoetin alpha, epoetin beta, darbepoetin	Published data only	NR	NR	0 events in both arms
Restricted to chemotherapy trials, license indication, or other populations							
Ross et al. [8]	1980–2005	Only studies within license indication, chemotherapy-induced anaemia	Epoetin alpha, epoetin beta, darbepoetin	Published data only	6	1,463	OR 1.41 (95% CI 0.81–2.47)
Ludwig et al. [18]	No literature search	Double-blind, placebo-controlled chemotherapy studies conducted by Amgen	Darbepoetin	Individual patient data	7	2,112	HR 1.57 (95% CI 1.10–2.26)

assumed to be treated within the license indication of the respective ESA [8] or to double-blind trials in patients receiving chemotherapy conducted by Amgen [18]. In general, cancer patients are at increased risk to develop thrombovascular events; nevertheless, it is a rare event. Therefore, a large sample size is needed to achieve sufficient power to detect differences between ESA and control if they exist. The first meta-analysis that evaluated thrombovascular events (TVEs) was based on 12 studies and 1,738 patients [4]. The overall estimate for the risk to develop TVEs was increased by factor 1.58 (95% CI 0.94–2.66) for patients receiving ESAs compared to controls [4]. However, the observed effect did not reach conventional levels of statistical significance. When this meta-analysis was updated in 2006 data from a total of 35 studies and 6,679 patients were analyzed. In this updated analysis the previously observed effect size was confirmed and statistical significance was reached (RR 1.69, 95% CI 1.35–2.06) [6]. With the exception of one meta-analysis that was restricted to studies within the license indication of ESAs [8] all subsequent meta-analyses confirmed the observed effect.

Main limitations of the literature-based meta-analysis are potential reporting and publication biases. Publications may highlight an increased risks of TVEs in ESA-treated patients compared to control but may be reluctant to report this if the opposite effect is observed, i.e. TVEs observed less frequently in the ESA group compared to controls. The published literature may therefore represent a biased sample. These biases can be detected with funnel plot and regression analyses, for a funnel plot from the Bohlius et al. [24] meta-analysis see Fig. 13.1. A regression analysis confirmed ($P = 0.00988$) statistically significant asymmetry, suggesting that negative results (in this case no thrombotic event) have been underreported [24].

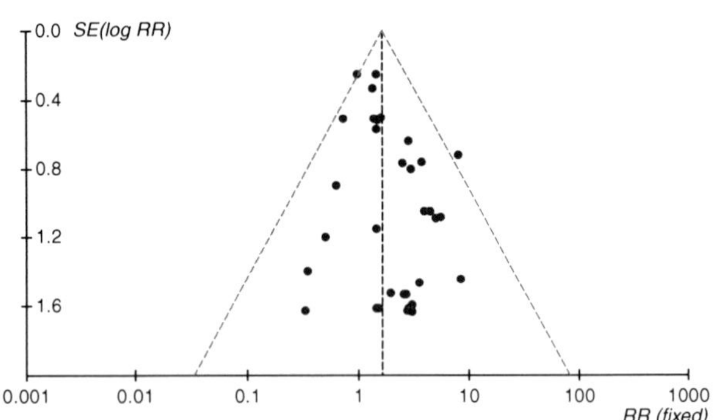

Fig. 13.1 Funnel plot TVEs, plot derived from Bohlius et al. [24]

However, the concern of reporting and publication biases may be less worrisome since two individual patient data meta-analyses confirmed the adverse effect of ESAs on thrombovascular events [17, 18]. Data for these meta-analyses were taken directly from the randomized controlled trials and not from publications or reports, thus, publication or reporting biases are less likely to occur. In these meta-analyses 7 trials including 2,112 patients [18] and 12 trials including 2,297 patients [17] were evaluated. The risk for thrombovascular events was increased by factor 1.57 (95% CI 1.10–2.26) [18] and 1.62 (95% CI 1.13–2.31) [17], respectively. Thus, these individual patient data meta-analyses confirm the findings from previous literature-based meta-analyses. Nevertheless, a detection bias cannot be excluded. None of the randomized studies evaluated in the systematic reviews and meta-analyses had an active screening programme for the detection of thrombovascular events in place. Physicians treating cancer patients with ESAs might be more observant towards thrombovascular events in patients receiving ESAs compared to control.

Number Needed to Treat

We applied the results generated by the Ludwig et al. [18] meta-analysis to a range of hypothetical populations to calculate numbers needed to treat to cause one additional harmful event (NNTH), see Table 13.5. With an assumed relative risk of 1.57 (95% CI 1.10–2.26) to develop thrombovascular events in patients receiving ESAs compared to controls, in a cancer population with low risk of TVEs (i.e. 1%) for every 175 (95% CI 79–1,000) patients treated with ESAs one additional patient might develop a TVE. In contrast, in a population with an underlying risk to develop TVEs of 20%, the NNTH is 9 (95% CI 4–50), thus, for every nine patients treated with ESAs one additional patient might develop a thrombovascular event.

Table 13.5 Number needed to treat to cause one additional thrombovascular event

Underlying risk for thrombovascular events (%)	RR for thrombovascular events, ESA vs control	NNTH (95% CI)
1	RR 1.57 (95% CI	175 (95% CI 79–1,000)
5	1.10–2.26)	35 (95% CI 16–200)
10		18 (95% CI 8–100)
20		9 (95% CI 4–50)

Abbreviations: RR, relative risk; NNTH, number needed to treat to cause one additional harmful event; CI, confidence interval.

Survival and Mortality

Survival and mortality were evaluated in 18 meta-analyses, see Table 13.6. Five of these were restricted to or reported separately results for studies within the license indication of respective ESAs [8] or patients receiving chemotherapy [18, 19]. Six of the meta-analyses were solely based on individual patient data [16–19], in one study some individual patient data for survival were retrieved [4]. Four of the studies were conducted or funded by pharmaceutical companies manufacturing ESAs [8, 16–18].

The results generated by these meta-analyses changed over time. While the first meta-analysis addressing survival showed an overall survival benefit for patients

Table 13.6 Survival and mortality

Meta-analysis	Period covered	Inclusion criteria	Drugs	Data source	Studies included	Patients included	On-study mortality[a]	Overall survival[a]	Survival/ mortality, not specified[a]
Bohlius et al. [4]	1985–2002	Cancer, MDS, chemotherapy, radiotherapy, no therapy	Epoetin alpha, epoetin beta	Published and unpublished data	19	2,805	NR	HR 0.84 (95% CI 0.69–1.02)[b]	NA
Wilson et al. [5]	1985–2004	Cancer, MDS, chemotherapy, radiotherapy, no therapy	Epoetin alpha, epoetin beta, darbepoetin	Published data only	26	5,308	NR	HR 1.03 (95% CI 0.92–1.16)	NA
Bohlius et al. [6]	1985–2005	Cancer, MDS, chemotherapy, radiotherapy, no therapy	Epoetin alpha, epoetin beta, darbepoetin	Published data only	42	8,167	NR	HR 1.08 (95% CI 0.99–1.18)	NA
Seidenfeld et al. [7] (Epoetin)	1985–2005	Cancer, chemotherapy, radiotherapy	Epoetin alpha, epoetin beta	Published data only	35	6,918	NR	HR 1.11 (95% CI 1.00–1.22)	NA
Seidenfeld et al. [7] (Darbepoetin)	1985–2005	Cancer, chemotherapy, radiotherapy	Darbepoetin	Published data only	4	973	NR	HR 0.96 (95% CI 0.78–1.17)	NA
Ross et al. [8]	1980–2005	Studies with and without chemotherapy-induced anaemia	Epoetin alpha, epoetin beta, darbepoetin	Published data only	17	3,048	HR 1.14 (95% CI 0.90–1.45)	NR	NR

Table 13.6 (continued)

Meta-analysis	Period covered	Inclusion criteria	Drugs	Data source	Studies included	Patients included	On-study mortality[a]	Overall survival[a]	Survival/mortality, not specified[a]
Bennett et al. [10]	up to 2008	Cancer, chemotherapy, radiotherapy, no therapy	Epoetin alpha, epoetin beta, darbepoetin	Published data only	51	13,611	NR	NR	HR 1.10 (95% CI 1.01–1.20)[c]
Tonelli et al. [13]	1950–2007	Cancer, MDS, chemotherapy, radiotherapy, no therapy, surgery	Epoetin alpha, epoetin beta, darbepoetin	Published and unpublished reports	28	6,525	NR	NR	RR 1.15 (95% CI 1.03–1.29)[d]
Lambin et al. [20]	Up to 2009	Head and neck cancer	Epoetin alpha, epoetin beta	Published data only	5	1,397	NR	HR 0.73 (95% CI 0.58–0.91)[e]	NR
Aapro et al. [16].	No literature search conducted	RCTs conducted by Roche or Boehringer	Epoetin beta	Individual patient data	9	1,413	RR 0.97 (95% CI 0.69–1.36)[f]	NR	NR
Aapro et al. [17]	No literature search conducted	RCTs conducted by Roche or Boehringer	Epoetin beta	Individual patient data	12	2,297	HR 1.13 (95% CI 0.87–1.46)	HR 1.13 (95% CI 0.98–1.31)[a]	NA
Bohlius et al. [19]	1985–2008	Cancer, chemotherapy, radiotherapy, no therapy	Epoetin alpha, epoetin beta, darbepoetin	Individual patient data	53	13,933	HR 1.17 (95% CI 1.06–1.30)	HR 1.06 (95% CI 1.00–1.12)	NA

Table 13.6 (continued)

Meta-analysis	Period covered	Inclusion criteria	Drugs	Data source	Studies included	Patients included	On-study mortality[a]	Overall survival[a]	Survival/mortality, not specified[a]
Ross et al. [7]	1980–2005	MDS	Epoetin alpha, epoetin beta, darbepoetin	Published data only	NR	NR	NR	NR	OR 1.7 (95% CI 0.4–7.4)
Restricted to chemotherapy trials, license indication or other populations									
Hedenus et al. [15]	No literature search conducted	Double-blind, placebo-controlled chemotherapy studies conducted by Amgen	Darbepoetin	Individual patient data	4	1,129	HR 0.95 (95% CI 0.78–1.16)	NR	NA
Ross et al. [8]	1980–2005	Only studies within license indication, chemotherapy-induced anaemia	Epoetin alpha, epoetin beta, darbepoetin	Published data only	11	2,014	OR 0.99 (95% CI 0.72–1.36)	NR	NR
Ludwig et al. [18]	No literature search conducted	Double-blind, placebo-controlled chemotherapy studies conducted by Amgen	Darbepoetin	Individual patient data	7	2,122	HR 1.11 (95% CI 0.84–1.47)	HR 0.97 (95% CI 0.85–1.10)	NA

Table 13.6 (continued)

Meta-analysis	Period covered	Inclusion criteria	Drugs	Data source	Studies included	Patients included	On-study mortality[a]	Overall survival[a]	Survival/mortality, not specified[a]
Bohlius et al. [19]	1985–2008	Cancer, more than 70% of patients in a given study receiving chemotherapy	Epoetin alpha, epoetin beta, darbepoetin	Individual patient data	38	10,441	HR 1.10 (95% CI 0.98–1.24)	HR 1.04 (95% CI 0.97–1.11)	NA
Tonelli et al. [13] (subgroup analysis chemotherapy-induced anaemia)	1950–2007	Cancer, MDS, chemotherapy, radiotherapy, no therapy, surgery	Epoetin alpha, epoetin beta, darbepoetin	Published and unpublished reports	23	4,273	NR	NR	RR 1.04 (95% CI 0.86–1.26)[c]

[a]Effect estimate ESA versus control (fixed effects if not reported otherwise).
[b]Sensitivity analysis: when data from the Littlewood 2001 study were included adjusted for prognostic factors the overall result was HR 0.81 (95% CI 0.67–0.99).
[c]Based on random effects model.
[d]Based on random effects model, when excluding surgery trials HR 1.15 (95% CI 1.02–1.28).
[e]Lambin et al. [20] reported proportion of patients alive.
[f]Pooled analysis not stratified by study.

receiving ESAs [4], these results could not be confirmed in later meta-analyses. After the early meta-analyses, which included studies that had not been designed to assess survival as a primary or secondary study endpoint, new randomized controlled trials became available that had actually been designed to address survival as primary or secondary endpoint [25–27]. Unexpectedly, these trials showed detrimental effects for patients receiving ESAs compared to controls. Including these and other studies with detrimental effects on survival in the following updates and new meta-analyses, the overall survival estimates for patients receiving ESAs compared to control became worse. Literature-based meta-analyses reported effect estimates of 1.08 (95% CI 0.99–1.18) [6], 1.10 (95% CI 1.01–1.20) [10], 1.11 (95% CI 1.00–1.22) [7], and 1.15 (95% CI 1.03–1.29) [13] in favour of control patients not receiving ESAs. An independent individual patient data meta-analysis based on data from 53 studies with 13,933 patients reported an HR of 1.17 (95% CI 1.06–1.30) for on-study mortality (defined as mortality during study plus 30 days follow-up) and 1.06 (95% CI 1.00–1.12) for overall survival (defined as mortality during long-term follow-up) [19].

Not all of the meta-analyses conducted reached conventional levels of statistical significance which in part might be due to a lack of power. Another problem that hampers direct comparisons between different meta-analyses refers to divergent definitions of endpoints. Since literature-based meta-analyses have to analyze the data as reported in the literature, inconsistencies across studies may occur. For example, some studies reported on on-study mortality, others on long-term overall survival, some on both endpoints, and several studies on none of these. In some meta-analyses overall survival was chosen as outcome [5–7], others did not specify how different lengths of follow-up were handled [10, 13]. With individual patient data meta-analyses these limitations can be overcome, because all data can be handled and analyzed with the same analysis strategy. Results for on-study mortality reported in different individual patient data meta-analyses published since 2008 revealed similar results, with HRs ranging from 1.13 [28] to 1.17 [19] for all cancer patients and from 1.10 [19] to 1.11 [18] for patients undergoing chemotherapy.

Although it is now generally accepted that ESAs increase mortality in cancer patients receiving ESAs outside the license indication, there is an ongoing debate whether or not ESAs increase mortality in patients undergoing chemotherapy. Four individual patient data meta-analyses have addressed this issue [8, 15, 18, 19]. When comparing the two most recent individual patient data meta-analyses [18, 19], Ludwig et al. [18] found an increased risk for on-study mortality in cancer patients undergoing chemotherapy and receiving darbepoetin compared to controls (HR 1.11; 95% CI 0.84–1.47, $n = 2,112$). Bohlius et al. [19] detected a similar effect size in patients undergoing chemotherapy and receiving ESA compared to controls (HR 1.10; 95% CI 0.98–1.24; $n = 10,441$) [19]. In both meta-analyses the observed effect for on-study mortality was not statistically significant. However, assuming a mortality rate of 10% during a trial duration of 16 weeks in cancer patients receiving chemotherapy, an HR for on-study mortality of 1.10 converts into an absolute risk difference of 1%. In order to detect this difference in a single clinical study with an alpha level set at 5% and a beta level of 20%, about 36,000 patients would be needed to reach sufficient statistical power to detect this difference. Thus, even current individual patient meta-analyses including 2,122 [18] and 10,441 [19] patients do not provide sufficient power to detect this small difference. Therefore, from a statistical point of view an increased risk to die cannot be excluded in patients receiving ESAs and undergoing chemotherapy. From a clinical point of view patients receiving concurrent chemotherapy may reach lower hemoglobin levels under ESA treatment compared to patients not receiving chemotherapy which might translate into a lower risk for lethal thrombovascular events and impaired tumour control. However, the underlying pathophysiological mechanisms are not well understood yet and require further research.

Number Needed to Treat to Cause One Additional Harmful Event

When applying the results generated by the Bohlius et al. [19] meta-analysis to a range of hypothetical cancer populations based on the methods reported by Altman et al. [29], the following numbers needed to harm emerge, see Table 13.7. With an assumed relative risk of 1.17 (95% CI 1.06–1.30) to die when receiving ESAs compared to controls, in a cancer population with low mortality (i.e. survival at 1 year 90%) for every 63 (95% CI 36–176) patients treated with ESAs 1 additional patient might die. In a population with an underlying survival at 1 year of 70% the NNTH is 24 (95% CI 14–67). Thus, for every 24 patients treated with ESAs 1 additional patient may die.

Table 13.7 Number needed to treat to cause one additional death

Underlying chance for survival (%)	HR for on-study mortality, ESA vs control	NNT (95% CI)
90	HR 1.17 (95% CI 1.06–1.30)	NNTH 63 (95% CI NNTH 36–NNTH 176)
80		NNTH 34 (95% CI NNTH 19–NNTH 94)
70		NNTH 24 (95% CI NNTH 14–NNTH 67)
90%	HR 1.10 (95% CI 0.98–1.24)	NNTH 106 (95% CI NNTH 44–NNTB 527)
80%		NNTH 57 (95% CI NNTH 24–NNTB 279)
70%		NNTH 41 (95% CI NNTH 17–NNTB 200)

Abbreviations: NNT, number needed to treat; NNTH, number needed to treat to cause one harmful event; NNTB, number needed to treat to cause one beneficial event.

Discussion

Several reasons have been discussed that may explain the observed increased risk for death in cancer patients receiving ESAs. Some study authors and commentators have stressed flaws in the design of several of the major RCTs, which had detected detrimental effects in patients receiving ESAs. For example, baseline imbalances favouring controls were criticized. However, while these effects may occur by chance in single RCTs, they should be factored out in large meta-analyses. High hemoglobin concentrations induced by erythropoiesis-stimulating agents, particularly when greater than 15 g/dL, might impair tumour control or increase the risk of fatal thromboembolic and cardiovascular events [25, 30, 31]. Direct comparison of different target hemoglobin concentrations in patients with renal impairment showed increased mortality in patients treated to achieve high hemoglobin (Hb) concentrations and those treated with high doses of erythropoiesis-stimulating agents [32–34]. Unfortunately, similar studies have not been conducted in the setting of cancer patients. Ludwig et al. attempted to evaluate the effect of post-baseline Hb on mortality. He found that patients achieving high Hb levels independent of blood transfusions were at decreased risk to die compared to patients not achieving high Hb levels [18]. At the same time he found that patients achieving high Hb levels only by the means of transfusion are at increased risk to die, both in the ESA group and in the control group. Again, this underlines previous observations that anaemic patients and patients not responding to ESA have potentially more aggressive cancer and are at higher risk for dying. However, causality with respect to the effect of ESAs cannot be derived from these observations. Other explanations relate to effects of these drugs on the vascular system and tumour tissue. Increasing evidence suggests that erythropoiesis-stimulating agents might cause thromboembolic and cardiovascular events independent of haemoglobin concentrations [35–38]. Whether endogenous or exogenous erythropoietins stimulate proliferation of cancer cells expressing erythropoietin receptors is still undergoing debate [39, 40].

In conclusion, the findings of several meta-analyses on erythropoiesis-stimulating agents in cancer patients demonstrate that ESAs reduce the risk for red blood cell transfusions and increase the risk for thrombovascular events and mortality. There is an ongoing debate whether or not ESAs increase mortality in cancer patients receiving chemotherapy as well. However, the currently available data are insufficient to exclude an increased risk for death in cancer patients undergoing chemotherapy and receiving ESAs. In clinical practice, the increased risks of death and thrombovascular events should be balanced against the benefits of treatment with erythropoiesis-stimulating agents, taking into account each patient's clinical circumstances and preferences.

References

1. Marsh WA, Rascati KL. Meta-analyses of the effectiveness of erythropoietin for end-stage renal disease and cancer. Clin Ther. 1999;21:1443–55.

2. Seidenfeld J, Piper M, Flamm C, et al. Epoetin treatment of anemia associated with cancer therapy: a systematic review and meta-analysis of controlled clinical trials. J Natl Cancer Inst. 2001;93:1204–14.

3. Jones M, Schenkel B, Just J, Fallowfield L. Epoetin alfa improves quality of life in patients with cancer: results of metaanalysis. Cancer. 2004;101:1720–32.

4. Bohlius J, Langensiepen S, Schwarzer G, et al. Recombinant human erythropoietin and overall survival in cancer patients: results of a comprehensive meta-analysis. J Natl Cancer Inst. 2005;97:489–98.

5. Wilson J, Yao GL, Raftery J, et al. A systematic review and economic evaluation of epoetin alfa, epoetin beta and darbepoetin alfa in anaemia associated with cancer, especially that attributable to cancer treatment. Health Technol Assess. 2007;11:1–220.

6. Bohlius J, Wilson J, Seidenfeld J, et al. Recombinant human erythropoietins and cancer patients: updated meta-analysis of 57 studies including 9353 patients. J Natl Cancer Inst. 2006;98:708–714.

7. Seidenfeld, J, Piper, M, Bohlius, J, Weingart, O, Trelle, S, Engert, A, Skoetz, N, Schwarzer, G, Wilson, J, Brunskill, S, Hyde, C, Bonnell, C, Ziegler, KM, Aronson, N. Comparative effectiveness of epoetin and darbepoetin for managing anemia in patients undergoing cancer treatment. 3. Rockville, MD: Agency for Healthcare Research and Quality; 2006.

8. Ross SD, Allen IE, Henry DH, et al. Clinical benefits and risks associated with epoetin and darbepoetin in patients with chemotherapy-induced anemia: a systematic review of the literature. Clin Ther. 2006;28:801–31.

9. Ross SD, Allen IE, Probst CA, et al. Efficacy and safety of erythropoiesis-stimulating proteins in myelodysplastic syndrome: a systematic review and meta-analysis. Oncologist. 2007;12:1264–73.

10. Bennett C.L., Silver S.M., Djulbegovic B, et al. Venous thromboembolism and mortality associated with recombinant erythropoietin and darbepoetin administration for the treatment of cancer-associated anemia. JAMA. 2008;299:914–24.

11. Minton O, Richardson A, Sharpe M, Hotopf M, Stone P. A systematic review and meta-analysis of the pharmacological treatment of cancer-related fatigue. J Natl Cancer Inst. 2008;100:1155–66.

12. Mundle S, Lefebvre P, Vekeman F, et al. An assessment of erythroid response to epoetin alpha as a single agent versus in combination with granulocyte- or granulocyte–macrophage-colony-stimulating factor in myelodysplastic syndromes using a meta-analysis approach. Cancer. 2009;115:706–15.

13. Tonelli M, Hemmelgarn B, Reiman T, et al. Benefits and harms of erythropoiesis-stimulating agents for anemia related to cancer: a meta-analysis. CMAJ. 2009;180(11):E62–71.

14. Cella D, Kallich J, McDermott A, Xu X. The longitudinal relationship of hemoglobin, fatigue and quality of life in anemic cancer patients: results from five randomized clinical trials. Ann Oncol. 2004;15:979–86.

15. Hedenus M, Vansteenkiste J, Kotasek D, Austin M, Amado RG. Darbepoetin alfa for the treatment of chemotherapy-induced anemia: disease progression and survival analysis from four randomized, double-blind, placebo-controlled trials. J Clin Oncol. 2005;23:6941–8.

16. Aapro M, Coiffier B, Dunst J, Osterborg A, Burger HU. Effect of treatment with epoetin beta on short-term tumour progression and survival in anaemic patients with cancer: a meta-analysis. Br J Cancer. 2006;95:1467–73.

17. Aapro M, Scherhag A, Burger HU. Effect of treatment with epoetin-beta on survival, tumour progression and thromboembolic events in patients with cancer: an updated meta-analysis of 12 randomised controlled studies including 2301 patients. Br J Cancer. 2008;99:14–22.

18. Ludwig H, Crawford J, Osterborg A, et al. Pooled analysis of individual patient-level data from all randomized, double-blind, placebo-controlled trials of darbepoetin alfa in the treatment of patients with chemotherapy-induced anemia. J Clin Oncol. 2009;27:2838–47.

19. Bohlius J, Schmidlin K, Brillant C, et al. Recombinant human erythropoiesis-stimulating agents and mortality in patients with cancer: a meta-analysis of randomised trials. Lancet. 2009;373:1532–42.

20. Lambin P, Ramaekers BL, van Mastrigt GA, et al. Erythropoietin as an adjuvant treatment with (chemo) radiation therapy for head and neck cancer. Cochrane Database Syst Rev. 2009;3:CD006158.
21. Quirt I, Micucci S, Moran LA et al. Erythropoietin in the management of patients with nonhematologic cancer receiving chemotherapy. Systemic Treatment Program Committee. Cancer Prev Control. 1997;1:241–8.
22. Couture F, Turner AR, Melosky B et al. Prior red blood cell transfusions in cancer patients increase the risk of subsequent transfusions with or without recombinant human erythropoietin management. Oncologist 2005;10:63–71.
23. Clark O, Adams JR, Bennett CL et al. Erythropoietin, uncertainty principle and cancer related anaemia. BMC Cancer 2002;2:23.
24. Bohlius J, Wilson J, Seidenfeld J, et al. Erythropoietin or darbepoetin for patients with cancer. Cochrane Database Syst Rev. 2006;3:CD003407.
25. Henke M, Laszig R, Ruebe C, et al. Erythropoietin to treat head and neck cancer patients with anaemia undergoing radiotherapy: randomised, double-blind, placebo-controlled trial. Lancet. 2003;362:1255–60.
26. Leyland-Jones B. Breast cancer trial with erythropoietin terminated unexpectedly. Lancet Oncol. 2003;4:459–60.
27. Leyland-Jones B., Semiglazov V., Pawlicki M., et al. Maintaining normal hemoglobin levels with epoetin alfa in mainly nonanemic patients with metastatic breast cancer receiving first-line chemotherapy: a survival study. J Clin Oncol. 2005;23:5865–8.
28. Aapro M., Spivak J.L. Update on erythropoiesis-stimulating agents and clinical trials in oncology. Oncologist. 2009;14(Suppl 1):6–15.
29. Altman D.G., Andersen P.K. Calculating the number needed to treat for trials where the outcome is time to an event. Br Med J. 1999;319:1492–5.
30. Vaupel P., Thews O., Hoeckel M. Treatment resistance of solid tumors: role of hypoxia and anemia. Med Oncol. 2001;18:243–59.
31. Vaupel P, Thews O, Mayer A, Hockel S, Hockel M. Oxygenation status of gynecologic tumors: what is the optimal hemoglobin level? Strahlenther Onkol. 2002;178:727–31.
32. Besarab A, Bolton WK, Browne JK, et al. The effects of normal as compared with low hematocrit values in patients with cardiac disease who are receiving hemodialysis and epoetin. N Engl J Med. 1998;339:584–90.
33. Singh AK, Szczech L, Tang KL, et al. Correction of anemia with epoetin alfa in chronic kidney disease. N Engl J Med. 2006;355:2085–98.
34. Phrommintikul A, Haas SJ, Elsik M, Krum H. Mortality and target haemoglobin concentrations in anaemic patients with chronic kidney disease treated with erythropoietin: a meta-analysis. Lancet. 2007;369:381–8.
35. Vaziri ND. Mechanism of erythropoietin-induced hypertension. Am J Kidney Dis. 1999;33:821–8.
36. Fisher JW. Erythropoietin: physiology and pharmacology update. Exp Biol Med (Maywood). 2003;228:1–14.
37. Stohlawetz PJ, Dzirlo L, Hergovich N, et al. Effects of erythropoietin on platelet reactivity and thrombopoiesis in humans. Blood. 2000;95:2983–9.
38. Wun T, Law L, Harvey D, et al. Increased incidence of symptomatic venous thrombosis in patients with cervical carcinoma treated with concurrent chemotherapy, radiation, and erythropoietin. Cancer. 2003;98:1514–20.
39. Arcasoy MO. Erythropoiesis-stimulating agent use in cancer: preclinical and clinical perspectives. Clin Cancer Res. 2008;14:4685–90.
40. Sinclair AM, Rogers N, Busse L, et al. Erythropoietin receptor transcription is neither elevated nor predictive of surface expression in human tumour cells. Br J Cancer. 2008;98:1059–67.

Chapter 14
Clinical Practice Guidelines for the Use of Erythroid-Stimulating Agents: ASCO, EORTC, NCCN

Alan E. Lichtin

Three organizations spent a great amount of time, effort, and money writing clinical practice guidelines for the use of erythroid-stimulating agents (ESAs). The American Society of Hematology and American Society of Clinical Oncology (ASH/ASCO) panel was convened by these respective professional societies in the United States and a guideline was written in 2002 [1] and an update was published January 1, 2008 (called the 2007 update) [2]. The European equivalent professional society, European Organization for Research and Treatment of Cancer (EORTC), wrote their original guideline in 2004 and updated their ESA guideline in January 2007 [3]. The National Comprehensive Cancer Network (NCCN), a collaborative organization of major comprehensive cancer centers in the United States, published an update of their ESA guideline in July 2008 [4]. (The reader of this chapter in this book must realize that much has transpired in this field since these guideline updates have been written. New data have been published very recently which have led the FDA in the United States and the European Medicine Agency (EMEA) in Europe to recommend curtailment of the use of ESAs. Thus, much in this chapter is of "historical" interest. By the time this chapter is published, more changes may occur, leading to newer pronouncements from the regulators on both sides of the Atlantic.)

All three documents are similar. Indeed, there are three individuals who are co-authors on two of these three manuscripts in the United States. Two authors of the ASH/ASCO guideline then wrote subsequent major meta-analyses, one with 8,167 subjects and another with 13,933 subjects. These meta-analyses are covered in the previous chapter of this book.

Indeed, all three updates reflect growing concern of the potential harms of ESAs when given to cancer patients with anemia, especially those who are not receiving concomitant chemotherapy. Each organization's original guideline had a more liberal application of ESAs applied to patients. The updates reflect new FDA black-box warnings, which were promulgated in 2007. These black-box warnings cautioned

A.E. Lichtin (✉)
Department of Medicine, Cleveland Clinic Lerner College of Medicine, Cleveland, OH 44195, USA; Taussig Cancer Center, Cleveland Clinic Health Systems, Cleveland, OH 44195, USA
e-mail: lichtia@ccf.org

G.H. Lyman, D.C. Dale (eds.), *Hematopoietic Growth Factors in Oncology*, Cancer Treatment and Research 157, DOI 10.1007/978-1-4419-7073-2_14, © Springer Science+Business Media, LLC 2011

against raising the hemoglobin level too high because the incidence of venous thromboembolic disease (VTE) rises the higher the hemoglobin level. Also, admonitions against using ESAs in the setting of curative intent chemotherapy were given by the FDA. This reflects the emergence of data suggesting shortened survival and more rapid growth of tumor cells with exposure to ESAs.

Another major change in all three guideline updates reflects hemoglobin levels at which the clinician should initiate ESA therapy, as well as the hemoglobin level at which to suspend ESA therapy once the hemoglobin level starts to rise. The FDA black-box warning of August 2007 states that ESAs should not be initiated at hemoglobin levels $\geq$ 10 g/dL. Also, FDA clarified that 12 g/dL is not an appropriate goal or upper target for hemoglobin level, but rather the clinician should aim for the lowest level of hemoglobin to avoid transfusion.

The EORTC guideline update, having been written prior to August 2007, still advises initiating ESAs when patients undergoing chemotherapy or X-ray therapy have hemoglobin levels of "9–11 g/dL." The EORTC update still states a target hemoglobin of 12–13 g/dL. The ASH/ASCO and the NCCN guidelines are more in line with the FDA black-box warning. Indeed, the NCCN guideline discusses "asymptomatic" and "symptomatic" anemias recognizing that some individuals can tolerate lower hemoglobin levels than others, without noting a reduced sense of well being.

Initiating ESAs

The NCCN guideline update has eliminated any reference to hemoglobin levels for consideration of treatment with ESAs and target hemoglobin ranges were removed throughout the guidelines. The ASH/ASCO guideline update still considers a hemoglobin < 10 g/dL as a starting point for considering ESAs *as an option* for ameliorating anemia associated with chemotherapy. Because the NCCN guideline update was published in July 2008, there is stronger language in it, reflecting the most up-to-date FDA black-box warnings, especially as far as not administering ESAs in the setting of curative chemotherapy. Only the NCCN guideline update incorporates that language explicitly.

The NCCN guideline has a helpful algorithm for approaching the anemic cancer patient on or off chemotherapy. It dissects out factors that are important for making the decision whether to encourage or discourage the use of ESAs in these populations of patients. An advantage of the NCCN guideline, in particular, is the specification of cardiopulmonary factors, which tip the balance toward or away from ESA treatment. It divides anemia into mild (hemoglobin 10–11 g/dL), moderate (hemoglobin 8–10 g/dL), and severe (hemoglobin < 8 g/dL). It specifies physiologic symptoms of cardiopulmonary distress ("peripheral edema, sustained tachycardia and tachypnea, as well as subjective physical symptoms [which] may include chest pain, dyspnea on exertion, orthostatic lightheadedness/near syncope or syncope, and fatigue").

A "shared decision approach" is applied more widely in the 2007 ASH/ASCO update. Once the hemoglobin level falls toward or below 10 g/dL, ESAs are *an option* for raising hemoglobin levels, as are transfusions. There is less explicit language about cardiopulmonary symptoms as they relate to recommending the use of ESAs. It is implicit that clinicians should discuss the options with their patients and come to a mutual decision as to what is best for the patient. An individual who is anemic from chemotherapy, but who is phobic about getting blood, or for religious reasons refuses blood transfusion, may wish to receive an ESA treatment. A clinician who is concerned with how a patient might physiologically handle a transfusion (previous allergic reactions to blood products, a person with a history of producing antibodies to other individuals' blood, a patient with very poor venous access, etc.) may come to a mutual decision with a patient to receive ESAs.

The authors of the ASH/ASCO guideline "recognize that there is a subset of patients for whom initiating ESAs at a higher hemoglobin [>10 g/dL] may be worth considering." These include the elderly with "limited cardiopulmonary reserve, those with underlying coronary artery disease or symptomatic angina, those with impaired physical functioning due to decreased energy or exercise capacity." Then, a statement is made about quality-of-life (QOL) studies. Without referencing any specific study but noting the field of QOL research as it pertains to the ESAs, it states, "the best clinical opinion of the Update Committee is that a trial of ESAs may be warranted for such patients" [2].

The NCCN guideline reflects upon QOL research and states, "Data indicate that ESAs may improve fatigue in a small percentage of patients, however more research is needed." Then, there are references to four articles that relate to this statement [5–8].

CMS reimbursement policy and the present FDA black-box warning do not give clinicians or patients this leeway [9]. To be reimbursed, one must observe a hemoglobin < 10 g/dL before using ESAs. Certainly a future update to the ASH/ASCO update will be published where the reality of the new FDA black-box warning will be integrated into new recommendations. As it is now, at the time of the writing of this chapter, if a clinician has a patient with a hemoglobin of 10–11 g/dL, who had started non-curative chemotherapy for cancer with a hemoglobin of, say, 14 g/dL, and who has limited cardiopulmonary reserves [for example, begins having true angina between hemoglobin 10 and 11 g/dL] the only option, unless the patient is wealthy enough to afford paying for ESAs out of pocket or who has a more generous insurance program than Medicare, is transfusion. Many clinicians are bothered that the option of using ESAs for such a patient has been made so problematic [10].

The EORTC 2007 update appears to be the most "out of date" of the guidelines. They state "that in cancer patients receiving chemotherapy and/or radiotherapy, treatment with erythropoietic proteins should be initiated at a hemoglobin level of 9–11 g/dL based on anemia related symptoms rather than a fixed hemoglobin concentration. Early intervention with erythropoietic proteins may be considered in asymptomatic anemic patients with hemoglobin levels 11.9 g/dL, provided that individual factors like intensity and expected duration of chemotherapy are reconsidered." Based on the new FDA black-box warning, there would be contraindication to the majority of the above quote. Even more against present FDA labeling is the following quote from the EORTC: "The target hemoglobin concentration should be 12–13 g/dL. Once this level is achieved, maintenance doses should be titrated individually" [3]. Again, the present FDA recommendation is not to aim for any particular ceiling hemoglobin level [e.g., 12 g/dL], rather the FDA directs the clinician to "give the lowest dose. . . to avoid transfusion. This is generally in the range of 9–10 g/dL of Hemoglobin" [9].

The European Medicines Agency (EMEA) website contains a press office release entitled "Questions and answers on epoetins and the risk of tumour growth and blood clots in the veins" [11]. It states the agency is closely monitoring the safety of epoetin-containing medicines. "In 9/07, the Agency finalized a full safety review of all epoetins, which has resulted in changes to the prescribing information for all the medicines, to ensure they are only used in patients whose anaemia is causing symptoms, such as weakness or a lack of energy." The EMEA proceeds to quote the Bennett meta-analysis [12] and the Thomas Gynecologic Oncology Group Trial [13]. Then, they describe a meeting of an oncology scientific advisory group, during which "the experts stated that in cancer patients with a reasonably long life expectancy, the benefit of using epoetins to avoid blood transfusions does not balance the risks of tumour progression and shorter survival." The Committee for Medicinal Products for Human Use (CHMP) of EMEA stated that "the product information for all epoetics that are authorized for use in cancer patients should be updated to include a warning that transfusion should be the preferred method for correcting anemia in cancer patients, especially those with a long life expectancy. The committee also recommended that the companies who make epoetin-containing medicines should carry out, as a priority, additional studies to clarify the risks and benefits of epoetins used in the treatment of cancer patients as currently recommended."

The consequences of the EMEA action for patients and doctors include the following:

- Doctors who prescribe epoetin-containing medicines for the treatment of anemia in cancer patients must remember that they should use them only in patients when their anemia is causing symptoms and is having an impact on their state of health.
- Doctors are warned that blood transfusion is the preferred option for treating anemia in cancer patients with a good prognosis. Epoetins should only be used when the benefit in terms of patient preference clearly outweighs the risk of the cancer getting worse.

A contrast between the FDA and EMEA may be in their use of terms. FDA warns doctors not to use ESAs when the chemotherapy being given is with "curative intent" or in the adjuvant setting, and EMEA states not to give ESAs when the patient "has a good prognosis." There is some room for interpretation in both of these statements. Certainly, though, adjuvant chemotherapy is an easier term to define.

Venous Thromboembolic Disease

A new topic in the ASH/ASCO guideline update which was not present in the 2002 original was the understanding that some chemotherapy regimens in certain cancer scenarios are more likely to be complicated by thromboembolic disease (VTE). Between 2002 and 2007, there were reports of myeloma patients receiving thalidomide and lenalidomide having a higher risk of VTE [14]. The NCCN guideline expanded this VTE risk to include other risk factors, such as prior history of VTE, heritable mutation, hypercoagulability, elevated pre-chemotherapy platelet count, recent surgery, hormonal agents, prolonged inactivity by hospitalization, steroids, as well as co-morbidities such as hypertension [4].

Iron

There is an entire new section in the 2007 ASH/ASCO update on iron monitoring and supplementation. Several studies during the 2000s demonstrated greater rises in hemoglobin for ESA-treated patients receiving intravenous (IV) iron compared with those receiving no or oral iron supplementation [15–17]. There have been further studies reported since all three guideline updates were published, as well [18, 19]. The ASH/ASCO guideline discussed methodologic flaws in the studies and did not really make a definitive statement encouraging doctors to use IV iron along with ESAs. The NCCN guideline states, "IV iron products are recommended for iron repletion in cancer patients with absolute iron deficiency (ferritin <30 ng/mL, transferrin saturation <15%) or in patients receiving erythropoietic drugs" [4]. Both guidelines discuss adverse events with IV iron. NCCN encourages low molecular weight iron dextran. EORTC quotes some of these same studies yet does not make a definite statement encouraging IV iron use with ESAs. A comment might be made, however, that iron deficiency corrected with well-tolerated oral iron can be a most gratifying experience for doctor and patient. It is very inexpensive and consumes very little time. Cancer patients who are iron deficient often are losing blood through their GI tract and the different studies describe very different methodologies for finding the source of blood loss and putting an end to the hemorrhage.

Survival

The most worrisome aspect of ESA use is whether it may shorten survival of cancer patients. Since the EORTC guideline is the oldest update and since the survival question has been a relatively newer phenomenon, it misses out on discussing the weight of this issue. Since NCCN's ESA guideline update is the most up-to-date, it includes a more thorough discussion of this topic.

The first important notation of this problem came from Henke [20] and Leyland-Jones [21]. Henke conducted a radiation therapy trial in head and neck cancer patients receiving XRT. The objective of that trial was to see if ESAs could cause radio-sensitization and lead to better survival. Starting hemoglobin values for women were <12 g/dL and men were <13 g/dL and target (stopping) values were $\geq$ 14 g/dL for women and $\geq$ 15 g/dL for men. There was decreased overall survival for ESA-treated individuals (hazard radio for death 1.39, $p = 0.02$, and for locoregional progression, the hazard ratio was 1.69, $p = 0.007$). Leyland-Jones authored the BEST study (Breast Cancer Erythropoietin Survival Trial): 939 patients with metastatic breast cancer who received chemotherapy, X-ray therapy and/or hormones were randomized to receive weekly erythropoietin alfa or placebo. Study drug was started if baseline hemoglobin was <13 g/dL or when hemoglobin decreased below that level during the study. It should be remembered that the study aimed to keep the hemoglobin normal and these patients were kept non-anemic. The study was terminated early by the Data Monitoring Committee when a higher mortality in the ESA arm was discovered. "Final analysis showed reduced 1 year survival of patients who received ESA versus those who received placebo (70% vs. 76%, respectively, HR=1.37; $p = 0.01$"). There was an increased number of venous thromboembolic events in the ESA group, but this did not explain all of the survival differences.

Two other chemotherapy trials [22, 23] and one other X-ray therapy trial [24] described similar observations of decreased survival in ESA-treated cancer patients. The Hedenus trial randomized ESA use in lymphoid malignancy subjects and the PREPARE study was in breast cancer patients, like the Leyland-Jones study. A combined chemo-radiotherapy trial from the Gynecologic Oncology Group, by Thomas [13] demonstrated a decreased overall survival and decreased progression-free survival in darbepoetin-treated subjects. Finally, in cancer patients not receiving active chemotherapy or X-ray therapy, there are two studies showing more rapid tumor growth and decreased overall survival. One was the EPO-CAN-20 [22], which was a study of 70 non-small cell lung cancer patients, receiving epoetin alfa 40,000 U/week for 12 weeks versus placebo. There was decreased overall survival in the ESA-treated group with a hazard ratio for death of 1.84, $p = 0.04$. The Amgen 103 trial, by Smith [25] used darbepoetin in non-myeloid cancer patients at a dose of 6.75 μg/kg/4 weeks. Starting hemoglobin $\leq$ 11 g/dL and stopping value was >13 g/dL. Decreased overall survival was noted in the darbepoetin group with a hazard ratio for death of 1.3 with $p = 0.003$.

It was this litany of worrisome studies which led the manufacturers to add black-box warnings to their ESAs. The NCCN update states, "In keeping with the FDA product labels of ESAs, the panel recommends transfusion as the only appropriate treatment for anemia in patients with solid tumors who are not undergoing chemotherapy; ESAs are not indicated for these patients" [26].

Myelodysplasia (MDS)

The EORTC document does not have any special mention of ESA use in MDS. Both the ASH/ASCO and NCCN guidelines do specifically separate out this special population. An early Italian randomized controlled trial showing benefit and less transfusions in low-risk MDS patients seems to have stood the test of time [27]. The NCCN document refers readers to the NCCN Clinical Practice Guidelines in Oncology: Myelodysplastic Syndrome for ESA use in this population.

Conflict of Interest

It is hard to be silent on this topic as it relates to clinical practice guidelines. The level of conflict tolerated by the three guidelines is a little eye-opening. Four of eight (50%) of the EORTC authors had disclosed financial interests with the companies, which make ESAs. Also, the authors did not only just receive research support, but also served on advisory boards, received honoraria, and participated in speaker's bureaus for Amgen, Hoffman-LaRoche, and Johnson & Johnson. The ASH/ASCO guideline writing committee had 8 of 13 with no financial relationship with pharmaceutical companies. The other 5 of 13 received research support from Amgen or Johnson & Johnson, or were consultants, both compensated and uncompensated. The NCCN guideline committee had 25 members and 2 had a financial relationship with Amgen. One author who was on both the NCCN guideline committee and the ASH/ASCO guideline committee had different disclosures. He noted he was either a speaker, consultant, expert witness, or advisor to Sanofi-Aventis US on the NCCN guideline, but was a consultant (compensated) and received honoraria and research funding from Amgen on the ASH/ASCO guideline. The time course was similar for both documents, so one might query why the disclosure was different in the two documents.

Professional societies (and academic centers) have evolved over the past few years toward increasing transparency as it relates to conflict of interest. Practice guideline writing committees of professional societies such as ASH and ASCO are under increasing scrutiny, and there is a trend toward having at least <50% of a guideline writing membership being non-conflicted and chairs or co-chairs having no conflicts. The day may come when practice guideline committees will tolerate zero conflicts with the pharmaceutical companies about whose drugs they are writing guidelines. Indeed, on April 1, 2009, a distinguished group of academics wrote a "Special Communication" in the *Journal of the American Medical Association* [28], advocating such a zero tolerance for practice guideline writing committees. They state, "Professional medical associations (PMA) should be encouraged to appoint to these committees only individuals with no ties to industry. At a minimum, PMA's must exclude from such committees persons with any conflict of interest ($0 threshold) involving direct salary support, research support, or additional income from a company whose product sales could be affected by the guidelines."

A criticism of this zero tolerance might be that such a position prevents individuals who are highly qualified from participating in promulgating guidelines. These academics proceed to comment: "One concern might be that such restrictions will exclude the most qualified individuals from guideline committees. However, there is a tendency to confuse the most qualified with the most visible. Moreover, any difficulties can be easily circumvented by circulating drafts of guidelines widely for comment, but leaving the drafting of the final document to a group of knowledge-able professionals who are free of conflict of interest insofar as a particular class of drugs or devices is concerned."

Since the three guidelines discussed in this chapter do not pass this new test of freedom from conflicts, are they at all believable? Perhaps, in the spirit of supreme and pragmatic caution, the use of ESAs should be curtailed until a new generation of guidelines is written by non-conflicted guideline writing committees.

A summary table covering key points in this chapter is shown in Table 14.1.

Table 14.1 Key differences in the three larger clinical practice guideline updates for ESA use in cancer patients

	EORTC	ASH/ASCO	NCCN
Date of publication	January, 2007	January 1, 2008	July, 2008
Trigger to start ESAs (treatment related)	9–11 g/dL	<10 g/dL (ESAs are an option)	Symptom assessment
Target hemoglobin once ESAs are initiated	12–13 g/dL	Raise hemoglobin level to avoid transfusions	Titrate dosage to avoid red blood cell transfusion
Conflict of interest disclosures (number with conflicts/total number of authors)	4/8 (50%)	5/13 (38%)	2/25[a] (8%)

[a]Conflicts with pharmaceutical manufacturers who do not make ESAs are listed for five other authors.

References

1. Rizzo JD, Lichtin AE, Woolf SH, et al. Use of epoetin in patients with cancer: evidence based clinical practice guidelines of the American Society of Clinical Oncology and the American Society of Hematology. J Clin Oncol. 2002;20:4083–107.
2. Rizzo JD, Somerfield MR, Hagerty KL, Seidenfeld J, Bohlius J, Bennett CL, Cella DF, Djulbegovic B, Goode MJ, Jakubowski AA, Rarick MU, Regan DH, Lichtin AE. Use of epoetin and darbepoetin in patients with cancer: 2007 American Society of Clinical Oncology/American Society of Hematology clinical practice guideline update. J Clin Oncol. 2008;26(1):132–49.
3. Bokemeyer C, Aapro MS, Courdi A, Foubert J, Link H, Osterborg A, Repetto L, Sonbeyran P. European Organization for Research and Treatment of Cancer [EORTC] guidelines for the use of erythropoietin proteins in anaemic patients with cancer; 2006 update. Eur J Cancer. 2007;43(2):258–70. [E pub 2006 Dec 19].
4. Rodgers GM, Becker PS, Bennett CL, Cella D, Chavan-klian A, Chesney C, Cleeland C, Coccia PF, Djubegovic B, Garet J, Gilreath JA, Kraut E, Lin WC, Matulovis U, Millensor M, Reinke D, Rosenthal J, Sabbatini P, Schwartz RN, Stein R, Vij R. Cancer and chemotherapy induced anemia [clinical practice guidelines in oncology]. J Natl Compr Canc Netw. 2008;6(6):536–64.
5. Minton O, Stone P, Richardson A, et al. Drug therapy for the management of cancer related fatigue. Cochrane Database Syst Rev. 2008:CD006704.

6. Cella D, Eton DT, Lai J-S, et al. Combining anchor and distribution based methods to derive minimal clinically important differences on the Functional Assessment of Cancer Therapy anemia and fatigue scales. J Pain Symptom Manage. 2002;24:547–61.

7. Cella D, Dobrez D, Glaspy J. Control of cancer-related anemia with erythropoietic agents: a review of evidence for improved quality of live and clinical outcomes. Ann Oncol. 2003;14:511–19.

8. Fallowfield L, Gagnon D, Cella D, et al. Multivariate regression analyses of data from a randomized, double-blind, placebo-controlled study confirmed quality of life benefit of epoetin alfa in patients receiving non-platinum chemotherapy. Br J Cancer. 2002;87:1341–53.

9. Hagerty K. Continued regulatory actions affecting the use of erythropoiesis-stimulating agents. J Oncol Pract. 2008;4(6):267–70.

10. Glaspy JA. Erythropoiesis-stimulating agents in oncology. J Natl Compr Canc Netw. 2008;6(6):565–84.

11. European Medicines Agency Document. Doc Ref EMEA/CHMP/333962/2008, Jun 26 2008.

12. Bennett CL, Silver SM, Djulbegovic G, et al. Venous thromboembolism and mortality associated with recombinant erythropoietin and darbepoetin administration for the treatment of cancer associated anemia. J Amer Med Assn. 2008;299(8):914–24.

13. Thomas G, Ali S, Hoebers FJ, et al. Phase III trial to evaluate the efficacy of maintaining hemoglobin levels above 12 g/dL with erythropoietin vs. above 10 g/dL without erythropoietin in anemic patients receiving concurrent radiation and cisplatinum for cervical cancer. Gynecol Oncol. 2008;108:317–25.

14. Bennett CL, Angelotta C, Yarnold PR, et al. Thalidomide and lenolidomide-associated thromboembolism among patients with cancer. J Amer Med Assn. 2006;296:2558–60.

15. Auerbach M, Ballard H, Trout JR, et al. Intravenous iron optimizes the response to recombinant human erythropoietin in cancer patients with chemotherapy-related anemia: a multicenter open-label, randomized trial. J Clin Oncol. 2004;22:1301–7.

16. Henry DH, Dahl NV, Auerbach M, et al. Intravenous ferric gluconate significantly improves response to epoetin alfa versus oral iron or no iron in anemic patients with cancer receiving chemotherapy. Oncologist. 2007;12:231–42.

17. Hedenus M, Birgegard G, Nasman P, et al. Addition of intravenous iron to epoetin beta increases hemoglobin response and decreases epoetin dose requirement in anemic patients with lymphoproliferative malignancies: a randomized multicenter study. Leukemia. 2007;21:627–32.

18. Bastit L, Vanderbroek A, Altintas S, et al. Randomized, multicenter, controlled trial comparing the efficacy and safety of darbepoetin alfa administered every 3 weeks with or without intravenous iron in patients with chemotherapy-induced anemia. J Clin Oncol. 2008;26(10):1611–18.

19. Pedrazzoli P, Farris A, Del Prete S, et al. Randomized trial of intravenous iron supplementation in patients with chemotherapy-related anemia without iron deficiency treated with darbepoetin alfa. J Clin Oncol. 2008;26(10):1619–25.

20. Henke M, Laszig R, Rube C, et al. Erythropoietin to treat head and neck cancer patients with anemia undergoing radiotherapy: randomized, double-blind, placebo-controlled trial. Lancet. 2003;362:1255–60.

21. Leyland-Jones B, Semiglozov V, Pawliki M, et al. Maintaining normal hemoglobin levels with epoetin alfa in mainly non anemic patients with metastatic breast cancer receiving first line chemotherapy. A survival study. J Clin Oncol. 2005;23:5960–72.

22. Wright JR, Ung YC, Julian JA, et al. Randomized double-blind, placebo-controlled trial of erythropoietin in non-small cell lung cancer with disease related anemia. J Clin Oncol. 2007;25:1027–32.

23. Hedenus M, Adriansson M, San Miguel J, et al. Efficacy and safety of darbepoetin alfa in anemic patients with lymphoproliferative malignancies: a randomized, double-blind, placebo-controlled study. Br J Haematol. 2003;122:394–403.

24. Overgaard J, Hoff C, San Hansen H. Randomized study of the importance of novel erythro-poiesis stimulating protein (Aranesp) for the effect of radiotherapy in patients with primary squamous cell carcinoma of the head and neck (HNSCC): the Danish Head and Neck Cancer Group (DAHANCA 10 [Abstract]). Eur J Cancer Suppl. 2007;5(6):7. Abstract 6LB.
25. Smith RE Jr, Aapro MS, Ludwig H, et al. Darbepoetin alfa for the treatment of anemia in patients with active cancer not receiving chemotherapy or radiotherapy: results of a phase III, multicenter randomized, double-blind, placebo-controlled study. J Clin Oncol. 2008;26: 1040–50.
26. U.S. Food and Drug Administration. Press release: FDA receives new data on risks of anemia drugs consistent with previous data on tumor growth and death. 3 Jan 2008. Available at http://www.fda.gov/lls/topics/NEWS/2008/NEW01769.html
27. Anonymous. A randomized double-blind placebo-controlled study with subcutaneous recombinant human erythropoietin in patients with low risk myelodysplastic syndromes: Italian Cooperative Study Group for rHuEpo in Myelodysplastic Syndromes. Br J Haematol. 1998;103:1070–4.
28. Rothman DJ, McDonald WJ, Berkowitz CD, et al. Professional medical associations and their relationships with industry. JAMA 2009;301(13):1367–72.

Part IV
The Thrombopoietic Agents

Chapter 15
Thrombocytopenia and Platelet Transfusions in Patients with Cancer

Jason Valent and Charles A. Schiffer

Abstract Platelet transfusions are a critical component of the supportive care for patients receiving intensive therapy for hematologic malignancies. The platelet count "triggering" prophylactic transfusion has decreased over the years, and studies comparing a prophylactic versus a therapeutic transfusion approach are in progress. The evidence supporting the need for platelet transfusions prior to different invasive procedures is reviewed. Lastly, studies evaluating the use of thrombopoietic stimulating agents to reduce hemorrhage and decrease the need for platelet transfusions are discussed. To date, there is no evidence that this approach is of clinical utility.

Initial reports in the mid-1960s by Hersh et al. [1] and Han et al. [2] suggested that allogeneic prophylactic platelet transfusion could reduce hemorrhagic deaths in patients with leukemia. Currently it is estimated that 9 million equivalent units of platelet concentrate are transfused in the United States each year [3] with the majority of platelet transfusions supporting patients with cancer diagnoses. Platelet transfusion strategies used in the supportive care of cancer patients can be grouped into two categories. The first is a prophylactic transfusion approach using a predefined minimum accepted platelet count as a trigger for transfusion. The second is a therapeutic transfusion policy using clinically significant bleeding as the indication for platelet transfusion. Despite the lack of randomized trials comparing prophylactic and therapeutic platelet transfusion in the modern era of antimicrobials and chemotherapy, prophylactic transfusion of platelets to patients receiving intensive chemotherapy has been widely accepted as standard of care [4–6].

C.A. Schiffer (✉)
Division of Hematology/Oncology, Karmanos Cancer Institute, Wayne State University School of Medicine, Detroit, MI 48201, USA
e-mail: schiffer@karmanos.org

G.H. Lyman, D.C. Dale (eds.), *Hematopoietic Growth Factors in Oncology*, Cancer Treatment and Research 157, DOI 10.1007/978-1-4419-7073-2_15, © Springer Science+Business Media, LLC 2011

Prophylactic Transfusion Strategy

The prophylactic platelet transfusion strategy uses a minimum platelet count as a prompt for platelet transfusion in patients despite the lack of signs or symptoms of bleeding. A landmark retrospective analysis in 1962 by Gaydos et al. established a quantitative relationship between platelet count and both severity and frequency of hemorrhagic episodes in thrombocytopenic patients with acute leukemia [7]. While hemorrhage was not consistently observed at lower platelet counts, grossly visible hemorrhage rarely occurred when platelet counts were above 20,000/μL. Of note is that the authors pointed out that a specific platelet count threshold for increased bleeding risk could not be identified. In an early small double-blind study from Higby et al., 12 patients were randomized to receive platelet transfusions and 9 to receive platelet-poor plasma transfusions when the platelet count fell to less than 30,000/μL [8]. Hemorrhage occurred in only 5 of the 12 patients transfused with platelets versus 8 of the 9 transfused with platelet-poor plasma.

The prophylactic transfusion strategy was then validated in two trials in the pediatric acute leukemia population. Roy et al. demonstrated that the risk of bleeding in a historical control group that did not receive platelet transfusions for thrombocytopenia was much higher than in prospectively analyzed patients receiving prophylactic platelet transfusion (56% in controls compared to 7% in transfused) [9]. A second prospective study by Murphy et al. compared the prophylactic to therapeutic transfusion strategy [10]. The threshold of 20,000 platelets/μL was used as the trigger for prophylactic platelet transfusion. For patients in the prophylactic transfusion arm, the number of days with hemorrhage was significantly less than in the therapeutic transfusion arm. This is not necessarily surprising, since for patients in the "therapeutic" arm, signs of hemorrhage were the indication for transfusion. There was no significant difference in survival between the two arms.

All of these studies were performed in the 1970s and earlier, at a time when the quality of antibiotic support, chemotherapy, and possibly the platelet transfusions themselves were inferior to current practice. In addition, aspirin was used as an antipyretic in the earlier years and Gram-negative bacteremia was much more common. Nonetheless, based on these studies, the 20,000 platelets/μL threshold for prophylactic transfusion became widely accepted as the trigger for transfusion thereafter until further studies were published in the 1990s.

Four studies at the end of the last century helped to revise the appropriate threshold for prophylactic platelet transfusions in patients undergoing intensive chemotherapy. Gmür et al. reported experience with 103 leukemia patients in 1991 that suggested the transfusion threshold of 10,000 platelets/μL was equivalent in safety to a transfusion threshold of 20,000 platelets/μL [11]. The initial publication of a randomized study demonstrating the safety of the 10,000 platelets/μL threshold came from Heckman et al. in a single institution trial at the University of Iowa [12]. Thirty-seven patients were randomized to the $\leq$10,000 platelets/μL arm and 41 to the $\leq$20,000 platelets/μL arm. No hemorrhagic deaths were observed in either arm and the number of transfusions on average was decreased from 11 in the 20,000 platelets/μL arm to 7 in the 10,000 platelets/μL arm although this was not statistically significant, perhaps due to the small sample size.

Rubella et al. published the results of a multicenter randomized trial of 276 patients in 1997 providing further support for the 10,000 platelets/μL threshold [13]. In this trial, platelet use was significantly decreased by 21.5% without an increase in packed red blood cell transfusion use or mortality when comparing transfusion thresholds of 20,000 and 10,000 platelets/μL. Safety of the 10,000 platelets/μL threshold was further confirmed in a study by Wandt et al. in 1998 [14]. This study again compared 20,000 and 10,000 platelets/μL as the thresholds for transfusion. Results showed no difference in bleeding episodes and a decrease in platelet use by 33%. Based on these results, a platelet count of $\leq$10,000/μL is recommended by the American Society of Clinical Oncology [4], the British Committee for Standards in Hematology [5], and the American Society of Hematology [6] as the trigger for prophylactic platelet transfusion in patients undergoing intensive chemotherapy.

It must be stressed that several studies have indicated that factors such as fever, serious infections, hypoalbuminemia, uremia, rapid falls in platelet count, recent hemorrhage, the presence of other coagulation abnormalities, hyperleukocytosis in patients with acute leukemia, the need for invasive procedures, and hemodynamic instability can be associated with increased risks of bleeding and may necessitate prophylactic platelet transfusion at thresholds higher than 10,000 platelets/μL [3, 7, 15]. Notably in the small series by Higby et al. mentioned above, fever preceded hemorrhage in 77% of patients with bleeding episodes [8]. These clinical factors should be considered when evaluating individual patients for platelet transfusion and indeed, all the randomized trials permitted transfusions at platelet counts higher than 10,000/μL in these clinical circumstances. In addition, patients with acute promyelocytic leukemia, serious infection, and coagulation abnormalities were not included in the above trials using $\leq$10,000 platelets/μL as the transfusion threshold.

Significance of Transfusion Dose

More recent studies have examined whether the dose of platelets transfused can safely be lowered to decrease the total number of platelets needed during treatment with intensive chemotherapy. A single unit of random donor platelets contains a minimum of 5.5×10^{10} platelets and an apheresis unit of single-donor platelets contains a minimum of 3×10^{11} platelets [16]. Endogenous thrombopoietin is adsorbed onto the surface of transfused platelets, effectively lowering the circulating levels of thrombopoietin in the thrombocytopenic patient [17]. It therefore might be theoretically desirable to limit the number of platelets per transfusion to maximize circulating levels of endogenous thrombopoietin at the time of megakaryocyte recovery.

The results of the PLADO study, a multicenter randomized trial with 1,351 patients, were reported at the 2008 American Society of Hematology annual meeting [18]. This study evaluated the use of low, standard, and high doses of platelet transfusion based on body surface area in patients undergoing chemotherapy for hematologic malignancies or in conjunction with stem cell transplant. The trigger for prophylactic transfusion was a morning platelet count of $\leq$10,000 platelets/μL.

The primary endpoint was episodes of World Health Organization (WHO) grade 2 or higher bleeding and more than 90% of the patients were transfused based on their treatment arm assignment. According to the WHO, grade 0 is no bleeding; grade 1 is petechiae, mucosal, or retinal bleeding without vision impairment; grade 2 is clinically significant minor blood loss such as melena, hematochezia, hematuria, or hemoptysis; grade 3 is gross blood loss requiring transfusion; grade 4 is debilitating blood loss, retinal bleeding with vision impairment, cerebral bleeding with neurologic sequelae, or hemorrhagic death. Results demonstrated no difference in episodes of grade 2, 3, or 4 bleeding among the three arms. Episodes of grade 3 or higher bleeding were only seen in about 10% of patients and episodes of grade 4 bleeding were only seen in about 2% of patients. Transfusion of packed red blood cells was the same in each arm and transfusion of platelets was reduced by 9% using the low-dose compared to the standard-dose strategy.

A second recently analyzed multicenter, multinational, randomized, non-inferiority trial also evaluated if the dose of platelet transfusion used in a prophylactic strategy could be lowered. The SToP study randomized patients, most of whom were receiving chemotherapy for acute leukemia, into low-dose or standard-dose arms for prophylactic platelet transfusions at a morning platelet count prompt of 10,000/μL [19]. The primary outcome was WHO grade 2 or higher bleeding episodes. After enrollment of 130 patients, the Data Safety Monitoring Board stopped the study early due to increased grade 4 bleeding in the low-dose arm. Three patients in this arm experienced grade 4 bleeding compared to none in the standard-dose arm, although fever or infection was present at the time of bleeding in all three patients. Two of the patients had retinal bleeding with vision impairment and one patient had a subdural hemorrhage with neurologic sequelae. Analysis of the 130 evaluable patients did not show any difference in rates of grade 2 or higher bleeding between the two arms. Due to the early discontinuation of the SToP study, it could not be determined if the grade 4 bleeding episodes seen only in the low-dose arm occurred by chance alone. Based on these results, it remains uncertain as to the role of lower-dose platelet transfusions in patients with hematologic malignancies.

There are potential drawbacks to utilizing lower doses of platelet transfusion. This approach generally increases the frequency of transfusion and thus, the work load required for blood bank and nursing staff, thereby possibly increasing the overall cost. In addition, lower transfusion dose would likely be insufficient to provide adequate platelet levels over the course of a weekend necessitating additional clinic visits. Given the available data, lower-dose platelet transfusions cannot be recommended routinely at this time.

Therapeutic Transfusion Strategy

Few studies in the modern era of supportive care have addressed the use of a therapeutic versus prophylactic platelet transfusions in thrombocytopenic patients. The therapeutic strategy mandates platelet transfusion only for clinically significant bleeding episodes. Supporting further investigation into this strategy, retrospective data in 2,942 adult oncology patients demonstrated no relationship between the lowest recorded platelet count for the day and risk of hemorrhage [15]. The therapeutic strategy was examined by Wandt et al. in 106 autologous peripheral blood stem cell transplant patients with stable clinical conditions [20]. No severe or life-threatening bleeding was reported and one-third of the patients did not require transfusion. These findings were confirmed by Wandt et al. in a randomized trial of 171 patients comparing a therapeutic to prophylactic platelet transfusion strategy in patients undergoing autologous stem cell transplantation [21]. Despite longer duration of thrombocytopenia in the therapeutic arm, no life-threatening or fatal bleeding occurred, presumably because of the rapid and predictable platelet count recovery using peripheral blood stem cells. Platelet transfusion usage was decreased by 27% in the therapeutic arm and 46% of the patients in this arm did not require platelet transfusion. There was no statistically significant difference in the number of red blood cell transfusions between the two arms.

Currently ongoing in the United Kingdom, the TOPPS study is a two-arm non-inferiority study of 600 patients comparing prophylactic versus therapeutic transfusion of platelets in patients being treated for hematologic malignancies with or without hematopoietic stem cell support [22]. Major bleeding ($\geq$WHO grade 2) is the primary outcome to be assessed. Results from this study are expected in 2011 and will better define whether a therapeutic transfusion strategy is as safe as the prophylactic strategy in a large group of patients with hematologic malignancies.

Platelet Transfusion for Invasive Procedures

Conducting prospective randomized trials comparing the safety of performing procedures at various platelet counts is difficult and perhaps not feasible. Retrospective analyses of rather older data and expert opinions do provide guidance as to the need for platelet transfusion prior to invasive procedures. More contemporary descriptive analyses in the era of fine needle aspirates, CT and ultrasound-guided biopsies, and ultrasound-guided catheter insertions would be welcomed.

Bone marrow biopsy: Based on expert opinion, bone marrow biopsy and aspiration can be performed safely at counts less than 20,000 platelets/μL [3].

Lumbar puncture: Retrospective data from two studies in adults suggest that lumbar punctures should be performed with platelet counts >20,000/μL [23, 24]. Both spinal subdural and spinal subarachnoid hematomas occurred more frequently in patients with pre-procedure platelet counts less than 20,000/μL. Retrospective analysis of lumbar punctures performed in a pediatric acute lymphoblastic leukemia population at St. Jude Children's Research Hospital found no serious complications in 5,223 procedures [25]. Patients in this study ranged in age from 1 month to 18 years (median 5.5 years). Twenty-nine procedures were performed in patients with platelet counts of 10,000/μL or less, 170 procedures were performed at platelet counts between 11,000 and 20,000/μL, and another 742 procedures were performed at platelet counts between 21,000 and 50,000/μL. The authors concluded that pre-procedure platelet transfusion was not necessary in this pediatric population if the platelet count was above 10,000/μL. It is not clear whether this can be directly extrapolated to larger, sometimes obese adults. There is little information available about the appropriate threshold when lumbar punctures are done with fluoroscopic guidance, but one would surmise that this approach substantially improves the safety of the procedure at lower platelet counts.

Surgery: Even for surgical procedures as extensive as craniotomy and laparotomy performed under direct visualization, retrospective data suggest that platelet counts of greater than 50,000/μL are sufficient to prevent undue bleeding risk [26]. Other consensus statements support the threshold of 50,000 platelets/μL for the performance of surgical procedures [27, 28] and retrospective data also support this threshold for non-image-guided liver biopsy [29]. The same 50,000 platelets/μL threshold is also recommended for the performance of dental extraction [30, 31] and central venous catheter placement [32, 33]. However, personal experience would suggest that central venous catheters placed into compressible vessels can be safely performed at platelet counts far below this threshold.

Gastrointestinal endoscopy and bronchoscopy: Endoscopy and bronchoscopy/bronchioalveolar lavage without biopsies can be safely performed at platelet counts less than 50,000/μL based on data from Chu et al. and Weiss et al. [34, 35]. Should biopsies be required at the time of endoscopy or bronchoscopy, available data would suggest transfusing the patient to a platelet count above 50,000/μL prior to the procedure [36].

One area in which contemporary data are lacking is in the performance of CT or ultrasound-guided core biopsies and fine needle aspirations. Based on data from transjugular liver biopsies reported by Wallace et al. [37], one can extrapolate that the threshold for pre-procedure platelet transfusion in these settings is below 30,000 platelets/μL. In this retrospective analysis of 51 transjugular liver biopsies in thrombocytopenic cancer patients, the post-procedure platelet count remained below 30,000 platelets/μL in 24 patients. Fifteen of these 24 patients were identified as refractory to platelet transfusion. There were no hemorrhage-related complications in this review. Based on these results, image-guided or transjugular liver biopsies can be safely performed with platelet counts below the current recommendation of 50,000/μL for non-image-guided liver biopsies.

Patients with coagulation abnormalities in addition to thrombocytopenia represent another population requiring consideration for pre-procedure platelet transfusion. In a study by Kluge et al. reviewing percutaneous tracheostomy under bronchoscopic control in 42 thrombocytopenic patients with a mean pre-procedure platelet count of 26,400/μL (range 1,000–47,000/μL), post-procedural bleeding occurred in only 2 patients, both of whom were receiving therapeutic heparin [38]. The majority of the patients in this study were either stem cell transplant recipients or undergoing treatment for hematologic malignancies. Nearly half of the patients in this study had a prolonged aPTT prior to the procedure and all but two patients had platelet transfusion prior to the tracheostomy. The authors concluded that this procedure could be safely performed in thrombocytopenic patients after platelet transfusion but coagulation abnormalities should be corrected prior to the procedure.

It is very important that the post-transfusion platelet count is checked prior to performing procedures in which a particular platelet count is desired. This can generally be done by checking a platelet count 10 min post-transfusion [39]. It is also important to have platelets available should unexpected bleeding occur during or shortly after the procedure. If patients require HLA or cross-matched platelets for transfusion, these also need to be available *prior* to the initiation of the procedure. When possible, it is imperative to correct all coagulation abnormalities prior to performing procedures in thrombocytopenic patients. Finally, the most experienced operator should perform the procedure.

The Use of Exogenous Thrombopoietin in Patients with Cancer

Given the limited availability and short shelf-life of allogeneic platelets, it would be desirable to identify therapeutic agents that could decrease the need for platelet transfusions in patients being treated for cancer. Two novel thrombopoietic growth factors able to stimulate the thrombopoietin (TPO) receptor were evaluated in the 1990s: recombinant human TPO and pegylated recombinant human megakaryocyte growth and development factor (PEG-rHuMGDF). Several studies in cancer patients were performed to examine if these agents could reduce the need for platelet transfusion.

Solid Tumors

Initial studies of TPO-stimulating agents were performed in patients with solid tumors. Basser et al. administered PEG-rHuMGDF in a placebo-controlled study at varying doses 1 day after chemotherapy with carboplatin and cyclophosphamide to patients with various solid tumors [40]. No difference in median platelet count nadir was observed and furthermore, the median platelet count nadirs in the control group were far above levels at which transfusion would be considered.

Another trial from Vadhan-Raj et al. used recombinant human TPO at various dosing schedules in sarcoma patients treated with doxorubicin and ifosfamide [41]. Previous data with this regimen without the use of recombinant human TPO demonstrated that thrombocytopenia was cumulatively more severe with subsequent cycles of chemotherapy. With the use of recombinant human TPO prior to and within 4 days after the administration of cycle 2 of chemotherapy, mean platelet count nadirs were higher in patients treated with recombinant human TPO when compared to cycle 1 in which no recombinant human TPO was administered. Furthermore over the course of four cycles of chemotherapy administration, a significant reduction in the number of platelet transfusions (23% vs 55%) was seen in patients who received optimal schedules of recombinant human TPO compared to those subjects who were determined to receive suboptimal dosing schedules.

Vadhan-Raj et al. also reported that the administration of recombinant human TPO attenuated carboplatin-induced thrombocytopenia in patients treated for gynecologic malignancies [42]. This study used the first cycle of chemotherapy as the control arm in which no recombinant human TPO was given and compared platelet counts with the second cycle which included the administration of recombinant human TPO on days 2, 4, 6, and 8. The mean platelet count nadir was significantly higher and the duration of clinically meaningful thrombocytopenia (defined by a platelet count < 20,000/μL) was significantly shorter in the cycle of chemotherapy given with recombinant human TPO.

A third placebo-controlled study reported by Fanucchi et al. in 1997 used PEG-rHuMGDF in patients undergoing treatment with carboplatin and paclitaxel for non-small cell lung cancer [43]. Treatment arms received varying doses of PEG-rHuMGDF daily starting with the day of chemotherapy. Patients treated with PEG-rHuMGDF had a significantly more rapid return to baseline platelet count (14 days in treatment arm compared to more than 21 days in placebo arm), a significantly earlier nadir of the platelet count (7 days in treatment arm compared to 15 days in placebo arm), and a higher median platelet count nadir (188,000/μL in treatment arm compared to 111,000/μL in placebo arm). The range of nadir platelet count in the placebo arm of this study was 21,000–307,000/μL. One patient in the placebo arm received a platelet transfusion for hemoptysis when the platelet count was 21,000/μL and this was the only platelet transfusion given in this study. As evidenced by the median platelet count nadir in the patients receiving placebo, this chemotherapy regimen could not demonstrate any potential clinical benefit from a TPO-stimulating agent as the level of thrombocytopenia was not severe. Indeed, there are few, if any, standard regimens used for patients with solid tumors which predictably require repeated platelet transfusions.

Transplantation and Acute Myeloid Leukemia

Three double-blind, placebo-controlled studies using PEG-rHuMGDF were performed in patients undergoing myeloablative chemotherapy regimens prior to autologous stem cell transplant and in patients undergoing induction and consolidation chemotherapy for acute myeloid leukemia [44–46]. The study drug was administered on day 0 either as a onetime dose or daily until platelet count recovery in the transplant study and after the completion of chemotherapy on a daily basis until platelet count recovery in the two AML studies. Identical doses of the study drug were administered during induction and consolidation chemotherapy in both AML trials. A subsequent trial in patients with AML evaluated the addition of a loading dose of PEG-rHuMGDF given prechemotherapy [47]. Unfortunately, there was no effect on platelet count nadir, time to platelet recovery, and the number of platelet transfusions required in patients treated with PEG-rHuMGDF, although patients receiving the PEG-rHuMGDF had significantly higher platelet counts at the time of count recovery.

There are several explanations for the inability of exogenous TPO to shorten the duration of severe thrombocytopenia and therefore decrease the number of platelet transfusions required in patients undergoing myeloablative chemotherapy.

- Myeloablative chemotherapy regimens rapidly produce an aplastic bone marrow devoid of megakaryocytes. Both endogenous and exogenous TPO require megakaryocytes or their precursors to be present in the marrow to have an effect [48] and thus, even pharmacologic doses of exogenous TPO would not be able to increase the platelet count when administered during marrow aplasia.
- Endogenous TPO levels are markedly elevated during periods of thrombocytopenia [49]. Emmons et al. demonstrated serum or plasma TPO levels in patients with aplastic bone marrows to be roughly 20-fold higher than normal controls. Thus, any residual or regenerating megakaryocytes may already be exposed to a maximal stimulus for growth and differentiation and additional exogenous stimulation with a TPO receptor agonist might not have an additive effect.
- Another confounding factor is the delay between initial exposure to TPO and the production of circulating platelets. Even in healthy volunteers there is a 1-week lag between TPO administration and an increase in platelet count because TPO does not stimulate the release of platelets from the megakaryocyte and marrow, but rather promotes growth and differentiation of less mature megakaryocyte precursors [50].

Myelodysplasia

Limited data from Komatsu et al. suggested that PEG-rHuMGDF could be effective in some thrombocytopenic patients with myelodysplastic syndromes [50]. Of the 21 patients in this study with platelet counts < 30,000/μL, daily PEG-rHuMGDF for 14 days produced an average doubling of the platelet counts with responses in one-third of the patients. The peak effect on platelet counts occurred approximately 5 weeks after initiation of treatment. However, one would predict that in many patients with myelodysplastic syndromes, and particularly those with more advanced disease, the dysplastic megakaryocytes would be incapable of responding to even pharmacologic doses of exogenous TPO. Indeed, this has been the experience with the use of erythropoietic-stimulating agents in this population. Furthermore, it is unusual to have isolated severe thrombocytopenia as the predominant abnormality in patients with myelodysplastic syndromes.

Other Uses for TPO-Stimulating Agents

Another potential use for TPO-stimulating agents would be to increase the yield of harvested platelets from whole blood and platelet donors. As these normal individuals have ample megakaryocytes, one would expect treatment responses to be similar to those seen in patients treated for solid tumors. In 2001, Kuter et al. published the results of a placebo-controlled trial examining the effects of PEG-rHuMGDF on platelet yields in healthy platelet donors [51]. Compared with placebo, a nearly threefold increase in the number of harvested platelets was seen in patients treated with a 3-μg/kg dose of PEG-rHuMGDF without apparent toxicity. Another randomized study using PEG-rHuMGDF was undertaken assessing the post-treatment platelet count in paid healthy volunteers receiving this agent compared to placebo. Treated subjects had platelet counts that essentially doubled when compared to baseline; however, 13 of the 538 subjects on the PEG-rHuMGDF arm developed thrombocytopenia and in some patients this persisted for months to years. The thrombocytopenia proved to be due to the development of antibodies to PEG-rHuMGDF that cross-reacted with endogenous TPO. This finding ended study of recombinant human TPO and PEG-rHuMGDF in normal human subjects [52].

There were also some practical concerns about using TPO agents in healthy blood and platelet donors. Two visits to the blood donation center would be required, the first for the administration of the drug and the second for the platelet donation 12 days later at the time of maximal platelet count [51, 53]. This could discourage potential donors from volunteering. Another theoretical concern is the increased risk of arterial thrombosis in patients with thrombocytosis as a result of the TPO-stimulating agent, potentially "unmasking" previously undetected atherosclerotic disease resulting in myocardial infarction or stroke. While uncommon, platelet counts over 1,000,000/μL were seen in patients treated in solid tumor studies using TPO-stimulating agents [51, 53].

Other Pharmacologic Agents in the Treatment of Chemotherapy-Induced Thrombocytopenia

The only FDA approved agent to treat thrombocytopenia secondary to chemotherapy is oprelvekin (recombinant human interleukin-11). In a small trial, patients receiving non-myeloablative chemotherapy regimens who required platelet transfusion with the preceding cycle of chemotherapy were randomized to receive oprelvekin or placebo during the subsequent cycle administered at the same dose [54]. Oprelvekin was administered subcutaneously daily for 14–21 days starting 1 day after the completion of chemotherapy or until the platelet count was ≥100,000/μL. In the 50-μg/kg treatment arm, 30% of the patients were able to tolerate the next cycle of chemotherapy without platelet transfusion compared to only 4% of the patients in the placebo arm. Side effects were mostly grade 1 or 2 in severity although edema, headache, tachycardia, and palpitations occurred significantly more often in the treatment arms. In another trial using myeloablative chemotherapy for treatment of breast cancer prior to autologous stem cell transplantation, oprelvekin was administered at two dose levels with statistically insignificant reductions in platelet transfusions when compared to placebo [55].

Recently two TPO receptor agonists, romiplostim [56] and eltrombopag [57], have been FDA approved for the treatment of chronic immune thrombocytopenic purpura. These agents have not exhibited immunogenicity and there have been no reports of thrombocytopenia due to the formation of cross-reacting antibodies against endogenous TPO.

Initial results from two trials using romiplostim to support thrombocytopenia in patients with myelodysplastic syndromes have recently been presented in abstract form. The first was a multicenter, double-blind, placebo-controlled study of 40 patients using romiplostim to offset thrombocytopenia associated with azacytidine treatment [58]. The incidence of platelet transfusions was 69% for the placebo group compared to 46 and 36% for the groups receiving 500 and 750 μg of romiplostim subcutaneously per week, respectively. Two serious adverse events were reported in the treatment arms (one arthralgia and one rash and hypersensitivity). One patient in the treatment arm had progression to AML. Two patients in the placebo group had episodes of grade 3 or higher bleeding compared to one in the 500-μg arm (epistaxis) and none in the 750-μg arm. The second trial was a phase 2, multicenter, single-arm, open-label study evaluating the ability of romiplostim to offset thrombocytopenia in 28 patients with baseline platelet counts $\leq$ 50,000/μL [59]. Sixty-eight percentage of patients had received a platelet transfusion in the last year prior to enrollment. Patients received romiplostim 750 μg by weekly or biweekly subcutaneous injection or biweekly intravenous injection. Mean duration of exposure to romiplostim was 12 weeks. For patients completing 8 weeks of treatment 61% did not require a transfusion during treatment. Two patients had disease progression to AML. Given these results it does not appear that romiplostim has clinical utility in thrombocytopenic patients with myelodysplastic syndromes not undergoing chemotherapy.

Clinical trials are currently recruiting patients to evaluate the utility of romiplostim to offset thrombocytopenia in patients undergoing treatment with carboplatin, doxorubicin/ifosfamide, and high-dose ifosfamide as well as in patients with aggressive non-Hodgkin's lymphoma treated with the rituximab + Hyper-CVAD regimen. These trials include treatment arms that administer romiplostim 5 days prior to the start of a cycle of chemotherapy. Eltrombopag is currently being evaluated in patients undergoing treatment with doxorubicin and ifosfamide for sarcoma and in thrombocytopenic patients with myelodysplastic syndromes or secondary AML who are not candidates for intensive treatment. The same significant caveats mentioned earlier when discussing the use of recombinant human TPO and PEG-rHuMGDF will be pertinent in these studies.

No studies with either romiplostim or eltrombopag are currently registered with the United States National Institutes of Health in patients undergoing chemotherapy for acute leukemia or stem cell transplantation. Because of the theoretic concern about stimulation of leukemia growth in patients with myeloid malignancies and MDS, careful monitoring of complete remission and relapse rates will be required if such studies are undertaken. This complication was not evident in the earlier trials in patients with AML, although these were relatively small exploratory studies.

Summary

Therapeutic platelet transfusions should be administered to bleeding patients with thrombocytopenia. In contrast, data and extensive clinical experience are supportive of withholding transfusion in clinically stable patients with counts below 10,000 platelets/μL. Other clinical factors that may alter the decision about when to transfuse platelets include the need for invasive procedures, ongoing anticoagulation or the presence of coagulation abnormalities, active infection, and hemodynamic instability.

Previous studies with recombinant human TPO and PEG-rHuMGDF have shown little, if any, clinical benefit in the prevention of severe thrombocytopenia. The goal of any pharmacologic intervention used in the treatment of chemotherapy-induced thrombocytopenia must be to shorten the period of severe thrombocytopenia and therefore decrease the number of platelet transfusions. By decreasing the number of transfusions, one would anticipate decreased costs, lower rates of transfusion-related infections, and transfusion reactions. It is unlikely that there will be any effect on the rate of alloimmunization which has been decreased substantially by the use of leukoreduced blood products and which is not directly related to the number of platelet transfusions [60, 61].

Although it is conceivable that TPO receptor agonists could result in higher post-platelet counts at the time of count recovery permitting earlier administration of the next course of treatment, it is not clear that any such increase in "dose intensity" will have an impact on survival in most tumors. Furthermore, most regimens used to treat solid tumors in adults do not cause significant thrombocytopenia and bleeding rates are low.

New TPO receptor agonists have been approved and others are in development. Currently no data are available about whether these agents shorten the period of severe thrombocytopenia in patients undergoing intensive chemotherapy. Further research in this area is ongoing in patients with sarcoma, non-Hodgkin's lymphoma, and myelodysplastic syndromes. However, based on previous trials using first-generation TPO-stimulating agents and initial trials with second-generation agents, one would expect minimal impact on transfusion requirements in most of these circumstances.

References

1. Hersh EM, Bodey GP, Nies BA, et al. Causes of death in acute leukemia. JAMA. 1965;193:105–9.
2. Han T, Stutzman L, Cohen E, et al. Effect of platelet transfusion on hemorrhage in patients with acute leukemia. Cancer. 1966;19:1937–42.
3. Sullivan MT, Wallace EL. Blood collection and transfusion in the United States in 1999. Transfusion. 2005;45:141–8.
4. Schiffer CA, Anderson KC, Bennett CL, et al. Platelet transfusion for patients with cancer: clinical practice guidelines of the American Society of Clinical Oncology. J Clin Oncol. 2001;19:1519–38.
5. British Committee for Standards in Haematology, Blood Transfusion Task Force (Chairman P. Kelsey). Guidelines for the use of platelet transfusions. Br J Haematol. 2003;122:10–23.

6. Slichter SJ. Evidenced-based platelet transfusion guidelines. Hematology. 2007;2007:172–8.
7. Gaydos LA, Freireich EJ, Mantel N. The quantitative relation between platelet count and hemorrhage in patients with acute leukemia. N Engl J Med. 1962;266:905–9.
8. Higby DJ, Cohen E, Holland JF, et al. The prophylactic treatment of thrombocytopenic leukemic patients with platelets: a double blind study. Transfusion. 1974;14:440–6.
9. Roy AJ, Jaffe N, Djerassi I. Prophylactic platelet transfusions in children with acute leukemia: a dose response study. Transfusion. 1973;13(5):283–90.
10. Murphy S, Litwin S, Herring LM, et al. Indications for platelet transfusion in children with acute leukemia. Am J Hematol. 1982;12:347–56.
11. Gmür J, Burger J, Schanz U, et al. Safety of stringent prophylactic platelet transfusion policy for patients with acute leukaemia. Lancet. 1991;338:1223–6.
12. Heckman KD, Weiner GJ, Davis CS, et al. Randomized study of prophylactic platelet transfusion threshold during induction therapy for adult acute leukemia: 10,000/μL versus 20,000/μL. J Clin Oncol. 1997;15(3):1143–9.
13. Rebulla P, Finazzi G, Marangoni F, et al. The threshold for prophylactic platelet transfusions in adults with acute myeloid leukemia. N Engl J Med. 1997;337:1870–5.
14. Wandt H, Frank M, Ehninger G, et al. Safety and cost effectiveness of a 10×10^9/L trigger for prophylactic platelet transfusions compared with the traditional 20×10^9/L trigger: a prospective comparative trial in 105 patients with acute myeloid leukemia. Blood. 1998;91:3601–6.
15. Friedmann AM, Sengul H, Lehmann H, et al. Do basic laboratory tests or clinical observations predict bleeding in thrombocytopenic oncology patients? A re-evaluation of prophylactic platelet transfusions. Transfus Med Rev. 2002;16:34–45.
16. Rudmann SV. Textbook of blood banking and transfusion medicine, Chapter 14. Philadelphia, PA: W.B. Saunders an Co; 2005. p. 380.
17. Folman CC, de Jong SM, de Haas M, et al. Analysis of the kinetics of TPO uptake during platelet transfusion. Transfusion. 2001;41:517–21.
18. Slichter S, Kaufman R, Assmann S, et al. Effects of prophylactic platelet dose on transfusion outcomes (PLADO trial). Blood (ASH Annual Meeting Abstracts). 2008;112. Abstract 285.
19. Heddle N, Cook R, Tinmouth A, et al. A randomized controlled trial comparing standard- and low-dose strategies for transfusion of platelets (SToP) to patients with thrombocytopenia. Blood (ASH Annual Meeting Abstracts). 2009;113:1564–73.
20. Wandt H, Schaefer-Eckart K, Frank M, et al. A therapeutic platelet transfusion strategy is safe and feasible in patients after autologous peripheral blood stem cell transplantation. Bone Marrow Transplant. 2006;37:387–92.
21. Wandt H, Wendelin K, Schaefer-Eckart K, et al. A therapeutic platelet transfusion strategy without routine prophylactic transfusion is feasible and safe and reduces platelet transfusion numbers significantly: preliminary analysis of a randomized study in patients after high dose chemotherapy and autologous peripheral blood stem cell transplantation. Blood (ASH Annual Meeting Abstracts). 2008;112. Abstract 286.
22. Blajchman M, Slichter S, Heddle N, et al. New strategies for the optimal use of platelet transfusions. Am Soc of Hematol Educ Program. 2008;198–204.
23. Edelson RN, Chernik NL, Posner JB. Spinal subdural hematomas complicating lumbar puncture. Arch Neurol. 1974;31:134–7.
24. Breuer AC, Tyler R, Marzewski DJ, et al. Radicular vessels are the most probable source of needle induced blood in lumbar puncture. Cancer. 1982;49:2168–72.
25. Howard SC, Gajjar A, Ribeiro RC, et al. Safety of lumbar puncture for children with acute lymphoblastic leukemia and thrombocytopenia. JAMA. 2000;284(17):2222–4.
26. Bishop JF, Schiffer CA, Aisner J, et al. Surgery in acute leukemia: a review of 167 operations in thrombocytopenic patients. Am J Hematol. 1987;26:147–55.
27. National Institutes of Health Consensus Conference. Platelet transfusion therapy. Transfus Med Rev. 1987;1:195–200.

28. Norfolk DR, Ancliffe PJ, Contreras M, et al. Consensus conference on platelet transfusion. Royal College of Physicians of Edinburgh, 27–28 November 1997. Br J Haematol. 1998;101:609–17.
29. McVay PA, Toy PT. Lack of increased bleeding after liver biopsy in patients with mild hemostatic abnormalities. Am J Clin Pathol. 1990;94:747–53.
30. Williford SK, Salisbury PL III, Peacock JE Jr, et al. The safety of dental extractions in patients with hematologic malignancies. J Clin Oncol. 1989;7:798–802.
31. Overholser CD, Peterson DE, Bergman SA, et al. Dental extractions in patients with acute nonlymphocytic leukemia. J Oral Maxillofac Surg. 1982;40:296–8.
32. Doerfler ME, Kaufman B, Goldenberg AS. Central venous catheter placement in patients with disorders of hemostasis. Chest. 1996;110:185–8.
33. Stellato TA, Gauderer MW, Lazarus HM, et al. Percutaneous isoelastic catheter insertion in patients with thrombocytopenia. Cancer. 1985;56:2691–3.
34. Chu DZJ, Shivshanker K, Stroehlein JR, et al. Thrombocytopenia and gastrointestinal hemorrhage in the cancer patient: prevalence of unmasked lesions. Gastrointest Endosc. 1983;29:269–72.
35. Weiss SM, Hert RC, Gianola FJ, et al. Complications of fiberoptic bronchoscopy in thrombocytopenic patients. Chest. 1993;104:1025–8.
36. Papin TA, Lynch JP III, Weg JG. Transbronchial biopsy in the thrombocytopenic patient. Chest. 1985;88:549–52.
37. Wallace MJ, Narvios A, Lichtiger B, et al. Transjugular liver biopsy in patients with hematologic malignancy and severe thrombocytopenia. J Vasc Interv Radiol. 2003;14(3):323–7.
38. Kluge S, Meyer A, Kühnelt P, et al. Percutaneous tracheostomy is safe in patients with severe thrombocytopenia. Chest. 2004;126(2):547–51.
39. O'Connell BA, Lee EJ, Schiffer CA. The value of 10-minute post transfusion platelet counts. Transfusion. 1988;26:66–7.
40. Basser RL, Rasko JEJ, Clarke K, et al. Randomized, blinded, placebo-controlled phase I trial of pegylated recombinant human megakaryocyte growth and development factor with filgrastim after dose-intensive chemotherapy in patients with advanced cancer. Blood. 1997;89:3118–28.
41. Vadhan-Raj S, Patel S, Bueso-Ramos C, et al. Importance of predosing of recombinant human thrombopoietin to reduce chemotherapy-induced early thrombocytopenia. J Clin Oncol. 2003;21:3158–67.
42. Vadhan-Raj S, Verschraegen CF, Bueso-Ramos C, et al. Recombinant human thrombopoietin attenuates carboplatin-induced severe thrombocytopenia and the need for platelet transfusions in patients with gynecologic cancer. Ann Intern Med. 2000;132:364–8.
43. Fanucchi M, Glaspy J, Crawford J, et al. Effects of polyethylene glycol-conjugated recombinant human megakaryocyte growth and development factor on platelet counts after chemotherapy for lung cancer. N Engl J Med. 1997;336:404–9.
44. Schuster MW, Beveridge R, Frei-Lahr D, et al. The effects of pegylated recombinant human megakaryocyte growth and development factor (PEG-rHuMGDF) on platelet recovery in breast cancer patients undergoing autologous bone marrow transplantation. Exp Hematol. 2002;30:1044–50.
45. Archimbaud E, Ottmann OG, Liu-Yan JA, et al. A randomized, double-blind, placebo controlled study with pegylated recombinant human megakaryocyte growth and development factor (PEG-rHuMGDF) as an adjunct to chemotherapy for adults with de novo acute myeloid leukemia. Blood. 1999;94:3694–701.
46. Schiffer CA, Miller K, Larson RA, et al. A doubleblind, placebo-controlled trial of pegylated recombinant human megakaryocyte growth and development factor as an adjunct to induction and consolidation therapy for patients with acute myeloid leukemia. Blood. 2000;95:2530–5.
47. Stone RM, Larson RA, Miller K, et al. A randomized, placebo-controlled, double-blind trial of a loading dose of pegylated recombinant human megakaryocytic growth and development factor (MGDF) as an adjunct to chemotherapy for acute myeloid leukemia (AML). ASCO. 2000;19:14.

48. Kaushansky K. Thrombopoietin: the primary regulator of platelet production. Blood. 1995;86:419–31.
49. Emmons RVB, Reid DM, Cohen RL, et al. Human thrombopoietin levels are high when thrombocytopenia is due to megakaryocyte deficiency and low when due to increased platelet destruction. Blood. 1996;87:4068–71.
50. Komatsu N, Okamoto T, Yoshida T, et al. Pegylated recombinant human megakaryocyte growth and development factor (PEG-rHuMGDF) increased platelet counts (plt) in patients with aplastic anemia (AA) and myelodysplastic syndrome (MDS) [abstract]. Blood. 2000;96:296a.
51. Kuter D, Goodnough L, Romo J, et al. Thrombopoietin therapy increases platelet yields in healthy platelet donors. Blood. 2001;98:1339–45.
52. Li J, Yang C, Xia Y, et al. Thrombocytopenia caused by the development of antibodies to thrombopoietin. Blood. 2001;98:3241–8.
53. Vadhan-Raj S, Murray LJ, Bueso-Ramos C, et al. Stimulation of megakaryocyte and platelet production by a single dose of recombinant human thrombopoietin in patients with cancer. Ann Intern Med. 1997;126:673–81.
54. Tepler I, Elias L, Smith J II, et al. A randomized placebo-controlled trial of recombinant human interleukin-11 in cancer patients with severe thrombocytopenia due to chemotherapy. Blood. 1996;87:3607–14.
55. Vredenburgh J, Hussein A, Fisher D, et al. A randomized trial of recombinant human interleukin-11 following autologous bone marrow transplantation with peripheral blood progenitor cell support in patients with breast cancer. Biol Blood Marrow Transplant. 1998;4:134–41.
56. Bussel JB, Kuter DJ, George JN, et al. AMG 531, a thrombopoiesis stimulating protein, for chronic ITP. N Engl J Med. 2006;355:1672–81.
57. Bussel JB, Cheng G, Saleh MN, et al. Eltrombopag for the treatment of chronic idiopathic thrombocytopenic purpura. N Engl J Med. 2007;357:2237–47.
58. Kantarjian H, Giles F, Greenberg P, et al. Effect of romiplostim in patients with low or intermediate risk myelodysplastic syndrome receiving azacytidine. Blood (ASH Annual Meeting Abstracts). 2008;112. Abstract 224.
59. Sekeres M, Kantarjian H, Fenaux P, et al. Subcutaneous or intravenous administration of romiplostim in thrombocytopenic patients with myelodysplastic syndrome. J Clin Oncol (ASCO Annual Meeting Proceedings) 2009;27:(15S). (May 20 Supplement). Abstract 7009.
60. The Trial to Reduce Alloimmunization to Platelets Study Group. Leukocyte reduction and ultraviolet B irradiation of platelets to prevent alloimmunization and refractoriness to platelet transfusions. N Engl J Med. 1997;337:1861–9.
61. Dutcher J, Schiffer CA, Aisner J, Wiernik PH. Alloimmunization following platelet transfusion: the absence of a dose response relationship. Blood. 1980;57:395–8.

Chapter 16
Romiplostim

David J. Kuter

Abstract Thrombocytopenia is a common clinical problem associated with a wide range of medical conditions including immune thrombocytopenia (ITP), chemotherapy-induced thrombocytopenia (CIT), hepatitis C-related thrombocytopenia, and myelodysplastic syndromes (MDS). Until recently, the only treatments for thrombocytopenia were to alleviate the underlying cause or to provide platelet transfusions. With the discovery and recent clinical availability of thrombopoietin (TPO) mimetics, a new treatment option has emerged. Two TPO mimetics are currently clinically available for treating ITP: romiplostim (an injectable peptide TPO mimetic) and eltrombopag (a non-peptide, orally available TPO mimetic). This chapter reviews the development, biology, and clinical trials with romiplostim. With few adverse effects, romiplostim is effective in raising the platelet count in over 80% of ITP patients, allowing them to discontinue other therapies, reduce the need for splenectomy, and improve their quality of life. Long-term theoretical side effects of romiplostim treatment include reticulin formation, thromboembolism, and antibody formation to romiplostim. A practical way of using romiplostim is provided: a higher starting dose of 3 mg/kg is recommended along with efforts to avoid withholding the dose. Future studies will assess the utility of romiplostim in CIT, hepatitis-C related thrombocytopenia, and MDS.

Introduction

Thrombocytopenia is a common medical condition that is due to increased platelet destruction (e.g., heparin-induced thrombocytopenia), decreased platelet production (e.g., chemotherapy), or some combination of both processes (e.g., immune thrombocytopenia [ITP]). With a decline in platelet count, the risk for bleeding

D.J. Kuter (✉)
Hematology Division, Massachusetts General Hospital, Boston, MA 02114, USA
e-mail: kuter.david@mgh.harvard.edu

G.H. Lyman, D.C. Dale (eds.), *Hematopoietic Growth Factors in Oncology*,
Cancer Treatment and Research 157, DOI 10.1007/978-1-4419-7073-2_16,
© Springer Science+Business Media, LLC 2011

increases and therapy for the thrombocytopenia is often necessary. Such therapy may involve the treatment of the underlying cause (e.g., chemotherapy dose reduction, splenectomy for ITP) or the administration of platelet transfusions to correct the thrombocytopenia. Until very recently, there has been no effective drug that increased platelet production to ameliorate thrombocytopenia.

Thrombopoietin (TPO) receptor mimetics are now available for the treatment of some forms of thrombocytopenia. Although first proposed to exist in 1958 [1], almost 40 years of arduous investigation passed before TPO was finally purified and cloned by five separate groups in 1994 [2–6]. It was identified by laborious purification methods from thrombocytopenic plasma or by innovative cloning schemes and called thrombopoietin, megapoietin, megakaryocyte growth and development factor, or c-mpl ligand. The last name, c-mpl ligand, indicated that it bound the c-mpl receptor, a hematopoietic cytokine receptor of unclear function that had previously been identified in 1991 [7]. We now know that the c-mpl receptor is the TPO receptor and that it binds the c-mpl ligand, TPO.

The long lag-time between discovery and approval of a molecule for patient care is attributed to the development of antibodies against one of the "first-generation" recombinant thrombopoietins. Two recombinant TPO molecules, recombinant human TPO (rhTPO) and pegylated recombinant human megakaryocyte growth and development factor (PEG-rHuMGDF), entered clinical trials in 1995 but further development was stopped in 1998 when antibodies formed against PEG-rHuMGDF cross-reacted with endogenous TPO and caused thrombocytopenia [8]. Subsequently, a number of non-immunogenic TPO peptide mimetics (romiplostim, PEG-TPOmp, Fab59), TPO non-peptide mimetics (eltrombopag, AKR-501, LGD-4665, NIP-004, NIP-022, butyzamide), and TPO receptor agonist antibodies (TPO minibody [VB22B sc(Fv)2], domain subclass-converted TPO agonist antibody [MA01G4344]) have been developed [9–11]. Two of these, romiplostim and eltrombopag, are now FDA-approved for treating thrombocytopenia in ITP. This chapter will review the biology, preclinical studies, and clinical development of romiplostim.

Romiplostim Structure

In 1997 a 14-amino acid peptide with no sequence homology with TPO was identified that bound and activated the TPO receptor [12]. Given its novel sequence, this peptide became of potential utility in that if antibodies developed to it in vivo, they might not cross-react with endogenous TPO and cause thrombocytopenia as had occurred with PEG-rHuMGDF [8]. Given the requirement that any TPO bind simultaneously to two TPO receptor molecules, it was found that dimerization of this peptide increased its specific activity by about 10,000-fold (Fig. 16.1). Unfortunately, the short circulatory half-life of peptides usually makes them poor pharmacologic agents. A solution to this problem is to stabilize the peptide (yet preserving a dimeric structure) by (a) pegylation [13], (b) incorporation into the complementarity-determining region (CDR) of immunoglobulin carrier molecules [14], or (c) attaching the peptides to a modified Fc receptor ("peptibody") [15].

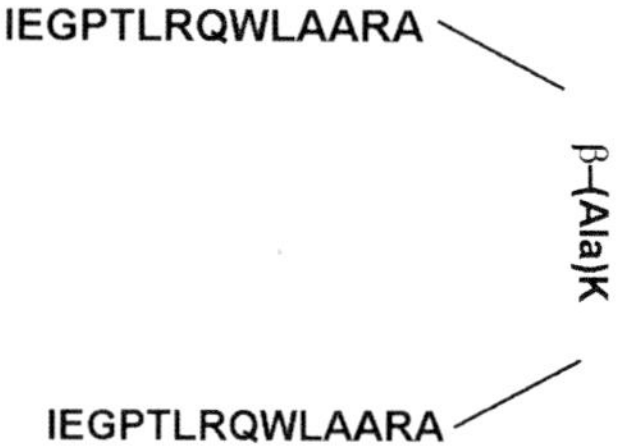

Fig. 16.1 Basic TPO peptide mimetic structure. The 14-amino acid TPO mimetic peptide (shown here as a dimeric peptide formed by an alanine bridge) serves as the basis for many of the TPO peptide mimetics that have been developed. Without dimerization, this peptide has approximately 10,000-fold less activity [12]

Pegylation of the dimeric 14-amino acid structure described above (pegylated TPO mimetic peptide [Peg-TPOmp]) produced a molecule that stimulated TPO-dependent cell lines at pM concentrations (the same as rhTPO) and produced a dose-dependent increase in platelet count in rats, mice, and dogs. Phase I studies of a single IV bolus of Peg-TPOmp (0.375, 0.75, 1.5, 2.25, 3 μg/kg) or placebo in 40 (randomized 6:2) healthy humans showed a mean peak platelet count on days 10–12 of 315 × 10^9/L with 0.375 μg/kg and 685 × 10^9/L with 3 μg/kg [13]. There were no untoward effects and endogenous TPO levels rose. There are no further reports of development of this molecule.

Recognizing that the CDR region of IgG is rarely itself antigenic, the 14-amino acid TPO peptide described above was inserted into each arm of the CDR region of a well-described IgG Fab$_2$ (called Fab59) with its activity optimized by careful modification of the flanking amino acids and the distance between the two peptides [14]. Fab59 had the same specific activity as rhTPO in stimulating cell lines and increased the platelet count in mice. It has not been developed further.

Initially named Amgen Megakaryopoiesis Protein-2 (AMP-2), and subsequently developed as AMG-531, romiplostim (Nplate®) is a 60-kDa structure composed of four 14-amino acid peptides attached by glycine bridges to a novel IgG1 heavy chain Fc construct called a peptibody (Fig. 16.2) [15]. To each arm of the Fc region are attached two TPO mimetic peptides, again creating a dimeric molecule capable of activating the TPO receptor. The peptides have no sequence homology with endogenous TPO such that if antibodies were to form against romiplostim, they would not cross-react with endogenous TPO. The peptibody structure conserved the CH2 and CH3 domains of the IgG-Fc which enable romiplostim to bind to and be recycled by the endothelial FcRn receptors providing it with a circulatory half-life of 120–160 h. Romiplostim is eventually cleared by the reticuloendothelial system [16].

Romiplostim Function

Romiplostim seems to function just like native TPO (Fig. 16.3). It binds to TPO receptors that appear to be exclusively present on non-lymphoid hematopoietic tissues (from stem cells to platelets) but not on non-hematopoietic tissues. TPO

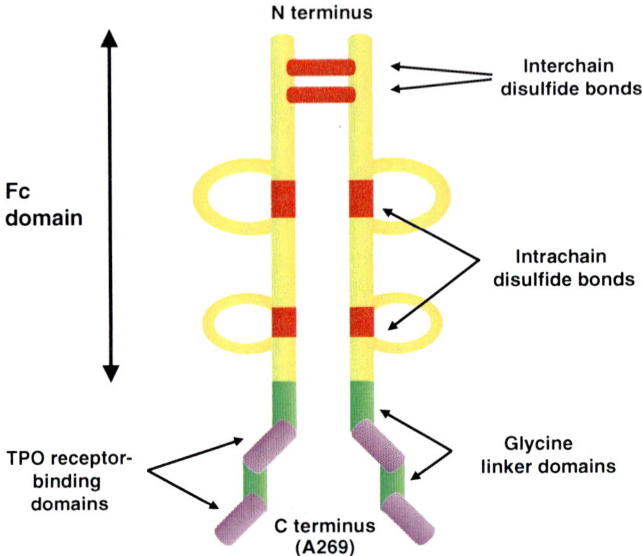

Fig. 16.2 Structure of romiplostim. Romiplostim (~60 kDa) is composed of the Fc (fragment "crystallized") portion of IgG1 to which two 14-amino acid TPO peptides are coupled via glycine bridges at the carboxy terminus of each IgG heavy chain. Interchain (at cysteines C7 and C10) and intrachain (cysteines C42–C102, C148–C206) disulfide bridges are as indicated (figure courtesy of Amgen, Inc., Thousand Oaks, CA)

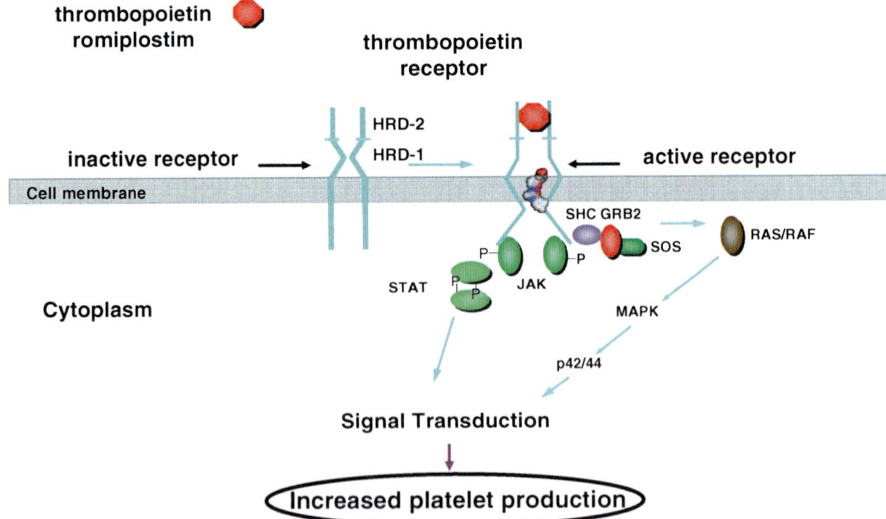

Fig. 16.3 Activation of the TPO receptor. The TPO receptor has been proposed to exist as an inactive preformed dimer (*left*) with a proximal (HRD-1) and distal (HRD-2) hematopoietic receptor domain (HRD). Upon binding of thrombopoietin or romiplostim to the distal HRD-2, the receptor (*right*) conformation changes and a number of signal transduction pathways are activated that increase platelet production

receptors on these target hematopoietic cells probably exist as preformed but inactive dimers. Each TPO receptor has two repetitive hematopoietic receptor domains (HRDs) and it is suggested that the two distal HRDs of the preformed TPO receptor dimer sterically interact to prevent receptor activation (since loss of the distal, but not the proximal HRDs creates a constitutively activated receptor) [17]. Upon binding of one romiplostim molecule, the positions of the distal HRDs are probably altered and the receptor dimer is activated. This initially involves activation by phosphorylation of JAK2 and STAT5 as well as autophosphorylation of the TPO receptor. These in turn activate a large variety of signaling pathways that promote cell viability, cell growth, megakaryocyte endomitosis, megakaryocyte maturation, and platelet production [10, 11, 18, 19].

TPO produces a wide range of effects in hematopoietic cells. It increases the viability of multipotential stem cells (absence of TPO or its receptor leads to aplastic anemia). It increases the mitotic rate and number of megakaryocyte colony-forming cells (Meg-CFC). It increases the ploidy and maturation rate of maturing megakaryocytes. Studies with romiplostim have been conducted to confirm most of these aspects of its TPO activity.

Romiplostim binds to the TPO receptor on platelets and TPO-dependent cell lines such as BaF3-Mpl. However, it binds to the platelet TPO receptor 17-fold less avidly than rhTPO (J. Li, unpublished data, 2002). Nonetheless, treatment of BaF3-Mpl cells with romiplostim resulted in rapid tyrosine phosphorylation of Mpl, JAK2, and STAT5 just like TPO. Romiplostim stimulated Meg-CFC growth in a dose-dependent manner and acted in concert with erythropoietin, stem cell factor, interleukin-3, and interleukin-6 to enhance Meg-CFC growth, similar to parallel experiments with TPO. In serum-free liquid cultures, romiplostim supported the development of mature polyploid megakaryocytes with a predominant DNA content of 32 N and 64 N, identical to that of parallel TPO-stimulated cultures. Competitive binding experiments showed that romiplostim effectively competed with ^{125}I-TPO for binding to BaF3-Mpl cells or normal platelets [20].

Preclinical Animal Studies with Romiplostim

Although varying in the extent of its effect, romiplostim showed activity in all animal species tested (mice, rats, rhesus monkeys, humans). Tests for competitive binding of romiplostim and ^{125}I-rhTPO demonstrated specific binding to rat, rabbit, cynomolgus monkey, and human platelets but with marked differences in affinity. In mice, single doses of 0.1–10 µg/kg were tested and platelet count increases were demonstrated at doses of ≥3 µg/kg. At a dose of 10 µg/kg the peak platelet count was $3,500 \times 10^9$/L versus $1,500 \times 10^9$/L for control mice. There was no effect on the white blood cell or red blood cell counts. What is unusual about the mice experiments is that the platelet counts rose much sooner than was seen in subsequent experiments in rhesus monkeys or humans: platelet counts started to rise on day 3 and peaked on day 6; falling back to baseline by day 10. This may be related to the short maturation time of megakaryocyte precursors in mice.

Single intravenous and subcutaneous doses of 0.5, 2.0, and 5.0 mg/kg (note the approximately 1,000-fold dose increase relative to the mice) were tested in 18 rhesus monkeys (Fig. 16.4). There was a dose-dependent rise in platelet count with a peak at day 9. At the highest dose the platelet count rose to about $1,200 \times 10^9$/L versus 400×10^9/L in control animals. PK modeling suggested a minimally effective dose of 0.1 mg/kg. Intravenous and subcutaneous dosing gave the same platelet response. The terminal $T_{1/2}$ of romiplostim was 107–143 h when given intravenously and 110 h (at low dose) or 169–196 h (at higher doses) when given subcutaneously. There was no effect on the white blood cell or red blood cell counts. No animal developed antibodies against romiplostim and no animal subsequently developed thrombocytopenia.

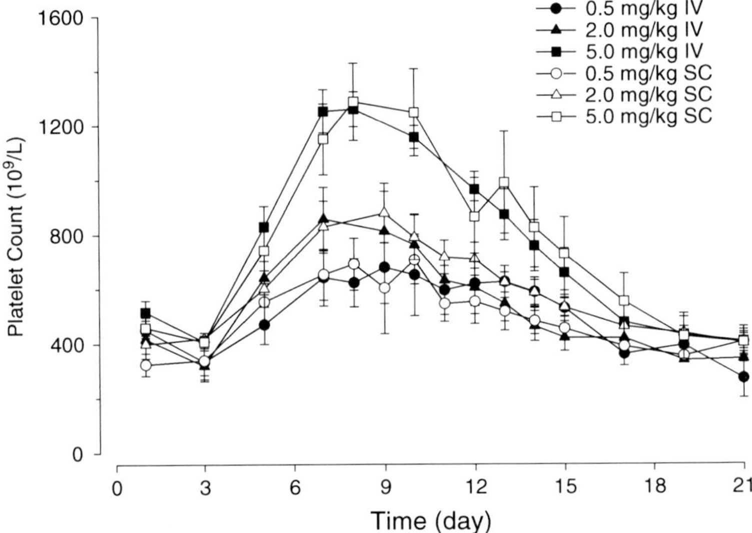

Fig. 16.4 Dose-dependent platelet count rise in rhesus monkeys. Single doses of romiplostim were injected on day 1 and the platelet count (±SD) followed. Platelet count begins to rise on day 5 and reaches a peak at day 9. Intravenous and subcutaneous doses are as indicated (figure courtesy of Amgen, Inc., Thousand Oaks, CA)

In rhesus monkeys treated with romiplostim three times a week for 4 weeks with subcutaneous doses of 0.5, 1.0, or 5 mg/kg, there was no accumulation of romiplostim. A dose-dependent rise in platelet count reached its peak at day 15 and maintained a plateau platelet count until sacrifice at day 28. Intravenous and subcutaneous dosings were compared at the highest dose and showed no difference in platelet response; for both routes the peak plateau platelet count was $2,500 \times 10^9$/L versus 500×10^9/L for the control animals. Clearance was unaffected in splenectomized mice but was higher in FcRn knockout mice.

Standard toxicity studies in animals at a wide range of doses uncovered no significant ocular, hepatic, cardiac, neurological, or muscular toxicity. Prolonged administration to rats for a month produced a sustained increase in platelet count and bone marrow megakaryocytes along with a marked dose-dependent increase in bone marrow fibrosis. There were minimal effects on the white blood cell or red blood cell counts. In rats treated with romiplostim for 1 month followed by a 1-month drug-free recovery, there were no bone marrow or blood abnormalities; indicating complete resolution of the fibrosis [21].

Phase I Studies in Healthy Humans

The first human studies involved 48 healthy human subjects randomized 1:2 to receive single doses of placebo or romiplostim in cohorts of 6 [16]. Using pharmacokinetic allometric scaling and in vitro potency testing from the animal experiments, it was anticipated that 10 μg/kg would be the "no effect" dose in humans; dose ranges from 10 to 1,000 μg/kg were planned. However, the 10 μg/kg dose increased platelet counts in all four healthy subjects so treated to over 1,000 $\times$ 10^9/L.[1] Subsequently doses of 0.1–2.0 μg/kg were then tested. At all doses tested, platelet counts started to rise on day 5 and reached a peak on day 15. Intravenous and subcutaneous administration produced the same platelet count response and showed identical non-linear pharmacokinetics. A minimal clinically effective subcutaneous dose of 1.0 μg/kg was established. There was no thrombocytopenia after administration and no antibody formation against romiplostim.

Platelet aggregation testing was performed on platelet-rich plasma obtained from untreated healthy volunteers and showed that addition of romiplostim to the test sample did not directly activate platelets. But, like rhTPO, the presence of romiplostim did lower the threshold for ADP activation by $\sim$50%. The concentration of ADP that half-maximally aggregated platelets (ADP50) was approximately 3.0 mM in untreated platelets and dropped to approximately 2.3, 1.6, and 1.1 mM when romiplostim was added at 1, 10, or 100 ng/mL, concentrations that can be attained after in vivo subcutaneous administration.

Studies of Romiplostim in ITP

Although ITP has long been known to be a disease of increased platelet destruction [22], recent studies have shown that ITP is also a disease of inappropriately low platelet production [23–25]. Platelet kinetic studies have shown that platelet production is normal or reduced in over 75% of ITP patients [23]. The current explanation for this is that the antiplatelet antibody (and possibly cytotoxic bone marrow lymphocytes) reduce the proliferation of megakaryocyte precursors and cause apoptosis [24, 25]. Since TPO can prevent apoptosis of megakaryocyte precursors and

---

[1] The probable explanation for this unexpected high response at this dose in humans versus rhesus monkeys is the twofold to threefold higher binding affinity of romiplostim for the human TPO receptor (J. Li, unpublished data, 2002).

megakaryocytes, it was hypothesized that TPO treatment might enhance platelet production and increase the platelet count.

Phase I–III studies in ITP have been completed with romiplostim; there is also a recently completed extension study that has treated subjects with romiplostim for up to 6 years. In most studies, patients were required to have a baseline platelet count of 30×10^9/L or less and have failed a prior ITP therapy; both splenectomized and non-splenectomized patients were studied.

Phase I studies: In the Phase I trial with romiplostim, 24 subjects with ITP and platelets $\leq 30 \times 10^9$/L ($\leq 50 \times 10^9$/L if on corticosteroids) were treated with two subcutaneous doses of romiplostim on days 1 and 15 [15]. There were 17 female and 7 male patients with a mean age of 44 ± 13 years and 79% had undergone splenectomy. Cohorts of four patients were treated with doses of 0.2, 0.5, 1, 3, 6, and 10 of µg/kg. The primary endpoint was safety and the secondary endpoint was response (platelet count double the baseline and $50–450 \times 10^9$/L). Doses of 0.2–1.0 µg/kg were ineffective but doses of 3.0–10.0 µg/kg were effective. All 12 patients at 3.0–10.0 µg/kg doubled their platelet count; 7/12 had their platelet count rise to over 50×10^9/L; and 4/12 had platelet count double the baseline and $50–450 \times 10^9$/L (efficacy endpoint of the study). The peak platelet count was dose-dependent: 163×10^9/L, 309×10^9/L, and 746×10^9/L for the 3, 6, and 10 µg/kg cohorts, respectively. No subject developed rebound thrombocytopenia and no anti-romiplostim antibodies were detected.

Phase II study: In a subsequent small, placebo-controlled, blinded Phase II study, patients with ITP were treated with romiplostim (1 or 3 µg/kg) or placebo weekly for 6 weeks. The primary efficacy endpoint was the same as the Phase I study (platelet count double the baseline and $50–450 \times 10^9$/L). Patient characteristics were comparable to those in the Phase I study. Mean peak platelet counts were 135×10^9/L, 241×10^9/L, and 81×10^9/L for the 1, 3 µg/kg, and placebo groups, respectively [15]. The primary endpoint (platelet count double baseline and $50–450 \times 10^9$/L) was attained in 1/4 (25%) of placebo patients and 10/16 (63%) of romiplostim patients. The platelet count doubled in 1/4 (25%) of placebo patients and 15/16 (94%) of romiplostim patients.[2]

Phase III studies: Two large randomized, placebo-controlled, 24-week trials of romiplostim have been completed; 1 in 63 splenectomized and 1 in 62 non-splenectomized ITP patients [26]. They were run concurrently and differed only in whether subjects had been splenectomized. Patients were treated for 24 weeks with romiplostim or placebo and had their weekly doses adjusted to attain a platelet count target of $50–200 \times 10^9$/L. All started at a dose of 1 µg/kg (romiplostim or placebo). Rescue therapy (IVIG, anti-D, increased steroid dose, platelet transfusion) was allowed if patients developed symptomatic bleeding or were felt to be at risk for this. A very rigid primary endpoint was designed to meet regulatory specifications:

---

[2]A single patient in the placebo group developed a delayed platelet response 6 weeks after the 6-week active treatment period ended and accounted for the only response seen in the placebo group.

a durable platelet response (defined as a weekly platelet count $\geq$ 50,000 on 6 of the last 8 weeks of study; no rescue medications used at any time). Additional efficacy and safety endpoints are described below.

Table 16.1 shows the characteristics of the patients enrolled in both studies. Both arms of each study were well balanced for patient characteristics. The major difference between the splenectomized group and the non-splenectomized group was the number of prior therapies (splenectomized group had a median of five or six prior therapies [including splenectomy] vs two or three for the non-splenectomized group) and the median duration of ITP (8 years for splenectomized group vs 2 years for the non-splenectomized group).

Table 16.1 Romiplostim Phase III trials – patient demographics [26]

	Splenectomized patients		Non-splenectomized patients	
	Romiplostim ($n = 42$)	Placebo ($n = 21$)	Romiplostim ($n = 41$)	Placebo ($n = 21$)
Median age (years)	51	56	52	46
Females, n (%)	27 (64%)	11 (52%)	27 (66%)	16 (76%)
Median duration of ITP (years since diagnosis)	7.75	8.50	2.20	1.60
$\geq$3 prior treatments, n (%)	39 (93%)	20 (95%)	15 (37%)	5 (24%)
Median platelet count (10^9/L)	14	15	19	19
Median TPO level (pg/mL)[a]	113	124	94	81
Receiving concurrent ITP treatment, n (%)	12 (29%)	6 (29%)	11 (27%)	10 (48%)
Median prior therapies, n	6	5	3	2

[a]Normal TPO levels range from 32 to 246 pg/mL.

The platelet count response to romiplostim therapy is shown in Fig. 16.5. Splenectomized patients reached the target platelet count by week 4 while the non-splenectomized patients did so by weeks 2–3. An overall platelet response (platelet count $\geq$ 50 $\times$ 10^9/L during 4 or more weeks of the 24-week study) was found in 79% (33/42) of splenectomized and 88% (36/41) of non-splenectomized patients compared to 0% (0/21) and 14% (3/21) of the respective placebo subjects ($p < 0.0001$). The responses were of significant duration in that during the 24 weeks of study, a platelet count of $\geq$50 $\times$ 10^9 was attained during 12.3 weeks for splenectomized subjects and 15.2 weeks for non-splenectomized subjects, versus 0.2 and 1.3 weeks, respectively, for the placebo subjects ($p < 0.0001$). The use of rescue medication was markedly reduced for the combined studies: 22% for romiplostim-treated versus 60% for placebo-treated patients ($p < 0.0001$). Romiplostim allowed more subjects (*splenectomized*: romiplostim – 100%, placebo – 17%; *non-splenectomized*: romiplostim – 73%; placebo – 50%) who had been on concomitant steroids to reduce or discontinue these medications. The primary endpoint (durable platelet response) was found in 38.1% (16/42) of splenectomized

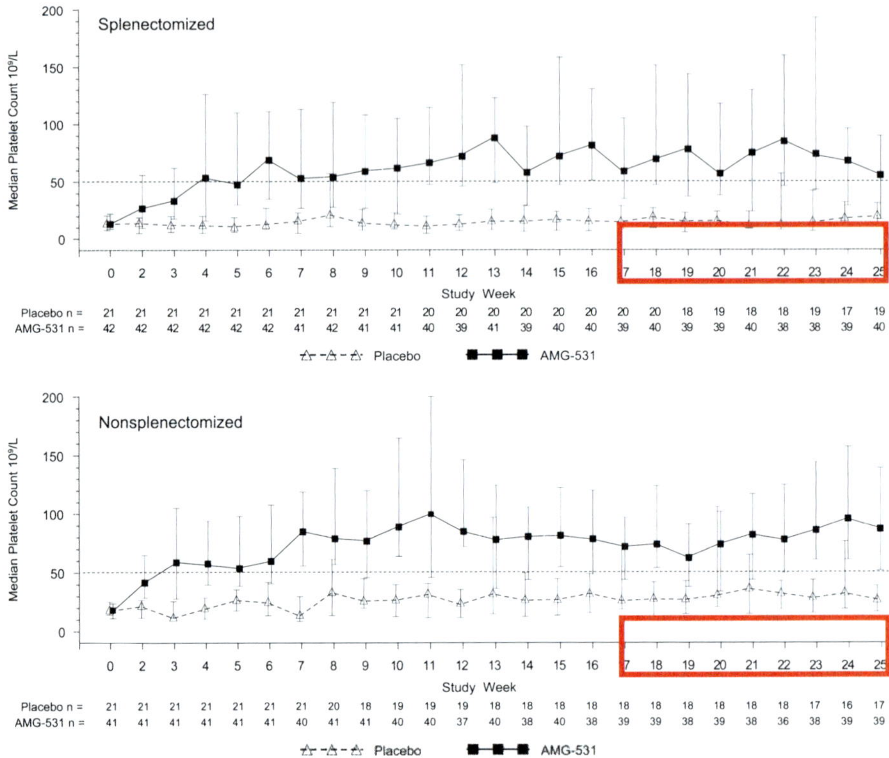

Fig. 16.5 Platelet count responses in splenectomized (*top*) and non-splenectomized (*bottom*) ITP patients treated with either romiplostim (AMG-531) or placebo. Mean platelet counts (*error bars* denote the range from the first to the third quartile) are plotted over 24 weeks of the study. The 50×10^9/L target platelet count is denoted by the *horizontal line*. The boxes encompass the last 8 weeks of the study during which the durable platelet response was measured [26]. The number (*n*) of subjects in each treatment group for each week is shown at the *bottom* of each figure

patients and 61.0% (25/41) of non-splenectomized patients compared with 0% (0/21) and 4.8% (1/21) of the respective placebo-treated patients ($p < 0.0001$).

The mean dose of romiplostim was slightly higher in the splenectomized patients compared with those not splenectomized (4 μg/kg vs 3 μg/kg). The only variables that were associated with a reduced durable platelet response rate were prior splenectomy and increased weight. Pretreatment thrombopoietin levels were usually normal and unrelated to response.

A post-hoc assessment of bleeding in these studies showed that romiplostim treatment was associated with many fewer ≥Grade 2 bleeding events than placebo treatment (15% vs 34%) as well as fewer ≥Grade 3 bleeding events (7% vs 12%). All ≥Grade 2 bleeding events occurred at platelet counts $<50 \times 10^9$/L and all ≥Grade 3 bleeding events occurred at platelet counts $<20 \times 10^9$/L.

Another Phase III study has just been concluded [27]. It compared the effect of romiplostim versus standard of care (SOC) for 1 year in subjects who had not undergone splenectomy. Eligible patients were required to have a platelet count $\leq 50 \times 10^9$/L and have had one prior ITP treatment. Patients were enrolled 1:2 to receive either SOC or romiplostim. The starting romiplostim dose was 3 µg/kg and doses were adjusted weekly or monthly. The first primary endpoint was the incidence of splenectomy or study discontinuation. The second primary endpoint was the incidence of treatment failure (defined as platelet count $\leq 20 \times 10^9$/L for 4 consecutive weeks at the highest recommended dose and schedule, or major bleeding event, or change in therapy due to intolerable side effect or bleeding symptoms) or study discontinuation. In total, 234 patients were randomized (SOC, 77; romiplostim, 157). In romiplostim-treated patients, there was a significantly lower incidence of splenectomy or study discontinuation (OR, 0.169; 95% CI 0.081, 0.351; $p < 0.0001$) and treatment failure or study discontinuation (OR, 0.374; 95% CI 0.188, 0.744; $p = 0.0039$) than in patients receiving SOC.

Long-term extension study: ITP subjects from the above Phase I–III studies were allowed to enroll in an open-label extension study of treatment with romiplostim with doses adjusted weekly or monthly per the platelet count. To be eligible subjects had to have completed a prior romiplostim trial (placebo-treated or romiplostim-treated), have no change in their clinical status, and have a platelet count $\leq 50 \times 10^9$/L. Some patients have been treated on this study for up to 6 years. The primary objective was to assess safety; secondary objectives were to assess long-term response, bleeding events, and the ability to reduce other ITP therapy such as steroids. Interim analyses of this study after up to 3 years (142 patients) [28] and after up to 4 years (223 patients) [21] have recently been presented.

Analysis of 223 patients after up to 4 years of study showed that 215 did and 8 did not receive romiplostim [21]. Thirty-seven discontinued the study for a wide variety of reasons; 186 remained on study. The patients in the study reflected a wide variety of patients with chronic ITP: 61% (137/223) were women; mean age was 50 ± 20 years; median baseline platelet count was 24×10^9/L (range 12–43 $\times 10^9$/L); 44% (99/223) had undergone splenectomy; the median time since diagnosis was 5 years (range 1–46 years); 15% (34/223) were on other concurrent ITP treatment.

After 4–8 weeks of dose adjustment and changes in concurrent ITP therapies (i.e., steroids), a mean plateau platelet count was attained and was relatively stable for up to 204 months (Fig. 16.6). The starting dose (1 µg/kg for patients previously on placebo or the last dose level for those previously on romiplostim) was changed per the platelet count and most patients attained a stable platelet count target (50–250 $\times 10^9$/L) at a stable dose of 6–8 µg/kg. Of the 164 patients on romiplostim for over 15 weeks, 77% had ≥ 10 weeks with a platelet count of $\geq 50 \times 10^9$/L. Of the 141 patients on romiplostim for over 30 weeks, 67% had ≥ 25 weeks with a platelet count of $\geq 50 \times 10^9$/L. Of the 116 patients on romiplostim for over 57 weeks, 41% had ≥ 52 weeks with a platelet count of $\geq 50 \times 10^9$/L.

Of the 34 patients entering the study on concurrent ITP therapies, 50% were able to discontinue that therapy and 24% could reduce their dose by more than 25%. The need for rescue therapies declined over the course of the study. The frequency of bleeding events also declined over the course of the study.

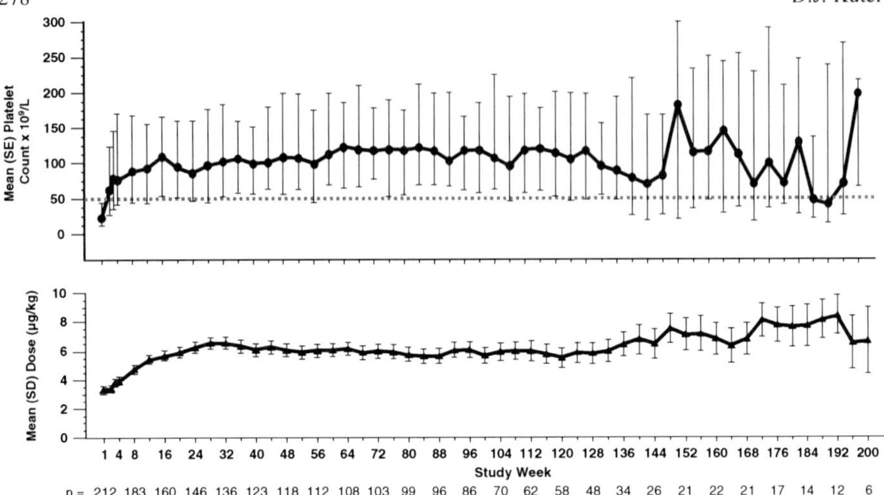

Fig. 16.6 Long-term response of platelet count to romiplostim treatment for up to 204 weeks. Mean platelet counts ($\pm$ SE) are in the upper panel and the mean romiplostim dose ($\pm$ SD) in the *lower panel* [21]. *Horizontal line* denotes the 50×10^9/L target platelet count. The number (*n*) of subjects at each time point is indicated at the *bottom*

One hundred and thirty-five subjects were trained to self-inject romiplostim and allowed to treat themselves at home (with monthly platelet count monitoring) and 132 found this form of therapy suitable. Analysis of the success of home therapy showed that the mean dose, mean platelet count, and rate of adverse events were the same for the 8-week period before and the 8-week period after starting self-injection.

Pediatric ITP study: Thrombocytopenia in pediatric patients is often related to viral infections and usually lasts less than 6 months [29, 30]. Under 15% of patients go on to have chronic ITP. Nonetheless the bleeding risk in such young and active patients is real and multiple therapies (corticosteroids, IV anti-D, IVIG) are commonly employed. A Phase I/II study of romiplostim in pediatric ITP patients has been completed and the platelet count rises are the same as in adults.

Clinical Studies of Romiplostim in Myelodysplastic Syndromes (MDS)

Thrombocytopenia is a common finding in patients with all forms of MDS. Modest responses to the first-generation TPO molecules have prompted studies with romiplostim [31]. In one study 84 patients with low-risk MDS (receiving only supportive care) and platelet counts less than 50×10^9/L were to receive 4 weekly treatments with romiplostim at fixed doses of 300, 700, 1,000, or 1,500 mg and then could enter an extension phase with weekly romiplostim treatments. In the interim analysis of the first 28 patients enrolled (median baseline count = 25×10^9/L), 17/23

(61%) had a platelet response (platelet count $\geq$50 $\times$ 10^9/L) with the median peak platelet count rising to 130 $\times$ 10^9/L over the 4-week treatment period [32]. In the extension phase, 11/23 (48%) achieved a durable response of at least 8 consecutive weeks. There were 16 bleeding events (defined as bleeding $\pm$ transfusions) in 6 of 11 subjects with a durable response (6 events during the durable response period) and 74 bleeding events in 11 subjects without a durable response.

A subsequent interim analysis of this study was performed after 44 subjects were enrolled and included 40 subjects who entered the extension phase [33]. The mean duration of exposure to romiplostim was 23 $\pm$ 16 weeks; 41% (18/44) achieved a durable platelet response (at least 8 weeks of platelet response); durable responses were seen in 41% (12/29) of those with platelets < 20 $\times$ 10^9/L and 40% (6/15) of those with platelets $\geq$ 20 $\times$ 10^9/L. The mean duration of platelet response was 22.8 ($\pm$13.3) weeks. A total of 104 platelet transfusions were given to 39% (17/44) of the patients; only 17% (3/18) were given to those patients with a durable response. Two patients transformed to acute leukemia. Of the six patients with temporary increases in peripheral blast count, all had their blast counts fall after romiplostim was stopped.

A second MDS study analyzed the effect of romiplostim on the incidence of thrombocytopenia in patients with low- or intermediate-risk MDS receiving azacytidine. Patients were randomized 1:1:1 (and stratified by platelet count $\geq$ or <50 $\times$ 10^9/L) to placebo or romiplostim at 500 or 750 mg weekly. Patients received azacytidine 75 mg/m^2/day by subcutaneous injection for the first 7 days of each month. The primary endpoint was significant thrombocytopenic events (defined as platelet count < 50 $\times$ 10^9/L after study week 3 or platelet transfusion at any time) and secondary endpoints were platelet nadir and platelet transfusions. Significant thrombocytopenic events occurred in 85% of placebo patients and 62 and 71% of the romiplostim 500- and 750-mg groups, respectively. Platelet transfusions were performed in 69, 46, and 36% of the placebo, 500-, and 750-mg groups, respectively. Nadir platelet counts were lower in the placebo group than in the two romiplostim groups. Only one patient showed disease progression to AML; the patient was in the 500-mg group [34].

Clinical Studies of Romiplostim in Chemotherapy-Induced Thrombocytopenia

Grade 4 thrombocytopenia is a relatively uncommon finding in patients treated with non-myeloablative chemotherapy for solid tumors; it is uniformly present in all patients undergoing myeloablative chemotherapy for leukemia or stem cell transplantation. Studies with the first-generation thrombopoietins (rhTPO and PEG-rHuMGDF) demonstrated a modest effect in reducing the need for platelet transfusions and an increased ability to maintain dose density and schedule for some chemotherapy regimens [11, 18]. However, results with these first-generation thrombopoietins showed no effect in myeloablative settings. Studies have been initiated with romiplostim in non-myeloablative chemotherapy but results are not yet available.

Clinical Studies of Romiplostim in Hepatitis C Thrombocytopenia

The thrombocytopenia associated with chronic infection with hepatitis C is largely due to decreased hepatic production of TPO as well as an ITP-like increased rate of platelet destruction [35]. Since a platelet count $< 70 \times 10^9/L$ is felt to limit effective antiviral treatment with interferon and ribavirin, attempts to increase the platelet count by replacing the TPO deficiency have been considered [36]. Since the underlying bone marrow in such patients is usually normal, platelet count increases comparable to those seen in healthy volunteers can be expected when such patients are treated with romiplostim. Studies with romiplostim may be initiated in this area.

Potential Complications of Romiplostim Treatment

Human exposure to romiplostim has been rather limited. No more than 400 subjects have been exposed to treatment in controlled trials for up to 250 weeks. Over 1,000 subjects are currently receiving commercial romiplostim through the NEXUS Program (see below) and are being followed for adverse effects.

In the placebo-controlled studies, short-term exposure risks have been minimal for 24 weeks of romiplostim. Headache, ecchymoses, and epistaxis were noted; all mild. These common adverse effects of romiplostim have been analyzed for all ITP subjects treated with romiplostim versus those treated with placebo. An exposure-adjusted assessment (adverse effect rate adjusted for duration of exposure to romiplostim or placebo) for risks shows that there is little difference between the groups except for higher rates of dizziness, insomnia, and myalgia in the romiplostim-treated patients (Table 16.2). Although mild, there is no clear explanation for these differences other than possibly the withdrawal of corticosteroids from the romiplostim-treated patients. When the rate of adverse events was analyzed in the long-term study with romiplostim, the adverse event rate decreased over time on study and no new types of adverse events were uncovered.

Since romiplostim may be used for a prolonged time in ITP patients, attention must be paid to potential, albeit uncommon, long-term risks of exposure. To date, the following issues have been identified:

- *Rebound thrombocytopenia*: Romiplostim is a treatment for the thrombocytopenia in ITP but does not affect the underlying rate of platelet destruction. Upon stopping romiplostim after 24 weeks of treatment in the Phase III studies, platelet counts returned to the prior low baseline in most patients. Within 2 weeks of

Table 16.2
Duration-adjusted rate of frequently reported adverse events [40]

	Placebo Pt-yr $= 19.8^a$ $N = 46$ n (rate[b])	Romiplostim Pt-yr $=$ 186.5[a] $N = 204$ n (rate[b])
Headache	32 (161.6)	270 (144.8)
Epistaxis	18 (90.9)	136 (72.9)
Arthralgia	13 (66.7)	95 (51.5)
Dizziness	1 (5.1)	49 (26.3)
Insomnia	3 (15.2)	49 (26.3)
Myalgia	1 (5.1)	42 (22.5)
Pain in extremity	4 (20.2)	51 (27.3)
Abdominal pain	0 (0)	9 (6.0)
Shoulder pain	0 (0)	14 (7.5)
Dyspepsia	3 (15.2)	21 (11.3)
Paraesthesia	0 (0)	17 (9.1)

[a]Pt-yr, total subject years on study.
[b]Rate, study duration-adjusted event rate per 100 subject-years (n/Pt-yr $\times$ 100).

discontinuation of romiplostim, 37 of 51 (73%) patients who responded on the study had platelet counts less than 50×10^9/L. Only 7 of the 83 patients given romiplostim (2 splenectomized and 5 non-splenectomized patients) maintained a platelet count of 50×10^9/L or more 12 weeks after discontinuation of the drug. In most of these patients the thrombocytopenia eventually returned.

Moreover, some patients have their platelet counts transiently drop below their prior baseline values. In the Phase I/II studies, romiplostim was stopped after 2–6 weeks and the platelet count fell in almost all patients. However, the post-treatment platelet count transiently fell by more than 10×10^9/L below the prior baseline in 4 of 41 patients. All four returned to their prior baseline within 4 weeks but two subjects required rescue therapy [15].

These studies suggest that upon discontinuation of romiplostim, the platelet count returns to its prior low value and sometimes below that. Careful monitoring of platelet counts is important upon discontinuation of romiplostim treatment.

- *Reduced platelet activation threshold.* None of the recombinant TPO molecules or TPO mimetics directly activates platelets. However, all recombinant TPO and TPO peptide mimetics, but none of the TPO non-peptide mimetics, reduce the threshold for platelet activation by 50% (vide supra). This is unlikely to provoke thrombosis since the first-generation TPO mimetics had the same properties, but even in cancer patients caused no increased risk of thrombosis.
- *Thromboembolic complications*: Recent studies have suggested that ITP (and/or its treatments) creates a prothrombotic state and an increased risk for arterial and venous thromboembolism [37]. A potential mechanism for this is the large number of healthy new platelets being formed. Arterial and venous thromboembolic

events have been reported in clinical trials with romiplostim, but in the placebo-controlled Phase III ITP studies have been no more frequent than in the placebo group.

- *Increased bone marrow reticulin*: Bone marrow reticulin is a normal component of the bone marrow and may be increased in patients with ITP and many other autoimmune disorders [38]. It is distinct from collagen fibrosis. Although bone marrow examination was rarely performed in studies of ITP patients, reticulin was found in 10 of 271 subjects treated with romiplostim. Of five patients for whom pretreatment bone marrow samples were available, four showed increased reticulin on treatment [21]. Only one showed a small area of collagen fibrosis. In those patients who had a repeat bone marrow examination after romiplostim was discontinued, the reticulin staining intensity became reduced. No patient showed any evidence of any myeloproliferative disease.

  In a small prospective study of ten subjects who had bone marrow biopsies performed before and during romiplostim treatment, six patients provided adequate paired samples for reticulin staining. Reticulin staining was within the normal range in all patients and only one of six evaluable patients showed an increase in bone marrow reticulin staining while on treatment with romiplostim [21].

  Increased reticulin is a well-described (and reversible) effect of TPO; eight of nine AML patients treated with rhTPO and filgrastim developed increased bone marrow reticulin versus only two of six who received GM-CSF alone; upon discontinuation of rhTPO, the reticulin fully reversed within an average of 30 days (range 13–42 days) [39].

- *Increased blast count*: Increased blasts were seen in some MDS patients treated with romiplostim [32, 33]. In these uncontrolled studies, there was no placebo group to assess if this was due to the natural history of MDS or an effect of treatment. Similar blood cell effects have been seen with exposure to filgrastim and were reversible. In AML patients treated with first-generation TPO molecules, there was no acceleration of blasts and no change in remission rates [11, 18].

  In the ITP studies, two subjects were noted to have transiently increased immature cells in the peripheral blood. Both stopped romiplostim and the findings abated. The appearance of these cells might simply be a reflection of the asplenic state in these two subjects. One also had bone marrow chromosomal abnormalities prior to treatment [21]. In the studies of MDS patients receiving supportive care only, transient increases in blasts were seen in 6 of 44 patients; all reversed upon discontinuation of romiplostim.

- *Antibody formation*: Given the prior problems with antibody development to PEG-rHuMGDF, careful attention has been given to screening patients for the possible development of anti-romiplostim and anti-TPO antibodies. Of over 271 patients exposed, only two have shown evidence of formation of antibody against romiplostim. Both antibodies reacted only with romiplostim (and not with TPO), were transient, and did not appear to exacerbate thrombocytopenia.

- *Pregnancy*: Although ITP during pregnancy can be difficult to treat, there are no studies of romiplostim in pregnancy. Romiplostim is bound and transported by the FcRn receptor and should cross the placenta via that mechanism. Since

fetal megakaryocyte precursor cells have increased responsiveness to TPO, even small amounts of romiplostim could cause a rapid rise in fetal platelet counts. Until further studies assess the potential fetal risk of romiplostim, other therapies should be used to treat pregnant patients with ITP.
- *Cataract formation*: This has not been described in animals or humans exposed to romiplostim.

Using Romiplostim

Romiplostim (Nplate®) is now FDA-approved for the treatment of ITP. The exact wording of its approval is as follows:

- Nplate® is indicated for the treatment of thrombocytopenia in patients with chronic immune (idiopathic) thrombocytopenic purpura (ITP) who have had an insufficient response to corticosteroids, immunoglobulins, or splenectomy.
- Nplate® should be used only in patients with ITP whose degree of thrombocytopenia and clinical condition increase the risk for bleeding.
- Nplate® should not be used in an attempt to normalize platelet counts.

Romiplostim is produced by recombinant DNA technology in *Escherichia coli* (*E. coli*). Romiplostim is supplied as a sterile, preservative-free, lyophilized, solid white powder for subcutaneous injection after reconstitution with sterile water. Two vial presentations are available which contain a sufficient amount of active drug to provide either 250 or 500 mg of deliverable romiplostim, respectively. Each single-use 250-mg vial of romiplostim contains the following: 375 mg romiplostim, 30 mg mannitol, 15 mg sucrose, 1.2 mg L-histidine, 0.03 mg polysorbate 20, and sufficient HCl to adjust the pH to a target of 5.0. Each single-use 500-mg vial of romiplostim contains the following: 625 mg romiplostim, 50 mg mannitol, 25 mg sucrose, 1.9 mg L-histidine, 0.05 mg polysorbate 20, and sufficient HCl to adjust the pH to a target of 5.0 [16]. The usual initial dose in ITP subjects is 1 μg/kg with weekly dose escalations of 1–2 μg/kg up to 10 μg/kg. After attaining a stable target platelet count (50–100 $\times$ 10^9/L) by weekly titration of the romiplostim dose, platelet counts should be measured at least monthly.

As part of the new post-approval FDA requirements, a vigorous REMS (Risk Evaluation and Mitigation Strategy) program called the Nplate® NEXUS (Network of Experts Understanding and Supporting Nplate® and Patients) Program has been established to help assure the safe and appropriate use of romiplostim. Romiplostim is available only through the restricted distribution Nplate® NEXUS Program. Under the Nplate® NEXUS Program, only prescribers and patients registered with the program are able to prescribe, administer, or receive romiplostim. Under current guidelines, the weekly injections are to be administered by a healthcare professional. Given the current data from the long-term extension study, self-administration by patients will hopefully be available in the future.

It should be noted that even though approved only for treatment of ITP, neither FDA requirements nor the Nplate® NEXUS Program is empowered to restrict physician use of romiplostim to any one thrombocytopenic disorder. Romiplostim is currently being reimbursed for the treatment of ITP. An ITP Reimbursement Assistance program is available through the Nplate® NEXUS Program.

This reviewer has had considerable experience with the dosing of romiplostim in patients with ITP. Like other ITP treatments, dosing must be individualized and no dosing algorithm fits all clinical settings. A number of treatment issues deserve comment.

- The usual starting dose is 1 μg/kg and should be increased by 1 μg/kg weekly to attain the target platelet count. While this may be a conservative approach for the stable, non-bleeding patient who is being transitioned from corticosteroids to romiplostim, it is too slow for patients who need a more rapid increase in counts. In the Phase III studies of romiplostim versus standard of care, a starting dose of 3 μg/kg was used [27]. Furthermore, in the Phase III studies of romiplostim versus placebo the starting dose was 1 μg/kg but was increased by 2 μg/kg every week for platelet counts $\leq 10 \times 10^9$/L and every 2 weeks for platelet counts $11–50 \times 10^9$/L until the target platelet count was attained [26].
- The target platelet count is usually $50–100 \times 10^9$/L. There is usually no need (and indeed may be a risk) to increase the platelet count into the normal range. The data from the Phase III studies suggest that the bleeding risk returns to normal when the platelet count is $>50 \times 10^9$/L. Given the worry that higher platelet counts might be associated with an increased risk of thrombosis, a stable platelet count of $50–100 \times 10^9$/L is all that is required in most ITP patients. At these levels, most patients have adequate hemostasis and can take prophylactic warfarin or aspirin. In some patients requiring major orthopedic or neurological surgery, a temporary increase in target platelet count to $>100 \times 10^9$/L may be indicated.
- There is a synergy between corticosteroids and romiplostim in many ITP patients. Upon weaning corticosteroids, there is usually a need to increase the romiplostim dose to maintain a stable platelet count. Conversely, the administration of corticosteroids will increase the platelet count and (if being used chronically) will mandate a reduction in the dose of romiplostim. Transient administration of corticosteroids, though temporarily raising the platelet count, should usually not require change in romiplostim dose to avoid creating cycles of rapidly rising and then falling platelet counts.
- ITP patients often drop their platelet counts during times of viral or bacterial infection. To avoid creating cycles of rapidly falling and then rising platelet count, it is prudent not to increase the dose of romiplostim during such acute events. For most chronic patients, these falls can be ignored or, if bleeding or $<10 \times 10^9$/L, given a brief course of steroids.
- Withholding a weekly dose of romiplostim may cause a serious and potentially life-threatening drop in platelets. Since romiplostim does not affect the underlying rate of platelet destruction, stopping weekly treatment usually results in the platelet count falling; in some individuals this may be to a platelet count below

their prior baseline ("rebound thrombocytopenia") as was seen in the Phase I/II trials.

- What should be done if the platelet count goes too high? At platelet counts of $200\text{--}600 \times 10^9$/L, reduction of the weekly dose by 1 μg/kg should usually be considered. At platelet counts $>600 \times 10^9$/L, a reasonable option is to hold the drug and monitor the platelet count every 3–4 days; restart romiplostim at a dose 1 μg/kg less when the platelet count is $<250 \times 10^9$/L. For a few patients (those with headaches or at increased risk of thrombosis) with platelet counts $>600 \times 10^9$/L, administration of 81 mg of aspirin should be considered.

- Once a stable dose and platelet count have been attained, do not make frequent dosing changes. Romiplostim is a very potent stimulator of platelet production. Too frequent changes in dose (increasing 1 week and reducing or holding the dose the next week) will create great fluctuations in the platelet count. Dose changes should usually be contemplated only when several consecutive weekly counts have validated that the platelet count is out of the target range.

- How will I know if the patient still has ITP? For most patients ITP does not just disappear and will remain a chronic illness. Since the target treatment count is below the normal values, if a patient develops a normal platelet count it may be due to disease remission or, more likely, to an excessive dose of romiplostim. To assess this situation, the weekly dose should be reduced by 1 μg/kg weekly and the platelet count monitored. If at 1 μg/kg the platelet count is still in the normal range, weekly dosing can be stopped and the platelet count monitored closely. Most such patients will have a return of their thrombocytopenia and require reinstitution of romiplostim. Some will continue to have a normal platelet count and would appear to be in remission from their disease.

- What if a patient wants to discontinue therapy? Again, given the concern for rebound thrombocytopenia such patients need to be closely monitored (at least weekly) and other rescue therapies be available. This is true whether the patient has responded or not to romiplostim. If possible, the weekly dose should be slowly tapered by 1 μg/kg weekly rather than simply stopping treatment.

Conclusions

The long quest to develop a clinically effective and safe therapy to increase platelet production now appears to be ended. Romiplostim is a potent stimulator of platelet production and has shown marked efficacy in treating thrombocytopenia due to ITP. It has shown the highest response rates for any ITP therapy before or after splenectomy; it decreased the need for splenectomy. The common adverse effects seem mild and easily dealt with. The major issue of rebound thrombocytopenia upon discontinuation can usually be managed by encouraging patient compliance and closely monitoring platelet counts if the drug is stopped. The increase of bone marrow reticulin or even collagen remains the subject of ongoing studies but to date has been reversible and not associated with any long-term hematological consequences.

A wide range of other thrombocytopenic conditions should also respond to romiplostim. These disorders include drug-induced thrombocytopenia, hepatitis C-related thrombocytopenia, liver failure patients awaiting liver transplantation, presurgical patients with mild (30–50×10^9/L) thrombocytopenia, chemotherapy-induced thrombocytopenia, and possibly routine platelet apheresis donors. Short-term exposure in ITP patients might also be used to prepare patients for splenectomy or treat pediatric ITP (where the duration of disease is usually less than 6 months). Post-marketing surveillance of ITP subjects as well as new studies in a number of these other areas should allow a clearer understanding of the additional benefits and risks of romiplostim.

References

1. Kelemen E, Cserhati I, Tanos B. Demonstration and some properties of human thrombopoietin in thrombocythaemic sera. Acta Haematol. 1958;20:350–5.
2. Lok S, Foster DC. The structure, biology and potential therapeutic applications of recombinant thrombopoietin. Stem Cells. 1994;12:586–98.
3. Kuter DJ, Beeler DL, Rosenberg RD. The purification of megapoietin: a physiological regulator of megakaryocyte growth and platelet production. Proc Natl Acad Sci USA. 1994;91:11104–8.
4. de Sauvage FJ, Hass PE, Spencer SD, Malloy BE, Gurney AL, Spencer SA, Darbonne WC, Henzel WJ, Wong SC, Kuang WJ. Stimulation of megakaryocytopoiesis and thrombopoiesis by the c-Mpl ligand. Nature. 1994;369:533–8.
5. Bartley TD, Bogenberger J, Hunt P, Li YS, Lu HS, Martin F, Chang MS, Samal B, Nichol JL, Swift S, Johnson MJ, Hsu RY, Parker VP, Suggs S, Skrine JD, Merewether LA, Clogston C, Hsu E, Hokom MM, Hornkohl A, Choi E, Pangelinan M, Sun Y, Mar V, McNinch J, Simonet L, Jacobsen F, Xie C, Shutter J, Chute H, Basu R, Selander L, Trollinger D, Sieu L, Padilla D, Trail G, Elliott G, Izumi R, Covey T, Crouse J, Garcia A, Xu W, Del Castillo J, Biron J, Cole S, Hu MCT, Pacifici R, Ponting I, Saris C, Wen D, Yung YP, Lin H, Bosselman RA. Identification and cloning of a megakaryocyte growth and development factor that is a ligand for the cytokine receptor Mpl. Cell. 1994;77:1117–24.
6. Kato T, Ogami K, Shimada Y, Iwamatsu A, Sohma Y, Akahori H, Horie K, Kokubo A, Kudo Y, Maeda E. Purification and characterization of thrombopoietin. J Biochem. 1995;118: 229–36.
7. Wendling F, Tambourin P. The oncogene V-MPL, a putative truncated cytokine receptor which immortalized hemtopoietic progenitors. Nouv Rev Fr Hematol. 1991;33:145–6.
8. Li J, Yang C, Xia Y, Bertino A, Glaspy J, Roberts M, Kuter DJ. Thrombocytopenia caused by the development of antibodies to thrombopoietin. Blood. 2001;98:3241–8.
9. Kuter DJ. Thrombopoietin and thrombopoietin mimetics in the treatment of thrombocytopenia. Annu Rev Med. 2009;60:193–206.
10. Kuter DJ. New drugs for familiar therapeutic targets: thrombopoietin receptor agonists and immune thrombocytopenic purpura. Eur J Haematol Suppl. 2008;69:9–18.
11. Kuter DJ. New thrombopoietic growth factors. Blood. 2007;109:4607–16.
12. Cwirla SE, Balasubramanian P, Duffin DJ, Wagstrom CR, Gates CM, Singer SC, Davis AM, Tansik RL, Mattheakis LC, Boytos CM, Schatz PJ, Baccanari DP, Wrighton NC, Barrett RW, Dower WJ. Peptide agonist of the thrombopoietin receptor as potent as the natural cytokine. Science. 1997;276:1696–9.
13. Cerneus D, Brown K, Harris R, End D, Molloy C, Yurkow E, Koblish H, Franks C, Moolenaar M, Burggraaf K. Stimulation of platelet production in healthy volunteers by a novel pegylated peptide-based thrombopoietin (TPO) receptor agonist. Blood. 2005;106:363a–4a.

14. Frederickson S, Renshaw MW, Lin B, Smith LM, Calveley P, Springhorn JP, Johnson K, Wang Y, Su X, Shen Y, Bowdish KS. A rationally designed agonist antibody fragment that functionally mimics thrombopoietin. Proc Natl Acad Sci USA. 2006;103:14307–12.

15. Bussel JB, Kuter DJ, George JN, McMillan R, Aledort LM, Conklin GT, Lichtin AE, Lyons RM, Nieva J, Wasser JS, Wiznitzer I, Kelly R, Chen CF, Nichol JL. AMG 531, a thrombopoiesis-stimulating protein, for chronic ITP. N Engl J Med. 2006;355:1672–81.

16. Wang B, Nichol JL, Sullivan JT. Pharmacodynamics and pharmacokinetics of AMG 531, a novel thrombopoietin receptor ligand. Clin Pharmacol Ther. 2004;76:628–38.

17. Sabath DF, Kaushansky K, Broudy VC. Deletion of the extracellular membrane-distal cytokine receptor homology module of Mpl results in constitutive cell growth and loss of thrombopoietin binding. Blood. 1999;94:365–7.

18. Kuter DJ, Begley CG. Recombinant human thrombopoietin: basic biology and evaluation of clinical studies. Blood. 2002;100:3457–69.

19. Kaushansky K. Thrombopoietin. N Engl J Med. 1998;339:746–54

20. Broudy VC, Lin NL. AMG531 stimulates megakaryopoiesis in vitro by binding to Mpl. Cytokine. 2004;25:52–60.

21. Kuter DJ, Bussel J, Newland A, de Wolf JT, Guthrie TH, Jr, Wasser JS, Gehl L, Nie K, Berger D. Long-term treatment with romiplostim in patients with chronic immune thrombocytopenic purpura (ITP): 3-year update from an open-label extension study. Blood. 2008;112:154a.

22. Harker LA, Finch CA. Thrombokinetics in man. J Clin Invest. 1969;48:963–74.

23. Ballem PJ, Segal GM, Stratton JR, Gernsheimer T, Adamson JW, Slichter SJ. Mechanisms of thrombocytopenia in chronic autoimmune thrombocytopenic purpura. Evidence of both impaired platelet production and increased platelet clearance. J Clin Invest. 1987;80:33 40.

24. McMillan R, Wang L, Tomer A, Nichol J, Pistillo J. Suppression of in vitro megakaryocyte production by antiplatelet autoantibodies from adult patients with chronic ITP. Blood. 2004;103:1364–9.

25. Houwerzijl EJ, Blom NR, van der Want JJ, Esselink MT, Koornstra JJ, Smit JW, Louwes H, Vellenga E, de Wolf JT. Ultrastructural study shows morphologic features of apoptosis and para-apoptosis in megakaryocytes from patients with idiopathic thrombocytopenic purpura. Blood. 2004;103:500–6.

26. Kuter DJ, Bussel JB, Lyons RM, Pullarkat V, Gernsheimer TB, Senecal FM, Aledort LM, George JN, Kessler CM, Sanz MA, Liebman HA, Slovick FT, de Wolf JT, Bourgeois E, Guthrie TH, Jr, Newland A, Wasser JS, Hamburg SI, Grande C, Lefrere F, Lichtin AE, Tarantino MD, Terebelo HR, Viallard JF, Cuevas FJ, Go RS, Henry DH, Redner RL, Rice L, Schipperus MR, Guo DM, Nichol JL. Efficacy of romiplostim in patients with chronic immune thrombocytopenic purpura: a double-blind randomised controlled trial. Lancet. 2008;371:395–403.

27. Rummel M, Boccia R, Macik G, Pabinger I, Selleslag D, Gehl L, Wang X, Berger DP, Kuter DJ. Efficacy and safety of romiplostim versus standard of care as chronic therapy for nonsplenectomized patients with immune thrombocytopenia (ITP). Haematologica. 2009;94(Supp 2):425 abs 1059.

28. Bussel J, Kuter DJ, Pullarkat V, Lyons RM, Guo M, Nichol JL. Safety and efficacy of long-term treatment with romiplostim in thrombocytopenic patients with ITP. Blood. 2009;113:2161–71.

29. George JN, Raskob GE. Idiopathic thrombocytopenic purpura: a concise summary of the pathophysiology and diagnosis in children and adults. Semin Hematol. 1998;35:5–8.

30. George JN. Treatment options for chronic idiopathic (immune) thrombocytopenic purpura. Semin Hematol. 2000;37:31–4.

31. Komatsu N, Okamoto T, Yoshida T, Nakeo S, Urabe A, Nagasawa T, Yonemura Y, Takeshita A, Ikeda Y, Sawada K, Hotta T, Kanamaru A, Bessho M, Minami N, Okamura T, Jinnai I, Kanakura Y, Mizoguchi H. Pegylated recombinant human megakaryocyte growth and development factor (PEG-rHuMGDF) increased platelet counts (plt) in patients with aplastic anemia (AA) and myelodysplastic syndrome (MDS). Blood. 2000;96:296a.

32. Kantarjian H, Giles F, Fenaux P, Becker P, Boruchov A, Bowen D, Hellstrom-Lindberg E, Larson R, Lyons R, Muus P. Evaluating safety and efficacy of AMG 531 for the treatment of thrombocytopenic patients with myelodysplastic syndrome (MDS): preliminary results of a phase 1/2 study. J Clin Oncol. 2007;25:365a.

33. Kantarjian H, Fenaux P, Sekeres MA, Becker P, Boruchov A, Bowen D, Larson R, Lyons R, Muus P, Shammo J, Ehrman M, Hu K, Nichol J. Phase 1/2 study of AMG 531 in thrombocytopenic patients (pts) with low-risk myelodysplastic syndrome (MDS): update including extended treatment. Blood. 2007;110:81a.

34. Kantarjian H, Giles F, Greenberg P, Paquette RL, Wang E, Gabrilove JL, Garcia-Manero G, Gray J, Hu K, Franklin, J. Effect of romiplostim in patients (pts) with low or intermediate risk myelodysplastic syndrome (MDS) receiving azacytidine. Blood. 2008;112:89a.

35. Rajan SK, Espina BM, Liebman HA. Hepatitis C virus-related thrombocytopenia: clinical and laboratory characteristics compared with chronic immune thrombocytopenic purpura. Br J Haematol. 2005;129:818–24.

36. McHutchison JG, Dusheiko G, Shiffman ML, Rodriguez-Torres M, Sigal S, Bourliere M, Berg T, Gordon SC, Campbell FM, Theodore D, Blackman N, Jenkins J, Afdhal NH. Eltrombopag for thrombocytopenia in patients with cirrhosis associated with hepatitis C. N Engl J Med. 2007;357:2227–36.

37. Aledort LM, Hayward CP, Chen MG, Nichol JL, Bussel J. Prospective screening of 205 patients with ITP, including diagnosis, serological markers, and the relationship between platelet counts, endogenous thrombopoietin, and circulating antithrombopoietin antibodies. Am J Hematol. 2004;76:205–13.

38. Kuter DJ, Bain B, Mufti G, Bagg A, Hasserjian RP. Bone marrow fibrosis: pathophysiology and clinical significance of increased bone marrow stromal fibres. Br J Haematol. 2007;139:351–62.

39. Douglas VK, Tallman MS, Cripe LD, Peterson LC. Thrombopoietin administered during induction chemotherapy to patients with acute myeloid leukemia induces transient morphologic changes that may resemble chronic myeloproliferative disorders. Am J Clin Pathol. 2002;117:844–50.

40. ODAC Meeting Briefing Document. 2008. http://www.fda.gov/ohrms/dockets/ac/08/briefing/2008-4345b1-02-AMGEN.pdf. Amgen, Inc.

Chapter 17
Eltrombopag

James B. Bussel and Mariana P. Pinheiro

Abstract The current concepts and the management of ITP have significantly changed in the past decade. Decreased use of cytotoxic therapy and the introduction of new selective modalities of drug such as TPO-r mimetics are the landmarks of this change. Discovered in the middle of last decade, followed by experiments in mice and then approved in humans, Eltrombopag is the first TPO-r mimetic available. It has been used and validated in several clinical studies in different etiologies of thrombocytopenia, including primary ITP (chronic Immune ThrombocytoPenia) and secondary ITP, due to hepatitis C and more recently in bone marrow failure as myelodysplastic syndromes. Good tolerability and low side effects are the strengths of this drug, contrasted with issues regarding administration (it must be taken every day apart from specific meals containing high levels of calcium, which leads to problems with compliance). We review the first clinical studies with this agent, emphasizing the significant findings.

Introduction

Human use of eltrombopag (SB-497115-GR, Promacta®) was first reported in 2007 in normal volunteers. Subsequently a number of studies have pursued its use in patients with ITP and in those with thrombocytopenia associated with liver disease caused by hepatitis C. Thus far three large, randomized controlled trials have been reported and an additional such trial in ITP has been presented in abstract form only. Of note, published animal data are limited since eltrombopag is only known to be active in humans and chimpanzees and, therefore, safety data are only available for a small number of chimps in whom the platelet count increased (J. Jenkins, personal communication).

J.B. Bussel (✉)
Division of Pediatric Hematology–Oncology, Department of Pediatrics in Obstetrics and Gynecology and in Medicine, Weill Cornell Medical College, New York Presbyterian Hospital, Weill Cornell Medical Center, New York, NY 10044, USA
e-mail: jbussel@med.cornell.edu

G.H. Lyman, D.C. Dale (eds.), *Hematopoietic Growth Factors in Oncology*, Cancer Treatment and Research 157, DOI 10.1007/978-1-4419-7073-2_17,
© Springer Science+Business Media, LLC 2011

Biochemistry

Eltrombopag ($C_{25}H_{22}N_4O_4$) (Fig. 17.1) is a small molecule (molecular weight 442 Da), member of the biarylhydrazone class of compounds, which are non-peptide agonists of the thrombopoietin receptor (TpoR). The activation of TpoR occurs as eltrombopag associates with metal ions (Zn^{2+}) and specific amino acid domains in the juxtamembrane and transmembrane portions of the receptor. When bound to TpoR, eltrombopag initiates a sequence of events through phosphorylation and activation of the receptor. Once the TpoR is phosphorylated, it triggers activation of the cytoplasmatic tyrosine kinases as Janus Kinases (JAK)2 and tyrosine kinase 2, which in turn activate signal transducers and activators of transcription (STAT)5, phosphoinositide-3 kinase, and Ras-mitogen-activated protein kinase (MAPK) thereby promoting megakaryocyte duplication and differentiation into platelets.

Fig. 17.1 Structure of eltrombopag

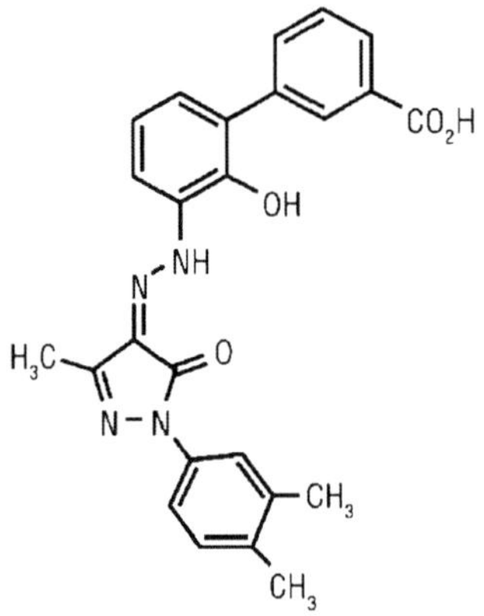

Preclinical Activity of Eltrombopag

Previous in vitro studies have demonstrated that the activity of eltrombopag is dependent on expression of TpoR and that a selective interaction with TpoR is responsible for the thrombopoietic activity of the drug. Erickson-Miller et al. [1] analyzed the molecular structure of the drug and the specificity of binding and activation of the TpoR, including second messenger signaling pathways (Fig. 17.2). They also investigated possible anti-apoptotic activity through lowering caspase-3 and caspase-7 cleavage activity. Effects such as induction of stimulation, proliferation, and differentiation in mammalian cells were compared with those seen with rhTpo.

Eltrombopag is known to have specificity for the TpoR and it is unable to activate JAK/STAT signaling pathways on cells expressing other hematopoietic growth

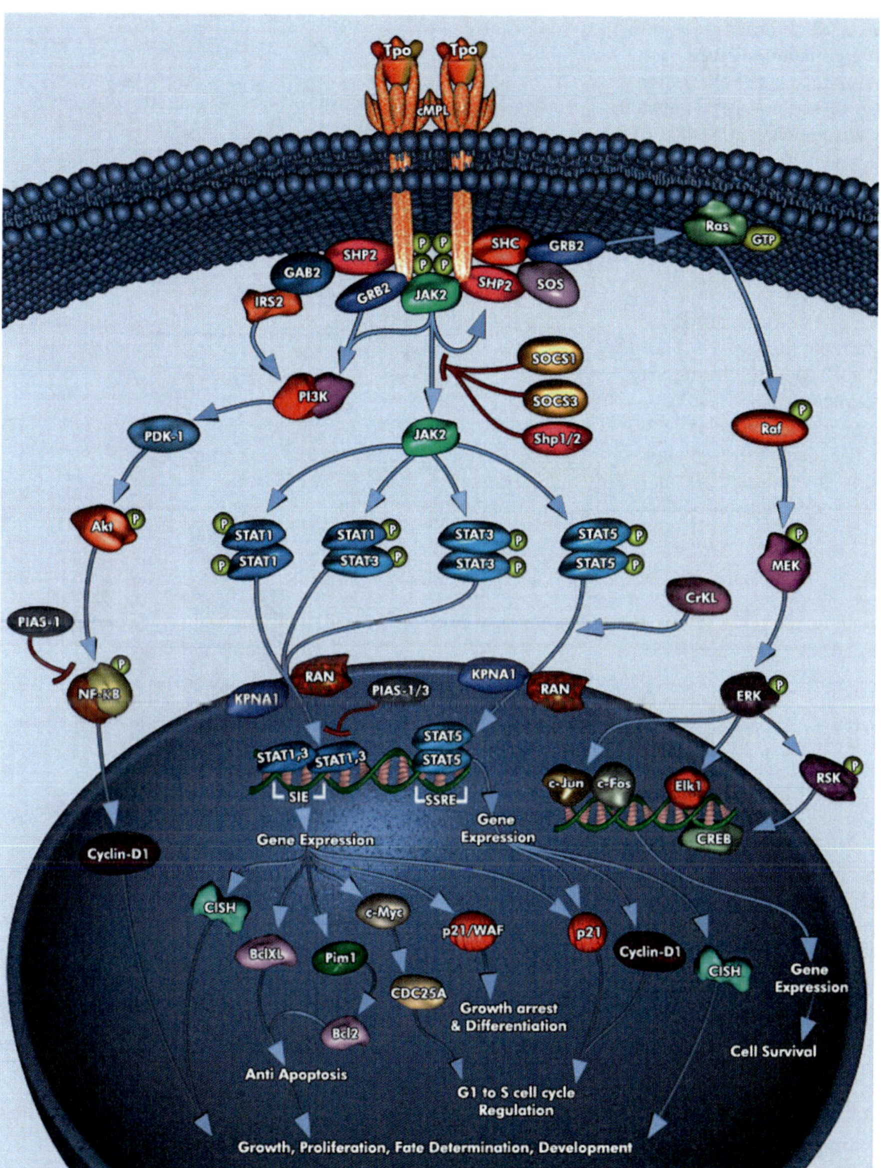

Fig. 17.2 Thrombopoietin signaling pathway

factor receptors (such as receptors for cytokines as EPO, G-CSF, INF-α, INF-γ, and IL-3). Similarly, studies with Tpo-dependent human cell lines (N2C-Tpo cells that endogenously express the TpoR) incubated with eltrombopag demonstrated that the proliferative effect was dependent on the expression of the TpoR.

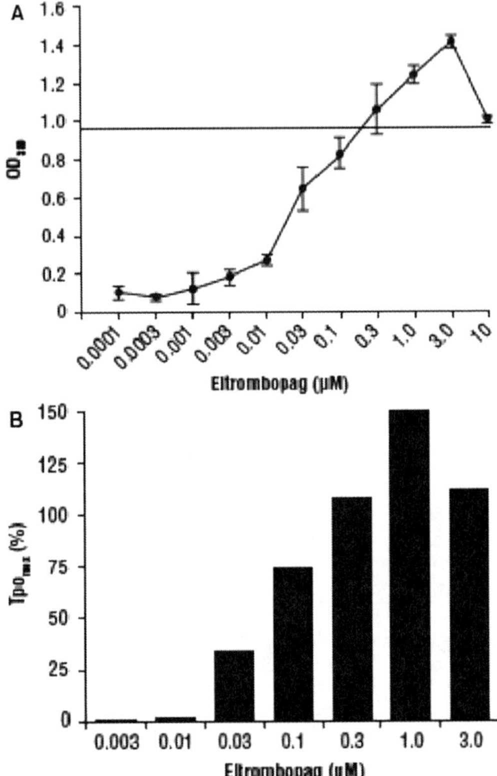

Fig. 17.3 Proliferation and differentiation induced by eltrombopag. **a** Proliferation of BAF3/hTpoR cells induced by eltrombopag after 48 h of treatment; the *dotted line* represents the activity of cells treated with 100 ng/mL of recombinant human thrombopoietin. OD, optical density. **b** Representative example of megakaryocyte differentiation of CD34+ cells after 10 days of eltrombopag treatment; similar results were obtained with six independent marrow samples. **Panel b** was printed from Duffy and Erickson-Miller [2]

Eltrombopag was able to promote the proliferation and differentiation of CD34-selected bone marrow stem cells into committed megakaryocyte lineage CD41+ cells in a dose-dependent manner (Fig. 17.3).

Eltrombopag lowered caspase cleavage to a similar degree as rhTpo illustrating an anti-apoptotic mechanism. The same study demonstrated that eltrombopag is able to activate Tpo signaling pathways (STAT5 and p42/44 MAPK) with kinetics similar to rhTpo, although to a lesser degree. When combined with rhTpo, eltrombopag displayed an additive rather than antagonistic effect (Fig. 17.4).

This additive effect was observed when eltrombopag was added to either suboptimal amount of rhTpo or in the presence of rhTpo at a concentration that causes a plateau in cell proliferation rates. These data suggest that Tpo and eltrombopag have different binding sites on the TpoR and may have an additive effect on cell signaling.

Their conclusions were that eltrombopag has a Tpo mimetic activity that is dose-dependent, has an agonistic effect additive to that of rhTpo, and, similarly to thrombopoietin, interacts specifically with the Tpo receptor triggering initially the JAK/STAT and subsequently, activating the MAPK signaling pathways.

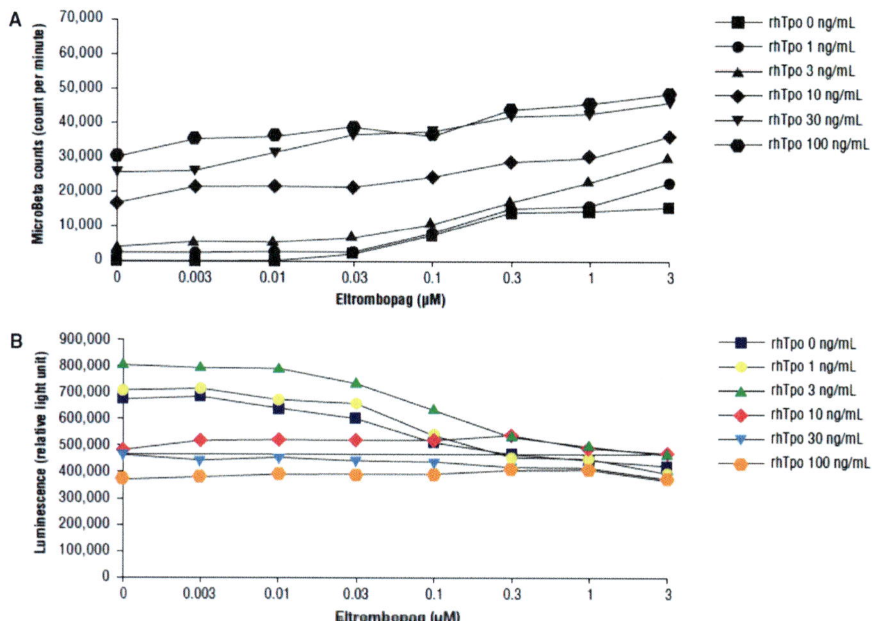

Fig. 17.4 Additive effects of eltrombopag and rhTpo. **a** Proliferation, as measured by thymidine incorporation, of N2C-Tpo cells by eltrombopag (0.003–3 µM) in combination with recombinant human thrombopoietin (rhTpo 1–100 ng/mL). **b** Activation of caspase-3 and caspase-7 by eltrombopag (0–3 µM) in combination with rhTpo (0–100 ng/mL) in N2C-Tpo cells

First Phase 1 Clinical Study of Eltrombopag

Eltrombopag was first analyzed in terms of safety, tolerability, pharmacokinetics, and pharmacodynamics in a phase 1 placebo-controlled clinical trial performed in healthy human volunteers by Jenkins et al. [3] (published in *Blood*, February, 2007). The results of this phase 1 trial set the stage for the subsequent randomized controlled trials described below.

In this study eltrombopag was administered as an oral capsule once-daily for 10 days at escalating doses of 5, 10, 25, 30, 50, and 75 mg in 73 healthy male volunteers who were blinded to medication. The investigator and sponsor were not blinded. The mean baseline platelet count was 239,000/mm^3 (range 134,000–347,000/mm^3). Safety, tolerability, pharmacokinetic, and pharmacodynamic assessments were made at several time points during and after the 10-day dosing phase.

The preclinical data were confirmed as eltrombopag was shown to have oral bioavailability with a serum concentration displaying a dose-dependent and linear pattern. Despite limited clinical activity, increase in platelet counts were seen at 30 mg daily and a platelet count 20% above the baseline was achieved in all patients who took 50 mg and 75 mg daily. The mean platelet count increase was 42.9% and 50.4%, respectively.

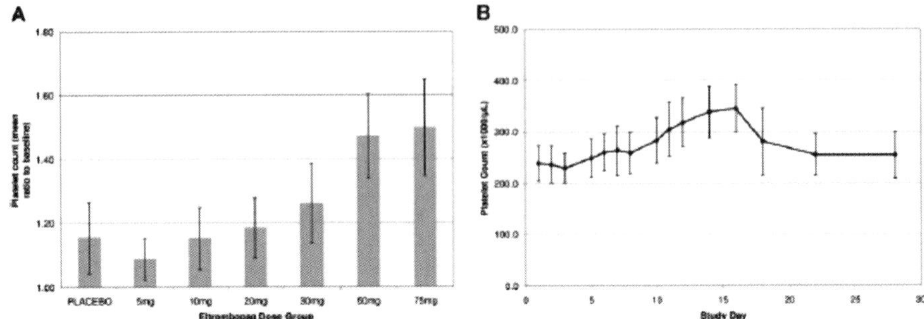

Fig. 17.5 Eltrombopag pharmacodynamics in normal volunteers. Pharmacodynamic data. **a** Platelet response in healthy male subjects following oral dosing with eltrombopag (once per day) for 10 days. Increases are apparent at 30, 50, and 75 mg. Values in graph indicate mean and 1 SD. **b** Kinetics of platelet response in healthy male subjects following 10 days oral dosing of 75 mg eltrombopag. The platelet number began rising at 5 days and peaked at day 15. Values in graph indicate mean and 1 SD

A consistent increase in platelet count started after 8 days of repeated doses of 75 mg of eltrombopag, with a peak on the 16th day returning to baseline values 12 days after the last dose (Fig. 17.5). Following discontinuation of treatment, there was no evidence of rebound thrombocytopenia, as platelet counts remained above baseline levels. Neither abnormal platelet function nor side effects of the administration of drug were reported in the normal controls.

Eltrombopag Use for the Treatment of Chronic Idiopathic Thrombocytopenic Purpura

The first multicenter, randomized, placebo-controlled trial in ITP [4] assessed whether and at what dose eltrombopag could increase platelet counts in patients with chronic disease. In this trial eltrombopag was administered to 117 subjects with at least a 6-month history of ITP, a platelet count of less than 30,000/mm^3 at enrollment and at least one prior treatment for ITP. The patients were at least 19 years old, with a median age of 50 years old. 38% were men and 79% were white. The four groups of patients received either placebo or eltrombopag at doses of 30, 50, or 75 mg/day for up to 6 weeks.

All patients were assessed weekly for safety, tolerability, and efficacy of the treatment during the 6-week treatment period and at 2-week intervals for 6 weeks after the study medication had been discontinued. Patients receiving stable maintenance immunosuppressive regimens, primarily glucocorticoids, were eligible but the dose had to remain unchanged throughout the study. Any other treatment for ITP must have been completed at least 2 weeks before the enrollment. Values within the normal range were required for neutrophils, reticulocyte count, creatinine, and liver enzymes. Exclusion criteria included secondary causes of immune thrombocytopenia such as HIV, Hep C virus, or SLE; comorbidities such as hemoglobin levels less than 10 g/dL, congestive heart failure, arrhythmia, thrombosis within 1 year before enrollment, or myocardial infarction within 3 months before enrollment. Pregnant or nursing women were also excluded and contraception was required during the study if patients were of childbearing age. Treatment was discontinued when platelet counts exceeded 200,000/mm^3.

Forty-eight percent of patients had a platelet count of 15,000/mm^3 or less and 47% had undergone splenectomy. Seventy-four percent of patients had at least 2 previous treatments for ITP (e.g., glucocorticoids, intravenous immunoglobulins, or danazol); and 32% were taking concomitant medication for ITP.

The primary endpoint, a platelet count of 50,000/mm^3 on day 43, was achieved in 81% of patients given 75 mg, 70% given 50 mg, and 28% given 30 mg compared to 11% on placebo group. The median platelet count approached the normal range and remained relatively stable in the group who continued the drug (median between 100,000 and 200,000/mm^3). These counts returned to levels near baseline within 2 weeks after discontinuation of therapy. The increase in platelet counts happened in a time and dose-dependent manner because both the increase of platelet counts and the velocity at which the platelets increased were greater with 75 mg than with 50 mg. A small effect was seen in the 30-mg group and even less in placebo (Fig. 17.6).

Multiple variables such as race, age, presence of concomitant ITP medication, previous splenectomy, and baseline platelet count (>15,000/mm^3 vs ≤15,000/mm^3) had no significant effect on the response to treatment. Patients receiving concomitant ITP medication, usually corticosteroids, responded similarly to patients receiving eltrombopag alone. In particular, after discontinuation of eltrombopag but while continuing concomitant medication, the platelet counts returned to at or near the previous baseline in that group. These findings indicate that eltrombopag was the drug responsible for the increment in platelet counts.

In the patients receiving doses of 50 or 75 mg, the incidence of bleeding as assessed by the WHO bleeding scale, decreased and then gradually returned to baseline levels within the 6 weeks of follow-up as the platelet count also returned to baseline (Fig. 17.7). The incidence of bleeding was the lowerst (regardless of the grade or cause) in the 75-mg group (4% compared to 14% placebo) indicating hemostatic efficacy of the newly produced platelets.

The incidence and severity of adverse effects were similar in all study groups including placebo and the most common side effect was mild-to-moderate headache. There was no evidence of any dose-limiting toxicity.

Thrombopoietin levels (measured by ELISA) remained normal (26–209 ng/L) and unchanged regardless of treatment. Health-related quality of life (based on the physical and mental component scores of the SF36v2 survey) was similar at the baseline and remained unchanged at the end of the study.

From this dose-ranging study it can be concluded that, at doses of 50 and 75 mg, eltrombopag is an effective, apparently safe, short-term treatment for patients with chronic ITP.

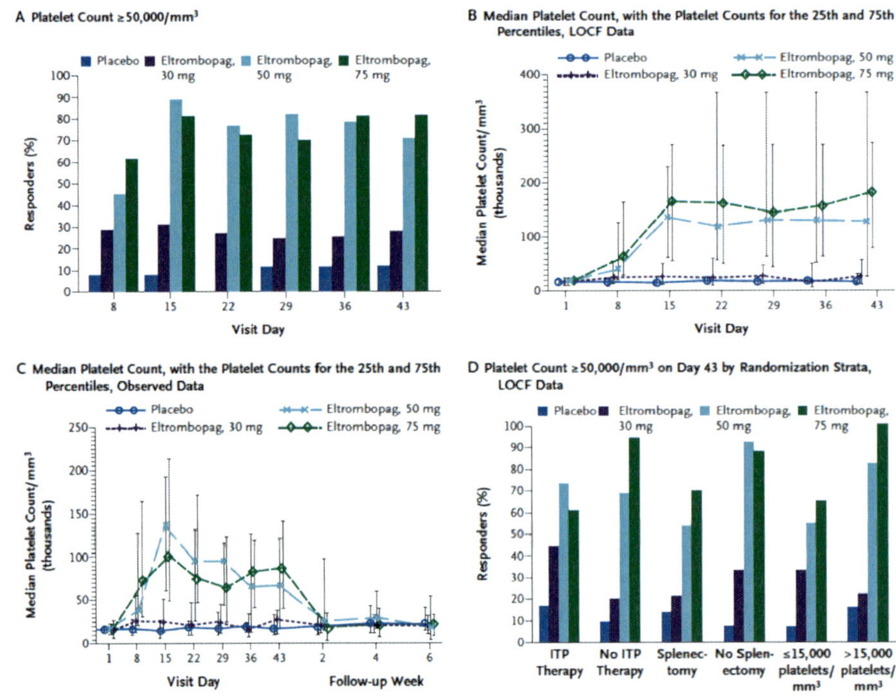

Fig. 17.6 Eltrombopag pharmacodynamics in chronic ITP patients **Panel a** shows the percentage of patients with a response in the four study groups at each weekly treatment visit, on the basis of last-observation-carried-forward (LOCF) data. On day 8, among patients treated with eltrombopag, 44 and 62% of patients receiving 50 and 75 mg, respectively, had a platelet count of more than 50,000/mm^3, and 88 and 81% of patients in these groups had a response by day 15. **Panel b** shows the median platelet counts at each visit, with the 25th and 75th percentiles shown as I bars, on the basis of LOCF data. By day 15, the median platelet counts for the groups receiving 50 and 75 mg of eltrombopag approached the normal range and remained there for the duration of the 6-week treatment period. **Panel c** shows the median platelet count at each weekly visit during the treatment period and at each biweekly visit after the treatment period on the basis of observed data. Patients who withdrew before day 43 were included in the follow-up. Discontinuation of treatment with 50 or 75 mg of eltrombopag before completion of the 6-week treatment period was primarily due to achievement of a platelet count of more than 200,000/mm^3. The median observed platelet counts remained elevated at 50,000 or more per mm^3 for the duration of the treatment in the groups receiving 50 and 75 mg of eltrombopag and returned to or were close to baseline levels within 2 weeks after the cessation of treatment. **Panel d** shows response rates according to the three stratification variables – use or non-use of concomitant ITP therapy (primarily prednisone or prednisolone), splenectomy status, and baseline platelet count (>15,000/mm^3 or ≤15,000/mm^3). A dose–response relationship was observed for each stratification variable

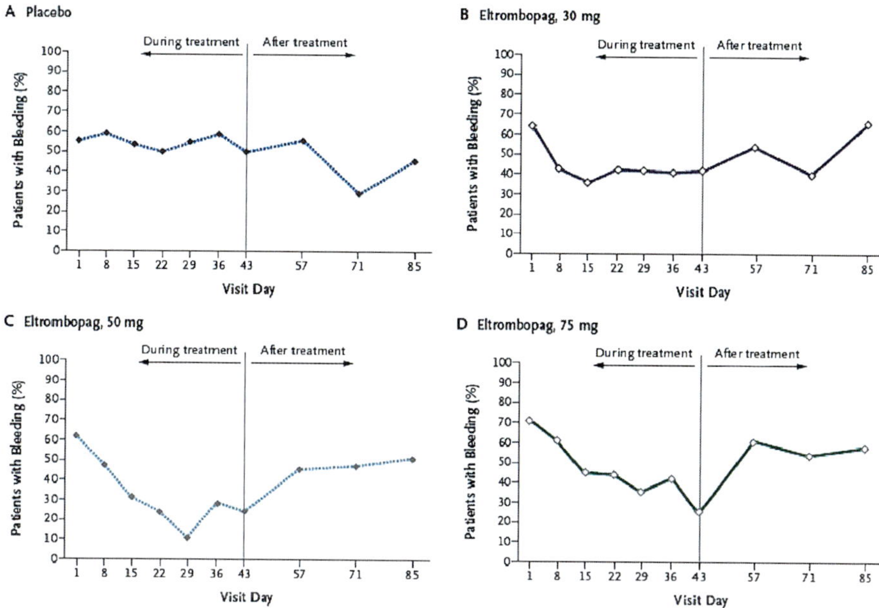

Fig. 17.7 Incidence of bleeding symptoms during and after treatment according to treatment group. The incidence of bleeding symptoms (defined according to the World Health Organization bleeding scale) decreased as platelet counts increased during treatment for patients receiving 50 or 75 mg of eltrombopag. The occurrence of bleeding symptoms gradually returned to baseline levels during the 6 weeks of follow-up, as the platelet counts returned to near-baseline levels

Assessment of an Increased Dose of Eltrombopag in Non-responders

A follow-up study was then performed in order to assess whether using an initial dose of 50 mg with the possibility of an increased dose up to 75 mg in non-responders the outcomes of platelet responses could improve. Fifty milligrams was chosen in preference to 75 mg because of the high rate of patients who started with 75 mg, and subsequently discontinued therapy because their platelet counts exceeded 200,000/μL. Therefore, a phase III randomized double-blinded, placebo-controlled was initiated in which eltrombopag or placebo (2:1) was administered to 114 patients with a median age of 48 years, approximately two-thirds women and three-quarters white [5]. As in the previous study, platelet counts were less than 30,000/mm^3 and most patients had a baseline platelet count of 15,000/mm^3. Additional inclusion criteria were normal creatinine and liver enzyme levels and exclusion criteria were patients who were using drugs or vitamins containing calcium or magnesium because of interference with eltrombopag gastrointestinal absorption. The treatment period was up to 6 weeks and the dose of eltrombopag could be increased to 75 mg after 3 weeks, if platelet counts remained less than

50,000/mm^3. In addition, treatment was discontinued in patients with platelet counts greater than 200,000/mm^3.

Thirty-nine percent had undergone splenectomy, 43% received concomitant ITP medication (three quarters of them had prednisone on both the placebo and the active treatment arms), and 41% had ITP for at least 5 years. All of them also had received at least one previous treatment for ITP (half of them received 3 or more ITP therapies) including corticosteroids, IVIG, and rituximab. The most common cause for withdrawal from the study was a platelet count above 200,000/mm^3 which occurred in 75% of patients on the active drug arm. 72% of the patients completed the 6 weeks of treatment.

The primary endpoint of this study, responsiveness to the drug defined by an increase in platelet counts to at least 50,000/mm^3 at day 43 of treatment, was achieved in 59% of the treatment group (compared to 16% on placebo). The median peak count for eltrombopag responders ($n = 43$) was 144,000/mm^3 (IQR 92.50–268). The median platelet count increased to 53,000/mm^3 by the second week in the eltrombopag group and remained around this range for the 6-week duration of the treatment period (Fig. 17.8).

One week after the end of treatment platelet counts were still at this range in 51% of patients. However, the counts gradually returned to previous baseline levels by 2 weeks after the end of the treatment period.

Patients responded to eltrombopag irrespective of the number of previous ITP treatments ($p = 0.31$), use of concomitant ITP drugs ($p = 0.77$), splenectomy status ($p = 0.75$), or baseline platelet counts 15,000/mm^3 ($p = 0.45$). Age and sex did not effect the response to treatment. Significantly fewer patients in the eltrombopag group compared to placebo had bleeding symptoms (39% vs 18%) ($p = 0.029$). However, after discontinuation of eltrombopag, a gradual return of platelet counts to baseline followed with proportionally increasing bleeding events, as in the previous study.

Mean scores for health-related quality of life at baseline and at the end of study were similar in placebo and eltrombopag groups. The proportion of adverse events during the treatment phase was 59% ($n = 45$) for the eltrombopag arm compared to 37% ($n = 14$) observed on the placebo arm. The most common were headache 8% (11% placebo) and bleeding 9% (11% placebo). Nausea and vomiting were absent in placebo but present in 5% of patients on the treatment arm.

Rare causes of bleeding (i.e., cerebral hemorrhage, gastrointestinal hemorrhage, and hematuria) caused withdrawal of one patient from the placebo group and one from eltrombopag, both of whom were non-responders. Increase in liver transaminases levels twice the upper limit was found in 6 patients on eltrombopag compared to one control. Abnormal liver function caused withdrawal from the study in one patient on eltrombopag, who was treated concomitant with long-term danazol therapy. No deaths occurred on study. Cataracts have been previously reported in preclinical studies in mice but were found in only two patients on eltrombopag and one patient that took placebo; all three had been previously treated with steroids.

This study confirmed the results of the previous randomized 6-week study demonstrating both efficacy and safety of 6-week therapy of eltrombopag in patients with chronic ITP.

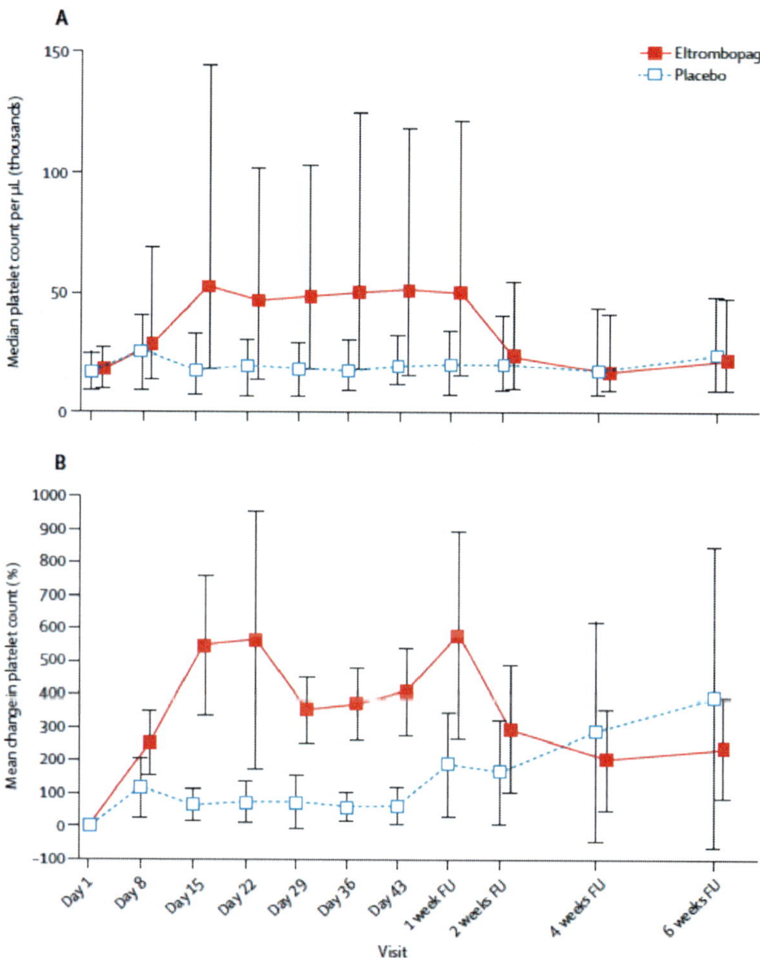

Fig. 17.8 Median platelet counts on ITP patients treated with eltrombopag. Median platelet counts (a) and mean changes in platelet counts (b) at every visit. (Median platelet counts at every visit are shown with IQR, and mean changes in platelet counts from baseline at every visit are shown with 95% CIs. FU = follow-up.) Four patients who received eltrombopag and two who received placebo were still receiving study medication on or within 3 days before the day 50 assessment and were included in this analysis

Eltrombopag for Secondary Thrombocytopenia Related to Hepatitis C Cirrhosis

McHutchinson, JG et al. published in 2007 a phase 2 clinical trial on eltrombopag in patients with hepatitis C [6]. This multicenter, randomized, double-blinded, placebo-controlled study of thrombocytopenia in patients with hepatitis C mediated liver disease using the same four doses as in the first ITP study. This study enrolled 74 patients with a median age of 51 years (range 30–74 years), with more than 2/3 men from 22 centers in the United States and Europe. These patients had chronic HCV infection (defined as the presence of anti-HCV antibodies and detectable HCV RNA levels) and thrombocytopenia with a baseline platelet count within a range of 26,000–94,000/mm^3 (median 55,000/mm^3). They were described as having compensated liver disease with cirrhosis confirmed by either a liver biopsy specimen or endoscopic evidence of portal hypertension. However, the severity of the liver disease was not formally graded in this study, for example, by Child-Pugh score (used to assess the severity and therefore the prognosis of chronic liver disease). Assessment of liver function monitoring was performed with eltrombopag treatment because the drug has been shown to increase liver transaminases in a small number of patients. Patients were excluded if they were pregnant, co-infected with human immunodeficiency virus or the hepatitis B virus or had a history of thrombosis.

This study consisted of two treatment phases. During the first 4-week treatment phase, prior to initiation of antiviral chemotherapy, the patients received eltrombopag once daily at doses of 30, 50, 75 mg or placebo. Hematologic, biochemical, and safety assessments were measured weekly. The treatment was interrupted when the platelet count was 200,000/mm^3 or more and restarted when this number was 100,000/mm^3 or less.

The second phase consisted of antiviral therapy if a patient had reached a predefined platelet count of 70,000/mm^3 or more for the use of peginterferon alfa-2a or 100,000/mm^3 or more for the use of peginterferon alfa-2b according to the package inserts for these two agents. Antiviral treatment with peginterferon and ribavirin was administered for 12 weeks concomitantly with eltrombopag or placebo. For safety, the dose of peginterferon was reduced by half if platelet counts had decreased to 25,000–50,000/mL^3 for peginterferon alfa-2a and 50,000–80,000 for peginterferon alfa-2b. The dose was stopped if platelet counts dropped below 25,000 and 50,000/mm^3, respectively.

Efficacy was defined by the ability of the drug to keep a consistent increase of platelet counts after the first 4 weeks (from the baseline value 20,000 to <70,000/mm^3) to 100,000/mm^3 or more and by the ability to continue peginterferon without a substantial decrease in the platelet count forcing an interruption or reduction in peginterferon/ribavirin therapy. The secondary endpoints included those related to safety and tolerability.

This study showed that eltrombopag increased platelet counts to 100,000/mm^3 or more in a dose-dependent manner. This effect was observed after each dose of the drug and was absent on the placebo group. An increase in platelet counts of 200,000/mm^3 or more was also observed on 25–52% of patients on eltrombopag (50–75 mg, respectively). These patients had their treatment interrupted until its platelet counts dropped to 100,000/mm^3 or fewer and at that point it was restarted.

The antiviral treatment phase could be initiated in two-thirds of patients, with the highest frequency of enrollment in the group receiving 75 mg of eltrombopag (91%) when compared to the 50-mg group (74%), 30-mg group (71%), or placebo (22%). In the 75-mg group, more patients (65%) were able to complete 12 weeks of the antiviral treatment phase, compared with patients in the groups receiving 50 mg (53%), 30 mg (36%), and placebo (6%). Despite the fact that platelet counts decreased in all eltrombopag patients during the antiviral treatment phase they remained consistently above baseline values with a nadir of more than 50,000/mm^3. No one in the placebo group had these results.

Platelet counts in the eltrombopag group were higher at all time points (Fig. 17.9) than placebo and remained higher than the level at which a reduction in the peginterferon dose is recommended (<50,000/mm^3), therefore no patient had their antiviral

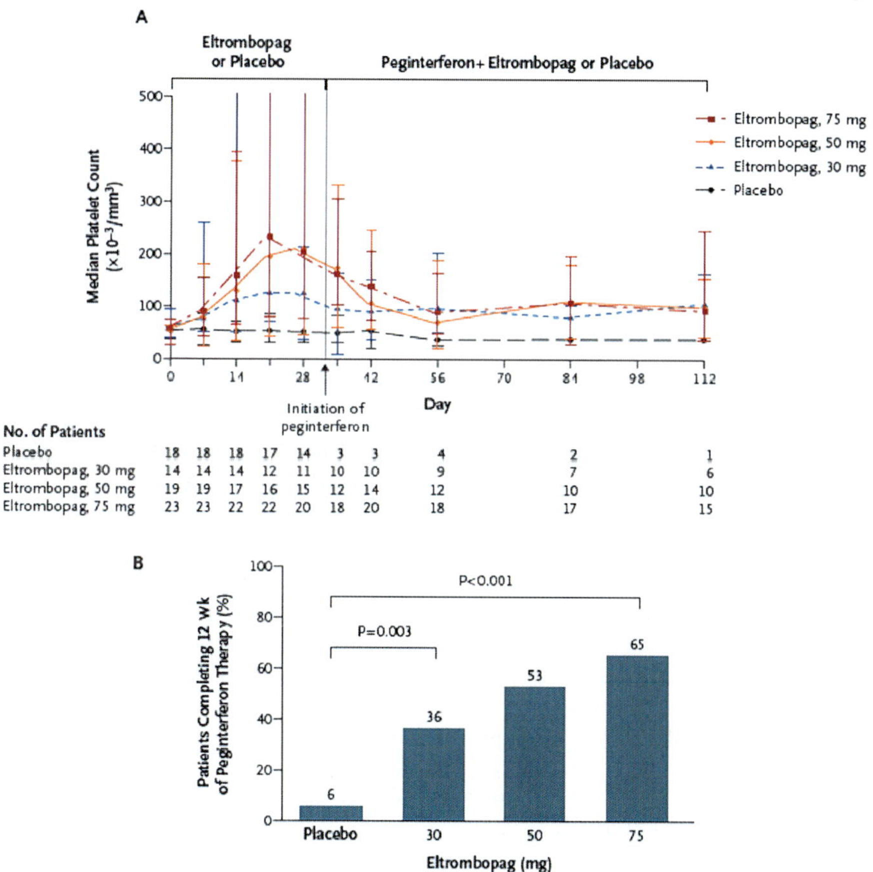

Fig. 17.9 Eltrombopag pharmacodynamics in hepatitis C patients. Median platelet counts and percentages of patients who completed the 12-week antiviral treatment phase. During the initial treatment phase, in which patients received eltrombopag or placebo, the median platelet count for each eltrombopag group was increased relative to the baseline value in a dose-dependent manner (**Panel a**). Counts reached a maximum at week 4, after which antiviral therapy was initiated while the administration of eltrombopag or placebo was continued. As expected, because of the marrow-suppressive effects of peginterferon, counts declined during the antiviral treatment phase and reached a nadir. However, platelet counts in the active treatment groups remained higher than those in the placebo group and those at baseline. I bars indicate the minimum and maximum values. **Panel b** shows the percentages of all patients randomly assigned to each group who completed the 12 weeks of antiviral therapy

treatment interrupted. Some of the patients in the treatment group had platelet counts higher than 200,000/mm^3 and required temporary interruption on eltrombopag therapy.

Side effects were observed, such as headaches (36% with 17% on placebo) and, less frequently, dry mouth, abdominal pain, and nausea, all in low grades of severity. Adverse events during the subsequent antiviral treatment phase were similar in all groups. The most common side effects related to interferon-based therapy were influenza-like symptoms, fatigue, chills, and headache.

In summary, eltrombopag therapy was able to increase platelet counts in patients with thrombocytopenia due to HCV-related cirrhosis, and, at the highest dose, to consistently maintain this effect even when combined with a potential thrombocytopenogenic drug, e.g., peginterferon. The combined use of a TpoR agonist and antiviral drugs including peginterferon and ribavirin would not only enable a greater number of patients to initiate antiviral treatment for hepatitis C, but would also allow a greater number to continue their treatment without dose interruption or reduction. There is a clear consensus that continuing antiviral therapy without interruptions or dose reductions substantially increases the chance of viral eradication.

RAISE Study and Ongoing EXTEND Phase III Study

Finally, the RAISE study [7] has not been published but has been presented in abstract form. It is a 6-month randomized placebo-controlled study of ITP in which standard of care was offered in addition to eltrombopag or placebo (2:1). It demonstrated that eltrombopag could be used for 6 months without loss of platelet effect and that no significant increase in thromboembolic events nor hepatic toxicity were seen. Platelet counts increased, bleeding decreased and health-related quality of life increased.

Similarly there is a large ongoing single-arm phase III study of the long-term treatment of patients with chronic ITP who have been on one of the previous eltrombopag ITP studies. This study, called Extend [8], has been presented in abstract form and suggests that development of tachyphylaxis is rare and that thrombotic and hepatic toxicities are infrequent.

The development of target TpoR agonists has been a landmark development in the management of thrombocytopenia from multiple causes. While the bulk of published data surrounding TPO-R agonists have focused on patients with chronic ITP (see also Chapter 16 by Dr. Kuter, this volume), it is clear that for patients with other diseases eltrombopag may benefit as well. In particular, the use of eltrombopag has been explored in patients with thrombocytopenia secondary to hepatitis C. In addition to the initial study summarized here, three large-scale trials are ongoing all with the intent of allowing better management of these patients. The focus has been on patients with thrombocytopenia prior to the initiation of antiviral therapy but in the future these agents will likely be used in patients who become thrombocytopenic on therapy. In contrast, studies demonstrating efficacy in chemotherapy-induced thrombocytopenia have not been forthcoming and it remains to be investigated whether TpoR agents, in particular eltrombopag have any important role in this setting.

In summary the availability of TpoR agents has already revolutionized the management of chronic ITP and potentially will do the same for hepatitis C-induced thrombocytopenia and may also prove to have clinical benefit in other thrombocytopenic conditions such as myelodysplastic syndrome, chemotherapy-induced thrombocytopenia, and stem cell transplanted patients. More studies are needed to assess the long-term impact and to address possible long-term risks of chronic exposure to this thrombopoietic drug such as cataracts, liver dysfunction, and a theoretical but potential effect on bone marrow fibrosis.

References

1. Erickson-Miller C, et al. Preclinical activity of eltrombopag (SB-497115), an oral, nonpeptide thrombopoietin receptor agonist. Stem Cells. 2009;27:424–30.
2. Duffy KJ, Erickson-Miller CL. The discovery of eltrombopag, an orally bioavailable TpoR agonist. In: Metcalf BW, Dillon S, editors. Target validation in drug discovery. Burlington, MA: Academic Press; 2007. pp. 241–254.
3. Jenkins JM, et al. Phase 1 clinical study of eltrombopag, an oral, nonpeptide thrombopoietin receptor agonist. Blood. 2007;109:4739–41.
4. Bussel JB, et al. Eltrombopag for the treatment of Chronic idiopathic thrombocytopenic purpura. N Engl J Med. 2007;357:2237–47.
5. Bussel JB, et al. Effect of eltrombopag on platelet counts and bleeding during treatment of chronic idiopathic thrombocytopenic purpura: a randomized, double-blind, placebo-controlled trial. Lancet. 2009;373:641–8.
6. McHutchinson JG, et al. Eltrombopag for thrombocytopenia in patients with cirrhosis associated with hepatitis C. N Engl J Med. 2007;357:2227–36.
7. Cheng G, et al. Eltrombopag for management of chronic immune thrombocytopenia (RAISE): a 6-month, randomized, phase 3 study. Lancet, 2010, in press.
8. EXTEND (Eltrombopag eXTENded Dosing Study): An extension study of eltrombopag olamine (SB-497115-GR) in adults, with idiopathic thrombocytopenic purpura (ITP) – EXTEND STUDY.

Part V
Special Considerations

Chapter 18
The Hematopoietic Growth Factors in Acute Leukemia: US Perspective

Olga Frankfurt and Martin S. Tallman

Introduction

The role of myeloid growth factors (GFs) in the management of acute leukemias has been evaluated extensively in multiple clinical trials. Granulocyte colony-stimulating factor (G-CSF) and granulocyte–macrophage colony-stimulating factor (GM-CSF) have been given prior to, concurrently with, and/or sequentially after the chemotherapy with the goal of reducing the duration of neutropenia and consequently, the incidence and severity of infections, as well as improving the rate of remissions and overall survival (OS). GFs have also been studied as chemotherapy-sensitizing agents, in an effort to recruit dormant myeloid stem cells into the sensitive phase of the cycle. Additionally, GFs, shown to stimulate proliferation and differentiation of leukemia cells in vitro, have been evaluated as monotherapy in patients with acute leukemia.

The majority of studies show modest reduction in the duration of the neutropenia, which does not consistently correlate with the severity of infection, rate, or duration of remissions, disease-free survival, and OS. Attempts to enhance the chemosensitivity of the leukemic cells and to decrease drug resistance failed to improve the rate of remission and survival in several large series. However, an improved outcome in younger AML patients with normal karyotype has been reported. Several anecdotal case reports showed that GF monotherapy is able to induce CR in patients with acute leukemia. Data from the published clinical trials do not appear to support emergence of drug-resistant leukemia, worsening toxicity and bone marrow failure with GF administration.

O. Frankfurt (✉)
Division of Hematology and Oncology, Feinberg School of Medicine, Robert H. Lurie Comprehensive Care Cancer, Northwestern University, Chicago, IL 60611, USA
e-mail: o-frankfurt@northwestern.edu

G.H. Lyman, D.C. Dale (eds.), *Hematopoietic Growth Factors in Oncology*,
Cancer Treatment and Research 157, DOI 10.1007/978-1-4419-7073-2_18,
© Springer Science+Business Media, LLC 2011

G-CSF, GM-CSF, and Their Receptors

Myeloid growth factors, although extensively used as pharmacological agents in clinical practice, are natural endogenous regulators of the innate immune response to infectious and inflammatory stimuli [1, 2]. Receptors for the G-CSF and GM-CSF are present on the neutrophil progenitors and mature cells, where they enhance production in the former and metabolic burst associated with the phagocytosis and the killing of the pathogens in the latter. When added to cultures of murine and human marrow cells in a semisolid medium G-CSF stimulates the growth of neutrophil colonies, whereas GM-CSF stimulates production and activation of neutrophils, eosinophils, basophils, monocytes, and dendritic cells [3]. Endotoxins, as well as inflammatory mediators, such as tumor necrosis factor (TNF) and IL-1, stimulate production of GM-CSF and G-CSF by the monocytes, macrophages, endothelial cells, and fibroblasts.

G-CSF, mapped to 17q11.2, is an 18-kDa glycoprotein that in addition to supporting survival, proliferation and differentiation of the neutrophil progenitors, causes the premature release of neutrophils from the bone marrow and enhances their phagocytic capacity. The administration of G-CSF results in toxic granulation of neutrophils in the peripheral blood, which is a morphological correlate of their heightened functional state. Activation of neutrophils by G-CSF in the bone marrow results in the release of matrix metalloproteases, which allows for the mobilization of hematopoietic stem cells. G-CSF receptor (G-CSFR), a homodimer, encoded by a single gene on chromosome 1p35–p34.3, is expressed by pluripotent and myeloid-committed progenitors as well as differentiated myeloid cell from the myeloblast to the mature neutrophil. G-CSFR may not be exclusively expressed by the myeloid cells, as its presence has been recently documented in a subset of lymphocytes and monocytes, vascular endothelial cells, human placenta, trophoblastic cells, and possibly neuronal and glial cells, although the biologic effect of its expression in non-myeloid tissues remains unclear [4–8]. Signaling pathways activated by the G-CSFR include activation of JAK tyrosine kinase and STAT factors [4, 9–11].

GM-CSF, mapped to 5q31.1, is an 18–28-kDa glycoprotein produced by T lymphocytes, monocytes, macrophages, endothelial cells, and fibroblasts [12]. Its receptor, a heterodimer, is expressed on neutrophils, monocytes, and fibroblasts among other cells. Similar to G-CSF, GM-CSF increases peripheral blood neutrophil counts and augments the neutrophil respiratory burst in vitro, resulting in enhanced bactericidal and antifungal activity [13]. Unlike G-CSF, GM-CSF raises the neutrophil count only by redistributing PMNLs and instead increases the number of circulating cells from other hematopoietic lineages. Knockout experiments in mice suggest that G-CSF is essential for the neutrophils' development whereas elimination of GM-CSF negatively impacts the number and function of alveolar macrophages, but does not result in neutropenia [14, 15].

Clinical trials aimed at evaluating the role of GFs in patients with acute leukemias were initiated in the early 1990s, after the G-CSF and GM-CSF were purified and molecularly cloned in 1984 and 1985, respectively, and recombinant GFs have been shown to shorten the duration of neutropenia in patients receiving intensive chemotherapy for lung cancer [16].

Formulations and Modifications of G-CSF and GM-CSF

Two recombinant forms of GM-CSF are utilized in clinical practice – sargramostim (yeast-expressed GM-CSF) and molgramostim (*Escherichia coli*-expressed GM-CSF), with only the former approved by the FDA for the clinical use in the United States. Besides filgrastim, a recombinant non-glycosylated G-CSF expressed in *E. coli*, approved by the FDA, and lenograstim, a glycosylated G-CSF expressed in mammalian cell lines, a pegylated filgrastim (pegfilgrastim) has been introduced for single-dose administration to the clinical use.

Various modifications of the GFs, including pegylation and glycopegylation, have been utilized to increase their size, delay renal clearance, and increase biologic potency. Pegylation, achieved by addition of polyethylene glycol (PEG), extends plasma half-life of the GFs and enhances their effectiveness, without causing immunogenicity. For example, pegylated G-CSF (pegfilgrastim; Neulasta, Amgen) is produced by adding a 20-kDa polyethylene glycol moiety to the N terminus of filgrastim [17]. Although this modification does not alter the in vivo or in vitro effects of the molecule, it prolongs renal clearance (elimination half-life) from 3.5 to 20–30 h in patients with normal renal function, hence prolonging the biological effect of GFs [17]. In a randomized clinical trial filgrastim (5 μg/kg) administered daily for up to 14 days, a single injection of pegfilgrastim (100 μg/kg) and fix-dose pegfilgrastim (6 mg) had similar efficacy and safety profiles in patients with breast cancer undergoing multiagent chemotherapy [18–20]. A retrospective case–control analysis suggested that a single administration of pegfilgrastim with hyper-CVAD chemotherapy in patients with ALL and NHL leads to similar kinetic of neutrophil recovery ($p = 0.75$), risk of febrile neutropenia ($p = 0.16$), frequency of documented infections ($p = 0.85$), and delay in the next cycle of chemotherapy ($p = 0.75$) as daily filgrastim [21].

Another pegylated form of G-CSF, differing by changes in the G-CSF gene sequence to create multiple new pegylation sites, has been shown to have similar effects to the clinically available pegylated G-CSF in animals studies and phase I and IIa human trials (MAXY-34; Maxygen, Redwood City, CA) [17].

Glycopegylation of G-CSF, a site-specific pegylation leading to selective attachment of pegfilgrastim to O-glycan sites, showed similar in vivo effects to other forms of pegylated G-CSF (BioGeneriX, Mannheim, Germany, and Neose, Horsham, PA) [17, 22]. Pegylated GM-CSF as well as multiple other alterations, such as modification of G-CSF with poloxamer 407, *and* hydroxypropyl methylcellulose, ionic copolymer pluronic F127 to make a slow released forms; production of recombinant G-CSF/IgG-Fc, G-CSF-albumin, SCF/IgG-Fc, diphtheria toxin-G-CSF are at the various stages of clinical development [23–28]. Other modifications, such as combinations of G-CSF/GM-CSF, G-CSF/IL-3, and GM-IL-3, although initially looked promising, were shown to be immunogenic and did not proceed to further clinical development [29–32].

GFs in Acute Myeloid Leukemia

GFs Decrease the Duration of Neutropenia

Bacterial and fungal infections are the major sources of morbidity and mortality, particularly in older patients with acute leukemia undergoing intensive chemotherapy [33, 34]. Therefore, it is not surprising that many clinical trials addressed the addition of GFs to induction and consolidation therapy in an attempt to decrease the incidence and severity of neutropenia-associated infection (Table 18.1). Additionally, it was anticipated that administration of GFs would minimize a delay in administration of subsequent cycles of consolidation chemotherapy and permit the delivery of more intensive regimen.

The most consistent outcome of clinical trials utilizing GFs is the reduction of the duration of neutropenia by approximately 2–7 days without significant effect on the frequency and length of severe fungal and bacterial infections [35–38]. Aside from the results of the European AML Cooperative Group, the Eastern Cooperative Oncology Group (ECOG), and European Organization for Research and Treatment of Cancer–Gruppo Italiano Malattie Ematologiche dell'Adulto (EORTC–GIMEMA) trials, the majority of these studies failed to show an improvement in rate of complete remission (CR) and OS.

Usuki and colleagues evaluated the influence of G-CSF administered after the induction therapy on the infection-related parameters and outcome of therapy in de novo AML patients. Patients older than 15 years, who achieved remission after the induction chemotherapy were randomized to receive G-CSF (120 patients) and no G-CSF (125 patients) until the recovery of blood counts. The median duration of the febrile neutropenia was significantly shorter (3 days vs 4 days, $p = 0.0001$) and time to neutrophils recovery significantly faster (12 days vs 18 days, $p = 0.0001$) in the G-CSF group than in the control group. However, the CR rates (80.8% vs 76.8%), 5-year probability of DFS (34.5% vs 33.6%), and OS (42.7% vs 35.6%) were similar between the groups [39]. Even though 40% of patients in the control group received the G-CSF after a documented infection, analysis performed on an "as-treated" basis failed to demonstrate CR improvement in G-CSF group. Similarly, in the Cancer and Leukemia Group B (CALGB) trial, patients older than 60 years with de novo AML were randomly assigned to receive GM-CSF (193 patients) or placebo (195 patients) the day after competing the standard "7 + 3" induction chemotherapy [36]. Although the median duration of neutropenia was shorter in GM-CSF arm (15 days vs 17 days, $p = 0.02$) compared to the placebo arm, the rate of CR and treatment-related mortality were similar in both groups.

Table 18.1 Prospective randomized trials evaluating the effect of growth factors on the neutropenia-related complications in AML

References	N	Age, type	GF type	Time of administration	Neutrophil recovery	Frequency of the documented infection	Length of hospitalization	CR	Survival (DFS, OS)
CALGB, Stone et al. [36]	388	>60 De novo, untreated	GM-CSF (*E. coli*) vs placebo	Day 8 Induction	Improved (15 days vs 17 days, $p = 0.02$)	Similar	Similar (28 days vs 30 days, $p = 0.11$)	Similar (5% vs 54%, $p = 0.61$)	Similar – OS (9.4 months)
ECOG, Rowe et al. [38]	124	55–70	GM-CSF (yeast) vs placebo	Day 11 Induction Consolidation	Improved (13 days vs 17 days, $p = 0.001$)	Improved ($p = 0.002$)	Similar (36 days vs 38 days, $p = 0.29$)	Similar (60% vs 44%, $p = 0.08$)	Improved – OS (10.6 months vs 4.8 months, $p = 0.048$) Similar – DFS (8.5 months vs 9.6 months, $p = 0.95$)
AML Cooperative Study Group, Dombret et al. [37]	233	>65 De novo, untreated	G-CSF (mammalian cell line) vs placebo	48 h after induction (day 9)	Improved (21 days vs 27 days, $p < 0.001$)	Similar (48%)		Improved (70% vs 47%, $p = 0.002$)	Similar – OS ($p = 0.76$)

Table 18.1 (continued)

References	N	Age, type	GF type	Time of administration	Neutrophil recovery	Frequency of the documented infection	Length of hospitalization	CR	Survival (DFS, OS)
EORTC–GIMEMA, Zittoun [95]	102	15–45	GM-CSF vs control	*GM-CSF (days 0–7 +/−) vs GM-CSF (days 8–28 −/+) vs GM-CSF (day 0–28 +/+) vs control (−/−)	Similar			Trend toward improvement in control arm	Similar (trend toward decreased OS in /+ compared to /−; OR 1.51 [95% CI 0.92–2.49])
HOVON and Swiss Group for clinical cancer research, Löwenberg et al. [56]	253	15–60 Untreated	GM-CSF vs control	*GM-CSF with chemo (+/−) vs during and after chemo (+/+) vs after chemo (−/+) vs control (−/−)	Improved in (−/+) (26 days vs 30 days, $p <$ 0.001)	Similar		Similar	Similar

Table 18.1 (continued)

References	N	Age, type	GF type	Time of administration	Neutrophil recovery	Frequency of the documented infection	Length of hospitalization	CR	Survival (DFS, OS)
International AML Leukemia Study Group, Heil et al. [99]	521	>16 De novo, untreated	G-CSF (*E. coli*) vs placebo	Day + 1 induction Consolidation	Improved (20 days vs 25 days, $p = 0.0001$)	Similar (37% vs 36%, $p = 0.85$)	Improved (20 days vs 25 days, $p = 0.0001$)	Similar (69% vs 68%, $p = 0.47$)	Similar (10.1 months vs 9.4 months, $p = -0.99$)
SWOG 9031, Godwin et al. [100]	234	>55 De novo/ secondary	G-CSF (*E. coli*) vs placebo	Day 10 after induction	Improved (15% reduction, $p = 0.014$)	Similar	Similar ($p = 0.27$)	Similar (41% vs 50%, $p = 0.89$)	Similar – DFS (6 months vs 9 months, $p = 0.71$) Similar – OS (12.5 months vs 14 months, $p = 0.83$)
GOELAM, Witz et al. [96]	240	55–75 Untreated	GM-CSF (*E. coli*) vs placebo	Days 1–28 Induction	Improved (24 days vs 29 days. $p = 0.0001$)	Similar (67% vs 72%, $p = 0.42$)	Similar ($p = 0.1$)	Similar (63% vs 60.5%, $p = 0.79$)	**Improved – 2-year DFS (48% vs 21%, $p = 0.003$) ***Similar – 2-year OS ($p = 0.08$)

Table 18.1 (continued)

References	N	Age, type	GF type	Time of administration	Neutrophil recovery	Frequency of the documented infection	Length of hospitalization	CR	Survival (DFS, OS)
GOELAM, Harousseau et al. [40]	194	15–60 De novo in CR	G-CSF (*E. coli*) vs control	Day 1 Consolidation (two cycles)	Improved (12 days vs 19 days, $p <$ 0.001 cycle 1; 20 days vs 28 days, $p < 0.001$ – cycle 2)	Similar (55% vs 66%, $p = 0.16$ – cycle 1; 40.5% vs 55.5%, $p = 0.07$ – cycle 2)	Improved (24 days vs 27 days, $p < 0.001$)	n/a	Similar – 2-year OS (64% vs 63%, $p = 0.24$) Similar – 2-year DFS (47% vs 43%, $p = 0.45$)
Australia Leukemia Study Group (ALSG), Bradstock et al. [101]	112	16–60 Untreated	G-SCF (mammalian cell line) vs control	Day 8 Induction	Improved (18 days vs 22 days, $p = 0.0005$)			Similar (81% vs 75%, $p = 0.5$)	Similar
MRC AML11, Goldstone et al. [102]	226	>56 De novo/ secondary, untreated	G-CSF vs placebo	Day 8 Induction	Improved by 5 days			Similar	Similar

Table 18.1 (continued)

References	N	Age, type	GF type	Time of administration	Neutrophil recovery	Frequency of the documented infection	Length of hospitalization	CR	Survival (DFS, OS)
Gran AML Study Group, Usuki et al. [39]	245	15–87 De novo, untreated	G-CSF (*E. coli*) vs control	48 h after induction	Improved (12 days vs 18 days, $p =$ 0.0001)	Similar (83% vs 91%, $p =$ 0.08)		Similar (80.8% vs 76.8%, $p =$ 0.532)	Similar –OS (20.8 months vs 18.8 months, $p =$ 0.59) Similar – 20 months DFS (14 months vs 12.5 months, $p =$ 0.94)
EORTC– GIMEMA, Amadori et al. [98]	722	61–80 De novo/ secondary, untreated	G-CSF (mammalian cell lines) vs control	G-CSF (+/–) vs G-CSF (+/+) vs G-CSF (–/+) vs control (–/–)	Improved with G-CSF given after chemotherapy (20 days vs 25 days, $p <$ 0.001)	Similar	Improved with G-CSF given after chemotherapy (27.2 days vs 29.7 days, $p < 0.001$)	Improved with G-CSF given with chemotherapy ($p =$ 0.009)	Similar

*+/+, GF administered concurrently and subsequently to chemotherapy; +/–, GF administered concurrently with chemotherapy; –/+, GF administered subsequently to chemotherapy; –/–, no GF administration.
**Highly significant in the cohort of patient ages 55–64 ($p = 0.002$), marginally significant in patients older than 60 years ($p = 0.22$).
***In younger patients (55–64), improvement of the OS was statistically significant.

Correspondingly, administration of the GFs after consolidation therapy to AML patients in remission failed to improve the overall outcome [40, 41]. In the study by the Harousseau and colleagues, patients with AML in remission were randomized to receive either a G-CSF (100 patients) or no G-CSF (94 patients) after each of the two cycles of intensive consolidation chemotherapy (ICC) [40]. The mean duration of neutropenia was dramatically reduced, both after the ICC 1 (12 days vs 19 days, $p < 0.001$) and after ICC 2 (20 days vs 28 days, $p < 0.001$) in the G-CSF group. The median duration of hospitalization (24 days vs 27 days, $p < 0.001$ after ICC 1; and 29 days vs 34 days, $p < 0.001$ after the ICC 2) and the median duration of intravenous antibiotics and antifungal therapy use were significantly reduced in G-CSF arm. However, the incidence of documented infections, the toxic death rate, and 2-year OS were not affected by the G-CSF administration. Furthermore, the median interval between ICC 1 and ICC 2 was reduced by only 2 days and proportion of patients undergoing ICC 2 was not increased in G-CSF arm.

A randomized study by Dombret and colleagues demonstrated improved CR rate, but not OS, whereas the ECOG study by Rowe and colleagues showed improved OS, but not CR rate (although a trend was present) in patients receiving GFs compared to placebo [37, 38]. In the ECOG double-blind, randomized clinical trial, patients with AML ages 55–70, who achieved aplasia after standard "7 + 3" induction regimen received yeast-derived GM-CSF (52 patients) or placebo (47 patients) until neutrophil recovery [38]. In the GM-CSF arm, the median duration of neutropenia ($p = 0.001$), overall treatment-related toxicity ($p = 0.049$), and infectious toxicity ($p = 0.015$) were shorter compared to the placebo arm. The median survival of patients on the GM-CSF arm was 10.6 months vs 4.8 months in the placebo arm ($p = 0.048$). However, the length of the hospital stay and the rate of CR were not significantly different. In the European AML Cooperative Group Study, lenograstim or placebo was randomly administered to the patients older than 65 years with AML on day 9 after completion of induction chemotherapy [37]. Although the median duration of neutropenia ($p < 0.001$) was significantly shorter and rate of CR was significantly higher (70% vs 47%, $p = 0.002$) in the G-CSF arm compared to placebo, the mortality rate at 8 weeks and OS did not differ between two groups.

Direct comparison of the various studies is difficult because of the variability in type, schedule, and dose of the chemotherapeutic agents, as well as type, timing, and duration of GF administration; difference in the patient population characteristics and the outcome of the placebo group; and the inconsistency in the schedule of antibiotic administration, hospitalization, and the blood counts monitoring [42]. For example, in the study by Rowe and colleagues, which was the only study that showed the benefit in terms of OS, the shorter than expected median survival in the placebo arm might have contributed to the outcome [38].

Several studies suggested that by virtue of reducing the length of hospital stay, duration of the parenteral antibiotics use, and time of febrile neutropenia, administration of GFs is of economical benefit [43–45]. According to the economical analysis of the ECOG trial, administration of GM-CSF resulted in the cost saving ($2,310), comparable to the one reported by the Lu and colleagues ($2,230). Similarly, cost-effectiveness analysis of GM-CSF administration in the GOELAM study showed significant cost savings and "in younger patients group saving were synonymous with GM-CSF" [45]. However, an analysis of the Southwest Oncology Group (SWOG) data showed no reduction in the overall costs of supportive care, despite the improvement of severity of the infection and duration of neutropenia [46]. The median cost of supportive care was similar in G-CSF ($8,768) and placebo arms ($8,616) in the report by Pui and colleagues [47]. The cost of therapy of placebo arm was significantly different in these trials suggesting that cost analysis could be institution specific.

Administration of GFs after the induction of chemotherapy in patients with AML is not a standard practice. It may be reasonable to administer G-CSF or GM-CSF shortly after the completion of induction chemotherapy to older patients (>55 years), with the goal of modestly decreasing the duration of neutropenia and possibly decreasing the risk of severe infection and length of the hospital stay. It is not anticipated that the GFs will have a favorable impact on the rate of CR, DFS, and OS.

Administration of GFs after the consolidation chemotherapy can be recommended in patients with AML to shorten the duration of neutropenia (more profound improvement compared to the after-induction administration) and decrease the rate of infections requiring antibiotic therapy. No effect on the duration of the CR and OS should be anticipated.

GFs as Chemotherapy-Sensitizing Agents

Despite the advances made in the field of acute myeloid leukemia, relapse due to the presence of minimal residual disease (MRD) and primary resistant leukemia remains the most important cause of treatment failure [48, 49]. A number of clinical trials have evaluated the safety and efficacy of G-CSF and GM-CSF as chemotherapy-sensitizing agents (Table 18.2). This strategy is based on the premise that GFs may recruit quiescent clonogenic leukemia cell into a sensitive phase of cell cycle, and hence potentiate the cytotoxic effect of chemotherapy [50]. Numerous in vitro and in vivo studies have demonstrated that there are receptors for the GFs on the leukemia cells and the simultaneous exposure to the GFs and chemotherapeutic drugs such as cytarabine may enhance the cytotoxic activity, increase intracellular level of the active cytarabine triphosphate (Ara-CTP), and increase DNA uptake of radiolabeled cytarabine [51–53]. Recently, G-CSF was shown to be a sensitizing agent to the gemtuzumab ozogamycin (GO) in cell lines and samples form patients with AML [54]. These preclinical studies, although varied in their methodology and the criteria of the cytotoxicity assessment, provided a rationale for the evaluation of the GFs as a means of modulating the myelosuppressive effects of chemotherapy in patients with AML. Despite the strong theoretical rationale, the majority of these studies did not show significant clinical benefit of GF administration in patients with either newly diagnosed or relapsed and refractory disease, in terms of CR, DFS, and OS.

Löwenberg and colleagues conducted a prospective multicenter clinical trial in which 640 patients with untreated AML, 18–60 years of age were randomized to

Table 18.2 Prospective randomized trials evaluating the "Priming" effect of growth factors in AML

References	N	Age, type	GF type	Time of administration	Neutrophil recovery	Infections	CR	OS, DFS
Heil et al. [94]	80	15–75 De novo	GM-CSF (*E. coli*) vs placebo	Day-1 Induction Consolidation	Similar	Similar	Similar (81% vs 79%, p = 0.57)	OS – similar (at 43 months 45% vs 49%, $p = 0.66$) RFS(relapse free survival) – similar (41 months 42% vs 41%, $p = 0.89$)
EORTC– GIMEMA, Zittoun et al. [95]	102	15–45 Untreated	GM-CSF (*E. coli*) vs control	GM-CSF (days 0–7 +/−) vs GM-CSF (days 8–28 −/+) vs GM-CSF (day 0–28 +/+) vs control (−/−)	Similar ($p = 0.28$)	Similar	Similar (trend toward improvement in control arm)	Similar (trend toward decreased OS in /+ compared to /−; OR 1.51 [95% CI 0.92–2.49])
EORTC– HOVON, Lowenberg et al. [56]	318	>60 De novo/ secondary	GM-CSF (*E. coli*) vs control	Induction Consolidation	Improved (23 days vs 25 days, $p = 0.0002$)	Similar	Similar (56% vs 55%, $p = 0.98$)	Similar (2 years: 15% vs 19% $p = 0.0.69$)
GOELAM, Witz et al. [96]	240	55–75 De novo	GM-CSF (*E. coli*) vs placebo	Days 1–28 Induction	Improved (24 days vs 29 days, $p = 0.0001$)	Similar	Similar (63% vs 60.5%, $p = 0.79$)	Similar ($p = 0.82$) Improved (2 years 49% vs 21%, $p = 0.003$)

Table 18.2 (continued)

References	N	Age, type	GF type	Time of administration	Neutrophil recovery	Infections	CR	OS, DFS
EMA91, Thomas et al. [59]	192	16–65 Relapsed/ refractory	GM-CSF (*E. coli*) vs placebo	Days 4–8 Induction	Similar (38 days vs 37 days)	Similar (45% vs 51%, $p > 0.1$)	Similar (65% vs 59%, $p = 0.35$)	Similar – OS (303 vs 254, $p=0.32$) Similar –DFS (251 days vs 240 days, $p=0.45$) Improved – Time to progression (median 152 days vs 115 days, $p=0.08$)
Hast et al. [97]	93	35–90	GM-CSF vs control	Start day-1 Induction Consolidation	Similar (18 days vs 21 days, $p=0.21$)	Similar (24 vs 29)	Similar (43%)	Similar
HOVON, Löwenberg et al. [55]	640	18–60 De novo/ secondary, untreated	G-CSF (mammalian cell line) vs control	Start day 0 Induction Consolidation	Similar	Similar	Similar (79% vs 83%, $p = 0.24$)	Improved DFS (4 years 42% vs 33%, $p = 0.02$) Reduced risk of relapse (relative risk 0.77 [95% CI 0.61–0.99]) OS–Similar ($p=0.16$)
Löfgren et al. [57]	110	>64 De novo	GM-CSF vs control	Start day 0 Induction Consolidation	Improved (17 days vs 25 days, $p = 0.03$)	Improved (39 vs 46, $p = 0.05$)	Similar (65% vs 64%)	Similar (9 months vs 14 months)

Table 18.2 (continued)

References	N	Age, type	GF type	Time of administration	Neutrophil recovery	Infections	CR	OS, DFS
ECOG Rowe et al. [60]	245	>55 Untreated	GM-CSF (*E. coli*) vs placebo	Day-1 Induction	–	–	Similar (38% vs 40% $p = 0.73$)	Similar (5.3 months vs 8.5 months, $p = 0.11$) Similar (6.9 months vs 5.1 months, $p = 0.73$)
EORTC–GIMEMA, Amadori et al. [98]	722	61–80	G-CSF (mammalian cell lines) vs control	G-CSF (+/−) vs G-CSF (+/+) vs G-CSF (−/+) vs control (−/−)	Improved with G-CSF given after chemotherapy (20 days vs 25 days, $p < 0.001$)	Similar	Improved with G-CSF given with chemotherapy ($p = 0.009$)	Similar
Thomas et al. [58]	259	15–50	GM-CSF vs control	Days 1–10 Induction Consolidation			Similar (91% vs 87%)	EFS – improved (42% vs 34%) OS – similar

receive G-CSF 1 day prior to and concurrently with the two cycles of chemotherapy [55]. Among the patients in CR, after a median follow up of 55 months, a higher rate of DFS was noted in the G-CSF group compared to the controls (at 4 years – 42% vs 33%, $p = 0.02$), attributable to a reduced probability of relapse (relative risk 0.77 [95% CI 0.61–0.99, $p = 0.04$]). Overall, however, OS and DFS were similar between the groups ($p = 0.16$). Subgroup analysis indicated that the major, if not the entire, benefit of G-CSF was in the subgroup of patients with standard risk disease (by cytogenetics) – 4-year OS 45% vs 35% (relative risk of death 0.75 [95% CI 0.59–0.95, $p = 0.02$]) and DFS 45% vs 33% (relative risk 0.70 [95% CI 0.55–0.90, $p = 0.006$]). The outcome of patients with unfavorable prognosis was not improved and the small number of patients in the favorable subgroup (~6%) limited the meaningful analysis.

A similarly designed randomized trial of GM-CSF in patients older than 60 years, conducted by the same group, failed to demonstrate the improvement in the rate of CR and DFS, possibly owing to the increased number of patients with abnormal cytogenetics (55%) [56]. A Swedish multicenter randomized trial tested addition of the GM-CSF to MEC (mitoxantrone, etoposide, cytarabine) chemotherapy in older patients with de novo AML. The CR rate was 65% with GM-CSF arm and 64% in patients without GM-CSF, the median CR duration was 6 months versus 13 months, median OS was 9 months versus 14 months, median time to neutrophils recovery was 17 days versus 25 days, and a number of positive blood cultures was 39 versus 46. Hence, addition of GM-CSF before, during, and after chemotherapy did not improve the outcome of *older* patients with AML [57].

In the recent multicenter prospective randomized trial conducted by the Acute Leukemia French Association (ALFA) Group, the role of GM-CSF priming on the outcome of 256 *younger* (15–50 years) patients with AML was evaluated [58]. GM-CSF was administered from day 1–10 of induction and consolidation chemotherapy. After the induction therapy, the CR rate was similar in both groups (91% with GM-CSF vs 87% without GM-CSF). After a median follow-up of 3 years there was a trend toward improvement of DFS in the GM-CSF group (42% vs 34%, $p = 0.06$) without improvement in OS. Subset analysis indicated that most of the benefit occurred in the patients with intermediate risk cytogenetics (3-year EFS 50% vs 35%, $p = 0.05$) owing in part to the lower risk of relapse (29% vs 47%, $p = 0.05$) and reduced treatment-related mortality (19% vs 23%) at 3 years. Administration of GM-CSF did not improve outcome of patients with favorable ($p = 0.8$) and unfavorable ($p = 0.3$) cytogenetics. Of interest, patients with abnormal intermediate-risk karyotype appeared to benefit more from GM-CSF administration (3-year EFS, 55% vs 19%, $p = 0.03$) compared to those with normal karyotype (3-year EFS, 47% vs 42%, $p = 0.4$).

Although multiple trials studied the efficacy of GFs as priming agents in a clinical setting, only a few correlative studies were conducted to establish if the recruitment of the leukemic blasts into the chemotherapy sensitive cell phase indeed occurred and if it correlated with the clinical outcome [59, 60]. Cell cycle studies, accompanying EMA91 (Etoposide, Mitoxantrone, Cytarabine) trial by Thomas and colleagues, showed increased recruitment of cells in the S phase between days 4 and

8 (days of administration of GM-CSF) in the GM-CSF group compared to placebo ($p = 0.006$). However, this finding did not correlate with the overall outcome of the group receiving GM-CSF. Similarly, in the ECOG trial reported by Rowe and colleagues, priming for 48 h with GM-CSF resulted in significant increase of leukemia cells in the S cycle compared to placebo (2.05% vs 0.25%, $p = 0.003$), which did not correlate with clinical benefit [60].

The use of GFs as priming agents in combination with chemotherapy for patients with AML raised the concern that stimulation of the residual normal precursors could increase their sensitivity to the chemotherapy, causing the prolonged bone marrow suppressions. This theory has not been substantiated by published data. Additionally, no evidence of in vivo stimulation of residual leukemia cells by GFs has been reported.

The use of the GFs as sensitizing agent in patients with AML (including de novo, secondary, high risk, younger patients or in elderly) is not recommended at this time, as it has no effect on DFS and OS.

GFs as Monotherapy in AML

Several case reports described achievement of CR with GF monotherapy in patients with the newly diagnosed and relapsed/refractory acute leukemia (14 AML, 3 APL, 2 ALL) [61, 62]. Majority of patients presented with pancytopenia and infection. The time to response (from 2 weeks to 3 months) and its duration (from 2 to 10 months) ranged widely. The mechanisms of remission induction are not clear. It is conceivable, that stimulation of the normal hematopoietic precursors more extensively than leukemia cells by G-CSF results in relative rather than the absolute reduction in the blasts count. However, the presence of durable responses and occasional cytogenetic remissions argues against this theory. It has been established that blasts from patients with AML express high procaspase protein levels, enhanced by the GM-CSF administration [63, 64]. In vitro data have shown that GM-CSF induces a dual effect: it stimulates cell proliferation (up-regulates Bcl-2, Bcl-XL) and, simultaneously, triggers pro-apoptotic signal in AML cells (up-regulates BAX, SOCS-2 and SOCS-3, procaspases 2 and 3, PARP cleavage). Faderl and colleagues have demonstrated that in the clonogenic assays, low dose of GM-CSF stimulates colony proliferation, whereas at concentration exceeding 0.05 μg/mL, the number of colonies decreases [64]. Differential expression of the high- and low-affinity GM-CSF receptors may have accounted for the difference in response.

Outside of context of a clinical trial, GF monotherapy to treat acute leukemia cannot be recommended.

GFs in Acute Lymphoblastic Leukemia

In the last 30 years, significant advances have been made in the management of adult ALL. Although the institution of high-intensity, multiagent pediatric regimens results in the CR rate of 80–90% in adult patients, the overall long-term DFS is only 35–50%. Multiple clinical trials evaluated the addition of GFs to the induction and/or consolidation chemotherapy with goals of improving the outcome of patients with ALL (Table 18.3). The aims of most of the studies were to determine if GFs are able to shorten the time of bone marrow recovery; reduce the incidences of febrile neutropenia, documented infections, and mortality due to the infection; minimize the hospital stay; and improve the rate and duration of CR. Since dose intensity appears to influence outcome, shortening the duration of neutropenia and infection by administering GFs may improve adherence to the treatment schedule.

Similar to the finding in AML patients, the most consistent outcome of prophylactic administration of GFs during induction and consolidation chemotherapy in ALL was a shortened duration of the neutropenia and earlier myeloid recovery [65, 66]. Some studies also showed an improvement of infection-related parameters, reduced hematologic toxicity of dose intensification, better compliance with the treatment schedule, and reduced infection-related mortality [65–67]. A few studies showed the increased rate of CR without improvement in OS [66]. Only a single small study demonstrated a positive impact of GFs on OS and DFS [68].

The study conducted by the Japan Adult Leukemia Study Group (JALSG) established the dose of 5 μg/kg administered intravenously, as the optimal dose to accelerate the neutrophil recovery after the intensive remission induction and consolidation chemotherapy [65]. In this small prospective clinical trial 41 adult patients with newly diagnosed ALL were randomized to receive 0, 2, 5, or 10 μg/kg of G-CSF. The neutrophil recovery after induction chemotherapy was significantly faster in the 5 ($p = 0.047$) and 10 μg/kg ($p = 0.011$) groups compared to the 2 μg/kg, but was similar between the two former groups. After the consolidation therapy, neutrophil recovery was significantly faster in the 2, 5, and 10 μg/kg groups than in no G-CSF group ($p < 0.001$), but did not differ in three former groups. Frequency of febrile neutropenia and incidence of documented infections appeared to be less in 5 and 10 μg/kg groups than in 0 and 2 μg/kg groups.

In a double-blind, randomized trial of 198 patients with de novo ALL conducted by the CALGB, administration of G-SCF, 5 μg/kg subcutaneously, on day 4 of *induction* chemotherapy appeared to shorten the duration of neutropenia (29 days vs 16 days, $p < 0.001$), decrease the duration of the hospital stay (28 days vs 22 days, $p = 0.02$), and reduce the induction mortality (11% vs 4%, $p = 0.04$). However, no significant decrease in the incidence or severity of infections, mucositis, or bleeding was observed. This discrepancy could potentially be explained by the fact that chemotherapy-induced complications tend to occur early in thecourse of the chemotherapy, at the nadir of WBC, prior to the bone marrow response to the GF stimulation. Nevertheless, the more rapid resolution of neutropenia may have led to a prompt resolution of toxicity, as patients who received GFs spent fewer days in the hospital during the induction course than did those receiving placebo. The CR rates were higher with G-CSF (90% vs 81%, $p = 0.04$), whereas DFS at 4.7 years was not affected (although study was not designed to detect significant difference) [66]. Of interest, the neutrophil recovery endpoints and the length of the hospitalization were similar between younger (<60) and older patients. Platelet recovery was

Table 18.3 Prospective randomized trials evaluating the role of growth factors in ALL

References	N	Age	GF type	Time of administration	Time to completion of chemotherapy	Neutrophil recovery	Episodes of febrile neutropenia	Frequency of the documented infection	Death during induction	CR	Survival (DFS, OS)
Ohno et al. [65]	41	15–65	G-CSF (0, 2, 5, 10 μg/kg)	Induction, at nadir Consolidation	Not addressed	Improved with higher dose of GFs	Improved	Improved	Similar	Not addressed	Not addressed
Ottmann et al. [69]	67	16–65	G-CSF vs control	Induction (second phase, week 4 of 8)	Improved ($p = 0.008$)	Improved (8 vs 12.5, $p < 0.002$)	Similar (35% vs 47%, $p = 0.28$)	Similar (43% vs 56%, $p = 0.25$); non-viral infections reduced by 50%	One death in control group	Similar	Similar
Welte et al. [91]	34	0.25–18	G-CSF vs control	Induction (from day 7)	Improved ($p = 0.007$)	Improved	Improved (17% vs 40%, $p = 0.007$)	Improved (8% vs 15%, $p = 0.04$)	Similar	Similar	Similar
Geissler et al. [92]	53	16–79	G-CSF vs control	Induction (from day 2)	Not addressed	Improved (16 days vs 26 days, $p < 0.001$)	Improved (12% vs 42%, $p < 0.05$)	Improved (40% vs 77%, $p < 0.05$)	Two in control group and one in G-CSF group	Similar	Similar

Table 18.3 (continued)

References	N	Age	GF type	Time of administration	Time to completion of chemotherapy	Neutrophil recovery	Episodes of febrile neutropenia	Frequency of the documented infection	Death during induction	CR	Survival (DFS, OS)
Pui et al. [47]	148	2 months–17 years	G-CSF vs placebo	Induction (from day 30)	Improved ($p < 0.001$)	Improved (5.3 days vs 12.7 days, $p = 0.007$)	Similar (58% vs 68%, $p = 0.23$)	Overall– improved (12 vs 27, $p = 0.009$); severe infection – similar (5 vs 6)	No death	Similar (99% vs 99%)	Similar
Larson et al. [66]	198	>15	G-CSF vs placebo	Induction (from day 4)	Similar	Improved (16 days vs 22 days, $p < 0.001$)	Similar (46% vs 45%, $p = 1$)	Similar	Similar <60: 10% vs 25%, $p = 0.24$ >60: 4% vs 8%, $p = 0.32$	Improved (87% vs 77%, $p = 0.04$)	Similar

Table 18.3 (continued)

References	N	Age	GF type	Time of administration	Time to completion of chemotherapy	Neutrophil recovery	Episodes of febrile neutropenia	Frequency of the documented infection	Death during induction	CR	Survival (DFS, OS)
Ifrah et al. [93]	67	15–55	GM-CSF vs placebo	Induction (from day 7)	Improved time to allo-BMT	Similar (16 days vs 18 days)	Similar (median, 9 days vs 10 days, $p = 0.07$)	Not addressed	No toxic death	Not addressed	Not addressed
Hoiowiecki et al [68]	64	16–58	G-CSF vs placebo	Induction (36 h after through 48 h before 4 weekly doses of chemotherapy) Consolidation (48 h after each dose)	Improved ($p = 0.005$)	Improved ($p < 0.05$)	Induction – similar Entire treatment – improved (60% vs 90%, $p = 0.04$)	Induction – similar (9% vs 21%, p-NS) Entire treatment – improved	Two in control group due to CNS bleed	Similar	OS – improved (59% vs 27%, $p = 0.048$)

Table 18.3 (continued)

References	N	Age	GF type	Time of administration	Time to completion of chemotherapy	Neutrophil recovery	Episodes of febrile neutropenia	Frequency of the documented infection	Death during induction	CR	Survival (DFS, OS)
Thomas et al [67]	148	15–55	GM-CSF vs G-CSF vs control	Induction (from day 9 or day 17)	Not addressed	Similar (22 vs 21, vs 22)	Similar (20 days vs 19 days vs 22 days)	Similar (15% vs 24% vs 22%)	Similar	Overall: improved (81% vs 72% vs 66%, $p = 0.008$)	Overall: similar (3-year DFS 28% vs 40% vs 23%; 5-year DFS 18% vs 32% vs 23%)
Thomas et al [67]	88	15–55	GM-CSF vs G-CSF vs control	Induction (from day 4)	Not addressed	Improved (18 days vs 16 days vs 23 days, $p < 0.05$)	Similar (20 days vs 17 days vs 20 days)	Improved (19% vs 3% vs 28%, $p = 0.01$)	Similar		

significantly faster in older patient group receiving G-CSF (17 days vs 26 days, p = 0.04). Additionally, in this patient group the rate of CR (81% vs 55%, p = 0.1) and mortality rate (10% vs 25%, p = 0.24) were in favor of patients who received G-CSF; the lack of statistical significance was likely due to the small number of patients. In addition, despite the improved response rate and fewer deaths during induction therapy, patients in the G-CSF arm were not able to complete their first 3 months of prescribed chemotherapy any more rapidly than those in the placebo group. Hence, it was not possible to increase the intensity of the leukemia therapy by shortening the time required to deliver the treatment. This conclusion was different from the results of the German ALL study group, in which 76 adults with de novo ALL were randomized to receive G-CSF or no G-CSF during the last 4 weeks of an 8-week remission induction regimen [69]. Although similar to the CALGB study, the duration of neutropenia (8 days vs 12.5 days, $p < 0.002$) was significantly reduced without an effect on the incidence of infections in the G-CSF arm, the prolonged interruptions of chemotherapy were less frequent; delays of more than 2 weeks occurred in 24% of patients receiving G-CSF versus 46% of patients in the control arm (p = 0.01). For this reason, the planned chemotherapy was completed more rapidly with the use of G-CSF (median, 39 days vs 44 days, p = 0.008), although the clinical significance of this improvement is uncertain.

The French Groupe d'Etude et de Traitement de la Leucemie Aiguë Lymphoblastique de l'Adulte (GET-LALA) group conducted two consecutive prospective, randomized, open-label multicenter phase III trials, comparing the G-CSF, GM-CSF, and no GFs administered with 4-week 4-drug LALA-94 induction regimen in adult patient with de novo ALL [67]. In the first trial, the GFs were administered from the last day of anthracycline infusion (day 9 in the idarubicin arm and day 17 in the daunorubicin arm) and in the second one, the GFs were started on the day 4 of induction chemotherapy until the neutrophil recovery. A total of 95 patients were in the G-CSF arm, 67 in GM-CSF, and 74 in the control group. Overall, there appeared to be a trend, which did not reach statistical significance, toward the reduction of the duration of neutropenia (21 days in control group, 18 days in GM-CSF, and 17 days in G-CSF), severity of the infection (16% with GFs vs 24% without), and duration of the antibiotic administration (median, 18 days with G-CSF, 19 days with GM-CSF, and 23 days without GFs) in the group that received GFs. However, if evaluated separately, the shortened duration of neutropenia (23 days in control group, 18 days in GM-CSF, and 16 days in G-CSF, $p < 0.05$) and decreased incidence of severe infection (3% vs 28%, p = 0.01) were only evident in the second study, while there was no difference between the groups in the first trial. Although there was a trend toward the improved CR rate in the GM-CSF group (69% in G-CSF, 81% in GM-CSF, and 66% in the control group, p = 0.08), there were no differences in terms of therapy-related mortality, DFS, and OS.

A randomized study by the Ibarra and colleagues compared the efficacy and side-effect profile of G-CSF and GM-CSF in 71 patients with acute leukemia (ALL and ANLL) undergoing induction and consolidation therapy [70]. Time to neutrophil recovery (19 days for G-CSF vs 16 days, p = 0.08), episodes of febrile neutropenia (85% vs 78%, p = 0.45), and frequency of side effects (gastrointestinal, cutaneous, and musculoskeletal manifestations) were similar between the groups.

A potential benefit of time-sequenced administration of GFs and chemotherapy with an intent to generate cell cycle-dependent protection of normal hematopoietic progenitors, based on the experimental model [71], has been explored in a randomized trial in patient with ALL [68]. G-CSF, administered daily starting 36 h after and 48 h prior to 4 weekly induction chemotherapy administrations, resulted in the reduction of the overall treatment duration (134 days vs 153 days, $p = 0.005$). The rate of CR (94% vs 87%) and infectious complications was similar between the groups, however, the duration of severe neutropenia, adherence to the therapy ($p = 0.04$), and length of the hospital stay were significantly better in patients receiving G-CSF compared to that of the controls.

The safety concerns regarding administration of GFs to the patients with ALL are similar to the ones raised in patients with AML. There was apprehension that addition of GFs may sensitize normal hematopoietic cells to the cytotoxic effect of cell cycle active chemotherapy and cause prolonged bone marrow suppression. Additionally, since the certain subgroups of ALL patients may express receptors for G-CSF (blasts co-expressing myeloid markers, patients with $t(9;22)$ ALL, and T-cell ALL), the theoretical possibility of stimulating the proliferation of leukemia had to be excluded [72]. Based on the clinical trials conducted to date in adult and pediatric patients with ALL, there is no evidence that administration of GFs stimulates proliferation of lymphoblasts or accelerates re-growth of leukemia [47, 69]. Subset analysis of patients randomized to receive G-CSF or placebo, such as patients with Ph+ ALL, showed no difference in the rate of hematologic recovery or overall outcome [66]. The cumulative incidence of developing AML at 3 years did not differ significantly between the two groups of pediatric ALL patients (G-CSF and placebo, administered after the completion of the induction therapy); 5.1% [95% CI 0.1–10] in the G-CSF arm and 3.9% [95% CI 0–8.4] in the placebo group ($p = 0.36$) [47]. However, no long-term analysis evaluating the risk of developing AML has been published.

In summary, results of the randomized controlled clinical trials demonstrated that GFs support results in a more rapid resolution of neutropenia, which consequently leads to modest improvements in incidence of severe infections, dose intensity of chemotherapy administration, and induction death rates. For patients with ALL undergoing intensive chemotherapy, the most significant impact of GF is likely to be on a subset of patients who are expected to sustain a delay in hematological recovery such as elderly, patients who received multiple courses of myelosuppressive chemotherapy, and patients with ongoing infection.

Other GFs

Multiple growth factors exhibiting various effects on myeloid, erythroid, and lymphoid precursors have been evaluated in acute leukemias.

Interleukin-3 (IL-3) mapped to the 5q31.1 is a multilineage factor produced by the T lymphocytes and mast cells. Its receptor, a heterodimer, has similar structure to that of GM-CSF. IL-3 deficiency is associated with delayed hypersensitivity but has no effect on hematopoiesis. Results of the initial trial combining IL-3 and induction chemotherapy (daunorubicin or mitoxantrone and cytarabine) in AML demonstrated acceptable toxicity [73]. Subsequent randomized study comparing low-dose cytarabine alone or in combination with GM-CSF or IL-3 in 180 patients with MDS (73 patient with RAEB-t) failed to show a statistically significant difference with regards to response rate and degree of cytopenia [74].

IL-5 located on the 5q31.1 is a 50–60-kDa glycoprotein produced by T lymphocytes. Its receptor is a heterodimer and shares structural similarities to that of GM-CSF and IL-3. IL-5 plays an important role in the production and deployment of eosinophils [75].

Keratinocyte growth factor (KGF), a 28-kDa heparin-binding member of the FGF (fibroblast GF) family, is primarily synthesized by fibroblasts [76, 77]. It has an important role in maintaining the barrier function of epithelium and the healing process after injury. KGF receptors are present on epithelial cells in the tongue, oral mucosa, GI tract as well as liver, lung, and pancreas, but absent on the surface of hematopoietic cells [78, 79]. Palifermin/KGF-1 mimics the action of endogenous KGF and is more stable due to the removal of 23 amino acids from the N-terminal domain. In a large randomized double-blinded trial of 212 patients with hematological malignancies undergoing autologous hematopoietic stem cell transplant, the incidence of grade 3–4 mucocytis (63% vs 98%, $p < 0.001$) as well as median duration of mucocytis (3 days vs 9 days, $p < 0.001$) were less in the KGF group. Use of total parenteral nutrition (31% vs 55%, $p < 0.001$) and cumulative dose of opioid analgesic (212 mg vs 535 mg, $p < 0.001$) were also significantly lower in the palifermin group [77]. The risk of side effects, primarily skin and oral toxicities, was slightly higher in the palifermin group as well. Several small clinical trials, only one of which was randomized, conducted in patients undergoing allogeneic stem cell transplant demonstrated the protective effect of palifermin in only certain subgroups [80–83]. Other clinical trials with palifermin, including a phase II clinical trial of patients with MDS and AML, as well as studies with another recombinant KGF repifermin, are ongoing [84].

Macrophage colony-stimulating factor (M-CSF), mapped to 1p21-p13, is a 40–90-kDa glycoprotein produced by monocytes, macrophages, and epithelial cells among others in response to endotoxins and inflammatory stimuli. Activation of M-CSF receptor, expressed on monocytes and macrophages, promotes proliferation and survival of these cells, whereas deficiencies lead to monocytopenia, decreased osteoclasts, and osteopetrosis [16]. Recombinant pegylated M-CSF has been evaluated in several randomized clinical trials [85–87]. Results of a study of 108 patients with AML randomized to receive two doses of M-CSF or placebo, failed to show statistical difference in median time to platelet and red cell transfusion independence as well as neutrophil recovery [85]. In another study, patients with newly diagnosed AML were randomized to receive either 2.5 or 5 μg of M-CSF or placebo after completion of chemotherapy [86]. Although higher platelet levels in remission were achieved by the group receiving M-CSF compared to that of a placebo group, there was no improvement in platelet transfusion requirement or rate of CR. Further development of the M-CSF was hindered by the reports of the development of neutralizing antibodies to thrombopoietin leading to cytopenias [88].

Interleukin-11 (IL-11), cytokine that is involved in various biological activities including hematopoiesis, is the only agent currently approved by the FDA for the management of the chemotherapy-induced thrombocytopenia. In a randomized clinical trial of 51 patients older than 60 years of age with AML or advanced MDS, addition of IL-5 to gemtuzumab ozogamicin (GO) was associated with increased CR rate, but without any survival benefit [89]. In a randomized, double-blinded study of 40 patients with hematological malignancies (21 AML and 14 ALL) undergoing chemotherapy, subcutaneous administration of human recombinant IL-11 was associated with reduced risk of developing bacterial infection ($p = 0.02$) [90]. However, the narrow therapeutic index of IL-11 significantly limits its use in clinical practice. Recently, a number of novel thrombopoietin (TPO) receptor agonists have been developed with promising clinical activity and lesser potential for immunogenicity. Several of these second-generation platelet-stimulating agents are currently in clinical development, including peptide (romiplostim, Nplate) and non-peptide (eltrombopag (Promacta) and AKR5 01) mimetics.

Stem cell factor (SCF or kit-ligand), mapped to 12q22–24, is a 40-kDa glycoprotein produced by fibroblasts, endothelial, and stromal cells and acts synergistically with myeloid growth factors to promote survival and proliferation. Deficiencies in kit, which is expressed on a wide variety of cells, lead to anemia, pigmentation abnormalities, and infertility; administration of SCF is associated with mast cell proliferation [16].

Development of the myeloid GFs, particularly G-CSF, has improved various aspects of care for patients with acute leukemias. Innovative drug development programs together with improved understanding of the neutrophil biology and design of novel GFs will lead to new clinical trials aimed at improving outcomes in patients with acute leukemias.

References

1. Hubel K, Dale DC, Liles WC. Therapeutic use of cytokines to modulate phagocyte function for the treatment of infectious diseases: current status of granulocyte colony-stimulating factor, granulocyte–macrophage colony-stimulating factor, macrophage colony-stimulating factor, and interferon-gamma. J Infect Dis. 2002;185(10):1490–501.
2. Christopher MJ, Link DC. Regulation of neutrophil homeostasis. Curr Opin Hematol. 2007;14(1):3–8.
3. Welte K, et al. Filgrastim (r-metHuG-CSF): the first 10 years. Blood. 1996;88(6):1907–29.
4. Demetri GD, Griffin JD. Granulocyte colony-stimulating factor and its receptor. Blood. 1991;78(11):2791–808.
5. Boneberg EM, et al. Human monocytes express functional receptors for granulocyte colony-stimulating factor that mediate suppression of monokines and interferon-gamma. Blood. 2000;95(1):270–6.
6. Franzke A, et al. G-CSF as immune regulator in T cells expressing the G-CSF receptor: implications for transplantation and autoimmune diseases. Blood. 2003;102(2):734–9.

7. Solaroglu I, et al. A novel neuroprotectant granulocyte-colony stimulating factor. Stroke. 2006;37(4):1123–8.

8. Kirsch F, Kruger C, Schneider A. The receptor for granulocyte-colony stimulating factor (G-CSF) is expressed in radial glia during development of the nervous system. BMC Dev Biol. 2008;8:32.

9. Avalos BR. Molecular analysis of the granulocyte colony-stimulating factor receptor. Blood. 1996;88(3):761–77.

10. Anderlini P, Champlin RE. Biologic and molecular effects of granulocyte colony-stimulating factor in healthy individuals: recent findings and current challenges. Blood. 2008;111(4):1767–72.

11. Kaushansky K. Lineage-specific hematopoietic growth factors. N Engl J Med. 2006;354(19):2034–45.

12. Hamilton JA. Colony-stimulating factors in inflammation and autoimmunity. Nat Rev Immunol. 2008;8(7):533–44.

13. Gil-Lamaignere C, et al. Interferon-gamma and granulocyte–macrophage colony-stimulating factor augment the activity of polymorphonuclear leukocytes against medically important zygomycetes. J Infect Dis. 2005;191(7):1180–7.

14. Lieschke GJ, et al. Mice lacking granulocyte colony-stimulating factor have chronic neutropenia, granulocyte and macrophage progenitor cell deficiency, and impaired neutrophil mobilization. Blood. 1994;84(6):1737–46.

15. Lieschke GJ, et al. Mice lacking both macrophage- and granulocyte–macrophage colony-stimulating factor have macrophages and coexistent osteopetrosis and severe lung disease. Blood. 1994;84(1):27–35.

16. Crawford J, et al. Reduction by granulocyte colony-stimulating factor of fever and neutropenia induced by chemotherapy in patients with small-cell lung cancer. N Engl J Med. 1991;325(3):164–70.

17. Dale DC. Neutrophil biology and the next generation of myeloid growth factors. J Natl Compr Canc Netw. 2009;7(1):92–8.

18. Holmes FA, et al. Blinded, randomized, multicenter study to evaluate single administration pegfilgrastim once per cycle versus daily filgrastim as an adjunct to chemotherapy in patients with high-risk stage II or stage III/IV breast cancer. J Clin Oncol. 2002;20(3):727–31.

19. Green MD, et al. A randomized double-blind multicenter phase III study of fixed-dose single-administration pegfilgrastim versus daily filgrastim in patients receiving myelosuppressive chemotherapy. Ann Oncol. 2003;14(1):29–35.

20. Kubista E, et al. Bone pain associated with once-per-cycle pegfilgrastim is similar to daily filgrastim in patients with breast cancer. Clin Breast Cancer. 2003;3(6):391–8.

21. Lane S, Crawford J, Kenealy M, Cull G. Pegfilgrastim compared to granulocyte colony stimulating factor (G-CSF) with hyper-CVAD chemotherapy regimen for aggressive lymphoid malignancy. Blood. 2005;106:11.

22. DeFrees S, et al. GlycoPEGylation of recombinant therapeutic proteins produced in *Escherichia coli*. Glycobiology. 2006;16(9):833–43.

23. Doherty DH, et al. Site-specific PEGylation of engineered cysteine analogues of recombinant human granulocyte–macrophage colony-stimulating factor. Bioconjug Chem. 2005;16(5):1291–8.

24. Robinson SN, et al. Hematopoietic progenitor cell mobilization in mice by sustained delivery of granulocyte colony-stimulating factor. J Interferon Cytokine Res. 2005;25(8): 490–500.

25. Cox GN, et al. Enhanced circulating half-life and hematopoietic properties of a human granulocyte colony-stimulating factor/immunoglobulin fusion protein. Exp Hematol. 2004;32(5):441–9.

26. Halpern W, et al. Albugranin, a recombinant human granulocyte colony stimulating factor (G-CSF) genetically fused to recombinant human albumin induces prolonged myelopoietic effects in mice and monkeys. Pharm Res. 2002;19(11):1720–9.

27. Erben U, Thiel E, Notter M. Differential effects of a stem cell factor-immunoglobulin fusion protein on malignant and normal hematopoietic cells. Cancer Res. 1999;59(12):2924–30.

28. Chadwick DE, et al. Cytotoxicity of a recombinant diphtheria toxin-granulocyte colony-stimulating factor fusion protein on human leukemic blast cells. Leuk Lymphoma. 1993;11(3–4):249–62.

29. MacVittie TJ, et al. Myelopoietin, an engineered chimeric IL-3 and G-CSF receptor agonist, stimulates multilineage hematopoietic recovery in a nonhuman primate model of radiation-induced myelosuppression. Blood. 2000;95(3):837–45.

30. Williams DE, Park LS. Hematopoietic effects of a granulocyte–macrophage colony-stimulating factor/interleukin-3 fusion protein. Cancer. 1991;67(10 Suppl):2705–7.

31. Vadhan-Raj S, et al. In vivo biologic effects of PIXY321, a synthetic hybrid protein of recombinant human granulocyte–macrophage colony-stimulating factor and interleukin-3 in cancer patients with normal hematopoiesis: a phase I study. Blood. 1995;86(6): 2098–105.

32. Lee AY, et al. A recombinant human G-CSF/GM-CSF fusion protein from *E. coli* showing colony stimulating activity on human bone marrow cells. Biotechnol Lett. 2003;25(3): 205–11.

33. Smith TJ, et al. 2006 update of recommendations for the use of white blood cell growth factors: an evidence-based clinical practice guideline. J Clin Oncol. 2006;24(19): 3187–205.

34. Baer MR, et al. Phase 3 study of the multidrug resistance modulator PSC-833 in previously untreated patients 60 years of age and older with acute myeloid leukemia: Cancer and Leukemia Group B Study 9720. Blood. 2002;100(4):1224–32.

35. Ohno R, et al. Effect of granulocyte colony-stimulating factor after intensive induction therapy in relapsed or refractory acute leukemia. N Engl J Med. 1990;323(13):871–7.

36. Stone RM, et al. Granulocyte–macrophage colony-stimulating factor after initial chemotherapy for elderly patients with primary acute myelogenous leukemia. Cancer and Leukemia Group B. N Engl J Med. 1995;332(25):1671–7.

37. Dombret H, et al. A controlled study of recombinant human granulocyte colony-stimulating factor in elderly patients after treatment for acute myelogenous leukemia. AML Cooperative Study Group. N Engl J Med. 1995;332(25):1678–83.

38. Rowe JM, et al. A randomized placebo-controlled phase III study of granulocyte–macrophage colony-stimulating factor in adult patients (>55–70 years of age) with acute myelogenous leukemia: a study of the Eastern Cooperative Oncology Group (E1490). Blood. 1995;86(2):457–62.

39. Usuki K, et al. Efficacy of granulocyte colony-stimulating factor in the treatment of acute myelogenous leukaemia: a multicentre randomized study. Br J Haematol. 2002;116(1): 103–12.

40. Harousseau JL, et al. Granulocyte colony-stimulating factor after intensive consolidation chemotherapy in acute myeloid leukemia: results of a randomized trial of the Groupe Ouest-Est Leucemies Aigues Myeloblastiques. J Clin Oncol. 2000;18(4):780–7.

41. Moore JO, et al. Granulocyte-colony stimulating factor (filgrastim) accelerates granulocyte recovery after intensive postremission chemotherapy for acute myeloid leukemia with aziridinyl benzoquinone and mitoxantrone: Cancer and Leukemia Group B Study 9022. Blood. 1997;89(3):780–8.

42. Estey EH. Growth factors in acute myeloid leukaemia. Best Pract Res Clin Haematol. 2001;14(1):175–87.

43. Bennett CL, et al. Economic analysis of a randomized placebo-controlled phase III study of granulocyte macrophage colony stimulating factor in adult patients (>55–70 years of age) with acute myelogenous leukemia. Eastern Cooperative Oncology Group (E1490). Ann Oncol. 1999;10(2):177–82.

44. Lu Z, Luo R, Erder H, et al. Cost impact of filgrastim as an adjunct to chemotherapy for patients with acute myeloid leukemia. Blood. 1996;88(10, Suppl 1):209a.

45. Woronoff-Lemsi M, Demoly P, Arveux P. Cost-effectiveness analysis of GOELEM SA3, a randomized placebo-controlled protocol of GM-CSF for elderly patients with acute myeloid leukemia. Blood. 1997;90(10, Suppl 1):72a.
46. Bennett CL, et al. Economic analysis of granulocyte colony stimulating factor as adjunct therapy for older patients with acute myelogenous leukemia (AML): estimates from a Southwest Oncology Group clinical trial. Cancer Invest. 2001;19(6):603–10.
47. Pui CH, et al. Human granulocyte colony-stimulating factor after induction chemotherapy in children with acute lymphoblastic leukemia. N Engl J Med. 1997;336(25):1781–7.
48. Lowenberg B, Downing JR, Burnett A. Acute myeloid leukemia. N Engl J Med. 1999;341(14):1051–62.
49. Schiffer CA. Hematopoietic growth factors and the future of therapeutic research on acute myeloid leukemia. N Engl J Med. 2003;349(8):727–9.
50. Hiddemann W, et al. Granulocyte–macrophage colony-stimulating factor and interleukin-3 enhance the incorporation of cytosine arabinoside into the DNA of leukemic blasts and the cytotoxic effect on clonogenic cells from patients with acute myeloid leukemia. Semin Oncol. 1992;19(2 Suppl 4):31–7.
51. Miyauchi J, et al. Growth factors influence the sensitivity of leukemic stem cells to cytosine arabinoside in culture. Blood. 1989;73(5):1272–8.
52. Cannistra SA, et al. Simultaneous administration of granulocyte–macrophage colony-stimulating factor and cytosine arabinoside for the treatment of relapsed acute myeloid leukemia. Leukemia. 1991;5(3):230–8.
53. Lowenberg B, Touw IP. Hematopoietic growth factors and their receptors in acute leukemia. Blood. 1993;81(2):281–92.
54. Rutella S, et al. Granulocyte colony-stimulating factor enhances the in vitro cytotoxicity of gemtuzumab ozogamicin against acute myeloid leukemia cell lines and primary blast cells. Exp Hematol. 2006;34(1):54–65.
55. Lowenberg B, et al. Effect of priming with granulocyte colony-stimulating factor on the outcome of chemotherapy for acute myeloid leukemia. N Engl J Med. 2003;349(8):743–52.
56. Lowenberg B, et al. Use of recombinant GM-CSF during and after remission induction chemotherapy in patients aged 61 years and older with acute myeloid leukemia: final report of AML-11, a phase III randomized study of the Leukemia Cooperative Group of European Organisation for the Research and Treatment of Cancer and the Dutch Belgian Hemato-Oncology Cooperative Group. Blood. 1997;90(8):2952–61.
57. Lofgren C, et al. Granulocyte–macrophage colony-stimulating factor to increase efficacy of mitoxantrone, etoposide and cytarabine in previously untreated elderly patients with acute myeloid leukaemia: a Swedish multicentre randomized trial. Br J Haematol. 2004;124(4):474–80.
58. Thomas X, Raffoux E, De Botton S, Pautas C. Effect of priming with granulocyte–macrophage colony-stimulating factor (GM-CSF) in younger adults with newly diagnosed acute myeloid leukemia (AML): a trial by the Acute Leukemia French Association (ALFA) Group. Blood. 2005;106(11):530a. Abstract 1862.
59. Thomas X, et al. Granulocyte–macrophage colony-stimulating factor (GM-CSF) to increase efficacy of intensive sequential chemotherapy with etoposide, mitoxantrone and cytarabine (EMA) in previously treated acute myeloid leukemia: a multicenter randomized placebo-controlled trial (EMA91 Trial). Leukemia. 1999;13(8):1214–20.
60. Rowe JM, et al. A phase 3 study of three induction regimens and of priming with GM-CSF in older adults with acute myeloid leukemia: a trial by the Eastern Cooperative Oncology Group. Blood. 2004;103(2):479–85.
61. Takamatsu Y, et al. Remission induction by granulocyte colony-stimulating factor in hypoplastic acute myelogenous leukemia complicated by infection. A case report and review of the literature. Acta Haematol. 1998;99(4):224–30.
62. Ferrara F, et al. Complete remission in acute myeloid leukaemia with t(8;21) following treatment with G-CSF: flow cytometric analysis of in vivo and in vitro effects on cell maturation. Br J Haematol. 1999;106(2):520–3.

63. Faderl S, et al. Caspase 2 and caspase 3 as predictors of complete remission and survival in adults with acute lymphoblastic leukemia. Clin Cancer Res. 1999;5(12):4041–7.
64. Faderl S, et al. Granulocyte–macrophage colony-stimulating factor (GM-CSF) induces antiapoptotic and proapoptotic signals in acute myeloid leukemia. Blood. 2003;102(2): 630–7.
65. Ohno R, et al. A randomized controlled study of granulocyte colony stimulating factor after intensive induction and consolidation therapy in patients with acute lymphoblastic leukemia. Japan Adult Leukemia Study Group. Int J Hematol. 1993;58(1–2):73–81.
66. Larson RA, et al. A randomized controlled trial of filgrastim during remission induction and consolidation chemotherapy for adults with acute lymphoblastic leukemia: CALGB study 9111. Blood. 1998;92(5):1556–64.
67. Thomas X, et al. Efficacy of granulocyte and granulocyte–macrophage colony-stimulating factors in the induction treatment of adult acute lymphoblastic leukemia: a multicenter randomized study. Hematol J. 2004;5(5):384–94.
68. Holowiecki J, et al. G-CSF administered in time-sequenced setting during remission induction and consolidation therapy of adult acute lymphoblastic leukemia has beneficial influence on early recovery and possibly improves long-term outcome: a randomized multicenter study. Leuk Lymphoma. 2002;43(2):315–25.
69. Ottmann OG, et al. Concomitant granulocyte colony-stimulating factor and induction chemoradiotherapy in adult acute lymphoblastic leukemia: a randomized phase III trial. Blood. 1995;86(2):444–50.
70. Ibarra M, Escoboza J, Lopez-Hernandez M. Neutrophil recovery time and adverse effects in acute leukemia patients treated with intensive chemotherapy and concomitant G or GM CSF. Rev Invest Clin. 1999;51(2):77–80.
71. Aglietta M, et al. Kinetics of human hemopoietic cells after in vivo administration of granulocyte–macrophage colony-stimulating factor. J Clin Invest. 1989;83(2):551–7.
72. Tsuchiya H, et al. Responses to granulocyte colony-stimulating factor (G-CSF) and granulocyte–macrophage CSF in Ph1-positive acute lymphoblastic leukemia with myeloid surface markers. Blood. 1991;77(2):411–13.
73. Wielenga JJ, et al. Recombinant human interleukin-3 (rH IL-3) in combination with remission induction chemotherapy in patients with relapsed acute myelogenous leukemia (AML): a phase I/II study. Leukemia. 1996;10(1):43–7.
74. Zwierzina H, et al. Low-dose cytosine arabinoside (LD-AraC) vs LD-AraC plus granulocyte/macrophage colony stimulating factor vs LD-AraC plus interleukin-3 for myelodysplastic syndrome patients with a high risk of developing acute leukemia: final results of a randomized phase III study (06903) of the EORTC Leukemia Cooperative Group. Leukemia. 2005;19(11):1929–33.
75. Riccioni R, et al. Interleukin (IL)-3/granulocyte macrophage-colony stimulating factor/IL-5 receptor alpha and beta chains are preferentially expressed in acute myeloid leukaemias with mutated FMS-related tyrosine kinase 3 receptor. Br J Haematol. 2009;144(3): 376–87.
76. Finch PW, Rubin JS. Keratinocyte growth factor/fibroblast growth factor 7, a homeostatic factor with therapeutic potential for epithelial protection and repair. Adv Cancer Res. 2004;91:69–136.
77. Spielberger R, et al. Palifermin for oral mucositis after intensive therapy for hematologic cancers. N Engl J Med. 2004;351(25):2590–8.
78. Spencer A, et al. Prospective randomised trial of amifostine cytoprotection in myeloma patients undergoing high-dose melphalan conditioned autologous stem cell transplantation. Bone Marrow Transplant. 2005;35(10):971–7.
79. Moroni E, et al. Fibroblast growth factors and their receptors in hematopoiesis and hematological tumors. J Hematother Stem Cell Res. 2002;11(1):19–32.
80. Blazar BR, et al. Phase 1/2 randomized, placebo-control trial of palifermin to prevent graft-versus-host disease (GVHD) after allogeneic hematopoietic stem cell transplantation (HSCT). Blood. 2006;108(9):3216–22.

81. Nasilowska-Adamska B, et al. The influence of palifermin (Kepivance) on oral mucositis and acute graft versus host disease in patients with hematological diseases undergoing hematopoietic stem cell transplant. Bone Marrow Transplant. 2007;40(10):983–8.

82. Langner S, et al. Palifermin reduces incidence and severity of oral mucositis in allogeneic stem-cell transplant recipients. Bone Marrow Transplant. 2008;42(4):275–9.

83. van der Velden WJ, Herbers AH, Blijlevens NM. Palifermin in allogeneic HSCT: many questions remain. Bone Marrow Transplant. 2009;43(1):85–6.

84. Freytes CO, et al. Phase I/II randomized trial evaluating the safety and clinical effects of repifermin administered to reduce mucositis in patients undergoing autologous hematopoietic stem cell transplantation. Clin Cancer Res. 2004;10(24):8318–24.

85. Archimbaud E, et al. A randomized, double-blind, placebo-controlled study with pegylated recombinant human megakaryocyte growth and development factor (PEG-rHuMGDF) as an adjunct to chemotherapy for adults with de novo acute myeloid leukemia. Blood. 1999;94(11):3694–701.

86. Schiffer CA, et al. A double-blind, placebo-controlled trial of pegylated recombinant human megakaryocyte growth and development factor as an adjunct to induction and consolidation therapy for patients with acute myeloid leukemia. Blood. 2000;95(8):2530–5.

87. Geissler K, et al. Prior and concurrent administration of recombinant human megakaryocyte growth and development factor in patients receiving consolidation chemotherapy for de novo acute myeloid leukemia – a randomized, placebo-controlled, double-blind safety and efficacy study. Ann Hematol. 2003;82(11):677–83.

88. Basser RL, et al. Development of pancytopenia with neutralizing antibodies to thrombopoietin after multicycle chemotherapy supported by megakaryocyte growth and development factor. Blood. 2002;99(7):2599–602.

89. Estey EH, et al. Gemtuzumab ozogamicin with or without interleukin 11 in patients 65 years of age or older with untreated acute myeloid leukemia and high-risk myelodysplastic syndrome: comparison with idarubicin plus continuous-infusion, high-dose cytosine arabinoside. Blood. 2002;99(12):4343–9.

90. Ellis M, et al. Recombinant human interleukin 11 and bacterial infection in patients with [correction of] haematological malignant disease undergoing chemotherapy: a double-blind placebo-controlled randomised trial. Lancet. 2003;361(9354):275–80.

91. Welte K, et al. A randomized phase-III study of the efficacy of granulocyte colony-stimulating factor in children with high-risk acute lymphoblastic leukemia. Berlin–Frankfurt–Munster Study Group. Blood. 1996;87(8):3143–50.

92. Geissler K, et al. Granulocyte colony-stimulating factor as an adjunct to induction chemotherapy for adult acute lymphoblastic leukemia – a randomized phase-III study. Blood. 1997;90(2):590–6.

93. Ifrah N, et al. Intensive short term therapy with granulocyte–macrophage-colony stimulating factor support, similar to therapy for acute myeloblastic leukemia, does not improve overall results for adults with acute lymphoblastic leukemia. GOELAMS Group. Cancer. 1999;86(8):1496–505.

94. Heil G, et al. GM-CSF in a double-blind randomized, placebo controlled trial in therapy of adult patients with de novo acute myeloid leukemia (AML). Leukemia. 1995;9(1):3–9.

95. Zittoun R, et al. Granulocyte–macrophage colony-stimulating factor associated with induction treatment of acute myelogenous leukemia: a randomized trial by the European Organization for Research and Treatment of Cancer Leukemia Cooperative Group. J Clin Oncol. 1996;14(7):2150–9.

96. Witz F, et al. A placebo-controlled study of recombinant human granulocyte–macrophage colony-stimulating factor administered during and after induction treatment for de novo acute myelogenous leukemia in elderly patients. Groupe Ouest Est Leucemies Aigues Myeloblastiques (GOELAM). Blood. 1998;91(8):2722–30.

97. Hast R, et al. No benefit from adding GM-CSF to induction chemotherapy in transforming myelodysplastic syndromes: better outcome in patients with less proliferative disease. Leukemia. 2003;17(9):1827–33.

98. Amadori S, et al. Use of glycosylated recombinant human G-CSF (lenograstim) during and/or after induction chemotherapy in patients 61 years of age and older with acute myeloid leukemia: final results of AML-13, a randomized phase-3 study. Blood. 2005;106(1):27–34.
99. Heil G, et al. A randomized, double-blind, placebo-controlled, phase III study of filgrastim in remission induction and consolidation therapy for adults with de novo acute myeloid leukemia. The International Acute Myeloid Leukemia Study Group. Blood. 1997;90(12):4710–8.
100. Godwin JE, et al. A double-blind placebo-controlled trial of granulocyte colony-stimulating factor in elderly patients with previously untreated acute myeloid leukemia: a Southwest Oncology Group study (9031). Blood. 1998;91(10):3607–15.
101. Bradstock K, et al. Effects of glycosylated recombinant human granulocyte colony-stimulating factor after high-dose cytarabine-based induction chemotherapy for adult acute myeloid leukaemia. Leukemia. 2001;15(9):1331–8.
102. Goldstone AH, et al. Attempts to improve treatment outcomes in acute myeloid leukemia (AML) in older patients: the results of the United Kingdom Medical Research Council AML11 trial. Blood. 2001;98(5):1302–11.

Chapter 19
The Hematopoietic Growth Factors in Acute Leukemia: A European Perspective

Michael Heuser, Arnold Ganser, and Dieter Hoelzer

Abstract Acute myeloid leukemia (AML) and acute lymphoblastic leukemia (ALL) are malignant clonal disorders of the blood system requiring intensive and long-term cytotoxic treatment. Current chemotherapy protocols not only target the malignant cell, but are also highly toxic to normal hematopoietic cells as well. Leukemia patients thus experience prolonged times of neutropenia, thrombocytopenia, and anemia, which increase the risk for secondary complications like infections and bleeding. Twenty years ago leukemia patients were considered the ideal candidates to benefit from accelerated recovery of cytopenias by treatment with recombinant cytokines. Moreover, based on in vitro data, it was hypothesized that myeloid growth factors may sensitize AML cells to cytotoxic agents. Numerous clinical trials have documented the biologic activity of granulocyte and granulocyte–macrophage growth factors to accelerate neutrophil recovery after chemotherapy. However, there is high-level evidence that these myeloid growth factors neither reduce the incidence of severe infections nor improve the outcome of AML patients. Evidence from ALL trials is mixed with some studies suggesting a reduction of severe infections by myeloid growth factors whereas others report no effect. Most studies of acute leukemia patients suggested that myeloid growth factors are safe to use, however, a negative impact on event-free survival was found in one trial and an increased risk for secondary AML was reported in pediatric ALL patients. Thrombopoietins have not led so far to a significant increase in platelet numbers in leukemia patients. Chemokine receptor antagonists are now being evaluated in clinical trials for synergistic effects with chemotherapy and will be discussed briefly. Cytokine development mirrors the great advances that have been achieved in the understanding of regulatory mechanisms in hematopoiesis. As this understanding grows, new drugs and new applications will emerge.

M. Heuser (✉)

Department of Hematology, Hemostasis, Oncology, and Stem Cell Transplantation, Hannover Medical School, 30625 Hannover, Germany
e-mail: heuser.michael@mh-hannover.de

G.H. Lyman, D.C. Dale (eds.), *Hematopoietic Growth Factors in Oncology*, Cancer Treatment and Research 157, DOI 10.1007/978-1-4419-7073-2_19,
© Springer Science+Business Media, LLC 2011

Introduction

Acute myeloid and lymphoblastic leukemias are malignant clonal disorders with a very high proliferative capacity that require intensive chemotherapy for several months. Current treatment regimens inevitably induce a decrease in white blood cell counts especially of the neutrophil granulocytic lineage (neutropenia). Neutropenia itself is not associated with symptoms and does not affect quality of life (QoL). However, it is a risk factor for infection typically associated with fever and accompanied by considerable morbidity and mortality. The risk of infection begins to increase as the absolute neutrophil count (ANC) declines below $1,000/\mu L$ and is especially high, if the ANC is below $100/\mu L$ [1]. The duration of severe chemotherapy-associated neutropenia is another important risk factor for infection. It is often impossible to detect the infectious agent in febrile neutropenic patients. Therefore "FN" (febrile neutropenia) has been used as an operating term to describe incidence, characteristics, and outcome of patients likely to have an active infection during neutropenia. FN is defined as a single temperature $\geq 38.3°C$ or $\geq 38°C$ for over 1 h and <500 or $<1,000$ neutrophils/μL and a predicted decline to ≤ 500 neutrophils/μL over the next 48 h [2]. FN itself does not necessarily stand for an adverse outcome. Rather, as a current standard of care it prompts treatment with IV antibiotics and hospitalization, each associated with its own risks and costs, and is associated with a certain risk of sepsis and septic death. Several options have been tried in cancer patients to prevent the adverse outcomes of FN, including use of colony-stimulating factors (CSFs), prophylactic antibiotic use, granulocyte transfusion, and dose reduction or delay of chemotherapy.

Two decades ago granulocyte colony-stimulating factor (G-CSF) and granulocyte–macrophage colony-stimulating factor (GM-CSF) rapidly entered the clinic and were evaluated in multiple clinical trials. Different strategies in the use of CSFs have been investigated to reduce the incidence of FN and its sequelae in patients undergoing cytotoxic therapy. CSFs were used as primary prophylaxis (i.e., directly after the first cycle of chemotherapy in treatment-naïve patients and without any episode of FN), as secondary prophylaxis (i.e., directly after subsequent cycles following an episode of FN), or therapeutically (i.e., after the onset of FN to reduce its duration and improve the outcome of infection). In addition, CSFs were used concurrently with chemotherapy in AML patients to sensitize leukemic blasts expressing functional CSF receptors to the effects of cytotoxic drugs, a concept generally referred to as "priming." The evaluation of the proper use of CSFs in acute leukemias is ongoing as shown in Figs. 19.1 and 19.2. We evaluated all clinical trials of AML and ALL patients registered in a large clinical trials registry (clinicaltrials.gov, March 2009) for the use of CSFs as interventional drug; 14.9% of all registered but closed phase II or III AML trials and 19.2% of all closed phase II or III ALL trials investigated the effects of CSFs in acute leukemias. Today fewer trials than in the past investigate the effects of CSFs in acute leukemia – 7.3% of all registered phase II or III AML trials currently recruiting patients and 10.8% of registered phase II or III ALL trials.

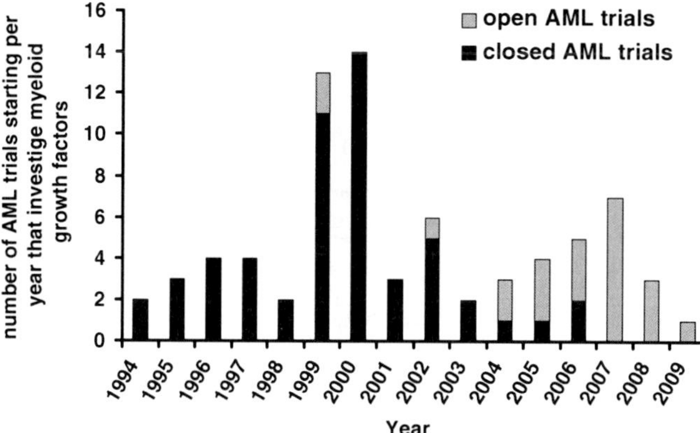

Fig. 19.1 Number of AML trials investigating myeloid growth factors. AML trials registered at clinicaltrials.gov (March 2009) that investigate filgrastim or sargramostim were selected and grouped by starting year and by trial status (open vs closed)

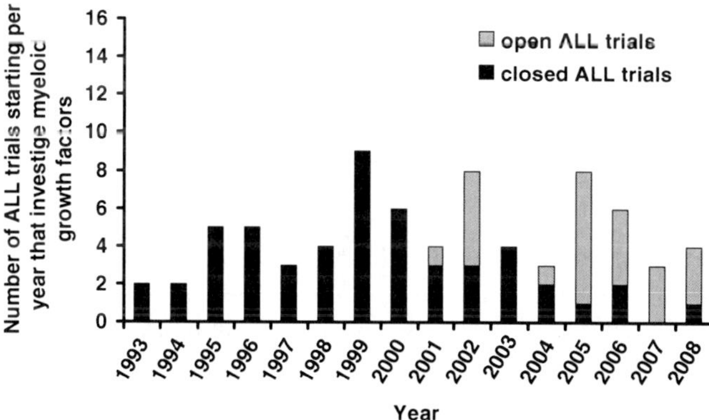

Fig. 19.2 Number of ALL trials investigating myeloid growth factors. ALL trials registered at clinicaltrials.gov (March 2009) that investigate filgrastim or sargramostim were selected and grouped by starting year and by trial status (open vs closed)

Filgrastim (G-CSF) is approved in the United States and Europe for use in adult AML patients following induction and consolidation chemotherapy and in patients with non-myeloid malignancies receiving myelosuppressive anticancer drugs associated with a significant incidence of severe neutropenia with fever. The pegylated long-acting form of filgrastim (pegfilgrastim) is only approved in patients with non-myeloid malignancies receiving myelosuppressive anticancer drugs associated with a significant incidence of severe neutropenia with fever. Use of lenograstim (gly-cosylated G-CSF) is approved in Europe in patients with malignancies receiving myelosuppressive anticancer drugs associated with a significant incidence of severe neutropenia with fever but is not approved in patients with refractory or relapsed AML, AML patients younger than 55 years of age, and AML patients with favorable cytogenetics (t(8;21) or t(15;17) or inv(16)). Sargramostim (GM-CSF) is approved in the United States for use after induction chemotherapy in older adults (55 years or older) with AML but is not licensed in Europe [3]. The following overview will summarize results of clinical trials investigating the use of CSFs in acute leukemia and highlight recommendations of current guidelines for the use of CSFs.

Safety of Myeloid Growth Factors in Acute Leukemias

The expression of functional CSF receptors on leukemic cells of the myeloid lineage raised concerns that CSF administration might be detrimental by accelerating leukemic progression or by promoting leukemic regrowth of AML cells when administered after chemotherapy. Moreover, it was speculated that premalignant myeloid cells expressing CSF receptors might proliferate and acquire additional mutations when stimulated with CSFs. These concerns have recently been fuelled by follow-up studies of breast cancer and pediatric ALL patients. In a large case–control study of 182 AML and MDS patients and 534 controls treated for breast cancer an increased risk of AML/MDS was found in patients who had received G-CSF (RR = 6.3, 95% CI 1.9–21) even when controlling for chemotherapy regimen and dose [4]. The median interval between the diagnosis of the first tumor and the onset of AML/MDS for all patients was 3.1 years (range 0.5–15 years). In 2,545 women receiving adjuvant therapy for operable breast cancer the national surgical adjuvant breast and bowel project found an increased risk to develop AML or MDS with cumulative doses of G-CSF higher than the median cumulative dose [5]. Relling et al. found an increased risk of myeloid leukemia or myelodysplastic syndrome in children treated with topoisomerase II inhibitors for acute lymphoblastic leukemia and G-CSF compared to treatment without G-CSF (median time to develop myeloid leukemia is 2.3 years) [6]. One trial of 102 younger AML patients treated with or without GM-CSF after chemotherapy found a significantly shorter EFS and a trend toward shorter OS ($P = 0.07$) in GM-CSF-treated patients compared to control patients [7]. Another trial of 110 older AML patients treated with GM-CSF during chemotherapy found a trend toward shorter OS in patients treated with GM-CSF compared to control patients ($P = 0.07$) [8]. Numerous other studies found no negative effect of myeloid growth factors on treatment outcome in acute myeloid or lymphoblastic leukemias.

Efficacy of CSFs to Prevent Infectious Complications in Acute Myeloid Leukemia

Induction and consolidation treatment in AML is associated with a high incidence of FN. CSFs have therefore been evaluated for their efficacy in reducing infectious complications in the induction and consolidation therapy of AML (Fig. 19.3).

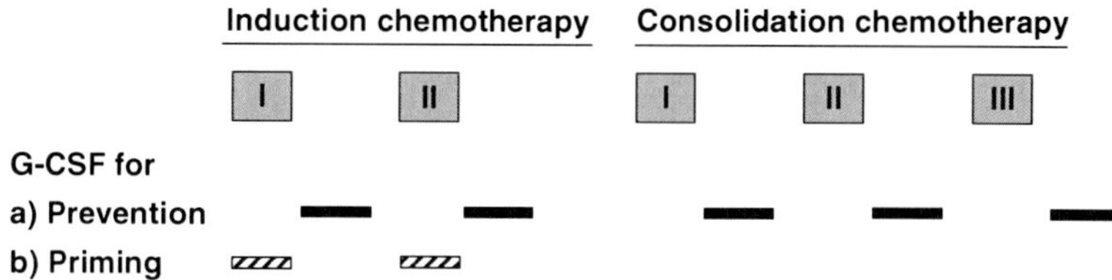

Fig. 19.3 Timing of myeloid growth factor application relative to chemotherapy cycles in AML patients for prevention of infectious complications or for priming of leukemic blasts to increase chemotherapy efficacy

Primary prophylactic use of CSFs in acute myeloid leukemias (CSF administration after chemotherapy prior to development of fever) has been investigated in numerous trials and is summarized in Table 19.1. In 12 trials reported between 1995 and 2005, 3,271 patients were investigated. Four trials included only patients younger than 60 years of age, 6 trials included only patients older than 55 years of age, and 2 trials included younger and older patients. All trials were randomized, six trials were placebo-controlled, and four trials were conducted double-blind. Four trials investigated the effects of GM-CSF, whereas eight trials used G-CSF. In 10 of 11 studies time to neutrophil recovery was significantly reduced by a median of 4.5 days. Six trials reported the incidence of documented infections and none of these six studies found a significant difference between CSF-treated and CSF-untreated patients. Five of the six remaining studies reported on grade 4–5 infectious complications and only one found a significant reduction of severe infectious complications in GM-CSF-treated patients compared to controls [9]. The length of hospitalization was reported in nine trials and only three trials found a significant reduction by 6, 3, and 2.5 days in GM-CSF-treated AML patients. Complete remission rate was not significantly different between CSF-treated versus control patients in ten trials, was significantly improved in one trial [10], and was significantly reduced in another trial [7]. EFS or DFS was reported in eight trials. Seven trials found no significant difference in EFS or DFS in GM-CSF-treated or control patients and one trial found a significantly worse EFS in the GM-CSF-treated group compared to the control group [7]. No difference in OS was found in 11 trials comparing GM-CSF versus control-treated patients, whereas one trial found a significantly improved OS in older patients treated with GM-CSF when the patient became aplastic [9]. Taken together, there is good evidence from well-controlled trials that prophylactic/supportive use of CSFs cannot improve clinically relevant endpoints in AML patients.

Efficacy of CSFs to Improve Outcome in AML (Priming)

In vitro studies proposed that CSFs may sensitize AML blasts to S-phase-specific agents such as cytarabine [11, 12]. Numerous studies investigated the "priming"

Table 19.1 CSF use after chemotherapy in AML

References	Patients (n)	Age (years), median (range)	Study design	Drug/dose	Time to neutrophil recovery (median, days) (drug vs control)	P	Incidence of infections (%) (drug vs control)	P	Hospitalization length (median days) (drug vs control)	P	CR rate (%) (drug vs control)	P	DFS/EFS (drug vs control)	P	OS (drug vs control)	P
Stone et al. [58]	388	69 (≥60)	Randomized, placebo-controlled, double-blind	GM-CSF, 5 μg/kg/d	15 vs 17 days[a]	0.02	18 vs 18[b]	1	28 vs 30	0.11	51 vs 54	0.61	n.d.	n.d.	Median 0.7 vs 0.9 years	0.1
Rowe et al. [9]	124	64 (55–70)	Randomized, placebo-controlled, double-blind	GM-CSF, 5 μg/kg/d	13 vs 17 days[a]	0.001	10 vs 36[b]	0.002	36 vs 38	0.29	60 vs 44	0.08	n.d.	n.d.	Median 10.6 vs 4.8 months	0.048
Dombret et al. [10]	173	71 (65–83)	Randomized, placebo-controlled	Lenograstim 5 μg/kg/d	21 vs 27[c]	<0.001	17 vs 20[b]	0.6	n.d.	n.d.	70 vs 47	0.002	EFS HR 0.87 (0.65–1.19)	0.39	HR 0.95 (0.69–1.31)	0.76
Zittoun et al. [7]	102	15–60	Randomized, open-label	GM-CSF, 5 μg/kg/d	22 vs 24.5[a]	n.s.	73 vs 81[d]	n.s.	No difference	n.s.	47.1 vs 74.5	0.008	EFS	0.02 favoring control	OR 1.51 (0.92 vs 2.49)	0.07
Löwenberg et al. [59]	253	42 (15–60)	Randomized, open-label	GM-CSF 5 μg/kg/d	26 vs 30[c]	0.001	77 vs 78	n.s.	No difference	n.s.	77 vs 77	n.s.	3-year DFS 41% vs 33%	n.s.	3-year OS 41% vs 35%	n.s.

Table 19.1 (continued)

References	Patients (n)	Age (years), median (range)	Study design	Drug/dose	Time to neutrophil recovery (median, days) (drug vs control)	P	Incidence of infections (%) (drug vs control)	P	Hospitalization length (median days) (drug vs control)	P	CR rate (%) (drug vs control)	P	DFS/EFS (drug vs control)	P	OS (drug vs control)	P
Heil et al. [60]	521	54 (16–89)	Randomized, placebo-controlled, double-blind	Filgrastim 5 μg/kg/d	20 vs 25[a]	<0.001	37 vs 35[d]	n.s.	23 vs 29	<0.001	69 vs 68	0.47	Median DFS 10.1 vs 9.4 months	0.99	Median 12.5 vs 14 months	0.89
Godwin et al. [61]	211	68 (56–88)	Randomized, placebo-controlled, double-blind	Filgrastim 400 μg/m^2/d	24 vs 27 days[a]	0.014	19 vs 14[b]	0.9	29 vs 29	0.27	41 vs 50	0.89	Median DFS 8 vs 9 months	0.38	Median 6 vs 9 months	0.71
Harousseau et al. [62]	194	47 (15–60)	Randomized, open-label	Filgrastim 5 μg/kg/d	12 vs 19 days[a]	<0.001	40 vs 43[d]	0.34	24 vs 27	<0.001	88 vs 87	0.95	2-year DFS 47% vs 43%	0.45	2-year OS 64% vs 63%	0.24
Goldstone et al. [63]	226	>55	Randomized, placebo-controlled	Lenograstim 293 μg/d	Reduction by 5 days[c]	n.d.	n.d.	n.d.	n.d.	n.d.	58 vs 51	n.s.	n.d.	n.d.	3-year OS 15% vs 18%	1

Table 19.1 (continued)

References	Patients (n)	Age (years), median (range)	Study design	Drug/dose	Time to neutrophil recovery (median, days) (drug vs control)	P	Incidence of infections (%) (drug vs control)	P	Hospitalization length (median days) (drug vs control)	P	CR rate (%) (drug vs control)	P	DFS/EFS (drug vs control)	P	OS (drug vs control)	P
Bradstock et al. [64]	112	43 (16–60)	Randomized, open-label	Lenograstim 5 μg/kg	18 vs 22 days[a]	<0.001	67 vs 69[d]	n.s.	28 vs 29.5	0.21	81 vs 75	0.5	n.d.	n.d.	HR 0.83 (0.49–1.4)	0.48
Usuki et al. [65]	245	49 (15–87)	Randomized, open-label	Filgrastim 200 μg/m^2/d	12 vs 18 days[a]	<0.001	47.5 vs 41.6[d]	0.37	n.d.	n.d.	80.0 vs 76.8	0.53	5-year DFS 34.5% vs 33.6%	0.94	5-year OS 42.7% vs 35.6%	0.59
Amadori et al. [14]	722	68 (61–80)	Randomized, open-label	Lenograstim 150 μg/m^2/d	20 vs 25[a]	<0.001	6.6 vs 6.7[b]	n.s.	27.2 vs 29.7	<0.001	50.6 vs 56.4	0.12	HR 1 (0.81–1.24)	n.s.	HR 0.98 (0.84–1.15)	n.s.

Abbreviations: n.s., not significant; n.d., no data; CR, complete remission; EFS, event-free survival; DFS, disease-free survival; OS, overall survival; OR, odds ratio; HR, hazard ratio.
[a]Neutrophils > 500/μL.
[b]Grade 4 infection or death from infection.
[c]Neutrophils > 1,000/μL.
[d]Documented infection.

effect of myeloid growth factors in previously untreated AML patients (Fig. 19.3) and are summarized in Table 19.2. In 13 trials reported between 1995 and 2007, the effects of CSFs given concurrently with chemotherapy were investigated in 4,172 AML patients. Three trials applied CSFs during chemotherapy only, seven trials continued CSF administration after chemotherapy until recovery of neutrophils, and three trials compared different application schedules during and/or after chemotherapy. Four trials included patients younger than 60 years of age, five trials included only patients older than 55 years of age, and four trials investigated both younger and older patients. All trials were randomized and three trials were placebo-controlled. Nine trials investigated GM-CSF and four trials investigated G-CSF. Seven trials reported on the time to neutrophil recovery and five found a significant reduction in the group treated with CSFs. In eight trials the incidence of documented infections is reported and only one trial found a trend for a reduced incidence of documented infections in patients treated with CSFs compared to control patients. In most studies CR rate was the primary endpoint. Ten trials did not find a significant difference for CR rate in patients treated with CSFs compared to control patients, whereas two trials found a significantly improved CR rate in patients treated with GM-CSF (one trial with patients younger than 50 years) [13] or G-CSF (one trial with patients older than 60 years) [14]. Both trials found a 10% increase of the CR rate. EFS or DFS was reported in 12 trials and was not significantly different in 10 trials. Two trials reported a significantly improved DFS in patients treated with G-CSF or GM-CSF. The proportion of disease-free patients at 4 years was 9% higher in patients treated with G-CSF compared to control patients [15] and 27% higher at 2 years in patients treated with GM-CSF compared to controls [16]. OS was not significantly different in patients treated with CSFs compared to controls in any of the 13 trials. One trial found a trend toward improved OS at 2 years in GM-CSF-treated patients (39% vs 27%) [16]. One trial using GM-CSF in older patients showed a trend toward worse OS in GM-CSF-treated patients ($P = 0.07$) [8]. One trial found a 10% increase in OS at 4 years in the subgroup of standard risk AML patients treated with G-CSF ($P = 0.02$) [15], however, two other trials found no difference in OS for this subgroup of AML patients [13, 17]. Overall, the majority of priming studies did not show any effect on outcome of AML patients. Only a few trials suggested a positive effect of CSFs on CR rate and DFS and only one trial suggested a favorable effect of G-CSF in the subgroup of AML patients with standard risk. It is generally agreed upon that use of CSFs during chemotherapy of AML patients cannot be recommended [18, 19].

Efficacy of CSFs to Prevent Infectious Complications in Acute Lymphoblastic Leukemia

Prophylactic use of CSFs beginning during or after chemotherapy in acute lymphoblastic leukemia patients has been investigated in several trials (Table 19.3). Eight trials included a total of 758 patients and were reported between 1993 and

Table 19.2 CSF use in AML during chemotherapy (priming)

References	Patients (n)	Age (years), median (range)	Study design	Drug/dose	CR rate (%) (drug vs control)	P	DFS/EFS (drug vs control)	P	OS (drug vs control)	P
Heil et al. [66]	80	55	Randomized, placebo-controlled, double-blind	GM-CSF 250 $\mu g/m^2/d$	81 vs 79	0.57	41 months DFS 42% vs 41%	0.89	43 months OS 45% vs 49%	n.s.
Zittoun et al. [7]	102	15–60	Randomized, open-label	GM-CSF, 5 $\mu g/kg/d$	67.3 vs 77.4	0.34	EFS	0.16	OR 1.26 (0.76 vs 2.07)	0.37
Löwenberg et al. [67]	318	68 (61–88)	Randomized, open-label	GM-CSF 5 $\mu g/kg$	56 vs 55	0.98	2-year DFS 15% vs 19%	0.69	2-year OS 22% vs 22%	0.55
Löwenberg et al. [59]	253	42 (15–60)	Randomized, open-label	GM-CSF 5 $\mu g/kg/d$	79 vs 76	n.s.	3-year DFS 32% vs 42%	n.s.	3-year OS 33% vs 44%	n.s.
Witz et al. [16]	240	66 (55–75)	Randomized, placebo-controlled	GM-CSF 5 $\mu g/kg/d$	63 vs 60.5	0.79	2-year DFS 48% vs 21%	0.003	2-year OS 39% vs 27%	0.082
Estey et al. [68]	215	65	Randomized, open-label	G-CSF 200 $\mu g/m^2/d$	57 vs 45	0.087	No difference	n.s.	No difference	n.s.
Hast et al. [69]	93	72 (35–90)	Randomized, open-label	GM-CSF 200 $\mu g/d$	43 vs 43	n.s.	n.d.	n.d.	No difference	0.95
Löwenberg et al. [15]	640	44 (18–60)	Randomized, open-label	Lenograstim 150 $\mu g/m^2/d$	79 vs 83	0.24	4-year DFS 42% vs 33%	0.02	4-year OS 40% vs 35%	0.16
					Standard risk: 87 vs 86	n.s.	Standard risk: 4-year DFS 45% vs 33%	0.006	Standard risk: 4-year OS 45% vs 35%	0.02

Table 19.2 (continued)

References	Patients (n)	Age (years), median (range)	Study design	Drug/dose	CR rate (%) (drug vs control)	P	DFS/EFS (drug vs control)	P	OS (drug vs control)	P
Rowe et al. [70]	245	67 (56–86)	Randomized, placebo-controlled	GM-CSF 250 $\mu g/m^2/d$	33 vs 40	n.s.	Median DFS 6.9 vs 5.1 months	0.73	Median OS 5.3 vs 8.5 months	0.11
Löfgren et al. [8]	110	77 (64–94)	Randomized, open-label	GM-CSF 200 $\mu g/m^2/d$	65 vs 64	n.s.	Median DFS 6 vs 13 months	n.s.	Median OS 9 vs 14 months	0.07 (favoring control)
Büchner et al. [17]	895	(16–83)	Randomized, open-label	G-CSF 150 $\mu g/m^2/d$	n.d.	n.d.	HR 0.96 (0.68–1.35) Standard risk: no difference	0.82 n.s.	HR 0.99 (0.77–1.3) Standard risk: no difference	0.99 n.s.
Amadori et al. [14]	722	68 (61–80)	Randomized, open-label	Lenograstim 150 $\mu g/m^2/d$	58.3 vs 48.6	0.009	HR 1.04 (0.84–1.3)	n.s.	HR 0.91 (0.78–1.02)	0.26
Thomas et al. [13]	259	27 (15–49)	Randomized, open-label	GM-CSF 5 $\mu g/kg/d$	88 vs 78	0.04	3-year EFS 42% vs 34%	0.06	3-year OS 54% vs 46%	0.2
							Standard risk: 3-year EFS 50% vs 35%	0.05	Standard risk OS: no difference	n.s.

Abbreviations: n.s., not significant; n.d., no data; CR, complete remission; EFS, event-free survival; DFS, disease-free survival; OS, overall survival; OR, odds ratio; HR, hazard ratio.

Table 19.3 CSF use in ALL patients

Previously untreated ALL

References	Patients (n)	Age (years), median (range)	Study design	Drug/dose	Time to neutrophil recovery (median, days) (drug vs control)	P	Incidence of infections (%) (drug vs control)	P	Hospitalization length (median days) (drug vs control)	P	CR rate (%) (drug vs control)	P	DFS/EFS (drug vs control)	P	OS (drug vs control)	P
Ohno et al. [71]	41	36 (13–78)	Randomized, open-label, after IND and CONS	G-CSF, 0 vs 2 vs 5 vs 10 µg/kg/d	8.5 vs 12 (2 vs 5 µg/kg)[a]	0.047	23 vs 50 (5 vs 2 µg/kg)[c]	0.38	n.d.	n.d.	80 vs 61.5 (5 vs 2 µg/kg)	0.225	n.d.	n.d.	n.d.	n.d.
Ottmann et al. [72]	76	(16–65)	Randomized, open-label, during IND 2	G-CSF 5 µg/kg/d	8 vs 12.5[a]	<0.002	45 vs 56[b]	0.25	n.d.	n.d.	n.d.	n.d.	20-month DFS 45% vs 43%	0.3	n.d.	n.d.
Papamichael et al. [73]	26	32 (15–49)	Non-randomized, sequential treatment groups, during chemo	GM-CSF 3 µg/kg/d	n.d.	n.d.	No difference[b]	n.s.	n.d.	n.d.	No differ-ence	n.s.	n.d.	n.d.	n.d.	n.d.
Geissler et al. [74]	53	(16–79)	Randomized, open-label, during IND 1 and 2	G-CSF 5 µg/kg/d	16 vs 26[a]	<0.001	40 vs 77[b]	<0.05	n.d.	n.d.	96 vs 80	0.19	24-month DFS 55% vs 46%	0.7	28-month OS 47% vs 39%	0.96

Table 19.3 (continued)

Previously untreated ALL

References	Patients (n)	Age (years), median (range)	Study design	Drug/dose	Time to neutrophil recovery (median, days) (drug vs control)	P	Incidence of infections (%) (drug vs control)	P	Hospitalization length (median days) (drug vs control)	P	CR rate (%) (drug vs control)	P	DFS/EFS (drug vs control)	P	OS (drug vs control)	P
Larson et al. [75]	198	35 (16–83)	Randomized, placebo-controlled, after IND	G-CSF 5 μg/kg/d	16 vs 22[a]	<0.001	78 vs 93[b]	0.13	22 vs 28	0.02	87 vs 77	0.04	Median DFS 2.3 vs 1.7 years	0.5	Median OS 2.4 vs 1.8 years	0.25
Ifrah et al. [76]	64	(15–55)	Randomized, placebo-controlled, after IND	GM-CSF 5 μg/kg/d	16 vs 18[c]	n.s.	n.d.	n.d.	n.d.	n.d.	77 vs 65.5	n.s.	n.d.	n.d.	n.d.	n.d.
Holowiecki et al. [20]	64	26.5 (16–58)	Randomized, open-label, during IND	G-CSF 150 μg/m^2	9 vs 19[c]	<0.05	9 vs 2 [d]	n.s.	36 vs 41	0.15	94 vs 87	n.s.	n.d.	n.d.	2-year OS 59% vs 27%	0.04
Thomas et al. [77]	236	33 (15–55)	Randomized, open-label, during IND	G-CSF 263 μg/d, GM-CSF 5 μg/kg/d	17/18 (G/GM-CSF) vs 21a (ctl)	n.s.	16/16 (G/GM-CSF) vs 24 (ctl)	n.s.	30/34 (G/GM-CSF) vs 34 (ctl)	n.s.	69/81 (G/GM-CSF) vs 66 (ctl)	0.08	5-year DFS 32%/18% vs 23%	n.s.	5-year OS 26%/28% vs 24%	n.s.

Table 19.3 (continued)

Early versus late start of CSFs in previously untreated ALL

Author/year	Patients (n)	Age (years), median (range)	Study design	Drug/dose	Time to neutrophil recovery (median, days) (early vs late)	P	Incidence of infections (%) (early vs late)	P	Hospitalization length (median days) (early vs late)	P
Bassan et al. [22]	65	(14–60)	Non-randomized, sequential treatment groups, during IND/early (d4) vs after IND/late (d15)	G-CSF 5 μg/kg/d	17 vs 21[c]	<0.002	35 vs 71[b]	0.007	n.d.	n.d.
Hofmann et al. [21]	55	34 (18–55)	Randomized, open-label, early (d12) vs late (d17) after CONS	G-CSF 263 μ/d	12 vs 12[c]	n.s.	47 vs 50[b]	n.s.	27 vs 29	n.s.
Weiser et al. [23]	199	(16–75)	Non-randomized, sequential treatment groups, early (d5) vs late (d10) during chemo	G-CSF 5 μg/kg/d	IND 18 vs 19[a]	0.04	23 vs 29[d]	n.s.	n.d.	n.d.
					CONS 12 vs 15[a]	<0.001				

Abbreviations: n.s., not significant; n.d., no data; CR, complete remission; EFS, event-free survival; DFS, disease-free survival; OS, overall survival; OR, odds ratio; HR, hazard ratio.
[a]Neutrophils > 1,000/μL.
[b]Documented infection.
[c]Neutrophils > 500/μL.
[d]Grade 4 infection or death from infection.

2004. Five trials only included patients younger than 65 years of age and three trials included both younger and older patients. Seven trials were randomized controlled studies, one compared sequential treatment groups, and two studies were placebo-controlled. G-CSF was investigated in five trials, GM-CSF in two trials, and one study compared G-CSF, GM-CSF, and control. The time to neutrophil recovery was reported in seven trials and five found a significant reduction in patients treated with CSFs. The incidence of documented infections was reduced in one of seven trials, and six studies did not find a significant difference between CSF and control group. The length of hospitalization was reported in three trials and one found a significant reduction in patients treated with CSFs compared to controls. CR rate was not significantly different in patients with CSFs or without in five trials, but increased in one trial of a total of six trials that reported CR rates. DFS was not different between treatment groups in four of four trials, and OS was not significantly different in three of four trials that reported OS, but significantly longer in one trial in patients treated with CSFs compared to controls [20].

In summary, CSFs during or after chemotherapy in untreated ALL patients reduce the duration of neutropenia but do not consistently reduce the incidence of infections. The majority of studies suggest that CSFs do not influence treatment outcome in ALL patients. Many studies included a relatively small number of patients and thus the evidence level of these studies is limited.

Three trials compared an early with a late treatment start of CSFs in previously untreated ALL patients. Duration of neutropenia and incidence of infections were similar whether G-CSF treatment was started on day 12 or 17 after consolidation chemotherapy [21]. Two non-randomized, sequential treatment group comparisons found that CSF treatment during induction chemotherapy (day 4 or 5) compared to a delayed start of CSFs (day 10 or 15) resulted in a significantly reduced neutropenia duration in both studies and a reduced infection rate in one study in the group treated early with CSFs [22, 23] (Table 19.3). These studies are inconclusive whether late CSF administration in ALL patients is as effective as early CSF administration to reduce the duration of neutropenia and the rate of infections.

CSFs in Refractory or Relapsed Acute Leukemias

Ohno et al. reported in 1990 about relapsed or refractory acute leukemia patients randomized to treatment with G-CSF or control [24]. Time to neutrophil recovery and the incidence of documented infections were significantly reduced. In a non-randomized, historically controlled trial with G-CSF in refractory or relapsed AML patients Kern et al. reported a significant reduction of time to neutrophil recovery by 4 days, but no significant reduction of severe infections [25]. In a third study, Thomas et al. investigated GM-CSF in 192 refractory or relapsed AML patients in a randomized, placebo-controlled, blinded study [26]. No difference was found for time to neutrophil recovery, incidence of infections, DFS, or OS. Milligan et al. investigated G-CSF priming during induction chemotherapy in refractory, relapsed, or AML patients with high-risk cytogenetics [27]. This randomized, controlled study with 356 patients aged 15–70 years did not find significant differences in the priming group compared to the control group for CR, DFS, and OS.

CSF administration in refractory or relapsed adult ALL patients has been studied in two non-randomized, historically controlled trials [28, 29]. Both trials found a significant reduction in time to neutrophil recovery. Only one trial reported on the incidence of infections, CR rate, and OS and did not find a difference for these parameters between CSF and control groups [28]. Taken together, studies are inconclusive whether CSFs can prevent infectious complications in refractory or relapsed AML patients.

Thrombopoietic Growth Factors

In addition to neutropenia, intensive chemotherapy for AML also results in severe thrombocytopenia in the vast majority of patients. Currently, platelet transfusions are the treatment of choice, and safe thresholds for platelet transfusions have been defined [30]. Nevertheless, platelet transfusions have potential risks with regard to transmission of infections, alloimmunization, and transfusion reactions [31]. Archimbaud et al. investigated pegylated recombinant human megakaryocyte growth and development factor (PEG-rHuMGDF) in 108 newly diagnosed AML patients at different dosage schedules. Biologic activity of PEG-rHuMGDF was demonstrated by higher peak platelet counts after regeneration as compared to the placebo group. However, there was no benefit of PEG-rHuMGDF in time to transfusion independence or total transfusion requirements [32]. Similar results were obtained by Schiffer et al. and Geissler et al. [33, 34].

In 2008, the US Food and Drug Administration (FDA) approved romiplostim for subcutaneous injection (Nplate, Amgen, Inc.) for the treatment of thrombocytopenia in patients with chronic immune (idiopathic) thrombocytopenic purpura (ITP) who had an insufficient response to corticosteroids, immunoglobulins, or splenectomy. Romiplostim is a thrombopoietin (TPO) receptor agonist that stimulates bone marrow megakaryocytes to produce platelets. No results from clinical trials have been reported so far for the use of romiplostim in patients with acute leukemia. In a single-arm trial investigating the use of romiplostim in myelodysplasic syndromes (MDS), 11 of 44 patients were reported as having possible disease progression, among whom 4 patients developed acute myelogenous leukemia. Thus, the use of romiplostim in AML or ALL patients has to be carefully considered (prescribing information, http://www.fda.gov/cder/foi/label/2008/125268lbl.pdf). In 2008, eltrombopag, a small molecule TPO receptor agonist, was approved by the US Food and Drug Administration for use in chronic immune thrombocytopenic purpura, however, it has not been tested in chemotherapy-induced thrombocytopenia.

Recommendations for the Use of CSFs in Acute Leukemias in Current Guidelines

Guidelines for the use of hematopoietic growth factors in cancer patients are available from the American Society of Clinical Oncology (ASCO) [18], the National Comprehensive Cancer Network (NCCN) [2], and the European Organization for Research and Treatment of Cancer (EORTC) [35]. Importantly, it is emphasized that guideline recommendations are understood as one of several treatment options. Specifically, dose reduction or delay of chemotherapy is the most common alternative.

ASCO published an update of their year 2000 guideline in 2006, where the use of CSFs is recommended for cancer patients with a high risk of FN based on age, medical history, disease characteristics, and myelotoxicity of the chemotherapy regimen if no other equally effective regimen with a lower incidence of FN is available. Definition of high risk has been changed from an incidence of FN of 40% or higher to 20% or higher [18]. Special recommendations are given for AML patients in induction, in consolidation, and in relapse. The ASCO guideline states that "CSF use following initial induction therapy is reasonable, although there has been no favorable impact on remission rate, remission duration or survival. Patients older than 55 years of age may be most likely to benefit from CSF use. CSF use can be recommended after the completion of consolidation chemotherapy because of the potential to decrease the incidence of infection and eliminate the likelihood of hos pitalization in some patients receiving intensive post-remission chemotherapy" [18]. ASCO does not recommend the use of CSFs to prime AML cells for increased susceptibility to chemotherapy and in relapsed or refractory AML patients. For ALL patients ASCO recommends CSFs "after the completion of the initial first few days of chemotherapy of the initial induction or first post-remission course" [18]. This very broad recommendation of CSF use in acute leukemia patients is based on the assumption that a reduction of the incidence of FN is a relevant endpoint. However, as discussed above, most AML trials failed to show a reduction in the clinically important endpoint of documented or severe infections in patients treated with CSFs compared to controls.

Guidelines of NCCN updated in 2009 recommend the use of CSFs for cancer patients with high risk (greater than 20%) of FN receiving treatment with curative intent, adjuvant therapy, or treatment expected to prolong survival and to improve QoL. It is stated that in the palliative setting, the use of high-risk chemotherapy is a difficult decision, but if high-risk chemotherapy is chosen, use of CSFs is reasonable. In patients with intermediate risk of FN (10–20%) individualized consideration of CSF use is recommended [2]. Regarding AML patients NCCN guidelines state that "growth factors may be considered in the elderly after chemotherapy is complete" [36].

Guidelines of the EORTC recommend use of CSFs for cancer patients at an overall risk of FN of 20% or greater. When using chemotherapy regimens associated with a FN risk of 10–20%, particular attention should be given to the assessment of patient characteristics that may increase the overall risk of FN [35]. No leukemia-specific recommendations of the EORTC exist.

Future Directions

Based on recent data several new strategies toward a more efficient way of using CSFs are at the horizon. First, it became evident that the frequency of FN is highest in the first cycle of chemotherapy [37]. This might be the result of confounding effects, e.g., that most patients with FN experience dose reductions in subsequent treatment courses or that normal hematopoiesis is most compromised during the first treatment course because of the large cell mass in the bone marrow of leukemia patients, however, it warrants further study. Administration of G-CSF only during the first cycle of chemotherapy in patients at risk of FN seems worth investigation as it will highly increase cost-effectiveness and reduce potential side effects in many patients. Bajorin et al. have investigated this approach in advanced or relapsed germ cell tumors. Patients were randomized to receive GM-CSF with either cycles 1 and 2 or cycles 3 and 4 of chemotherapy. Infections during neutropenia were significantly reduced in cycle 1 (22% vs 43%, $P = 0.03$), but not in the following cycles [38].

Second, risk factors for mortality during episodes of FN are now well documented [39], and CSF use could be tailored to patients with at least one or two of these factors. This approach will proof whether CSFs have the ability to reduce mortality from FN and may reduce overall costs associated with the broad use of CSFs.

Third, the efficacy and risk of antibiotic prophylaxis regarding development of antibiotic resistance might have to be weighed against the benefit and cost of CSFs in the future, as both efficacy in reducing mortality and a low risk of resistance has been shown recently for antibiotic prophylaxis [40, 41]. A revision of the guidelines for antibiotic prophylaxis in cancer patients by the Infectious Diseases Society of America is in progress. On a similar note, antifungal prophylaxis with posaconazole has been found effective in reducing the incidence of proven or probable invasive fungal infections in AML patients [42].

Fourth, new formulations of CSFs have been developed and licensed as the intellectual property of filgrastim is running out. Interestingly, the recombinant human keratinocyte growth factor palifermin, which has been shown to reduce grade 3 or 4 oral mucositis from 98% in the placebo group to 63% in the treatment group ($P < 0.001$), and reduced the incidence of FN in patients with hematologic malignancies undergoing autologous PBPC transplantation (75% vs 92% in controls, $P < 0.001$) [43]. Thus, protection of mucosal barrier as an entry site for infectious agents might become an additional treatment strategy to prevent adverse outcomes from FN.

New strategies for priming of AML cells have been suggested in the setting of novel targeted therapies such as gemtuzumab ozogamicin [44]. Simultaneous in vitro exposure of G-CSF and gemtuzumab ozogamicin was recently shown to augment apoptosis in primary AML samples and to render blast cells from refractory patients sensitive to the cytotoxic effects of gemtuzumab ozogamicin [45].

Currently, chemokine receptor (CXCR4) antagonists are explored in proof-of-principle studies in leukemia patients [46]. Stromal cell-derived factor-1 (SDF-1), now designated CXCL12 [47], is secreted by reticular stromal cells in the bone marrow and signals through the CXCR4 chemokine receptor [48, 49], expressed on hematopoietic and leukemia stem cells [50–52]. Through CXCL12, these stromal cells also attract circulating hematopoietic progenitor cells [53] or leukemia cells [54] for homing to the bone marrow. The CXCR4 antagonist plerixafor (AMD3100) rapidly induces stem cell mobilization to the peripheral blood and was recently approved for normal hematopoietic stem cell mobilization by the US Food and Drug Administration. The feasibility of using plerixafor for AML cell mobilization to the blood in an animal model and in AML patients was recently reported [55, 56]. Nervi et al. showed that treatment of leukemic mice with chemotherapy plus AMD3100 resulted in decreased tumor burden and improved overall survival in a model of acute promyelocytic leukemia compared to mice treated with chemotherapy alone [55]. Azab et al. showed that the interaction of multiple myeloma cells with their microenvironment can be disrupted by AMD3100 and that AMD3100 enhances bortezomib-induced tumor reduction [57]. Plerixafor is currently used in an ongoing clinical trial for mobilization of AML cells from the protective marrow microenvironment to the blood, where the AML cells are then targeted by conventional cytotoxic drugs.

Summary and Conclusions

The last two decades of extensive research on the myeloid growth factors G-CSF and GM-CSF for the treatment of patients with acute leukemia leave us with disappointing results. There is overwhelming evidence that the myeloid growth factors reduce the time to neutrophil recovery in neutropenic patients after chemotherapy. However, there is also high-level evidence from multiple studies that the incidence of severe infections and mortality from infections are not reduced by growth factor treatment in AML patients. Conflicting evidence exists in ALL patients whether the incidence of severe infections can be reduced by growth factor treatment. Multiple studies have investigated the concurrent use of CSFs with chemotherapy in AML patients to enhance efficacy of chemotherapy (priming), however, there is high-level evidence that this strategy is not effective in the majority of AML patients. Nevertheless, a significant number of current AML and ALL trial protocols make use of myeloid growth factors to prevent infectious complications and thus more evidence will be available in the future. The thrombopoietic growth factor rHuMGDF has not led to significantly accelerated recovery of platelet counts and its use has been discontinued. The majority of trials did not find leukemia promoting effects of myeloid growth factors in adult acute leukemia patients, however, two trials with adult AML patients, one trial in pediatric ALL patients, and two trials in breast cancer patients suggested that myeloid growth factors may have adverse effects. Novel players enter the arena of cytokine treatment in acute leukemias, and results from the combined use of antagonists of CXCR4 and chemotherapy in leukemia patients are anticipated with some optimism.

References

1. Rahman Z, Esparza-Guerra L, Yap HY, Fraschini G, Bodey G, Hortobagyi G. Chemotherapy-induced neutropenia and fever in patients with metastatic breast carcinoma receiving salvage chemotherapy. Cancer. 1997;79(6):1150–7.
2. Crawford J, Althaus B, Armitage J, et al. Myeloid growth factors. Clinical practice guidelines in oncology. J Natl Compr Canc Netw. 2007;5(2):188–202.
3. Heuser M, Ganser A. Colony-stimulating factors in the management of neutropenia and its complications. Ann Hematol. 2005;84(11):697–708.
4. Le Deley MC, Suzan F, Cutuli B, et al. Anthracyclines, mitoxantrone, radiotherapy, and granulocyte colony-stimulating factor: risk factors for leukemia and myelodysplastic syndrome after breast cancer. J Clin Oncol. 2007;25(3):292–300.
5. Smith RE, Bryant J, DeCillis A, Anderson S. Acute myeloid leukemia and myelodysplastic syndrome after doxorubicin–cyclophosphamide adjuvant therapy for operable breast cancer: the National Surgical Adjuvant Breast and Bowel Project Experience. J Clin Oncol. 2003;21(7):1195–204.
6. Relling MV, Boyett JM, Blanco JG, et al. Granulocyte colony-stimulating factor and the risk of secondary myeloid malignancy after etoposide treatment. Blood. 2003;101(10):3862–7.
7. Zittoun R, Suciu S, Mandelli F, et al. Granulocyte–macrophage colony-stimulating factor associated with induction treatment of acute myelogenous leukemia: a randomized trial by the European Organization for Research and Treatment of Cancer Leukemia Cooperative Group. J Clin Oncol. 1996;14(7):2150–9.
8. Lofgren C, Paul C, Astrom M, et al. Granulocyte–macrophage colony-stimulating factor to increase efficacy of mitoxantrone, etoposide and cytarabine in previously untreated elderly patients with acute myeloid leukaemia: a Swedish multicentre randomized trial. Br J Haematol. 2004;124(4):474–80.
9. Rowe JM, Andersen JW, Mazza JJ, et al. A randomized placebo-controlled phase III study of granulocyte–macrophage colony-stimulating factor in adult patients (>55 to 70 years of age) with acute myelogenous leukemia: a study of the Eastern Cooperative Oncology Group (E1490). Blood. 1995;86(2):457–62.
10. Dombret H, Chastang C, Fenaux P, et al. A controlled study of recombinant human granulocyte colony-stimulating factor in elderly patients after treatment for acute myelogenous leukemia. AML Cooperative Study Group. N Engl J Med. 1995;332(25):1678–83.
11. Miyauchi J, Kelleher CA, Wang C, Minkin S, McCulloch EA. Growth factors influence the sensitivity of leukemic stem cells to cytosine arabinoside in culture. Blood. 1989;73(5):1272–8.
12. Cannistra SA, Groshek P, Griffin JD. Granulocyte–macrophage colony-stimulating factor enhances the cytotoxic effects of cytosine arabinoside in acute myeloblastic leukemia and in the myeloid blast crisis phase of chronic myeloid leukemia. Leukemia. 1989;3(5):328–34.
13. Thomas X, Raffoux E, Botton S, et al. Effect of priming with granulocyte–macrophage colony-stimulating factor in younger adults with newly diagnosed acute myeloid leukemia: a trial by the Acute Leukemia French Association (ALFA) Group. Leukemia. 2007;21(3):453–61.
14. Amadori S, Suciu S, Jehn U, et al. Use of glycosylated recombinant human G-CSF (lenograstim) during and/or after induction chemotherapy in patients 61 years of age and older with acute myeloid leukemia: final results of AML-13, a randomized phase-3 study. Blood. 2005;106(1):27–34.

15. Lowenberg B, van Putten W, Theobald M, et al. Effect of priming with granulocyte colony-stimulating factor on the outcome of chemotherapy for acute myeloid leukemia. N Engl J Med. 2003;349(8):743–52.
16. Witz F, Sadoun A, Perrin MC, et al. A placebo-controlled study of recombinant human granulocyte–macrophage colony-stimulating factor administered during and after induction treatment for de novo acute myelogenous leukemia in elderly patients. Groupe Ouest Est Leucemies Aigues Myeloblastiques (GOELAM). Blood. 1998;91(8):2722–30.
17. Buchner T, Berdel WE, Hiddemann W. Priming with granulocyte colony-stimulating factor-relation to high-dose cytarabine in acute myeloid leukemia. N Engl J Med. 2004;350(21):2215–16.
18. Smith TJ, Khatcheressian J, Lyman GH, et al. 2006 update of recommendations for the use of white blood cell growth factors: an evidence-based clinical practice guideline. J Clin Oncol. 2006;24(19):3187–205.
19. Ottmann OG, Bug G, Krauter J. Current status of growth factors in the treatment of acute myeloid and lymphoblastic leukemia. Semin Hematol. 2007;44(3):183–92.
20. Holowiecki J, Giebel S, Krzemien S, et al. G-CSF administered in time-sequenced setting during remission induction and consolidation therapy of adult acute lymphoblastic leukemia has beneficial influence on early recovery and possibly improves long-term outcome: a randomized multicenter study. Leuk Lymphoma. 2002;43(2):315–25.
21. Hofmann WK, Seipelt G, Langenhan S, et al. Prospective randomized trial to evaluate two delayed granulocyte colony stimulating factor administration schedules after high-dose cytarabine therapy in adult patients with acute lymphoblastic leukemia. Ann Hematol. 2002;81(10):570–4.
22. Bassan R, Lerede T, Di Bona E, et al. Granulocyte colony-stimulating factor (G-CSF, filgrastim) after or during an intensive remission induction therapy for adult acute lymphoblastic leukaemia: effects, role of patient pretreatment characteristics, and costs. Leuk Lymphoma. 1997;26(1–2):153–61.
23. Weiser MA, O'Brien S, Thomas DA, Pierce SA, Lam TP, Kantarjian HM. Comparison of two different schedules of granulocyte-colony-stimulating factor during treatment for acute lymphocytic leukemia with a hyper-CVAD (cyclophosphamide, doxorubicin, vincristine, and dexamethasone) regimen. Cancer. 2002;94(2):285–91.
24. Ohno R, Tomonaga M, Kobayashi T, et al. Effect of granulocyte colony-stimulating factor after intensive induction therapy in relapsed or refractory acute leukemia. N Engl J Med. 1990;323(13):871–7.
25. Kern W, Aul C, Maschmeyer G, et al. Granulocyte colony-stimulating factor shortens duration of critical neutropenia and prolongs disease-free survival after sequential high-dose cytosine arabinoside and mitoxantrone (S-HAM) salvage therapy for refractory and relapsed acute myeloid leukemia. German AML Cooperative Group. Ann Hematol. 1998;77(3): 115–22.
26. Thomas X, Fenaux P, Dombret H, et al. Granulocyte–macrophage colony-stimulating factor (GM-CSF) to increase efficacy of intensive sequential chemotherapy with etoposide, mitoxantrone and cytarabine (EMA) in previously treated acute myeloid leukemia: a multicenter randomized placebo-controlled trial (EMA91 Trial). Leukemia. 1999;13(8):1214–20.
27. Milligan DW, Wheatley K, Littlewood T, Craig JI, Burnett AK. Fludarabine and cytosine are less effective than standard ADE chemotherapy in high-risk acute myeloid leukemia, and addition of G-CSF and ATRA are not beneficial: results of the MRC AML-HR randomized trial. Blood. 2006;107(12):4614–22.
28. Kantarjian HM, Estey EH, O'Brien S, et al. Intensive chemotherapy with mitoxantrone and high-dose cytosine arabinoside followed by granulocyte–macrophage colony-stimulating factor in the treatment of patients with acute lymphocytic leukemia. Blood. 1992;79(4):876–81.
29. Martino R, Bellido M, Brunet S, et al. Intensive salvage chemotherapy for primary refractory or first relapsed adult acute lymphoblastic leukemia: results of a prospective trial. Haematologica. 1999;84(6):505–10.

30. Wandt H, Frank M, Ehninger G, et al. Safety and cost effectiveness of a 10 × 10(9)/L trigger for prophylactic platelet transfusions compared with the traditional 20 × 10(9)/L trigger: a prospective comparative trial in 105 patients with acute myeloid leukemia. Blood. 1998;91(10):3601–6.

31. Kaushansky K. Thrombopoietin. N Engl J Med. 1998;339(11):746–54.

32. Archimbaud E, Ottmann OG, Yin JA, et al. A randomized, double-blind, placebo-controlled study with pegylated recombinant human megakaryocyte growth and development factor (PEG-rHuMGDF) as an adjunct to chemotherapy for adults with de novo acute myeloid leukemia. Blood. 1999;94(11):3694–701.

33. Schiffer CA, Miller K, Larson RA, et al. A double-blind, placebo-controlled trial of pegylated recombinant human megakaryocyte growth and development factor as an adjunct to induction and consolidation therapy for patients with acute myeloid leukemia. Blood. 2000;95(8):2530–5.

34. Geissler K, Yin JA, Ganser A, et al. Prior and concurrent administration of recombinant human megakaryocyte growth and development factor in patients receiving consolidation chemotherapy for de novo acute myeloid leukemia – a randomized, placebo-controlled, double-blind safety and efficacy study. Ann Hematol. 2003;82(11):677–83.

35. Aapro MS, Cameron DA, Pettengell R, et al. EORTC guidelines for the use of granulocyte-colony stimulating factor to reduce the incidence of chemotherapy-induced febrile neutropenia in adult patients with lymphomas and solid tumours. Eur J Cancer. 2006;42(15):2433–53.

36. Appelbaum FR, Baer MR, Carabasi MH, et al. NCCN Practice Guidelines for Acute Myelogenous Leukemia. Oncology (Williston Park). 2000;14(11A):53–61.

37. Heuser M, Ganser A, Bokemeyer C. Use of colony-stimulating factors for chemotherapy-associated neutropenia: review of current guidelines. Semin Hematol. 2007;44(3):148–56.

38. Bajorin DF, Nichols CR, Schmoll HJ, et al. Recombinant human granulocyte–macrophage colony-stimulating factor as an adjunct to conventional-dose ifosfamide-based chemotherapy for patients with advanced or relapsed germ cell tumors: a randomized trial. J Clin Oncol. 1995;13(1):79–86.

39. Kuderer NM, Dale DC, Crawford J, Cosler LE, Lyman GH. Mortality, morbidity, and cost associated with febrile neutropenia in adult cancer patients. Cancer. 2006;106(10):2258–66.

40. Gafter-Gvili A, Fraser A, Paul M, van de Wetering M, Kremer L, Leibovici L. Antibiotic prophylaxis for bacterial infections in afebrile neutropenic patients following chemotherapy. Cochrane Database Syst Rev. 2005;(4):CD004386.

41. Gafter-Gvili A, Paul M, Fraser A, Leibovici L. Effect of quinolone prophylaxis in afebrile neutropenic patients on microbial resistance: systematic review and meta-analysis. J Antimicrob Chemother. 2007;59(1):5–22.

42. Cornely OA, Maertens J, Winston DJ, et al. Posaconazole vs. fluconazole or itraconazole prophylaxis in patients with neutropenia. N Engl J Med. 2007;356(4):348–59.

43. Spielberger R, Stiff P, Bensinger W, et al. Palifermin for oral mucositis after intensive therapy for hematologic cancers. N Engl J Med. 2004;351(25):2590–8.

44. Tsimberidou AM, Giles FJ, Estey E, O'Brien S, Keating MJ, Kantarjian HM. The role of gemtuzumab ozogamicin in acute leukaemia therapy. Br J Haematol. 2006;132(4):398–409.

45. Rutella S, Bonanno G, Procoli A, et al. Granulocyte colony-stimulating factor enhances the in vitro cytotoxicity of gemtuzumab ozogamicin against acute myeloid leukemia cell lines and primary blast cells. Exp Hematol. 2006;34(1):54–65.

46. Burger JA, Peled A. CXCR4 antagonists: targeting the microenvironment in leukemia and other cancers. Leukemia. 2009;23(1):43–52.

47. Zlotnik A, Yoshie O. Chemokines: a new classification system and their role in immunity. Immunity. 2000;12(2):121–7.

48. Bleul CC, Farzan M, Choe H, et al. The lymphocyte chemoattractant SDF-1 is a ligand for LESTR/fusin and blocks HIV-1 entry. Nature. 1996;382(6594):829–33.

49. Oberlin E, Amara A, Bachelerie F, et al. The CXC chemokine SDF-1 is the ligand for LESTR/fusin and prevents infection by T-cell-line-adapted HIV-1. Nature. 1996;382(6594):833–5.

50. Sugiyama T, Kohara H, Noda M, Nagasawa T. Maintenance of the hematopoietic stem cell pool by CXCL12–CXCR4 chemokine signaling in bone marrow stromal cell niches. Immunity. 2006;25(6):977–88.

51. Mohle R, Bautz F, Rafii S, Moore MA, Brugger W, Kanz L. The chemokine receptor CXCR-4 is expressed on CD34$^+$ hematopoietic progenitors and leukemic cells and mediates transendothelial migration induced by stromal cell-derived factor-1. Blood. 1998;91(12):4523–30.

52. Tavor S, Petit I, Porozov S, et al. CXCR4 regulates migration and development of human acute myelogenous leukemia stem cells in transplanted NOD/SCID mice. Cancer Res. 2004;64(8):2817–24.

53. Peled A, Petit I, Kollet O, et al. Dependence of human stem cell engraftment and repopulation of NOD/SCID mice on CXCR4. Science. 1999;283(5403):845–8.

54. Sipkins DA, Wei X, Wu JW, et al. In vivo imaging of specialized bone marrow endothelial microdomains for tumour engraftment. Nature. 2005;435(7044):969–73.

55. Nervi B, Ramirez P, Rettig MP, et al. Chemosensitization of AML following mobilization by the CXCR4 antagonist AMD3100. Blood. 2009;113(24):6206–14.

56. Andreeff M, Konoplev S, Wang R, et al. Massive mobilization of AML cells into circulation by disruption of leukemia/stroma cell interactions using CXCR4 antagonist AMD3100: first evidence in patients and potential for abolishing bone marrow microenvironment-mediated resistance. Blood. (ASH Annual Meeting Abstracts) 2006;108. Abstract 568.

57. Azab AK, Runnels JM, Pitsillides C, et al. The CXCR4 inhibitor AMD3100 disrupts the interaction of multiple myeloma cells with the bone marrow microenvironment and enhances their sensitivity to therapy. Blood. 2009;113(18):4341–51.

58. Stone RM, Berg DT, George SL, et al. Granulocyte–macrophage colony-stimulating factor after initial chemotherapy for elderly patients with primary acute myelogenous leukemia. Cancer and Leukemia Group B. N Engl J Med. 1995;332(25):1671 7.

59. Lowenberg B, Boogaerts MA, Daenen SM, et al. Value of different modalities of granulocyte–macrophage colony-stimulating factor applied during or after induction therapy of acute myeloid leukemia. J Clin Oncol. 1997;15(12):3496–506.

60. Heil G, Hoelzer D, Sanz MA, et al. A randomized, double-blind, placebo-controlled, phase III study of filgrastim in remission induction and consolidation therapy for adults with de novo acute myeloid leukemia. The International Acute Myeloid Leukemia Study Group. Blood. 1997;90(12):4710–18.

61. Godwin JE, Kopecky KJ, Head DR, et al. A double-blind placebo-controlled trial of granulocyte colony-stimulating factor in elderly patients with previously untreated acute myeloid leukemia: a Southwest Oncology Group Study (9031). Blood. 1998;91(10):3607–15.

62. Harousseau JL, Witz B, Lioure B, et al. Granulocyte colony-stimulating factor after intensive consolidation chemotherapy in acute myeloid leukemia: results of a randomized trial of the Groupe Ouest-Est Leucemies Aigues Myeloblastiques. J Clin Oncol. 2000;18(4):780–7.

63. Goldstone AH, Burnett AK, Wheatley K, Smith AG, Hutchinson RM, Clark RE. Attempts to improve treatment outcomes in acute myeloid leukemia (AML) in older patients: the results of the United Kingdom Medical Research Council AML11 trial. Blood. 2001;98(5):1302–11.

64. Bradstock K, Matthews J, Young G, et al. Effects of glycosylated recombinant human granulocyte colony-stimulating factor after high-dose cytarabine-based induction chemotherapy for adult acute myeloid leukaemia. Leukemia. 2001;15(9):1331–8.

65. Usuki K, Urabe A, Masaoka T, et al. Efficacy of granulocyte colony-stimulating factor in the treatment of acute myelogenous leukaemia: a multicentre randomized study. Br J Haematol. 2002;116(1):103–12.

66. Heil G, Chadid L, Hoelzer D, et al. GM-CSF in a double-blind randomized, placebo controlled trial in therapy of adult patients with de novo acute myeloid leukemia (AML). Leukemia. 1995;9(1):3–9.

67. Lowenberg B, Suciu S, Archimbaud E, et al. Use of recombinant GM-CSF during and after remission induction chemotherapy in patients aged 61 years and older with acute myeloid leukemia: final report of AML-11, a phase III randomized study of the Leukemia Cooperative

Group of European Organisation for the Research and Treatment of Cancer and the Dutch Belgian Hemato-Oncology Cooperative Group. Blood. 1997;90(8):2952–61.
68. Estey EH, Thall PF, Pierce S, et al. Randomized phase II study of fludarabine + cytosine arabinoside + idarubicin +/− *all-trans* retinoic acid +/− granulocyte colony-stimulating factor in poor prognosis newly diagnosed acute myeloid leukemia and myelodysplastic syndrome. Blood. 1999;93(8):2478–84.
69. Hast R, Hellstrom-Lindberg E, Ohm L, et al. No benefit from adding GM-CSF to induction chemotherapy in transforming myelodysplastic syndromes: better outcome in patients with less proliferative disease. Leukemia. 2003;17(9):1827–33.
70. Rowe JM, Neuberg D, Friedenberg W, et al. A phase 3 study of three induction regimens and of priming with GM-CSF in older adults with acute myeloid leukemia: a trial by the Eastern Cooperative Oncology Group. Blood. 2004;103(2):479–85.
71. Ohno R, Tomonaga M, Ohshima T, et al. A randomized controlled study of granulocyte colony stimulating factor after intensive induction and consolidation therapy in patients with acute lymphoblastic leukemia. Japan Adult Leukemia Study Group. Int J Hematol. 1993;58(1–2):73–81.
72. Ottmann OG, Ganser A, Freund M, et al. Simultaneous administration of granulocyte colony-stimulating factor (filgrastim) and induction chemotherapy in acute lymphoblastic leukemia. A pilot study. Ann Hematol. 1993;67(4):161–7.
73. Papamichael D, Andrews T, Owen D, et al. Intensive chemotherapy for adult acute lymphoblastic leukaemia given with or without granulocyte–macrophage colony stimulating factor. Ann Hematol. 1996;73(6):259–63.
74. Geissler K, Koller E, Hubmann E, et al. Granulocyte colony-stimulating factor as an adjunct to induction chemotherapy for adult acute lymphoblastic leukemia – a randomized phase-III study. Blood. 1997;90(2):590–6.
75. Larson RA, Dodge RK, Linker CA, et al. A randomized controlled trial of filgrastim during remission induction and consolidation chemotherapy for adults with acute lymphoblastic leukemia: CALGB study 9111. Blood. 1998;92(5):1556–64.
76. Ifrah N, Witz F, Jouet JP, et al. Intensive short term therapy with granulocyte–macrophage-colony stimulating factor support, similar to therapy for acute myeloblastic leukemia, does not improve overall results for adults with acute lymphoblastic leukemia. GOELAMS Group. Cancer. 1999;86(8):1496–505.
77. Thomas X, Boiron JM, Huguet F, et al. Efficacy of granulocyte and granulocyte–macrophage colony-stimulating factors in the induction treatment of adult acute lymphoblastic leukemia: a multicenter randomized study. Hematol J. 2004;5(5):384–94.

Chapter 20
The Hematopoietic Growth Factors in the Myelodysplastic Syndromes

Jose Ortega, Rami Komrokji, and Alan F. List

Introduction

The myelodysplastic syndromes (MDSs) are a heterogeneous group of hematopoietic stem cell malignancies that are characterized by abnormal morphology and impaired bone marrow maturation resulting in progressive cytopenia(s) and a propensity to evolve into acute myeloid leukemia (AML) [1]. The biologic hallmark of the hematopoietic stem cells in MDS is a defective capacity for self-renewal and differentiation. Predisposition to MDS is amplified in the elderly because of senescence-associated depletion of stem cells and associated changes in the marrow microenvironment that may foster ineffective hematopoiesis and may also favor the development of secondary clones [2].

MDS Epidemiology and Etiology

MDS became reportable to the SEER (Surveillance, Epidemiology, and End Results: the United States cancer surveillance program) in 2001. SEER data from 2001 through 2003 showed that the risk of MDS increased with age, and approximately 86% of MDS cases were diagnosed in individuals aged $\geq$ 60 years (median age at diagnosis was 76 years). Men had a significantly higher incidence rate than women (4.5 vs 2.7/100,000/year). Among racial groups, white individuals had the highest incidence rate. Approximately 10,300 cases of MDS were diagnosed in the United States in 2003 [3].

MDS may occur at a delayed interval after exposure to alkylating agents, radiation, or both (secondary or therapy-related MDS). Primary or de novo MDS occurs without a known history of mutagen exposure. Possible risk-modifying factors from

R. Komrokji (✉)
H Lee Moffitt Cancer Center and Research Institute, Tampa, FL 33612, USA
e-mail: rami.komrokji@moffitt.org

G.H. Lyman, D.C. Dale (eds.), *Hematopoietic Growth Factors in Oncology*,
Cancer Treatment and Research 157, DOI 10.1007/978-1-4419-7073-2_20,
© Springer Science+Business Media, LLC 2011

epidemiologic studies include smoking and exposure to agricultural chemical or solvents [4].

Clinical Presentation and Diagnosis of MDS

Some patients are initially asymptomatic and thereby discovered incidentally on review of a routine complete blood count (CBC). The vast majority of patients present with symptoms related to cytopenia(s), most commonly a normocytic or macrocytic anemia. With time, many patients' red blood cells become transfusion-dependent. Neutropenia and/or thrombocytopenia may be found initially or may appear with progression of disease. Organomegaly is infrequently observed. The natural history of MDS ranges from a chronic course that may span years to a rapid course with progression to AML.

The initial approach to diagnosis should be to exclude the more common types of normocytic or macrocytic anemia as well as the more common causes of other unexplained cytopenias. The diagnosis of MDS relies on morphologic findings of dysplasia in a patient with clinical evidence of impaired hematopoiesis. Peripheral blood smears may reveal oval macrocytic red cells, hypogranular and hypolo-bated granulocytes (the pseudo-Pelger–Huët anomaly), and giant platelets. Bone marrow aspiration and biopsy are required in order to assess morphology, cyto-genetics, cellularity, and topography. Despite the presence of peripheral blood cytopenia(s), the bone marrow is typically normocellular or hypercellular (ineffec-tive hematopoiesis). The diagnosis of MDS requires demonstration of dysplastic features (abnormal morphology) in 10% or more of at least one cell lineage [5]. Morphologic manifestations of dysplasia in the bone marrow include megaloblas-tic red cell precursors with multiple nuclei or asynchronous maturation of the nucleus and the cytoplasm; ring sideroblasts (erythroid precursors with iron-laden mitochondria); predominance of immature myeloid cells; granulocytic precursors with asynchronous maturation of the nucleus and the cytoplasm; hypogranular and hypolobated granulocytes; megakaryocytes with few nuclear lobes; and small megakaryocytes (micromegakaryocytes) [5]. Dysplastic abnormalities in all lin-eages can include nuclear and cytoplasmic blebs, karyorrhexis, and misshapen nuclei. The number of myeloblasts may be increased.

Classification of MDS

The French–American–British classification of acute leukemias (FAB classifica-tion) was the first to define the myelodysplastic syndromes in 1976 [6]. The FAB classification was amended in 1982 to include five subtypes: RA (refractory anemia), RARS (refractory anemia with ringed sideroblasts), RAEB (refractory anemia with excess blasts), RAEB-t (refractory anemia with excess blasts in transformation), and CMML (chronic myelomonocytic leukemia).

The World Health Organization classification subsequently modified the MDS classification system in 2002 by adding more subtypes, thus making it more useful for prognosis and management decisions [7]. The MDS subtypes added were as follows: RCMD (refractory cytopenia with multilineage dysplasia, which served to distinguish between isolated erythroid and multilineage dysplasia), RCMD-RS (refractory cytopenia with multilineage dysplasia and ringed sideroblasts), RAEB-1 and RAEB-2 (refractory anemia with excess blasts-1 and -2, allowing for better discrimination of blast percentage), MDS unclassified, and MDS associated with isolated del(5q) recognizing this distinct group. RAEB-t was excluded in the WHO classification after the blast threshold for acute myeloid leukemia (AML) was changed from >30% blasts in the bone marrow to ≥20% blasts. CMML was assigned to a new category of MDS/MPD (myelodysplastic /myeloproliferative neoplasms).

The WHO classification for MDS was recently updated, with minor changes [8]. In the 2008 edition, MDS unclassified was redefined as refractory cytopenias with unilineage dysplasia, which include RA, refractory neutropenia, and refractory thrombocytopenia. The category of presumptive MDS with minimal cytogenetic criteria was introduced recognizing those cases with refractory cytopenia without dysplastic morphologic features that harbor a clonal cytogenetic abnormality characteristic of MDS (Table 20.1).

Cytogenetic studies are imperative for the evaluation of patients with MDS because of their invaluable contribution to assessment of prognosis and clonality. Clonal cytogenetic abnormalities are observed in approximately 50% of MDS cases. MDS associated with an isolated 5q deletion occurs more commonly in women and is characterized by megakaryocytes with hypolobated nuclei, refractory macrocytic anemia, normal or elevated platelet count, and a favorable clinical course. Complex karyotypes (≥3 abnormalities) usually include chromosome 5 and/or 7 abnormalities (−5, del(5q), −7, del(7q)) and are typically associated with an unfavorable clinical course. In the absence of morphological criteria, the clonal cytogenetic abnormalities −Y, +8, or del(20q) are not definitive evidence for MDS [9]. These patients should be followed carefully for emerging morphological evidence of MDS.

Prognosis and Risk Stratification of Patients with MDS

The International Prognostic Scoring System (IPSS) is useful for estimating the risk of leukemic transformation and overall survival in the absence of active treatment (Table 20.2) [10]. The IPSS separates patients into distinct subgroups of risk for 25% of patients to undergo evolution to AML: low (31% of patients), 9.4 years; INT-1 (intermediate-1, 39% of patients), 3.3 years; INT-2 (intermediate-2, 22% of patients), 1.1 years; and high (8% of patients), 0.2 year. These categories also separate patients into risk groups for median survival: low, 5.7 years; INT-1, 3.5 years; INT-2, 1.2 years; and high, 0.4 year. The IPSS was adopted as the primary prognostic scoring system in MDS and remains the most widely used scoring system to date.

Table 20.1 WHO 2008 MDS classification

Subtype	Dysplasia	Cytopenia	Peripheral blood blast (%)	Bone marrow blast (%)
RCUD (RA, RN, RT)	Unilineage dysplasia in one of the cell lines	Unicytopenia or bilineage	<1	<5
RARS	Erythroid dysplasia and more than 15% ringed sideroblasts	Anemia	<1	<5
RCMD	Dysplasia in two or more cell lines	Cytopenia(s)	<1	<5
MDS with isolated del5(q)	Erythroid dysplasia	Anemia	<1	<5
MDS-U	Variable or if no dysplasia must be accompanied by know MDS recurrent cytogenetic abnormality	Pancytopenia in case of unilineage dysplasia	Cases of RCMD and RCUD with 1% blasts are classified as MDS-U	<5
RAEB-1	Variable	Cytopenia(s)	2–4	5–9
RAEB-II	Variable	Cytopenia(s)	5–19	10–19

Abbreviations: RCUD, refractory cytopenia with unilineage dysplasia; RA, refractory anemia; RN, refractory neutropenia; RT, refractory thrombocytopenia; RARS, refractory anemia with ring sideroblasts; RCMD, refractory cytopenia with multilineage dysplasia; MDS-U, MDS unclassified; RAEB, refractory anemia with excess blasts.

Newer prognostic models have been proposed that take into account the WHO diagnostic criteria. In 2007, Malcovati and colleagues published a time-dependent prognostic scoring system for predicting survival and leukemic evolution in the MDS: the WHO classification-based prognostic scoring system (WPSS) [11]. The most important variables in this prognostic model included WHO subtype, karyotype (using the cytogenetic pattern according to the IPSS), and transfusion requirement. The WPSS is a dynamic prognostic scoring system, whereas IPSS has prognostic relevance only at the time of diagnosis.

Treatment Response Criteria

The heterogeneity of the MDS makes evaluating response to treatment a challenge. Various criteria have been used to assess response in therapeutic trials, making it difficult to compare studies and their results. In 2000, an International Working Group (IWG) proposed standardized response criteria for evaluating clinically significant

Table 20.2   The international prognostic scoring system[a]

Myelogenous risk subgroup risk[b]	Score	Median survival (years)	Acute leukemia (AML)
Low	0	5.7	
			9.4
Intermediate-1	0.5–1.0	3.5	3.3
Intermediate-2	1.5–2.0	1.2	1.1
High	≥2.5	0.4	0.2

The score is based on the following parameters

Prognostic variable	0	0.5	1.0	1.5	2.0
BM blasts (%) 21–30	<5	5–10		–	11–20
Karyotype	Good (normal or 5q- or 20q- or -Y)	Intermediate		Poor (≥3 abnormalities or monosomy 7)	
Cytopenias (hemoglobin < 10 g/dL, absolute neutrophil count (ANC) <1,500/μL, platelet count < 100,000/μL)	0/1	2/3			

[a]Modified from Greenberg et al. [10].
[b]Number of years for 25% of the patients to evolve into acute myelogenous leukemia.

responses in MDS. The criteria included measures of alteration in the natural history of disease, hematologic improvement, cytogenetic and pathologic response, and improvement in health-related quality of life (QOL). The criteria have been validated prospectively in MDS clinical trials. In 2006, the IWG recommended minor to address limitations of the initial proposal [8] (Table 20.3 summarizes the IWG criteria for hematological improvement).

Treatment Algorithm for MDS

For higher-risk MDS (IPSS INT-2/High), treatment options include methyltransferase inhibitors and allogeneic stem cell transplantation [12]. It is beneficial to pursue allogeneic stem cell transplantation early in the disease course (if the patient is a candidate), for higher-risk MDS [13]. For lower-risk MDS (IPSS low/INT-1), treatment options include hematopoietic growth factors, lenalidomide, immunosuppressive therapy (in young patients, hypocellular marrow, +/− HLA-DR15) [13–15], and methyltransferase inhibitors. Patients with lower-risk MDS are typically treated with the goal of improving hematopoiesis and reducing the negative consequences of ineffective hematopoiesis, such as managing transfusional iron

Table 20.3 IWG 2000 and 2006 hematological improvement criteria

	IWG 2000	IWG 2006
Hematological improvement (HI)	Hematologic improvement (HI) (improvements must last at least 8 weeks in the absence of ongoing cytotoxic therapy.) 1. *Erythroid response (HI-E)* *Major response*: for patients with pretreatment hemoglobin less than 11 g/dL, greater than 2 g/dL increase in hemoglobin; for RBC transfusion-dependent patients, transfusion independence *Minor response*: for patients with pretreatment hemoglobin less than 11 g/dL, 1–2 g/dL increase in hemoglobin; for RBC transfusion-dependent patients, 50% decrease in transfusion requirements 2. *Platelet response (HI-P)* *Major response*: for patients with a pretreatment platelet count less than 100,000/mm^3, an absolute increase of 30,000/mm^3 or more; for platelet transfusion-dependent patients, stabilization of platelet counts and platelet transfusion independence *Minor response*: for patients with a pretreatment platelet count less than 100,000/mm^3, a 50% or more increase in platelet count with a net increase greater than 10,000/mm^3 but less than 30,000/mm^3 3. *Neutrophil response (HI-N)* *Major response*: for absolute neutrophil count (ANC) less than 1,500/mm^3 before therapy, at least a 100%increase, or an absolute increase of more than 500/mm^3, whichever is greater *Minor response*: for ANC less than 1,500/mm^3 before therapy, ANC increase of at least 100%, but absolute increase less than 500/mm^3 4. *Progression/relapse after HI*: One or more of the following: a 50% or greater decrement from maximum response levels in granulocytes or platelets, a reduction in hemoglobin concentration by at least 2 g/dL, or transfusion dependence	*Erythroid response* (pretreatment, <11 g/dL) Hb increase by ≥1.5 g/dL Relevant reduction of units of RBC transfusions by an absolute number of at least four RBC transfusions/8 weeks compared with the pretreatment transfusion number in the previous 8 weeks. Only RBC transfusions given for a Hb of <9.0 g/dL pretreatment will count in the RBC transfusion response evaluation *Platelet response* (pretreatment, <100,000/mm^3) Absolute increase of ≥ 30,000/mm^3 for patients starting with <20/mm^3 Increase from <20,000 to >20,000/mm^3 and by at least 100% *Neutrophil response* (pretreatment, <1,000/mm^3) At least 100% increase and an absolute increase > 500/mm^3 *Progression or relapse after HI* At least one of the following: At least 50% decrement from maximum response levels in granulocytes or platelets Reduction in Hb by ≥ 1.5 g/dL Transfusion dependence

overload with iron chelation therapy. As a result, these patients may best be managed initially with a trial of growth factors. Usually, 2–3 months of therapy is necessary to determine if treatment will be effective. Subsequent therapy may involve lenalidomide or hypomethylating agents (5-azacytidine or decitabine) (HMTA) [16–19].

Supportive Care and Transfusion Therapy

Supportive care measures, including the administration of hematopoietic growth factors and antibiotics as well as the transfusion of blood products, remain the mainstay of management for patients with MDS. With supportive care, the treatment goal is to reduce the morbidity from ineffective hematopoiesis and to improve quality of life. Anemic patients who do not respond to treatment may be chronically transfused. Patients with chronic transfusion requirements should be transfused in order to ameliorate symptoms, improve tissue oxygenation, QOL, and physical and intellectual activities [16]. Typically, most patients become symptomatic at a hemoglobin level of 8 g/dL or lower; however, the hemoglobin threshold for transfusion will vary between patients due to differences in age, comorbidities, lifestyle, and physical activity level at work. Regarding management of chronic neutropenia and thrombocytopenia, there is no evidence that routine prophylaxis with cytokines, antibiotics, or pro-coagulants will improve outcomes in the MDS.

In order to collect data on the characteristics and treatment patterns of US patients with MDS, Sekeres and colleagues conducted six consecutive cross-sectional surveys among US hematology and medical oncology physicians [20]. A questionnaire collected data on the four–ten most recently seen MDS patients for each physician. A panel of 101 physicians characterized 614–827 patients per survey, for a total of 4,514 responses. Among recently diagnosed MDS patients, fewer patients with lower-risk disease than with higher-risk disease were dependent on either RBC transfusions (22% vs 68%) or platelet transfusions (6% vs 33%). More than 50% of all newly diagnosed and established patients used erythropoiesis-stimulating agents (ESAs). Few patients were considered for or received a bone marrow transplantation (recently diagnosed: 4%; established: ≤4%) or treatment on clinical trials (recently diagnosed: 1%; established: ≤4%). These data demonstrate that US MDS patients have substantial transfusion requirements as well as substantial use of ESAs.

Erythropoietic-Stimulating Agents (ESAs)

Erythropoietin (EPO; epoetin alfa, Epogen, Amgen/Procrit, Ortho) reduces transfusion requirements in 16% of unselected anemic MDS patients who receive the equivalent of 40,000–80,000 units weekly [21]. The addition of granulocyte colony-stimulating factor (G-CSF) to EPO nearly doubles the response rate by increasing recruitment of erythropoietin-responsive erythroid bursts. Furthermore, appropriate patient selection can substantially increase response rates. Darbepoetin (Aranesp, Amgen) is a hypersialated form of EPO with a prolonged serum half-life, allowing less frequent dosing. Preliminary results suggest that this agent is at least as effective as epoetin alfa.

Mechanism of Action

EPO and G-CSF promote growth and differentiation of hematopoietic progenitors. In MDS, they also potently inhibit apoptosis mediated by the mitochondria. Erythroblasts in lower-risk MDS constitutively release cytochrome c (a pro-apoptotic molecule) from the mitochondria to the cytoplasm [22]. It has been shown that in RARS, mitochondrial iron accumulates in the form of aberrant mitochondrial ferritin (MtF) [23]. Thus, in some subtypes of MDS, the mitochondrion appears to play a central role in the pathogenesis.

Erythropoietin

Attempts at using EPO to improve the anemia of patients with MDS dates back to the early 1990s. It was shown at that time that EPO had low efficacy in unselected anemic patients with MDS. A meta-analysis of the early trials by Hellstrom-Lindberg et al. included 17 original articles with a total of 205 patients with MDS who had been treated with EPO [21]. Thirty-three patients (16%) showed a significant response to treatment. Patients with RARS showed a significantly lower response rate than all other patients (7.5% vs 21%, $P = 0.010$). Also, patients who required transfusion showed a significantly lower response rate than patients without the need for transfusion (10% vs 44%, $P < 0.001$). Moreover, the serum EPO level was significantly lower in responding patients, but this parameter alone could not be used to identify patients with a favorable response. Patients with MDS other than RARS and without transfusion requirement showed a response rate of $\geq 50\%$, irrespective of their serum EPO level. In patients with RARS and serum EPO > 200 U/L, no responses were observed.

Single, Weekly Dosing of Erythropoietin

A single, weekly dose of 40,000 U of recombinant erythropoietin has been shown to be at least as effective as the more frequent (daily or thrice weekly) administrations of the growth factor. An Italian study reported on the treatment of 13 patients with low-to-intermediate risk MDS with a single, weekly dose of 40,000 U for at least 8 weeks [24]. Five patients (38.4%) achieved a major erythroid response (hemoglobin increase > 2 g/dL and/or transfusion independence), which was maintained after 3–11 months of follow-up, without modification of the dose. Single, weekly dosing has since been widely adopted as the preferred administration schedule of EPO and has been validated in numerous trials.

Erythropoietin Plus Granulocyte Colony-Stimulating Factor

G-CSF has been shown to nearly double the response rate to EPO in MDS. In vitro bone marrow progenitor culture data demonstrated that G-CSF synergizes with EPO to expand the production of EPO-responsive erythroid bursts. As a result, Negrin and colleagues treated 55 MDS patients with a combination of recombinant human EPO and recombinant human G-CSF in an attempt to investigate its potential clinical benefit [25]. Fifty-three (96%) had a neutrophil response and 21 (40%) had an erythroid response. An erythroid response was significantly more likely in the patients with low serum EPO level, higher absolute reticulocyte counts, and normal cytogenetics at study entry. Seventeen (81%) of the patients who responded to G-CSF + EPO continued to respond during an 8-week maintenance phase. G-CSF was then discontinued. Eight of 17 continued to have an erythroid response with EPO alone, whereas in 7 of the remaining 9 patients, resumption of G-CSF recaptured the erythroid response. The median duration of response to EPO + G-CSF was 11 months. Six patients had more durable responses (15–36 months). In summary, approximately one-half of responding patients require both G-CSF and EPO to maintain an effective erythroid response.

Hellstrom-Lindberg and colleagues conducted a randomized phase II study with long-term follow-up of 71 patients with MDS treated with G-CSF + EPO [26, 27]. Patients with MDS and anemia were randomized to treatment with G-CSF + EPO, according to one of the two schedules: arm A starting with G-CSF for 4 weeks followed by the combination for 12 weeks and arm B starting with EPO for 8 weeks followed by the combination for 10 weeks. Fifty evaluable patients (10 RA, 13 RARS, and 27 RAEB) were included in the study, 3 evaluable only for EPO therapy, and 47 for the combined treatment. The overall response rate to G-CSF + EPO was 38%, similar to the Negrin study. The response rates according to FAB subtype were RA 20%, RARS 46%, and RAEB 37%. Response rates were identical in the two treatment arms. This trial showed that initial treatment with G-CSF was not required for a response to the combination. Long-term follow-up of 71 evaluable patients treated with G-CSF + EPO (from this study and the previous study) demonstrated a median survival of 26 months. During a median follow-up of 43 months, the overall risk of AML transformation was 28%. Twenty patients entered long-term maintenance treatment, with median duration of response of 24 months. The IPSS had no impact on primary response rates, but was effective to predict survival, leukemia transformation, and to a lesser extent, duration of response.

The Nordic MDS Group investigated pretreatment variables from their clinical trials for their ability to predict erythroid responses to treatment with G-CSF + EPO [27], 98 patients with MDS (30 RA, 31 RARS, 32 RAEB, 5 RAEB-t) were treated with a combination of G-CSF (0.3–3.0 mcg/kg/day, s.c.) and EPO (60–300 U/kg/day, s.c.) for at least 10 weeks. Minimum criteria for erythroid response were as follows: elimination of RBC transfusion need or an increase in Hb $\geq$ 1.5 g/dL with 35 patients (36%) responding to treatment for a median duration of 11–24 months. In multivariate analysis, serum EPO level and initial RBC transfusion needs retained statistical significance ($P < 0.01$). Using pretreatment serum EPO levels (<100, 100–500, or >500 U/L) and RBC transfusion need (<2 or ≥2 units/month), a predictive score for erythroid response was developed. The score divides patients into three groups: one with a high probability of erythroid responses (74%), one intermediate group (23%), and one with poor responses to treatment (7%).

Decision Models for Treating Anemia in MDS with EPO +/− G-CSF

In 2003, the Nordic MDS group devised a validated decision model for treating the anemia of MDS with EPO + G-CSF [28] (Fig. 20.1). A total of 53 patients with MDS (15 RA, 21 RARS, 17 RAEB; 16 IPSS low, 26 IPSS INT-1, 5 IPSS INT-2) from a prospective study were included in the validation sample. Patients with good or intermediate probability of response were treated with G-CSF + EPO. The overall response rate was 42%, with 28.3% achieving a complete response and 13.2% a partial response to treatment. The response rates were 61% in the good predictive group and 14% in the intermediate predictive group. The model retained a significant predictive value in the evaluation sample ($P < 0.001$), and the observed response rates did not differ from those expected by the model, thus confirming the utility of the model. The authors proposed a practical recommendation for the use of treatment with G-CSF + EPO, recommending that treatment begins with EPO alone for non-RARS patients and in non-transfused RARS patients. A dose of 50,000 U/week is probably sufficient for the majority of patients. However, based on the results of Negrin et al. [25], Hellstrom-Lindberg et al. [26], and Mantovani et al. [29], an

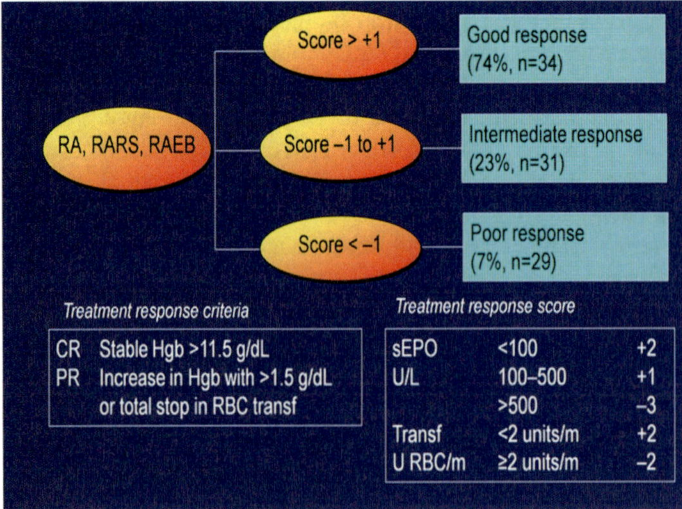

Fig. 20.1 Predictive model for erythroid-stimulating agents' response

increase in EPO dose up to 70,000 U or more could be considered, especially in cases with transfusion requirement and higher serum EPO levels. If there is still no response, then G-CSF could be added in a dose-adjusted manner to produce a clear rise in neutrophil count. RARS patients with pretreatment transfusion requirement should likely start therapy with the combination. It may also be possible that the addition of G-CSF may enable EPO doses to be lowered in some patients, which could lower the cost of the treatment.

In 2007, Sekeres and colleagues performed a Markov decision analysis that included 799 low-risk MDS patients treated with either growth factor (GF) or non-growth factor (NGF) therapies in an attempt to determine the appropriate initial therapy [30]. These treatment strategies were analyzed by categorizing patients into three different groups: either in the good GF predictive group (low-transfusion needs and low serum EPO levels), intermediate, or the poor GF predictive group (high-transfusion needs and high serum EPO levels). Patients receiving non-growth factor therapies were younger, with a median age of 65 years, compared with 69 years for patients receiving growth factors. Patients receiving NGF therapies had a lower response rate of 41.5%, compared with 46% for GF patients ($P < 0.05$), and were more likely to have received prior therapies ($P < 0.001$). Despite this, survival in the two groups did not differ, even after adjusting for age and baseline transfusion needs. After applying the decision model, life expectancies for the three GF predictive groups and the two treatment strategies were determined. In the good GF predictive group, initial therapy with GF improved survival compared with NGF therapies (3.38 vs 2.57 years). The advantage of GF to NGF therapies was lost when NGF therapies produced a response in $\geq$ 46% of patients. In the intermediate and poor GF predictive groups, NGF therapies maximized survival (2.57 vs 1.50 years and 2.57 vs 0.91 years, respectively), provided response rates for NGF were >14 and 4%, respectively, for each predictive group. The authors concluded that patients with low-risk MDS should be classified according to growth factor predictive models of response, with therapy tailored accordingly. Those in the good GF predictive group should almost always receive GFs, unless NGF approaches yield a high response rate. An example of this would be the use of lenalidomide for MDS associated with a 5q deletion cytogenetic abnormality, where response rates (defined as transfusion independence) are approximately two-thirds (Fig. 20.2).

Long-Term Outcome of Anemia Treatment in MDS with EPO and G-CSF

Jadersten et al. reported on long-term results of treatment of MDS with EPO and G-CSF [31]. A total of 129 patients were followed for up to 45 months after last inclusion in the Nordic MDS Group studies. Erythroid response rate was 39%. Median response duration was 23 months. Complete responders showed longer response duration than partial responders (29 vs 12 months, $P = 0.006$). IPSS groups' Low/INT-1 had longer response duration than INT-2/High (25 vs 7 months, $P = 0.002$). The time until 25% developed AML was longer in the good and intermediate predictive groups for erythroid response compared with the poor

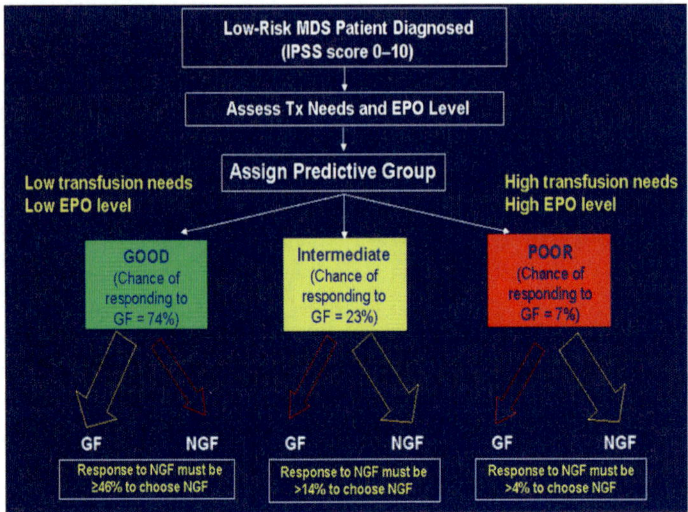

Fig. 20.2 Decision analysis of utilizing growth factors in lower-risk MDS

predictive group (52 vs 13 months, $P = 0.008$). Only 1 of 20 long-term responders developed AML. The effect on long-term outcome was then assessed by comparing treated patients with untreated patients selected from the IPSS database and adjusting for major prognostic variables. There was no difference in survival (OR, 0.9; $P = 0.55$) or risk of AML evolution (OR, 1.3; $P = 0.40$) between treated and untreated patients. The authors concluded that treatment with EPO and G-CSF does not affect overall survival or risk of AML evolution in comparison with supportive care only. Patients likely to benefit from treatment have high or intermediate probability of erythroid response according to the predictive model and belong to the IPSS categories Low or INT-1.

The same group subsequently conducted another analysis suggesting that treatment with EPO + G-CSF may improve survival in MDS [32]. They compared the long-term outcome of patients with MDS treated with EPO + G-CSF ($n = 121$) with untreated patients ($n = 237$) with MDS, adjusting for major prognostic variables. The EPO + G-CSF treated cohort included all patients from the three Nordic phase II trials. The control cohort was selected from an Italian cohort of consecutive untreated patients with MDS, based on the same criteria as for the EPO + G-CSF studies. The distribution of WHO groups, IPSS groups, transfusion-dependency, and predictive groups for response was all similar between the two cohorts. In the multivariate analysis, treatment was associated with improved overall survival (HR, 0.61; $P = 0.002$). This positive association was primarily observed in patients requiring < 2 units of RBCs per month. The authors emphasize that patients should be selected for this treatment carefully by excluding those in the poor predictive group for response. Also, EPO + G-CSF should be administered at the lowest possible dose. Furthermore, to avoid futility, treatment should be discontinued at the time of relapse of transfusion-dependency.

In the ECOG 1996 trial, Miller et al. evaluated the role of EPO +/− G-CSF for the treatment of anemic patients with MDS [33]. This was a phase III, prospective, randomized trial. One hundred and eighteen patients were enrolled and 105 were evaluable for response (RA, $n = 40$; RARS, $n = 36$; and RAEB, $n = 29$). Patients were initially randomized to either supportive therapy (ST) or EPO, 150 U/kg/day. Patients on the ST arm could cross over to the EPO arm if, after at least a 4-month period of observation, they had a $\geq 50\%$ increase in their transfusion requirement. In patients who did not respond to or did not maintain their response to EPO, G-CSF, 1 mcg/kg/day, was added. Patients who did not respond after 4 months received an increased dose of EPO (300 U/kg/day) + G-CSF. The response rate in the EPO arm was 35% versus 9% in the ST arm ($P = 0.002$). Of the 23 patients who crossed over from the ST arm, 30% responded to EPO. Six of 27 patients (22%) who received EPO 150 U/kg + G-CSF responded. Ten patients received EPO 300 U/kg + G-CSF and six (60%) responded. Transformation to acute leukemia occurred in 3.6 and 0% in the ST and EPO arms, respectively ($P = 0.50$). No difference in overall survival and AML transformation was seen between the EPO and ST arms, but there was a survival advantage for patients who had an erythroid response: median survival (MS) 53 months for responders versus 26 months for non-responders (P = 0.009). The pretreatment serum EPO level correlated with the response to treatment ($P = 0.004$): median EPO of 48 versus 140 μ/mL for responders versus non-responders. Responses were greater in RA > RARS > RAEB. These data suggest that survival is approximately doubled in anemic MDS patients who respond to treatment with EPO +/− G-CSF.

The French MDS group (GFM) analyzed prognostic factors of response, response duration, and possible impact on survival of treatment with EPO or DA +/− G-CSF in 403 MDS patients [34]. The erythroid response rate was 62% (40% major and 22% minor) using IWG 2000 criteria and 50% by IWG 2006 criteria. The median response duration was 20 and 24 months according to IWG 2000 and 2006 criteria, respectively. Significantly higher response rates were observed with <10% blasts, IPSS Low/INT-1, RBC transfusion independence, serum EPO level < 200 U/L, and, with IWG 2006 criteria only, shorter interval between diagnosis and treatment. Significantly longer response duration was associated with a major response (IWG 2000 criteria), IPSS Low/INT-1, <5% blasts, and absence of multilineage dysplasia. Multivariate-adjusted comparisons of survival between the French cohort and the untreated MDS cohort used to design the IPSS showed a comparable rate of progression to AML in both cohorts, but significantly better overall survival in the French cohort.

Darbepoetin

Darbepoetin alfa (DA) is a novel erythropoietic agent with greater sialic acid content, an approximately threefold longer terminal half-life, which allows for less frequent dosing, with a similar efficacy and safety profile and increased biological activity [35].

An Italian phase II study by Stasi and colleagues assessed the hematological changes associated with DA in anemic patients with previously untreated, IPSS Low/INT-1 MDS [36]. Fifty-three patients received DA s.c. once a week for 24 weeks. Treatment was initiated at 150 mcg fixed dose, and the dose was doubled if after the first 12 weeks, there was a suboptimal erythroid response. The final response rate was 24/53 (45%), with 21 major and 3 minor responses. Most responses were obtained at the 150 mcg dose. With a median follow-up of 9.4 months, 17 patients maintained their response. Treatment was well tolerated, with no relevant side effects. In multivariate analysis, only low serum EPO level (<200 U/L) predicted for response to therapy with DA.

The French MDS Group also conducted a phase II study with DA at a weekly dose of 300 mcg, s.c., in 62 anemic patients with MDS (with serum EPO level < 500 U/L) [37]. Most of the patients were classified as IPSS Low/INT-1. After 12 weeks, 44 (71%) patients had an erythroid response (34 major and 10 minor), including 8/13 patients who were previous non-responders to conventional EPO. The median dose of DA required to maintain response was 300 mcg every 14 days. Variables associated with favorable response to DA treatment were low serum EPO level and low or absent RBC transfusion need.

Gotlib and colleagues conducted a phase II intra-patient dose-escalation trial of weight-based DA +/− G-CSF in 24 patients with predominantly IPSS Low/INT-1 MDS [38]. Intra-patient dose escalation of DA was done in three 6-week dose cohorts until a major erythroid response was achieved: 4.5 mcg/kg/week, 9 mcg/kg/week, and 9 mcg/kg/week + G-CSF 2.5 mcg/kg twice weekly. RARS patients started on 9 mcg/kg/week. The weight-based dosing regimen resulted in a median starting DA dose of 390 mcg/week. Erythroid responses were observed in 16/24 patients (67%; 12 major and 4 minor). In major responders, the median response duration was 11 months. A major response was generated in 7/15 patients who suboptimally responded to DA alone with the addition of G-CSF. DA was well tolerated, except for one patient with diabetes who had worsening of mild baseline hypertension and renal insufficiency. The probability of erythroid response was increased by an IPSS score < 0.5 and RBC transfusion need of <2 units/month.

Efficacy of EPO Compared with that of Darbepoetin in the Treatment of Anemia in MDS?

A meta-analysis by Moyo and colleagues was performed to compare the erythroid response rates observed with EPO and darbepoetin in the treatment of anemic MDS patients [39]. The systematic review yielded 30 studies evaluating a total of 1,314 patients (EPO: 22 studies, 925 patients; darbepoetin: 8 studies, 389 patients). The pooled estimate of erythroid response rate was significantly higher for EPO IWG criteria studies (57.6%) versus non-IWG criteria studies (31.6%; $p < 0.001$). Study factors predictive of higher response rate in the EPO IWG criteria studies included a greater proportion of patients with RA/RARS ($p < 0.001$), lower mean baseline serum EPO level ($P = 0.007$), and fixed dosing regimen ($p < 0.001$). There was no difference in the pooled erythroid response rates between EPO (57.6%) and darbepoetin (59.4%; $P = 0.828$), suggesting that they have similar efficacy in MDS patients.

Adverse Effects of EPO and Darbepoetin

A meta-analysis of 57 studies including 9,353 cancer patients by Bohlius et al. showed that treatment with EPO or darbepoetin increases the risk of thromboembolic events, with a relative risk of 1.67 [40]. Among patients with chronic renal failure who were treated with ESAs to elevate hemoglobin levels into the normal range ($\geq$ 13.5 g/dL), as compared with those treated to achieve levels of 10.5–11.5 g/dL, an increased risk of death or cardiovascular or thromboembolic events has been demonstrated [41]. Flu-like symptoms, arthralgias, and cutaneous reactions may be seen at the initiation of treatment. Hypertension may also occur and should be monitored. In non-randomized clinical studies in MDS patients ESAs have been well tolerated with no reported increased risk of thrombosis or cardiovascular disease.

Combination Therapies with ESAs

In clinical practice, ESAs are often continued even if other lines of therapy are initiated. Ideally ESAs should be stopped after an adequate trial if ineffective.

Emerging data suggest the potential role of combining newer MDS therapies with ESAs. For example, lenalidomide, an approved immunomodulatory drug for treatment of MDS, enhances EPO receptor signaling in MDS erythroid precursors. In $CD34^+$ selected cells from normal marrow donors, treatment with lenalidomide or its analog, pomalidomide, induces the expansion of immature progenitors, and in particular, erythroid bursts. Both IMiDs delay erythroid maturation in vitro, while increasing the generation of immature erythroids that are erythropoietin responsive with coincident induction of hemoglobin transcription, with potent induction of hemoglobin-F [42, 43]. This provides a rational for testing combinations of lenalidomide and an ESA for treating MDS patients. In a pilot pharmacokinetic study in patients with Low and INT-1 risk who had failed prior ESA treatment, treatment with EPO 40,000 units/week was combined with lenalidomide in patients who did not respond to a 16-week trial of lenalidomide monotherapy. Forty patients were treated with lenalidomide monotherapy and 18 patients who did not respond to lenalidomide were treated with the lenalidomide and EPO combination. The major erythroid response rate was 35% with lenalidomide alone and 28% in patients with the combination therapy. Interestingly, these data suggest that lenalidomide can restore EPO responsiveness in a significant portion of patients. A high endogenous serum erythropoietin level prior to lenalidomide monotherapy was a predictor for response, whereas a low endogenous serum erythropoietin level before combination therapy was associated with response [44]. Based on this an ECOG sponsored phase III intergroup study for EPO-refractory patients with Low or INT-1 risk MDS will compare erythroid response rate to treatment with either lenalidomide monotherapy or combined with EPO.

Myeloid Growth Factors

Currently there is no evidence to support the routine use of either G-CSF or GM-CSF as monotherapy for the management of neutropenia in MDS patients. G-CSF and GM-CSF can increase the neutrophil counts in MDS patients. GM-CSF did neither affect hemoglobin levels nor the frequency of transformation to AML in two randomized clinical trials. In a randomized controlled trial in neutropenic MDS patients, G-CSF had no effect on survival, transformation to AML, or hemoglobin levels.

In our opinion, the myeloid growth factors, G-CSF or GM-CSF, have an established role in combination with ESA to improve erythropoiesis, for short-term use in cases of febrile neutropenia or recurrent infections and for interim management of drug-related neutropenia. In practice these growth factors are often used to treat or prevent neutropenia with newer agents such as hypomethylating agents or lenalidomide. Caution must be taken when these growth factors are used in the latter setting. Clonal evolution with emergence of chromosome 7 deletions, one of the most commonly acquired cytogenetic abnormality in MDS was reported in 3 of 12 deletion 5q patients treated in the MDS-001 trial in which myeloid growth factors were routinely applied [45]; whereas cytogenetic evolution involving this chromosome abnormality was rare in the MDS-003 and MDS-002 trials in which growth factors were used only sparingly. The G-CSF dependence of deletion 7/7q clones mandates restricted rather than prolonged growth factor administration [46].

Thrombopoietic Growth Factors

Thrombocytopenia and/or platelet dysfunction is common in MDS, with an estimated overall prevalence of non-treatment-related thrombocytopenia ranging from 40 to 65% [47]. Thrombocytopenia is more common in higher-risk disease and is frequently exacerbated by many of the therapies we use in MDS. The frequency of hemorrhagic death varies between 14 and 24% [47]. Thrombocytopenia remains the most challenging cytopenia to manage in MDS patients. Treatment is generally not lineage-specific and rather is part of the general treatment for MDS where, for example, hypomethylating agents may be considered. Thrombopoietic growth factors in the past had limited activity and excessive toxicity, which included agents such as interleukin-11 (oprelvekin) and interleukin-6. Development of recombinant thrombopoietin (TPO) was halted because of development of neutralizing antibodies that recognized the native protein with accompanied exacerbation of thrombocytopenia and in many cases, progression to severe aplastic anemia [47].

Oprelvekin (IL-11, Neumega®) was studied in two small safety and efficacy MDS trials with response rates of 38 and 27%, respectively. The duration of response was short but more importantly the side-effect profile of the drug and allergic reactions limited its further use in MDS. Similarly, IL-6 was studied in a small phase I study with a reported 36% response rate, however, like IL-11, rate adverse effects such as fever, fluid retention, and fatigue prevented prolonged administration [47].

More recently novel TPO receptor agonists have been developed for the treatment of ITP [48]. Romiplostim (AMG 531; Nplate®) is an Fc-peptide fusion protein (peptibody) linking two antibody Fc-domains with four TPO-R binding peptides that recognize the TPO receptor, c-mpl. In a phase I/II dose-escalating study, 44 thrombocytopenic patients ($\leq$50,000/μL) with low-risk MDS were treated with AMG 531. Doses ranged from 300 to 1,500 mcg 3 times/week. Platelet responses were observed in 41% of patients lasting a median duration of 22 weeks. The impact on the frequency of hemorrhagic events is not available. The clinical trial also raised safety concerns owing to an increased frequency of myeloblast stimulation with consequent elevation in bone marrow or peripheral blood blast percentage in more than 20% of patients [49]. Another TPO receptor ligand is eltrombopag, an oral small molecule TPO receptor agonist composed of four carbon-based rings containing both piperazine and hydrazine side chains. Eltrombopag binds to the TPO receptor at a site that is distinct from the binding site of the native TPO ligand and that of other receptor agonists [50]. In vitro, eltrombopag may have antileukemia and antiproliferative effects [51]. Eltrombopag is FDA-approved for the treatment of patients with ITP or thrombocytopenia associated with chronic hepatitis C infection. Plans for testing the safety and thrombopoietic potential of eltrombopag in treatment of thrombocytopenia in MDS are underway.

The Costs of Drugs Used to Treat MDS

As per an analysis performed by Greenberg et al., the estimated annual costs of growth factor therapy for MDS are significant: epoetin alfa (60,000–120,000 U/week, s.c.) = $26,076–$52,176; darbepoetin (300–500 mcg/week, s.c.) = $41,904–$87,300; and G-CSF (60 mcg 2–3 times/week) = $3,612–$5,424 [52]. In comparison, the annual cost of lenalidomide therapy (10 mg/day orally) is $94,584 and of iron chelation therapy with deferasirox (20 mg/kg/day orally) is $46,008. This analysis highlights the fiscal importance of proper patient selection for the appropriate therapies using the decision models described earlier.

Conclusions

If anemic MDS patients are carefully selected for treatment with EPO or darbepoetin +/− G-CSF, according to the decision model from the Nordic MDS group, approximately two-thirds of patients in the good predictive group (serum EPO $\leq$ 500 U/L and a transfusion need of <2 units/month) can be expected to experience an erythroid response, with the majority showing complete and durable responses, making them prime candidates for ESA treatment as initial therapy. It is recommended that treatment with either EPO or darbepoetin begins as monotherapy, at a dose of 40,000 U/week or 300 mcg/week, respectively. An escalation in EPO dose to 60,000 U or of darbepoetin to 400 mcg should be considered in non-responding patients. In the absence of response to dose adjustment, G-CSF can be added in a dose-adjusted manner to produce a discernable but not excess rise in neutrophil count. RARS patients are more likely to require the addition of G-CSF. It may also be possible that the addition of G-CSF may enable EPO doses to be lowered in some patients. Because of safety concerns pertaining to risk of thromboembolism, EPO + G-CSF should be administered at the lowest possible effective dose. Furthermore, because of cost and safety concerns, treatment should be discontinued at the time of relapse of transfusion-dependency. A role for the routine use of myeloid growth factors to manage persistent neutropenia is not established and their use should be limited to cases of neutropenic fever or infection- and treatment-induced neutropenia.

References

1. Greenberg P. The myelodysplastic syndromes. In: Hoffman R, Benz E, Shattil S, et al., editors. Hematology: basic principles & practice. 3rd ed. New York, NY: Churchill Livingstone; 2000. pp. 1106–29.
2. Cazzola M, Malcovati L. Myelodysplastic syndromes – coping with ineffective hematopoiesis. N Engl J Med. 2005;352(6):536–8.
3. Ma X, Does M, Raza A, et al. Myelodysplastic syndromes: incidence and survival in the United States. Cancer. 2007;109(8):1536–42.
4. Strom SS, Gu Y, Gruschkus SK, et al. Risk factors of myelodysplastic syndromes: a case–control study. Leukemia. 2005;19(11):1912–18.
5. Heaney M, Golde D. Myelodysplasia. N Engl J Med. 1999;340(21):1649–60.
6. Bennett JM, Catovsky D, Daniel MT, et al. Proposals for the classification of the acute leukaemias. French–American–British (FAB) co-operative group. Br J Haematol. 1976;33(4):451–8.
7. Vardiman JW, Harris NL, Brunning RD. The World Health Organization (WHO) classification of the myeloid neoplasms. Blood. 2002;100(7):2292–302.
8. Cheson BD, Greenberg PL, Bennett JM, et al. Clinical application and proposal for modification of the International Working Group (IWG) response criteria in myelodysplasia. Blood. 2006;108:419–25.
9. Swerdlow SH, Campo E, Harris NL, et al. WHO classification of tumours of haematopoietic and lymphoid tissues. 4th ed. 2008.
10. Greenberg P, Cox C, LeBeau MM, et al. International scoring system for evaluating prognosis in myelodysplastic syndromes. Blood. 1997;89(6):2079–88.
11. Malcovati L, Germing U, Kuendgen A, et al. Time-dependent prognostic scoring system for predicting survival and leukemic evolution in myelodysplastic syndromes. J Clin Oncol. 2007;25:3503–10.
12. Cutler CS, Lee SJ, Greenberg P, et al. A decision analysis of allogeneic bone marrow transplantation for the myelodysplastic syndromes: delayed transplantation for low-risk myelodysplasia is associated with improved outcome. Blood. 2004;104:579–85.
13. Saunthararajah Y, Nakamura R, Nam J, et al. HLA-DR15 (DR2) is overrepresented in myelodysplastic syndrome and aplastic anemia and predicts a response to immunosuppression in myelodysplastic syndrome. Blood. 2002;100(5):1570–4.

14. Molldrem JJ, Leifer E, Bahceci E, et al. Antithymocyte globulin for treatment of the bone marrow failure associated with myelodysplastic syndromes. Ann Intern Med. 2002;137(3): 156–63.
15. Shimamoto T, Iguchi T, Ando K, et al. Successful treatment with cyclosporine A for myelodysplastic syndrome with erythroid hypoplasia associated with T-cell receptor gene rearrangements. Br J Haematol. 2001;114(2):358–61.
16. Murphy MF, Wallington TB, Kelsey P, et al. British Committee for Standards in Haematology. Blood Transfusion Task Force. Guidelines for the clinical use of red cell transfusions. Br J Haematol. 2001;113:24–31.
17. Bowen D, Culligan D, Jowitt S, et al. UK MDS Guidelines Group. Guidelines for the diagnosis and therapy of adult myelodysplastic syndromes. Br J Haematol. 2003;120:187–200.
18. Leitch HA, Goodman TA, Wong KK, et al. Improved survival in patients with myelodysplastic syndrome (MDS) receiving iron chelation therapy. Blood. (ASH Annual Meeting Abstracts) 2006;108. Abstract 249.
19. Rose C, Brechignac S, Vassilief D, et al. Positive impact of iron chelation therapy (CT) on survival in regularly transfused MDS patients. A prospective analysis by the GFM. Blood. (ASH Annual Meeting Abstracts). 2007;110. Abstract 249.
20. Sekeres MA, Schoonen WM, Kantarjian H, et al. Characteristics of US patients with myelodysplastic syndromes: results of six cross-sectional physician surveys. J Natl Cancer Inst. 2008;100(21):1542–51.
21. Hellstrom-Lindberg E. Efficacy of erythropoietin in the myelodysplastic syndromes: a meta-analysis of 205 patients from 17 studies. Br J Haematol. 1995;89(1):67–71.
22. Tehranchi R, Fadeel B, Forsblom AM, et al. Granulocyte colony-stimulating factor inhibits spontaneous cytochrome *c* release and mitochondria-dependent apoptosis of myelodysplastic syndrome hematopoietic progenitors. Blood. 2003;101:1080–6.
23. Tehranchi R, Invernizzi R, Grandien A, et al. Aberrant mitochondrial iron distribution and maturation arrest characterizes early erythroid precursors in low-risk myelodysplastic syndromes. Blood. 2005;106:247–53.
24. Musto P, Falcone A, Sanpaolo G, et al. Efficacy of a single, weekly dose of recombinant erythropoietin in myelodysplastic syndromes. Br J Haematol. 2003;123(5):958.
25. Negrin RS, Stein R, Doherty K, et al. Maintenance treatment of the anemia of myelodysplastic syndromes with recombinant human granulocyte colony-stimulating factor and erythropoietin: evidence for in vivo synergy. Blood. 1996;87(10):4076–81.
26. Hellstrom-Lindberg E, Negrin R, Stein R, et al. Erythroid response to treatment with G-CSF plus erythropoietin for the anemia of patients with myelodysplastic syndromes: proposal for a predictive model. Br J Haematol. 1997;99(2):344–51.
27. Hellstrom-Lindberg E, Ahlgren T, Beguin Y, et al. Treatment of anemia in myelodysplastic syndromes with granulocyte colony-stimulating factor plus erythropoietin: results from a randomized phase II study and long-term follow-up of 71 patients. Blood. 1998;92(1):68–75.
28. Hellstrom-Lindberg E, Gulbrandsen N, Lindberg G, et al. A validated decision model for treating the anemia of myelodysplastic syndromes with erythropoietin + granulocyte colony-stimulating factor: significant effects on quality of life. Br J Haematol. 2003;120:1037–46.
29. Mantovani L, Lentini G, Hentschel B, et al. Treatment of anaemia in myelodysplastic syndromes with prolonged administration of recombinant human granulocyte colony-stimulating factor and erythropoietin. Br J Haematol. 2000;109(2):367–75.
30. Sekeres MA, Fu AZ, Maciejewski JP, et al. A decision analysis to determine the appropriate treatment for low-risk myelodysplastic syndromes. Cancer. 2007;109:1125–32.
31. Jadersten M, Montgomery SM, Dybedal I, et al. Long-term outcome of treatment of anemia in MDS with erythropoietin and G-CSF. Blood. 2005;106(3):803–11.
32. Jadersten M, Malcovati L, Dybedal I, et al. Erythropoietin and granulocyte-colony stimulating factor treatment associated with improved survival in myelodysplastic syndrome. J Clin Oncol. 2008;26:3607–13.
33. Miller KB, Kim HT, Greenberg P, et al. Phase III prospective randomized trial of EPO with or without G-CSF versus supportive therapy alone in the treatment of myelodysplastic

syndromes (MDS): results of the ECOG–CLSG trial (E1996). Blood. (ASH Annual Meeting Abstracts). 2004;104. Abstract 70.

34. Park S, Grabar S, Kelaidi C, et al. Predictive factors of response and survival in myelodysplastic syndrome treated with erythropoietin and G-CSF: the GFM experience. Blood. 2008;111(2):574–82.

35. Egrie JC, Dwyer E, Browne JK, et al. Darbepoetin alfa has a longer circulating half-life and greater in vivo potency than recombinant human erythropoietin. Exp Hematol. 2003;31(4):290–9.

36. Stasi R, Abruzzese E, Lanzetta G, et al. Darbepoetin alfa for the treatment of anemic patients with low- and intermediate-1-risk myelodysplastic syndromes. Ann Oncol. 2005;16:1921–7.

37. Mannone L, Gardin C, Quarre MC, et al. High-dose darbepoetin alpha in the treatment of anaemia of lower risk myelodysplastic syndrome: results of a phase II study. Br J Haematol. 2006;133:513–19.

38. Gotlib J, Lavori P, Quesada S, et al. A phase II intra-patient dose-escalation trial of weight-based darbepoetin alfa with or without granulocyte-colony stimulating factor in myelodysplastic syndromes. Am J Hematol. 2009;84:15–20.

39. Moyo V, Lefebvre P, Duh MS, et al. Erythropoiesis-stimulating agents in the treatment of anemia in myelodysplastic syndromes: a meta-analysis. Ann Hematol. 2008;87(7):527–36.

40. Bohlius J, Wilson J, Seidenfeld J, et al. Recombinant human erythropoietins and cancer patients: updated meta-analysis of 57 studies including 9353 patients. J Natl Cancer Inst. 2006;98(10):708–14.

41. Khuri FR. Weighing the hazards of erythropoiesis stimulation in patients with cancer. N Engl J Med. 2007;356:2445–8.

42. Moutouh-de Parseval LA, Verhelle D, Glezer E, et al. Pomalidomide and lenalidomide regulate erythropoiesis and fetal hemoglobin production in human CD34$^+$ cells. J Clin Invest. 2008;118(1):248–58.

43. Verhelle D, Corral LG, Wong K, et al. Lenalidomide and CC-4047 inhibit the proliferation of malignant B cells while expanding normal CD34$^+$ progenitor cells. Cancer Res. 2007;67(2):746–55.

44. List AF, Lancet JE, Melchert M, et al. Two-stage pharmacokinetic & efficacy study of lenalidomide alone or combined with recombinant erythropoietin (EPO) in lower risk MDS EPO-failures [PK-002]. Blood. (ASH Annual Meeting Abstracts) 2007;110(11):4626.

45. Bernasconi P, Catherine K, Marina B, et al. Has cytogenetic evolution any prognostic relevance in myelodysplastic syndromes (MDS)? A study on 153 patients. Blood. (ASH Annual Meeting Abstracts) 2007;110(11):2460.

46. Sloand EM, Yong AS, Ramkissoon S, Solomou E, et al. Granulocyte colony-stimulating factor preferentially stimulates proliferation of monosomy 7 cells bearing the isoform IV receptor. Proc Natl Acad Sci USA. 2006;103(39):14483–8.

47. Kantarjian H, Giles F, List A, et al. The incidence and impact of thrombocytopenia in myelodysplastic syndromes. Cancer. 2007;109(9):1705–14.

48. Bussel JB, Kuter DJ, George JN, et al. AMG 531, a thrombopoiesis-stimulating protein, for chronic ITP. N Engl J Med. 2006;355(16):1672–81.

49. Kantarjian H, Fenaux P, Sekeres MA, et al. Phase 1/2 study of AMG 531 in thrombocytopenic patients (pts) with low-risk myelodysplastic syndrome (MDS): update including extended treatment. Blood. (ASH Annual Meeting Abstracts) 2007;110(11):250.

50. Bussel JB, Cheng G, Saleh MN, et al. Eltrombopag for the treatment of chronic idiopathic thrombocytopenic purpura. N Engl J Med. 2007;357(22):2237–47.

51. Erickson-Miller CL, Delorme E, Tian SS, et al. Preclinical activity of eltrombopag (SB-497115), an oral, non-peptide thrombopoietin receptor agonist. Stem Cells (Dayton, Ohio). 2009 Feb;27(2):424–30.

52. Greenberg PL, Cosler LE, Ferro SA, et al. The costs of drugs used to treat myelodysplastic syndromes following national comprehensive cancer network guidelines. J Natl Compr Canc Netw. 2008;6(9):942–53.

Chapter 21
Hematopoietic Growth Factors in Older Cancer Patients

Michelle Shayne and Lodovico Balducci

Introduction

Approximately 80% of all malignancies arise in individuals over age 60 [1]. While evidence suggests that chemosensitivity of certain neoplasms may diminish with increasing age [2, 3], similar benefits from systemic chemotherapy have been observed regardless of age, provided adequate treatment doses are employed [4–8]. Nevertheless, older age remains an independent risk factor for substantial reductions in chemotherapy relative dose intensity (RDI) [9], potentially resulting in compromised outcomes. Reduction in chemotherapy dosing for elderly patients is not entirely unfounded. Dose reductions occur largely in response to the established association between older age and hematologic toxicity, particularly febrile neutropenia. Neutropenic complications in elderly patients are associated with prolonged hospitalization and higher mortality among hospitalized patients [10]. Myeloid growth factors have been employed in the setting of chemotherapy use in order to mitigate the precipitous decline in white blood cells associated with many chemotherapeutic regimens. Administration of myeloid growth factors may accordingly facilitate the delivery of full doses of chemotherapy in order to optimize parameters of survival. A positive impact of quality of life can be observed, as well, when neutropenic complications and their associated risks are minimized.

Red blood cell growth factors have been employed in older cancer patients in order to limit the need for transfusion due to chemotherapy-associated anemia and to limit anemia-related symptoms.

This chapter will address mechanisms for increased susceptibility of older patients to chemotherapy-related hematologic toxicities and strategies for employing hematopoietic growth factors to limit these toxicities and optimize quality of life for these patients. Current guidelines on the use of hematopoietic growth factors

M. Shayne (✉)
Division of Hematology/Oncology, University of Rochester, Rochester, NY 14607, USA
e-mail: michelle.shayne@urmc.rochester.edu

G.H. Lyman, D.C. Dale (eds.), *Hematopoietic Growth Factors in Oncology*,
Cancer Treatment and Research 157, DOI 10.1007/978-1-4419-7073-2_21,
© Springer Science+Business Media, LLC 2011

and economic considerations will be discussed, as well as controversies regarding erythroid growth factor use.

Myeloid Growth Factor Use in Older Cancer Patients

Hematologic complications of chemotherapy such as febrile neutropenia comprise one of the major chemotherapeutic dose-limiting toxicities. Since older age is associated with increased risk for developing neutropenic complications [10], the practice of employing significant chemotherapy dose reductions as a means of mitigating hematologic toxicities in older patients is common.

In a community-based study of 20,799 breast cancer patients, women of 65 years of age and older were more likely to receive significant reductions in chemotherapy dose intensity compared to younger patients and almost 15% of the older women received less than 50% of the reference-standard dose intensity [11]. The major reason for dose reductions in RDI is chemotherapy-related toxicity, particularly neutropenic complications [12]. Multiple risk models for neutropenic complications in cancer patients undergoing systemic chemotherapy have identified increasing age as a significant independent predictor of such risk [13]. The incidence of myelotoxicity increased after age 65 in the experience of the Breast Cancer International Research Group (BCIRG) and consequently, approximately 40% of the older women received a total dose of chemotherapy less than two-thirds of the planned dose [14]. The incidence of neutropenic infection in a study of 500 unselected large-cell lymphoma patients in the community treated with CHOP/CNOP (cyclophosphamide, adriamycin/mitoxantrone, vincristine, prednisone) was 38% for patients of 65 years of age and older as compared to 18% for younger patients. Duration of hospitalization for neutropenic complications was 25% (4 days) longer for the older patients [15]. Furthermore, more neutropenia-related deaths occur in older patients [16].

Effective dosing of chemotherapy need not be synonymous with compromised safety in older cancer patients. Aside from dose reduction, strategies to reduce risk of neutropenic complications include optimization of comorbid conditions, judicious use of prophylactic antibiotics, substitution of particularly myelotoxic agents with near equi-efficacious alternatives, as well as utilization of prophylactic myeloid growth factors when the risk of chemotherapy-induced neutropenic complications reaches or exceeds 10% [17]. Of these approaches, the use of prophylactic growth factors such as granulocyte colony-stimulating factors (G-CSF) and granulocyte–macrophage colony-stimulating factors (GM-CSF) is the strategy with the most consistent evidence for reducing risk of neutropenic complications in older cancer patients. Several randomized controlled studies have demonstrated significant risk reduction as high as 50% in development of neutropenic events for patients of 65 years of age and older as a result of CSF use [18–21]. Furthermore, some of the other previously listed prevention strategies are burdened by additional concerns, such as emergence of antibiotic resistance in the case of prophylactic antibiotic use, which in one study was reported at 60% [22]. In addition, the use of substituted chemotherapy agents may undermine outcome.

Risk Factors for Myelotoxicity in Older Cancer Patients

Several variables contribute to increasing risk of myelotoxicity in older patients undergoing systemic chemotherapy. In general, aging is associated with the potential for reduction in functional reserve, increased prevalence of comorbid medical conditions, as well as decline in cognitive, emotional, nutritional, and socioeconomic domains. While the effects of aging on the hematopoietic system in general are modest, these may become more pronounced after age 65 [23]. On the cellular level, older persons may have a limited ability to increase hematopoiesis in response to stressors such as infection or cytotoxic treatment as a result of fundamental dysregulation in cytokine production. The expression of GM-CSF among healthy patients of age 67–80 compared to young controls in one study was significantly decreased [24]. Increased circulating levels of proinflammatory cytokines in older persons may also impede hematopoietic progenitor response as well as interfere with hematopoietic growth factor precursors [25]. Nevertheless, evidence does suggest that older persons are responsive to growth factors such as G-CSF and GM-CSF [26].

Since the hematopoietic system is a major site of chemotherapy-induced collateral damage, we will review the influence of aging on hematopoiesis in further detail below.

Age and Hematopoiesis

Hematopoiesis involves the commitment of pluripotent hemopoietic stem cells (PHSC) into hematopoietic progenitors and the differentiation of these progenitors into marrow precursors from which mature circulating blood elements are derived [27] (Fig. 21.1). The PHSC are unique in their ability to enter different hematopoietic lineages, while hematopoietic progenitors may differentiate only into one lineage. The PHSC have a large capacity for self-replication, while this ability becomes progressively more reduced in progenitors and precursors. The proliferative rates of PHSC and of early progenitors are lower than that of differentiated precursors. It is this lower proliferation rate which shelters these elements from the damage of cycle-active chemotherapy. Commitment, differentiation, and maturation require an intact hematopoietic microenvironment, responsible for the homing of PHSC and for the production of hematopoietic cytokines [28, 29].

Hematopoiesis can be disrupted at several levels. These include a decline in PHSC reserve, due to exhaustion or loss of homing by the bone marrow microenvironment, reduced production of hematopoietic cytokines, decreased sensitivity of

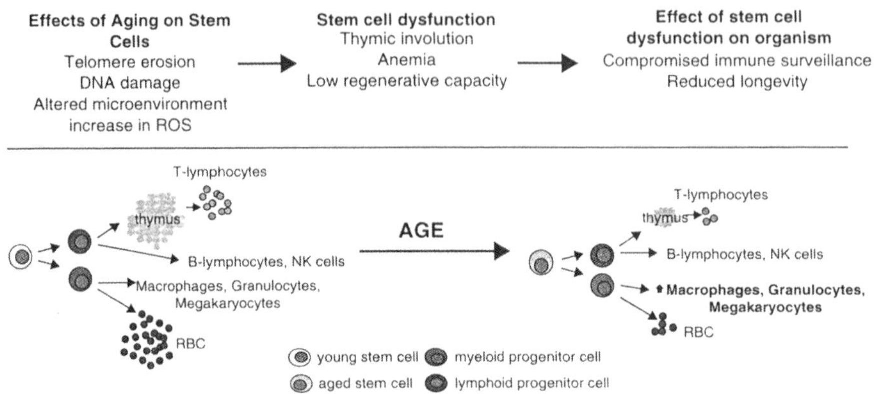

Fig. 21.1 Stem cell theory of aging

PHSC and hematopoietic progenitors to these cytokines, and microenvironmental alterations.

The reserve of PHSC may become reduced with age, as suggested by animal experiments and studies with humans. The self-replicative ability of murine hematopoietic stem cells is progressively reduced in serial transplants and recovery from hematopoietic injury is slower and less complete in older animals [30]. A progressive reduction of the telomere length and of telomerase activity in PHSC of older rodents further supports the increasingly limited self-replicative potential of PHSC with aging [27]. Hematopoietic stress produced by cage isolation or by injection of *Esherichia coli* endotoxin [31] has been shown to lead to a rapid reduction of the concentration of PHSC in older but not in younger animals. In humans, age-related reduction of hematopoiesis is suggested by: a) a progressive decline in hematopoietic tissue [32]; b) increased infection-related mortality [33]; c) a more limited proportion of circulating early hematopoietic precursors following injection of granulocyte–macrophage colony-stimulating factor (GM-CSF) [34]; d) increased incidence and prevalence of anemia of unknown origin [35]; and e) an increased risk of neutropenia, neutropenic infections, and thrombocytopenia following cytotoxic chemotherapy [36, 37]. Furthermore, the self-replicative ability of the early pluripotent hematopoietic progenitors CFU-GM declines progressively with age [38], as does the concentration of circulating CD34 cells [39].

Data regarding the production of hematopoietic cytokines in the aged are inconclusive. One study reported a decline in the production of GM-CSF by human monocytes "in vitro" [40], while other investigators reported "in vitro" decreased production of GM-CSF after phytohemoagglutinin stimulation from mononuclear cells obtained from healthy subjects aged 100 and older [38]. Interestingly, no difference was found between mononuclear cells obtained from patients aged 66–73 and those aged 30–45. In some cases of otherwise unexplained anemia, reduced circulating levels of erythropoietin were found in older patients [41, 42]. While it is possible that in at least some cases subclinical renal insufficiency may be responsible for this finding, a recent study revealed a primary deficiency in the production of erythropoietin in some older individuals [42]. These findings are limited to a small fraction of older individuals, however, and cannot be generalized to all the aged. Erythropoietin production in response to anemia does not appear affected by age, and some studies have demonstrated that the concentration of circulating erythropoietin was increased for persons over 70 as compared with younger persons with iron deficient anemia [41–43]. This observation may have been due to the development of anoxia for higher hemoglobin levels in older than in younger individuals. Age is associated with a chronic and progressive inflammatory status and increased circulating levels of catabolic cytokines including interleukin 6 (IL-6) and tumor necrosis factor (TNF) that may inhibit the production of hematopoietic growth factors [41].

Experimental studies are also inconclusive. In senescence-accelerated mice (SAM), the production of colony-inhibiting activity (CIA) in the bone marrow in response to lipopolysaccharide in one study was increased [44]. In young mice, lipopolysaccharide increased production of colony-stimulating activity, which in turn was followed by production of CIA.

The information related to age and sensitivity of hematopoietic elements to hematopoietic growth factors is limited and circumstantial. Decreased tolerance of hematopoietic stress by older rodents and older humans suggests impaired responsiveness of hematopoietic progenitors to hematopoietic cytokines [31]. In one study, the recovery of the original hematocrit was delayed in older polycythemic mice after phlebotomy, suggesting reduced responsiveness to erythropoietin [45].

Some authors have reported that the erythropoietic enhancement "in vitro" in the marrow of older individuals following indocin is reduced [46, 47]. Others have found that higher levels of erythropoietin were necessary to induce the same reticulocytic response in older than in younger anemic individuals [48, 49]. According to another study [38], "in vitro" responsiveness of pluripotent hematopoietic precursors to erythropoietin, G-CSF, and GM-CSF was well maintained even in persons aged 100 and older. Regardless of whether the sensitivity of early hematopoietic progenitors to physiologic amounts of growth factors is reduced, the response to pharmacologic doses of G-CSF, GM-CSF [50], and erythropoietin [51] appear to be unaffected by age.

Concerning changes in the hematopoietic microenvironment, most of the evidence comes from the bone marrow transplant literature. Age is a risk factor for reduced engraftment of allogeneic marrow, which suggests reduced ability to home hematopoietic stem cells [52]. The success of non-myeloablative transplants and of autologous stem cell rescues in patients over 70 indicates that the bone marrow microenvironment may still be able to home stem cells in older individuals [53, 54].

Age and Toxicity of Cancer Chemotherapy

A number of pharmacokinetic parameters change with increasing age [36] (Table 21.1). Aging is associated with a progressive decline in glomerular filtration rate. This can lead to toxicity in the setting of chemotherapy agents whose

Table 21.1 Pharmacokinetic parameters and consequences of aging

Parameter	Age-related effect
Absorption	• Decreased splanchnic circulation
	• Decreased gastric mobility and secretion
	• Decreased absorptive surface
Volume of distribution (Vd)	• Decreased lean body weight
	• Decreased albumin concentration
	• Decreased red blood cell mass
Hepatic metabolisms	• Decreased liver weight
	• Reduced splanchnic circulation
	• Reduced activity of p450 cytochrome reactions
	• Increased risk of drug interactions
Renal excretion	• Reduced glomerular filtration rate (GFR)
	• Reduced tubular reabsorption
Biliary excretion	• Appears well maintained

parent compounds are eliminated through the kidney (bleomycin, methotrexate, carboplatin) and drugs with active (idarubicinol, daunorubinol) or toxic (arauridine from high-dose cytarabine) metabolites eliminated by the kidneys. Risk modeling using a cohort of 1,449 cancer patients of 65 years of age and older treated in the community setting has demonstrated that an elevation in baseline GFR is an independent risk factor for neutropenic complications [37]. In addition, there may be increased limitations in hepatic uptake and metabolism of certain chemotherapeutic agents associated with aging. Hepatic metabolism of drugs decreases with increasing age due to a reduction in splanchnic circulation and hepatocyte mass. A baseline alkaline phosphatase level in excess of 120 U/L prior to initiation of chemotherapy is an independent risk factor for the development of neutropenic complications in cancer patients of 65 years of age and older [37].

The volume of distribution of water-soluble drugs is reduced in older persons. This can increase the serum concentration of these drugs and result in greater toxicity [55]. This occurs with aging due to progressive loss of body protein, a reduction in serum albumin [56], and decreased red cell mass [57].

Understanding these risk factors and how they contribute to chemotherapy-related hematologic toxicity in older cancer patients forms the basis for existing supportive care guidelines. A number of chemotherapy complications are more common in the elderly [36] (Table 21.2). We will discuss hematopoietic complications that are most common and/or most severe.

Table 21.2 Acute chemotherapy complications that become more common and severe with age

Myelodepression (virtually all chemotherapy drugs)
Mucositis (fluorinated pyrimidine, anthracyclines)
Cardiomyopathy (anthracyclines, trastuzumab)
Peripheral neuropathy (taxanes, vinca alkaloids, platinum derivatives)
Cerebellar dysfunction (cytarabine in high doses)

Table 21.3 Age and myelotoxicity of cancer chemotherapy: results of six retrospective trials

References	No. of patients	Patients ≥ 70 (%)	Source
Begg and Carbone [58]	5,459	780 (13%)	ECOG database
Gelman and Taylor [59]	231	31 (13%)	Dana Farber Cancer center: Patients over 65 years had been treated prospectively with dose-adjustment for cyclophosphamide and methotrexate and 2/3 FU dose and results compared with 161 fully evaluable younger patients Patients over 80 experienced shortened survival
Christman et al. [60]	170	70 (42%)	Piedmont Oncology Group database; high degree of patients selection
Giovannazzi-Bannon et al. [61]	672	• 65: 271 (40.3%) • 70: (25%)	Illinois cancer center phase II trials
Ibrahim et al. [62]	1,011	• 65: 244 (24%) • 70: (20%)	MD Anderson Hospital patients with metastatic breast cancer aged 50 and older
Ibrahim et al. [63]	390	• 65: 65 (18%) • 70: (< 10%)	MD Anderson Hospital patients with breast cancer receiving anthracycline-containing adjuvant chemotherapy

At least six clinical studies failed to demonstrate an increased risk and severity of myelotoxicity in patients of age over 65 or 70 as compared with younger patients (Table 21.3) [58–63].

These studies establish that chronologic age alone is not a contraindication to cytotoxic chemotherapy. These results do not necessarily apply to the general population of older patients because the studies are retrospective; include only a minority of patients of age over 75 and virtually no patient over the age 80; were conducted by major cooperative oncology groups or major cancer centers, including patients who were highly selected; and used older treatment regimens that were generally less aggressive than those currently in use.

A more realistic picture emerges from the overview of 500 patients with large-cell lymphoma treated in the community [64]. The risk of neutropenic infections was about 40% for those aged 65 and older and 18% for the younger ones. Furthermore, hospitalization for infections was 25% longer for the older individuals [65]. This finding is particularly troubling as hospitalization is a major cause of deconditioning and functional dependence for older individuals.

The association of aging with chemotherapy-induced myelosuppression is confirmed by a number of studies [66–76]. A number of trials have explored different forms of chemotherapy in elderly patients with non-Hodgkin's lymphoma [66, 70–76]. In all these studies the risk of severe neutropenia was higher than 50% and that of neutropenic infection was around 25%. The risk of death was between 5 and 30%. It is reasonable to assume that the risks of serious toxicity be even higher in the general population, as the patients involved in these studies were highly selected. The risk of more prolonged neutropenia, neutropenic infections, and neutropenic death is also increased among older patients (aged 60 and older) with acute myelogenous leukemia [77]. This may be, in part, due to the nature of the disease itself, as the PHSC itself may be abnormal in AML in the elderly.

The information related to the thrombocytopenia is more limited; in the lymphoma studies the incidence of grade III and IV thrombocytopenia was about 20%, which is higher than that reported in younger individuals.

Even less information related to chemotherapy-induced anemia exists. In older individuals anemia may be associated with a number of complications [78]. These include

- Fatigue that heralds increased functional dependence and mortality [79, 80].
- Increased risk of drug-related complications, especially delirium [81], and complications of cytotoxic chemotherapy [82].
- Increased risk of geriatric syndromes, including falls and dementia [83–85].

Indications for Growth Factor Use

Myelopoietic growth factors: The effectiveness of filgrastim in older patients is well established [20, 21, 86–88]. Price et al. administered G-CSF to young and old (≥70) healthy volunteers and found similar increase in neutrophil count and in the marrow neutrophil mitotic pool and similar reduction in the neutrophil marrow transit time [86]. Five studies [18, 20, 21, 87, 88] (Table 21.4) showed that prophylactic G-CSF reduced by 50–75% the risk of neutropenia and neutropenic infections in older individuals treated with CHOP. In a randomized controlled study of approximately 800 patients aged 65 and over, with lymphoma or metastatic breast, lung, or ovarian cancer, Balducci et al. demonstrated a 60% reduction in the risk of neutropenic infections [89].

The effectiveness of filgrastim and sarmograstim in AML is more controversial [90–98] (Table 21.5). It is clear that these cytokines do not increase the risk of leukemic relapse and reduce the risk of neutropenic infections when used following marrow aplasia during induction and after consolidation with high-dose cytarabine. It is less clear whether these drugs have an effect on early death, remission rate, and long-term survival. Only two studies, obtained a prolongation of overall survival and sarmograstim was used in both of them [90, 94].

Clearly, filgrastim and pegfilgrastim are the only agents of proven efficacy in solid tumors and lymphoma. In patients with AML both growth factors seem to

Table 21.4 Randomized and controlled studies demonstrating the benefits of hemopoietic growth factors in older patients with large-cell lymphoma receiving combination chemotherapy

Study	Patient number	Incidence of grade III and IV neutropenia (%)	Incidence of neutropenic infections (%)
Zinzani [71], VNCOP-B	350		
G-CSF		23	5
No G-CSF		56	21
Zagonel [87], CHOP			
G-CSF		4.8	4.8
No G-CSF		27.7	15.6
Bertini [88], VEPBC	90		
G-CSF		22	2
No G-CSF		44	9
Osby [74], CHOP and CNOP			
G-CSF		62	31
No G-CSF		91	47
Doorduijn [75], CHOP			
G-CSF			8
No G-CSF			14

reduce the risk of infections and hospitalizations and sarmograstim may improve survival.

Erythropoietin: Erythropoietin is effective in several forms of anemia including anemia associated with renal insufficiency [95] and anemia of inflammation that includes cancer-related anemia [96] and chemotherapy-related anemia [99, 100]. Both epoetin α and darbepoetin α appear effective in older individuals, in pharmacologic doses. Improvement of anemia has resulted in reduction of fatigue [101] that in older patient is harbinger of functional dependence [80]. The enthusiasm for these compounds has been tempered by a number of studies suggesting that they may increase the risk of thromboembolic diseases and the risk of cancer-related death in cancer patients [102, 103]. It should be emphasized that the risk of death does not appear increased when the levels of hemoglobin are maintained at ≤ 12 g/dL in patients receiving chemotherapy. Hopefully, once that the real risks of these preparations are established, important questions regarding red cell growth factor use in older cancer patients may be addressed such as whether these drugs may prevent functional dependence by relieving fatigue or mitigate chemotherapy-related dementia exacerbated in the presence of anemia.

Concerns about the use of hemopoietic growth factors: A number of concerns have been raised regarding hematopoietic growth factors. These include

Table 21.5 Hemopoietic growth factors in acute myeloid leukemia: randomized trials

References	No. of patients, ages	Conditions of use	RR (%)	Survival	Reduced days of neutropenia
Rowe et al. [90]	117, 55–75	After induction			5–6
GM-CSF			60	10.6 months	
No GM-CSF			44	4.8 months	
Heil et al. [91]	521, 16+	After induction and consolidation			−5
G-CSF			68	13 months	
No G-CSF			68	13 months	
Lowenberg et al. [92]	318, 61+	Induction; during and after chemotherapy			−2
GM-CSF			56	22	
No GM-CSF			55	22	
Zittoun et al. [93]	102	Induction			−1.5
GM-CSF		Before and during CT	77		
GM-CSF		After CT	48		
GM-CSF		Before, during and after CT	46		
No GM CSF			77		
Witz et al. [94]	240, 55–75	During induction and after			−6
GM-CSF			63	48	
No GM-CSF			60.5	21	
Stone et al. [95]	379, >55	Induction and consolidation		ND	−2
GM-CSF			51		
No GM-CSF			54		
Dombret et al. [96]	173, >65	Induction		ND	−6
GM-CSF			70		
No GM-CSF			41		
Ohno [97]	58, any age	Induction		ND	−12
G-CSF			50		
No G-CSF			37		
Godwin et al. [98]	234	Induction			−3 to 4
G-CSF			41	9 months	
No G-CSF			50	6 months	

ND = no data

- Administration-related discomfort, involving especially bone pain for G-CSF, and flu-like syndrome for GM-CSF. In our experience, the discomfort due to hematopoietic growth factors may be prevented by regular administration of acetaminophen and concern about discomfort should not prevent the administration of the drug.

- Hematopoietic exhaustion and stem cell competition: This concern is mostly theoretical. Hematopoietic exhaustion has not been observed in mice with accelerated hematopoiesis with G-CSF-producing tumors or in humans treated with filgrastim, lenograstim, or sarmograstim. Few cases of pure red blood cell aplasia were observed with epoetin α and β, in patients with renal insufficiency [104]. These complications occurred only in Europe and were ascribed to manufacturing problems.
- Stimulation of tumor growth: The concern that hematopoietic growth factors may lead to acute myeloid leukemia has never been conclusively supported by clinical experience. Two retrospective studies of a large group of women who had received adjuvant chemotherapy for breast cancer had suggested that the risk of AML was increased 10 years later as a result of the use of growth factor [105, 106]. The leukemogenic effect was more pronounced in older women. The effect, not confirmed in other studies [107, 108], appears to be relatively small. As such, it would not offset the potential benefits of these compounds. As already mentioned, enhanced growth of some tumors, particularly cancer of the breast and of the head and neck, has been ascribed to epoetin α and darbepoetin α use [106]. More studies are needed to confirm this effect and to establish its mechanism. Currently it appears prudent to use these compounds only when the hemoglobin levels are lower than 12 g/dL.

Timing of G-CSF Administration

The optimal timing of G-CSF administration has been investigated. Prophylactic use of pegfilgrastim in patients of 65 years of age and older has been shown to demonstrate a decrease in total number of neutropenic infections as well as neutropenic-related delay in chemotherapy administration or dose reduction [109]. Furthermore, most neutropenic events occur after the first cycle of chemotherapy for cancer patients [110, 111], including individuals of 70 years of age and older [37]. A population-based assessment of hospitalizations for chemotherapy-related neutropenia in older patients with non-Hodgkin's lymphoma demonstrated that 22% of the older patients in the cohort required hospitalization. Of these patients, 41% were hospitalized in cycle 1 and 22% in the second cycle [112]. These findings would support prophylactic use of growth factors, i.e., targeted use in high-risk patients early on in treatment as opposed to administration in reaction to a neutropenic-related event such as infection or myelosuppression necessitating chemotherapy dose reduction or delay. In a cohort of 999 cancer patients of age 70 and older receiving systemic chemotherapy, CSF was used in 33% of patients over the first four cycles of treatment, including 14% prophylactic CSF use in the first cycle [37]. In a prospective study of 117 randomly selected US community oncology practices that included 1,474 breast cancer patients, of whom 284 were of age 65 and older, significant differences were observed in the overall use of CSF over four cycles of 52.8 and 61.2%, between patients of age 65 and above and those under age 65, respectively ($p = 0.01$). Furthermore, prophylactic use between the age groups differed significantly as well with 27% of the younger breast cancer patients receiving CSF in cycle 1 as opposed to 19% of the older patients ($p < 0.01$) [113]. Although some of the apparent age-specific discrepancy in CSF use suggested by these data may be the result of less-frequent use of dose-dense breast cancer regimens in older women, further study is needed to better understand these practice trends.

Economic Analysis of CSF Use in Older Cancer Patients

Management of older cancer patients can be more costly than management of younger cancer patients. This is due to increased risk of treatment-related toxicities which, in the presence of increased number of comorbidities, result in greater risk for hospitalization. The development of fever in the setting of neutropenia, particularly in older cancer patients, often necessitates hospitalization for evaluation and administration of parenteral antibiotics. Neutropenic complications are more common and duration of hospitalization for management of these complications is longer in older cancer patients [15], which also drives overall cost. Strategies to reduce duration of hospitalization increase the potential for cost savings. In a multi-centered randomized controlled trial including 210 cancer patients hospitalized for fever and grade IV neutropenia, patients randomized to receive G-CSF experienced significantly decreased duration of severe neutropenia as compared to controls (median 2 days vs 3 days, $P < 0.0004$). Hospital stay was also shorter for those patients who received G-CSF (median 5 days vs 7 days, $P = 0.015$) with a resultant significant decrease in cost of hospitalization ($P = 0.01$) [114].

Benefits of cancer treatment are assessed in terms of disease-free and overall survival. Contributing to less cost-effective management in older patients is the reduced potential for benefit due to limited life expectancy and less treatment-responsive malignancy as compared to younger cancer patients [115]. In order to offset such intrinsic limitations in treatment benefits, significant gains must be had in reduction of treatment-related toxicity. In one study of early-stage breast cancer patients receiving adjuvant chemotherapy, targeted G-CSF for the women at highest risk of neutropenic complications was used to sustain dose intensity compared with women receiving a standard dose reduction. The estimated cost-effectiveness of targeted G-CSF use in the subgroup of patients at greatest risk for development of neutropenic complications was $34,000 per life-year gained [116]. This strategy proved to be effective not only in terms of cost-effectiveness but also regarding maintenance of chemotherapy standard dose intensity which has been shown to improve disease-free and overall survival [117].

The development and validation of risk models used to identify subgroups of individuals within the older cancer patient population who are at increased risk of incurring treatment-related neutropenic complications is crucial to maintaining cost-effective cancer care. Pretreatment variables associated with increased risk for developing first-cycle hematologic toxicity include a first-cycle absolute neutrophil count of <500 cells/mm^3, age over 65, Caucasian race, body surface area under 2 m [2], and use of anthracycline-containing regimens [118].

Guidelines on Use of Growth Factor Support for Older Cancer Patients

Several guidelines are available regarding use of primary prophylaxis in older cancer patients for whom systemic chemotherapy has been recommended. These include guidelines for the hematopoietic growth factors from the American Society of Clinical Oncology [119], the National Comprehensive Cancer Network (NCCN) [17], and the EORTC Cancer in the Elderly Task Force [120].

The NCCN guidelines for the chemotherapeutic management of older cancer patients include the following [17]:

1. Employ a form of geriatric assessment for persons of 70 years of age and older.
2. Adjust chemotherapy doses in accordance with GFR in patients of 65 years of age and older.
3. Utilize prophylactic filgrastim or pegfilgrastim for patients of 65 years of age and older who require chemotherapy regimens of dose intensity comparable to CHOP.
4. In select cases when considering erythropoietin, administer only if hemoglobin level is below 12 g/dL.
5. Consider substitution of fluorinated pyrimidines with capecitabine and implement preferential use of liposomal pegylated doxorubicin, weekly taxanes, vinorelbine, or gemcitabine.

Conclusions

- The risk of chemotherapy-related myelotoxicity increases with age.
- Chemotherapy-related myelotoxicity is the major cause of morbidity, mortality, and undertreatment in older cancer patients.
- The decision to initiate antineoplastic treatment should be based on physiologic rather than chronologic age.
- Prophylactic use of filgrastim or pegfilgrastim in patients with solid tumors receiving moderately toxic chemotherapy (such as CHOP or AC) significantly reduced the risk of neutropenic complications as well as the necessity for dose reduction.
- In older patients with AML both filgrastim and sarmograstin reduce the risk of infections and the duration of hospitalization. Sarmograstin may improve the survival of patients of 55 years of age and older.

- Anemia is a major cause of disability morbidity and mortality. The use of epoetin α or darbepoetin α may reduce these complications. These compounds may increase the risk of deep venous thrombosis but do not appear to increase cancer-related mortality if hemoglobin levels are maintained below 12 g/dL.
- The use of growth factors is cost-effective since their cost is offset by reductions in duration of hospitalization and other treatment-related costs associated with hematologic toxicity associated with chemotherapy use.
- The use of growth factors is supported by national guidelines as appropriate for use in older cancer patients.

References

1. Jemal A, Murray T, Samuels A, et al. Cancer statistics, 2003. CA Cancer J Clin. 2003;53: 5–26.
2. Extermann M. Acute leukemia in the elderly. Clin Geriatr Med. 1997;13:227–44.
3. O'Reilly SE, Connors JM, Howdel S, et al. Malignant lymphomas in the elderly. Clin Geriatr Med. 1997;13:251–64.
4. Dixon DO, Neilan B, Jones SE, et al. Effect of age on therapeutic outcome in advanced diffuse histiocytic lymphoma: the Southwest Oncology Group experience. J Clin Oncol. 1986;4:295–305.
5. Sargent DJ, Goldberg RM, Jacobson MD, et al. A pooled analysis of adjuvant chemotherapy for resected colon cancer in elderly patients. N Engl J Med. 2001;345:1091–7.
6. Early Breast Cancer Trialists Collaborative Group (EBCTCG). Effects of chemotherapy and hormonal therapy for early breast cancer on recurrence and 15 year survival: an overview of the randomized trials. Lancet. 2005;365:1687–717.
7. Elkin EB, Hurria A, Mitra D, et al. Adjuvant chemotherapy and survival in older women with hormone receptor-negative breast cancer: assessing outcome in a population-based, observational cohort. J Clin Oncol. 2006;24:2757–64.
8. Giordano SH, Duan Z, Kuo JF, et al. Use and outcomes of adjuvant chemotherapy in older women with breast cancer. J Clin Oncol. 2006;24:2750–6.
9. Lyman GH, Lyman CH, Agboola O. Risk models for predicting chemotherapy-induced neutropenia. Oncologist. 2005;10:427–37.
10. Kuderer NM, Dale D, Crawford J, Cosler L, Lyman GH. The morbidity, mortality and cost of febrile neutropenia in cancer patients. Cancer. 2006;106:2258–66.
11. Lyman GH, Dale D, Crawford J. Incidence, practice patterns, and predictors of low dose intensity in adjuvant breast cancer chemotherapy: results of a nationwide survey of community oncology practices. J Clin Oncol. 2003;21; 4524–4531.
12. Lyman GH, Dale DC, Friedberg J, et al. Incidence and predictions of low chemotherapy dose-intensity in aggressive non-Hodgkin's lymphomas. J Clin Oncol. 2004;22: 4302–11.
13. Lyman GH, Lyman C, Ogboola Y. Risk models for the prediction of chemotherapy-induced neutropenia. Neutropenia Oncol. 2001;1:2–7.
14. Crivellari D, Bonetti M, Castiglione-Gertsch M, et al. Burdens and benefits of adjuvant cyclophosphamide, methotrexate and fluorouracil and tamoxifen for elderly patients with breast cancer: The International Breast Cancer Study Group Trial VII. J Clin Oncol. 2000;18:1412–22.
15. Chrischilles E, Delgado DI, Stolshek BS, et al. Impact of age and colony stimulating factor use in hospital length of stay for febrile neutropenia in CHOP treated non-Hodgkin's lymphoma patients. Cancer Control. 2002;9:203–21.

16. Kuderer NM, Crawford J, Dale DC, et al. Impact of primary prophylaxis with granulocyte colony-stimulating factor (G-CSF) on febrile neutropenia and mortality in adult cancer patients receiving chemotherapy: a systematic review. J Clin Oncol. 2007;25:3158–67.

17. Crawford J, Armitage J, Balducci L et al: Myeloid Growth Factors v.1.2009. J Natl Comp Cancer Netw 2009; 7:64–83.

18. Zinzani PG, Storti S, Zaccaria A, et al. Elderly aggressive histology non-Hodgkin's lymphoma: first line VNCOP-B regimen experience on 350 patients. Blood. 1999;94:33–8.

19. Doorduijn JK, van der Holt B, van der Hem KG, et al. Randomized trials of granulocyte-colony stimulating factor (G-CSF) added to CHOP in elderly patients with aggressive non-Hodgkin's lymphoma. Blood. 2000;96:133a.

20. Osby E, Hagberg H, Kvaloy S, et al. CHOP is superior to CNOP in elderly patients with aggressive lymphoma while outcome is unaffected by filgrastim treatment: results of a Nordic Lymphoma Group randomized trial. Blood. 2003;101:3840–8.

21. Doorduijn JK, van der Holt B, van Imhoff GW, et al. CHOP compared with CHOP plus granulocyte colony-stimulating factor in elderly patients with aggressive non-Hodgkin's lymphoma. J Clin Oncol. 2003;21:3041–50.

22. Bucaneve G, Micozzi A, Menichetti F, et al. The Cruppo Italiano Malattie Ematologiche dell'Adulto (GIMEMA) Infection Program: Levofloxacin to prevent bacterial infections in patients with cancer and neutropenia. N Engl J Med. 2005;353:977–87.

23. Shayne M, Lichtman MA. Hematology in older persons. In: Lichtman MA, Beutler E, Kipps TJ, et al., editors. Williams hematology. 7th ed. New York, NY: McGraw-Hill Professional; 2005.

24. Ligthart GJ, Corberand JX, Fournier C, et al. Admission criteria for immunogerontological studies in man: The SENIEUR protocol. Mech Aging Dev. 1984;28:47.

25. Balducci L, Hardy CL, Lyman GH. Hemopoiesis and aging. Cancer Treat Res. 2005;124:109 34.

26. Shank WA Jr, Balducci L. Recombinant hemopoietic growth factors: comparative hemopoietic response in younger and older subjects. J Am Geriatr Soc. 1992;40:151.

27. Oakley E, Miller A, Waterstrat A, et al. Stem cell aging: potential effects on aging and mortality. In: Balducci L, Ershler WB, Bennett JN. Anemia in the elderly. New York, NY: Springer; 2007. pp. 1–20.

28. Haylock DN, Nilsson SK. Hematopoietic microenvironment and age. In: Balducci L, Ershler WB, DeGaetano G. Blood disorders in the elderly. Cambridge: Cambridge University Press; 2008. pp. 71–83.

29. Qualitative LF. Changes of hematopoiesis. In: Balducci L, Ershler WB, DeGaetano G, editors. Blood disorders in the elderly. Cambridge: Cambridge University Press; 2008. pp. 95–118.

30. Albright JW, Makinodan T. Decline in the growth potential of spleen-colonizing bone marrow stem cells of long-lived aging mice. J Exp Med. 1976;144:1204–13.

31. Balducci L, Hardy CL. Aging and hemopoietic stress. In: Balducci L, Ershler WB, DeGaetano G. Blood disorders in the elderly. Cambridge: Cambridge University Press; 2008. pp. 120–8.

32. Moscinski L. The aging bone marrow. In: Balducci L, Lyman GH, Ershler WB. Comprehensive geriatric oncology. London: Harwood Academic Publishers; 1998. pp. 414–23.

33. Htwe TH, Mushtaq A, Robinson SB, et al. Infection in the elderly. Infect Dis Clin N Am. 2007;21:711–43.

34. Chatta CS, Price TH, Allen RC, et al. Effects of "in vivo" recombinant methionyl human granulocyte colony-stimulating factor on the immune response and peripheral blood colony-forming cells in healthy young and elderly adult volunteers. Blood. 1994;84:2923–9.

35. Ferrucci L, Balducci L. Anemia of aging: the role of chronic inflammation and cancer. Sem Hematol. 2008;45:242–9.

36. Balducci L. Pharmacology of antineoplastic medications in older cancer patients. Oncology. 2009;23:78–85.

37. Shayne M, Culakova E, Poniewierski MS, et al. Dose intensity and hematologic toxicity in older cancer patients receiving systemic chemotherapy. Cancer. 2007;110:1611–20.

38. Marley SB, Lewis JL, Davidson RJ, et al. Evidence for a continuous decline in hemopoietic cell function from birth: application to evaluating bone marrow failure in children. Br J Haematol. 1999;106:162–6.

39. Bagnara GP, Bonsi L, Strippoli P, et al. Hemopoiesis in healthy old people and centenarian; well maintained responsiveness of CD34$^+$ cells to hemopoietic growth factors and remodeling of cytokine network. J Gerontol A Biol Sci Med Sci. 2000;55:B61–B70.

40. Baraldi-Junkins CA, Beck AC, Rothstein G. Hematopoiesis and cytokines. Relevance to cancer and aging. Hematol/Oncol Clin N Am. 2000;14:45–61.

41. Ferrucci L, Guralnik JM, Woodman RC, et al. Proinflammatory state and circulating erythropoietin in persons with and without anemia. Am J Med. 2005;118(11):1288–94.

42. Ferrucci L, Guralnik JM, Bandinelli S, et al. Unexplained anaemia in older persons is characterized by low erythropoietin and low levels of pro-inflammatory markers. Br J Haematol. 2007;136:849–55.

43. Tasaki T, Ohto H, Noguchi M, et al. Iron and erythropoietin measurements in autologous blood donors with anemia: implications for management. Transfusion. 1994;34:337–43.

44. Kumagai T, Morimoto K, Saitoh H, et al. Age-related changes in myelopoietic response to lipopolysaccaride in senescence-accelerated mice. Mech Ageing Dev. 2000;112:153–7.

45. Boggs DR, Patrene KD. Hematopoiesis and aging III: anemia and a blunted erythropoietic response to hemorrhage in aged mice. Am J Hematol. 1985;19:327–41.

46. Morra L, Moccia F, Mazzarello GP, et al. Defective burst-promoting activity of T lymphocytes from anemic and non-anemic elderly people. Ann Hematol. 1994;68:67–71.

47. Hyrota Y, Okamura S, Kimura N, et al. Hematopoiesis in the aged as studied by "in vitro" colony assay. Eur J Haematol. 1988;40:83–90.

48. Joosten E, Van Hove L, Lesaffre E, et al. Serum erythropoietin levels in elderly inpatients with anemia of chronic disorders and iron deficiency anemia. J Am Ger Soc. 1993;41:1301–4.

49. Nafziger J, Pailla K, Luciani L, et al. Decreased erythropoietin responsiveness to iron deficiency anemia in the elderly. Am J Hematol. 1993;43:172–6.

50. Chatta DS, Dale DC. Aging and haemopoiesis. Implications for treatment with haemopoietic growth factors. Drugs Aging. 1996;9:37–47.

51. Cascinu S, Del Ferro E, Fedeli A, et al. Recombinant human erythropoietin treatment in elderly cancer patients with cisplatin-associated anemia. Oncology. 1995;52:422–6.

52. Fields KK, Djulbegovic B. Hematopoietic stem cell transplantation in the older patient. In: Balducci L, Lyman GH, Ershler WB, Extermann M, editors. Comprehensive geriatric oncology. London: Taylor and Francis; 2004. pp. 489–500.

53. Kersting S, Verdonck LF. Successful outcome of nonmyeloablative allogeneic bone marrow transplant in patients with kidney dysfunction. Biol Blood Marrow Transplant. 2008;14:1312–16.

54. Kumar SK, Dingli D, Lacy MQ, et al. Autologous stem cell transplantation in patients of 70 years and older with multiple myeloma: results from a matched pair analysis. Am J Hematol. 2008;83:614–17.

55. Baker SD, Grochow L. Pharmacology of cancer: chemotherapy in the older person. Clin Geriatr Med. 1997;13:169–83.

56. Duthie EH. Physiology of aging: relevance to symptoms, perceptions, and treatment tolerance. In: Balducci L, Lyman GH, Ershler WB, editors. Comprehensive geriatric oncology. Amsterdam: Harwood Academic Publishers; 1998. pp. 247–62.

57. Balducii L, Hardy CH. Anemia of aging: a model of cancer-related anemia. Cancer Control JHLMCC. 1998;5(Suppl):17–21.

58. Begg CB, Carbone P. Clinical trials and drug toxicity in the elderly. The experience of the Eastern Cooperative Oncology Group. Cancer. 1983;52:1986–92.

59. Gelman RS, Taylor SG. Cyclophosphamide, methotrexate and 5-fluorouracil chemotherapy in women more than 65 year old with advanced breast cancer. The elimination of age trends in toxicity by using doses based on creatinine clearance. J Clin Oncol. 1984;2:1406–14.

60. Christman K, Muss HB, Case D, et al. Chemotherapy of metastatic breast cancer in the elderly. JAMA. 1992;268:57–62.

61. Giovannozzi-Bannon S, Rademaker A, Lai G, et al. Treatment tolerance of elderly cancer patients entered onto phase II clinical trials. An Illinois Cancer Center Study. J Clin Oncol. 1994;12:2447–52.

62. Ibrahim N, Frye DK, Buzdar AU, et al. Doxorubicin based combination chemotherapy in elderly patients with metastatic breast cancer. Tolerance and outcome. Arch Intern Med. 1996;156:882–8.

63. Ibrahim NK, Buzdar AU, Asmar L, et al. Doxorubicin based adjuvant chemotherapy in elderly breast cancer patients: The M.D. Anderson experience with long term follow-up. Ann Oncol. 2000;11:1–5.

64. Lyman GH, Dale DC, Friedberg J, et al. Incidence and predictors of chemotherapy low dose intensity in aggressive non-Hodgkin's lymphoma: a nationwide study. J Clin Oncol. 2004;22:4302–11.

65. Chrischilles EA, Link BK, Scott SD, et al. Factors associated with early termination of CHOP therapy and the impact on survival among patients with chemosensitive intermediate-grade non-Hodgkin's lymphoma. Cancer Control. 2003;10:396–403.

66. Kim YJ, Rubenstein EB, Rolston KV, et al. Colony stimulating factors (CSFs) may reduce complications and death in solid tumor patients with fever and neutropenia. Proc ASCO. 2000;19:612a. Abstract 2411.

67. Crivellari D, Bonetti M, Castiglione Gertsch M, et al. Burdens and benefits of adjuvant cyclophosphamide, methotrexate and fluorouracil and tamoxifen for elderly patients with breast cancer: the International Breast Cancer Study Group Trial VII. J Clin Oncol. 2000;18(7):1412–22.

68. Armitage JO, Potter JF. Aggressive chemotherapy for diffuse histiocytic lymphoma in the elderly. J Am Ger Soc. 1984;32:269–73.

69. Gomez H, Mas L, Casanova L, et al. Elderly patients with aggressive non-Hodgkin's lymphoma treated with CHOP chemotherapy plus granulocyte–macrophage colony-stimulating factor: identification of two age subgroups with differing hematologic toxicity. J Clin Oncol. 1998;16:2352–8.

70. Bastion Y, Blay J-Y, Divine M, et al. Elderly patients with aggressive non-Hodgkin's lymphoma: disease presentation, response to treatment and survival. A Groupe d'Etude des Lymphomes de l'Adulte Study on 453 patients older than 69 years. J Clin Oncol. 1997;15:2945–53.

71. Zinzani PG, Storti S, Zaccaria A, et al. Elderly aggressive histology non-Hodgkin's lymphoma: first Line VNCOP-B regimen experience on 350 patients. Blood. 1999;94:33–8.

72. Sonneveld P, de Ridder M, van der Lelie H, et al. Comparison of doxorubicin and mitoxantrone in the treatment of elderly patients with advanced diffuse non-Hodgkin's lymphoma using CHOP vs CNOP chemotherapy. J Clin Oncol. 1995;13:2530–9.

73. Tirelli U, Errante D, Van Glabbeke M, et al. CHOP is the standard regimen in patients ≥70 years of age with intermediate and high grade non-Hodgkin's lymphoma: results of a randomized study of the European organization for the Research and Treatment of Cancer Lymphoma Cooperative Study. J Clin Oncol. 1998;16:27–34.

74. Osby E, Hagberg H, Kvaloy S, et al. CHOP is superior to CNOP in elderly patients with aggressive lymphoma while outcome is unaffected by filgrastim treatment: results of a Nordic Lymphoma Group randomized trial. Blood. 2003;101:3840–8.

75. Doorduijn JK van derr Holt B, van der hem KG, et al. CHOP compared with CHOP plus granulocyte colony-stimulating factor in elderly patients with aggressive non-Hodgkin's lymphoma. J Clin Oncol. 2003;21:3041–50.

76. Meyer RM, Browman GP, Samosh ML, et al. Randomized phase II comparison of standard CHOP with weekly CHOP in elderly patients with non-Hodgkin's lymphoma. J Clin Oncol. 1995;13:2386–93.

77. Melchert M, Lancet J. Acute myeloid leukemia in the elderly. In: Balducci L, Ershler WB, DeGaetano G, editors. Blood disorders in the elderly. Cambridge: Cambridge University Press; 2008. pp. 237–55.

78. Balducci L. Consequences of chronic anemia in the older person. In: Balducci L, Ershler WB, DeGaetano G, editors. Blood disorders in the elderly. Cambridge: Cambridge University Press; 2008. pp. 192–202.

79. Hardy SE Studenski SA. Fatigue predicts mortality in older adults. J Am Ger Soc. 2008;56:1910–14.

80. Hardy SE, Studenski SA. Fatigue and function over 3 years among older adults. J Gerontol Med Sci. 2008;63:1389–92.

81. Marcantonio ER, Flacker JM, Michaels M, et al. Delirium is independently associated with poor functional recovery after hip fracture. J Am Ger Soc. 2000;48:618–24.

82. Schrijvers D. Role of red blood cells in pharmacokinetics of chemotherapeutic agents. Clin Pharmacokinet. 2003;42:779–91.

83. Atti AR, Palmer K, Volpato S, et al. Anaemia increases the risk of dementia in cognitively intact elderly. Neurobiol Aging. 2006;27:278–84.

84. Penninx BW, Pluijm SM, Lips P, et al. Late-life anemia is associated with increased risk of recurrent falls. J Am Ger Soc. 2005;53:2106–11.

85. Shah RC, Wilson RS, Tang Y, et al. Relation of hemoglobin to level of cognitive function in older persons. Neuroepidemiology. 2009;32:40–6.

86. Price TH, Chatta GS, Dale DC. Effect of recombinant granulocyte colony-stimulating factor on neutrophil kinetics in normal young and elderly humans. Blood. 1996;88:335–40.

87. Zagonel V, Babare R, Merola MC, et al. Cost-benefit of granulocyte colony-stimulating factor administration in older patients with non-Hodgkin's lymphoma treated with combination chemotherapy. Ann Oncol. 1994;5(Suppl 2):127–32.

88. Bertini M, Freilone R, Vitolo U, et al. The treatment of elderly patients with aggressive non-Hodgkin's lymphomas: feasibility and efficacy of an intensive multidrug regimen. Leukem Lymphoma. 1996;22:483–93.

89. Balducci L, Al-Halawani H, Charu V, et al. Elderly cancer patients receiving chemotherapy benefit from first-cycle pegfilgrastim. Oncologist. 2007;12:1416–24.

90. Rowe JM, Andersen JW, Mazza JJ, et al. Randomized placebo-controlled phase III study of granulocyte–macrophage colony stimulating factor in adult patients (>55–70 years of age) with acute myelogenous leukemia: a study of the Eastern Cooperative Oncology Group (E1490). Blood. 1995;86:457–62.

91. Heil D, Hoelzer D, Sanz MA, et al. A randomized double blind placebo controlled phase III study of filgrastim in remission induction and consolidation therapy for patients with "de novo" acute myeloid leukemia. The International Acute Leukemia Study Group. Blood. 1997;90:4710–18.

92. Lowenberg B, Suciu S, Archimbaud E, et al. Use of recombinant GM-CSF during and after remission-induction chemotherapy in patients aged 61 and older with acute non-lymphocytic leukemia: final report of AML-11 a phase III randomized study of the Leukemia Cooperative Group of European Organization for the Research and Treatment of Cancer and the Dutch Belgian Hematology Oncology Cooperative Group. Blood. 1997;90:2952–61.

93. Zittoun R, Suciu S, Mandelli F, et al. Granulocyte–macrophage colony stimulating factor associated induction treatment of acute myelogenous leukemia: a randomized study by the European Organization for Research and Treatment of Leukemia Cooperative Group. J Clin Oncol. 1996;14:2150–9.

94. Witz F, Sadoun A, Perrin MC. A placebo-controlled study of recombinant human granulocyte macrophage colony-stimulating factor administered during an induction treatment for "de novo" acute myelogenous leukemia in older patients. Blood. 1998;15:2722–30.

95. Stone RM, Berg DT, George SL, et al. Granulocyte–macrophage colony stimulating factor after initial chemotherapy for elderly patients with primary acute myelogenous leukemia. N Engl J Med. 1995;332:1671–7.

96. Dombret H, Chastang C, Fenaux P, et al. A controlled study of recombinant human granulocyte colony-stimulating factor in elderly patients after treatment for acute myelogenous leukemia. N Engl J Med. 1995;332:1678–83.

97. Ohno R, Naoe T, Kanamaru A, et al. A double-blind controlled study of granulocyte colony-stimulating factor started two days before induction chemotherapy in refractory acute myeloid leukemia. Blood. 1994;83:2086–92.

98. Godwin JE, Kapecky KJ, Head JR, et al. A double blind placebo controlled trial of granulocyte colony-stimulating factor in elderly patients with previously untreated acute myelogenous leukemia. Blood. 1998;91:3607–15.

99. Littlewood TJ, Bajetta E, Nortier JW, Vercammen E, Rapoport B. Effects of epoetin alfa on hematologic parameters and quality of life in cancer patients receiving nonplatinum chemotherapy: results of a randomized, double-blind, placebo-controlled trial. J Clin Oncol. 2001;19(11):2865–74.

100. Vansteenkiste J, Pirker R, Massuti B, et al. Double-blind, placebo-controlled, randomized phase III trial of darbepoetin alfa in lung cancer patients receiving chemotherapy. J Natl Cancer Inst. 2002;94(16):1211–20.

101. Curt GA, Breitbart W, Cella D, et al. Impact of cancer-related fatigue on the lives of patients: new findings from the Fatigue Coalition. Oncologist. 2000;5(5):353–60.

102. Bennett CL, Silver SM, Djulbegovic B, et al. Venous thromboembolism and mortality associated with recombinant erythropoietin and darbepoetin administration for the treatment of cancer-associated anemia. JAMA. 2008;299(8):914–24.

103. Bohlius J, Engert A, Schwarzer G. Erythropoiesis stimulating agents in the treatment of cancer-related anemia. JAMA. 2008;300:2854–2855.

104. Bennett CL, Luminari S, Nissenson AR, et al. Pure red blood cell aplasia and epoetin therapy. N Engl J Med. 2004;351:1403–8.

105. Hershman D, Neugut AI, Jacobson JS, et al. Acute myeloid leukemia or myelodysplastic syndrome following use of granulocyte colony-stimulating factors during breast cancer adjuvant chemotherapy. J Natl Cancer Inst. 2007;99(3): 196–205.

106. LeDeley MC, Suzan F, Cutuli B, et al. Anthracyclines, mitoxantrone, radiotherapy, and granulocyte colony-stimulating factor: risk factors for leukemia and myelodysplastic syndrome after breast cancer. J Clin Oncol. 2007;25:292–300.

107. Muss HB, Berry DA, Cirrincione C, et al. Toxicity of older and younger patients treated with adjuvant chemotherapy for node-positive breast cancer: the Cancer and Leukemia Group B experience. J Clin Oncol. 2007;25(24):3699–704.

108. Patt DA, Duan Z, Fang S, et al. Acute myeloid leukemia after adjuvant breast cancer therapy in older women: understanding risk. J Clin Oncol. 2007;25(25):3871–6.

109. Timmer-Bonte JN, de Boo TM, Smit AJ, et al. Prevention of chemotherapy-induced febrile neutropenia by prophylactic antibiotics plus or minus granulocyte colony-stimulating factor in small-cell lung cancer: a Dutch randomized phase III study. J Clin Oncol. 2005;23: 7974–84.

110. Lyman GH, Morrison VA, Dale DC, et al. Risk of febrile neutropenia among patients with intermediate-grade non-Hodgkin's lymphoma receiving CHOP chemotherapy. Leuk Lymphoma. 2003;44:2069–76.

111. Lyman GH, Delgado DJ. Risk and timing of hospitalization for febrile neutropenia in patients receiving CHOP, CHOP-R, or CHOP chemotherapy for intermediate-grade non-Hodgkin lymphoma. Cancer. 2003;98:2402–9.

112. Chen-Hardee S, Chrischilles EA, Voelker MS, et al. Population-based assessment of hospitalizations for neutropenia from chemotherapy in older adults with non-Hodgkin's lymphoma (United States). Cancer Causes Control. 2006;17:647–54.
113. Shayne M, Culakova E, Wolff DA, et al. Dose intensity and hematologic toxicity in older breast cancer patients receiving systemic chemotherapy. Breast Cancer Res Treat. 2006;100:S281.
114. Carcia-Carbonero R, Mayadomo JI, Tornamira MV, et al. Granulocyte colony-stimulating factor in the treatment of high-risk febrile neutropenia: a multicenter randomized trial. J Natl Cancer Inst. 2001;93:31–38.
115. Lyman GH, Kuderer N, Balducci L. Cancer care in the elderly: cost and quality of life considerations. Cancer Control. 1998;5:347–54.
116. Silber JH, Fridman M, DiPaula RS, et al. Modeling the cost-effectiveness of granulocyte-stimulating factor use in early-stage breast cancer. J Clin Oncol. 1998;16:2435–44.
117. Bonnadonna G, Valagussa P, Moliterni A, et al. Adjuvant cyclophosphamide, methotrexate, and fluorouracil in node-positive breast cancer: the results of 20 years of follow-up. N Engl J Med. 1995;332:901–6.
118. Lyman GH. Risk assessment in oncology clinical practice: from risk factors to risk model. Oncology. 2003;17:8–13.
119. Smith TJ, Khatcheressian J, Lyman GH, et al. 2006 update of recommendations for the use of white blood cell growth factors: an evidence-based clinical practice guideline. J Clin Oncol. 2006;24:3187–205.
120. Repetto L, Bigansoli L, Koehne CH, et al. EORTC Cancer in the Elderly Task Force guidelines for the use of the colony-stimulating factors in elderly patients with cancer. Eur J Cancer. 2003;39:2264–72.

Chapter 22
The Economics of the Hematopoietic Growth Factors

Adi Eldar-Lissai and Gary H. Lyman

Introduction

The last two decades have seen a dramatic increase in overall healthcare costs. Cancer treatment cost in the United States has increased by about 75% between 1995 and 2008, accounting for $93.2 billion in direct medical costs [1, 2]. Spending on cancer drugs has increased faster than spending on other areas of treatment (such as hospitalization), due to both increases in prices and in the rates of use. Of particular concern is that the magnitude of increase in prices exceeds the magnitude of their improvement in treatment efficacy [3].

The financial cost of cancer treatment is not only a burden to insurers, but also to people diagnosed with cancer and their caregivers, who may be facing substantial out-of-pocket costs [4]. Indirect cancer costs such as those associated with lost of productivity were estimated in the United States at $18.8 billion in 2008 [2].

Methods to evaluate and compare the costs and benefits of treatments are available and widely used by researchers and decision-makers. Cost-effectiveness analysis (CEA) provides a standard, well-accepted methodological technique for judging whether a medical innovation provides an acceptable value for money. A recent systematic review found that the number of studies evaluating the cost-effectiveness (CE) of cancer-related innovations has increased from an average of 7 studies a year prior to 2002 to 22 studies a year during 2006. Most of these CE analyses were conducted in the United States (53%) and were funded by government, foundation, or health organization (46%) [5].

The current chapter provides an overview of the economics and health outcomes pertaining to the utilization of growth factors. The first section will review current methods in evaluating costs and outcomes in healthcare. The second section reviews aspects in the cost of febrile neutropenia (FN) and colony-stimulating factors and the

G.H. Lyman (✉)
Duke University and the Duke Comprehensive Cancer Center, Durham, NC 27705, USA
e-mail: gary.lyman@duke.edu

G.H. Lyman, D.C. Dale (eds.), *Hematopoietic Growth Factors in Oncology,*
Cancer Treatment and Research 157, DOI 10.1007/978-1-4419-7073-2_22,
© Springer Science+Business Media, LLC 2011

third section reviews the associated health outcomes. Section four reviews cost and health outcomes considerations among special populations. The chapter concludes with a review of published economic analyses for colony-stimulating factors.

Costs and Outcomes Measure in Healthcare

Common Types of Economic Analyses

Cost-effectiveness analysis (CEA) is often used as a general term when referring to the use of an economic, analytic tool to evaluate and compare two or more treatment alternatives [6], in which a comparison between the cost and consequence of a given treatment to those of its alternatives is conducted. Clinical data are combined with the costs and outcomes of different events to calculate the cost-effectiveness (CE) of treatment strategies. There are several different types of such economic analyses: cost–benefit analysis, cost–utility analysis, cost-effectiveness analysis, and cost-minimization analysis. All analyses use similar methods and units to measure treatment cost, but they differ by the type of outcome they measure: quality-adjusted life years (QALYs) or life-years gained (LY) in cost–utility analysis, monetary value of treatment consequence in cost–benefit analysis, and common health effect (e.g., symptom-free days) of both treatments, achieved to a different degree, in cost-effectiveness analysis [7]. In cost-minimization analysis only the costs of the alternatives are being compared because it is known or expected that the effectiveness and safety of alternatives is identical. The different methods are summarized in Table 22.1.

Table 22.1 Summary of types of economic analyses [7]

Type of study	Cost measurement	Effectiveness measurement	Results measurement
Cost-minimization	Fiscal units	None	Monetary units
Cost-effectiveness	Fiscal units	Common outcome or effect of interest (e.g., FN episode avoided, life-year gained)	Cost per outcome
Cost–utility	Fiscal units	Utility measure (e.g., QALY)	Cost per QALY
Cost–benefit	Fiscal units	Monetary values of treatment outcome	Monetary units

FN, febrile neutropenia; QALY, quality adjusted life year.

A CEA has at least two comparisons (i.e., intervention of interest and a comparison group). Their difference in cost (incremental cost) is compared to their difference in effectiveness (incremental effectiveness) to calculate the following ratio, known as the Incremental Cost-Effectiveness Ratio (ICER):

$$ICER = \frac{Cost_{intervention} - Cost_{alternative}}{Effect_{intervention} - Effect_{alternative}} = \frac{Incremental\ Cost}{Incremental\ Effect}$$

If there are more than two alternatives, interventions are compared based on a pair-wise basis, ranking their costs in increasing order, and comparing their ICERs [8].

Estimating the overall cost of a program requires the consideration of both the activity levels (e.g., physicians' time cost) over time and the unit cost (e.g., drug cost). Direct medical costs refer to the cost of providing medical services by clinicians, diagnosis, treatment or prevention costs, follow-up, rehabilitation, and palliative care. These costs may occur in the hospital, physician office, or at the patient home. Direct non-medical costs represent those costs incurred while receiving treatment, such as the cost of transportation to and from the clinic or paying for a caregiver. Indirect non-medical costs include those associated with morbidity of disease, such as patient's time missed from work or unpaid caregiver [8, 9].

A commonly used health outcome measure is known as Quality-Adjusted Life Years (QALY). A QALY represents in a single measure the treatment effect on both the quality of life and changes in life expectancy (or duration of illness). To calculate QALY, a quality of life in a given disease state is measured on a preference scale (numeric rating with full health = 1 and dead = 0) and then multiplied by the duration of time the patient spends in that given stage. The advantage of QALY over other outcomes is that it is not disease-specific and therefore enables decision-makers to compare costs across diseases when making resource allocation decisions [8].

Perspective and Time Horizon of Economic Analyses

The decision which costs to include in an analysis primarily depends on the perspective and time horizon of the analysis. The perspective of the analysis refers to the viewpoint from which the analysis is being conducted and may include the individual patient, an institution, government, third-party payer, or society as a whole. A specific cost category will be included in the analysis if it is paid for by the entity whose perspective is being represented [10]. For example, when a patient's perspective is represented, time lost from work or amount paid for child care should be taken into account, but when the perspective is that of a third-party payer or an institution, these costs should be left out of the analysis.

The time horizon of the analysis represents the period of time over which costs and effects are being measured [6]. A CEA may be conducted over a short-term horizon, incorporating costs and effects occurring only during the treatment period, or it may be conducted over a long-term horizon and include costs that extend into the future to represent the lifetime costs and benefits. The challenge in performing a long-term horizon analysis is in correctly estimating future costs as well as life expectancy, as these data are not always available.

Uncertainty and Comparison Across Incremental Cost-Effectiveness Ratios

An intervention is considered to be cost-effective (i.e., its gains outweigh its cost) if the ICER is below a prespecified threshold. Such threshold should reflect society's willingness to pay (WTP) for the evaluated health benefit. The commonly used threshold of $50,000/QALY was suggested by Gold et al. [6] during the 1990s, but recent studies suggest that it no longer represents current WTP, and thresholds like $100,000/QALY or three times the GDP in the country where study is conducted are suggested [11, 12].

Uncertainty underlies any data, whether it is economic or clinical. Sensitivity analyses are performed to examine the effect of uncertainty on the study's results. The ultimate goal of sensitivity analysis is to examine whether under varying parameters' values, the ICER is still considered cost-effective given the prespecified threshold. This can be done by varying a single parameter at a time (one-way sensitivity analysis), few parameters at a time (multi-way sensitivity analysis), or by specifying a probability distribution for each parameter and repeating the analysis multiple times at a process known as a probabilistic sensitivity analysis and resulting in a 95% confidence interval of the ICER [6, 8].

The Cost of Febrile Neutropenia and Colony-Stimulating Factors

The Financial Burden of Neutropenia and FN on Overall Cancer Treatment

Randomized controlled trials (RCTs) have demonstrated that prophylactic granulocyte colony-stimulating factors (G-CSFs) initiated at the time or immediately following myelosuppressive chemotherapy are effective in reducing the incidence of FN by 50–90% [13–15]. Patients treated with a G-CSF have shorter lengths of hospitalization (LOS) and shorter time to neutrophil recovery than control subjects [16]. Thus, the use of G-CSFs holds the potential for cost-savings associated with decreases in FN and all-cause mortality and fewer, shorter, hospitalization.

In any cost analysis, the tradeoff between the additional cost of treatment and the potential savings in resources it holds should be considered. Similarly, the aforementioned potential savings associated with G-CSF should be compared to the relatively high cost of G-CSFs. Current price quotes based on Medicare Part B Average Price Sales are $2,243 for one pegfilgrastim injection and $208 and $322 for filgrastim 300 and 480 mL, respectively [17]. In RCTs, a single pegfilgrastim injection had efficacy comparable to 10–11 days of filgrastim in reducing the incidence of grade IV neutropenia (absolute neutrophil count (ANC) $< 0.5 \times 10^9$/L) but when taken collectively, these RCTs also suggest that prophylaxis pegfilgrastim provides higher rates of relative risk reduction than filgrastim [14].

The Economics of Colony-Stimulating Factors

Hospitalization for FN

It is estimated that in the United States, over 60,000 hospitalizations are neutropenia related, reflecting an incidence rate of 7.83 hospitalizations per 1,000 cancer patients [18]. Hospitalization incidence rates among patients who receive chemotherapy are even higher as this population group is at higher risk (for example: 178 cases per 1,000 chemotherapy treated non-Hodgkin's Lymphoma patients [18]) and hence, posing a great financial and medical burden in the overall care of cancer patients.

Two different studies estimated the national rates of hospital mean length of stay (LOS) for neutropenia-related hospitalization and found that for all cancer types, LOS ranges from 9.2 (SD = 10.4) to 11.5 (SD = 0.1) days [18, 19]. Both studies also show that duration and cost per total and day of hospitalization vary substantially by cancer type: for solid cancers mean LOS was 6.8 (SD = 6.5) to 8.13 (SD = 0.1) days, and between 16.9 (SD = 15.1) to 19.7 (SD = 0.4) days among leukemia patients. Hospitalization costs increase with increased LOS, severity of neutropenia, and the number of comorbidities. The mean cost per neutropenia hospitalization may vary from $13,400 (SD = $2,100) [18] to about $19,110 (SD = $350) among patients with various malignancies [19].

Variation in hospitalization costs exists not only among patients with different cancer types, but also among those patients who recover from FN and those experiencing in-hospital mortality (Fig. 22.1). The mean cost per day (patients with solid tumors only) for surviving patient is estimated at about $1,950 (SD = 1,040) and at $3,150 (SD = $2,000) for dying patients [20, 21].

Studies to evaluate the incidence and cost of FN-related hospitalization traditionally include the costs associated directly with hospitalization and neglecting to estimate the costs associated with any prior hospital encounter the patient had, namely, emergency department (ED) visit for triage and evaluation. While the literature is relatively thin a recent study by Courtney et al. [22] report a median per patient ED cost of $1,455 ($n = 57$ visits) and resulting from hospital/nursing activities, radiology, diagnostic tests, and antibiotic use.

In studies of G-CSF utilization patterns in community oncology practices, it was documented that not only that the addition of filgrastim to chemotherapy treatment reduces the incidence of FN and hospitalizations, but that each additional day of prophylaxis filgrastim is associated with hospitalization risk reduction (RR) of 15–19% for NHL patients, 17–23% RR for breast cancer patients, and 8–9% RR for those with lung cancer [23]. Similar results indicate that use of low-dose filgrastim compared with standard-dose filgrastim resulted in more patients developing FN (32% vs 7.5%, p-value = 0.0014) and more FN-related hospitalizations (32% vs 6.5%, p-value < 0.001) [24]. Comparing hospitalization risk among patients receiving filgrastim and pegfilgrastim in community settings shows that patients who received prophylaxis filgrastim had approximately 40% increase in the odds of developing FN compared to patients who received prophylaxis pegfilgrastim [25],

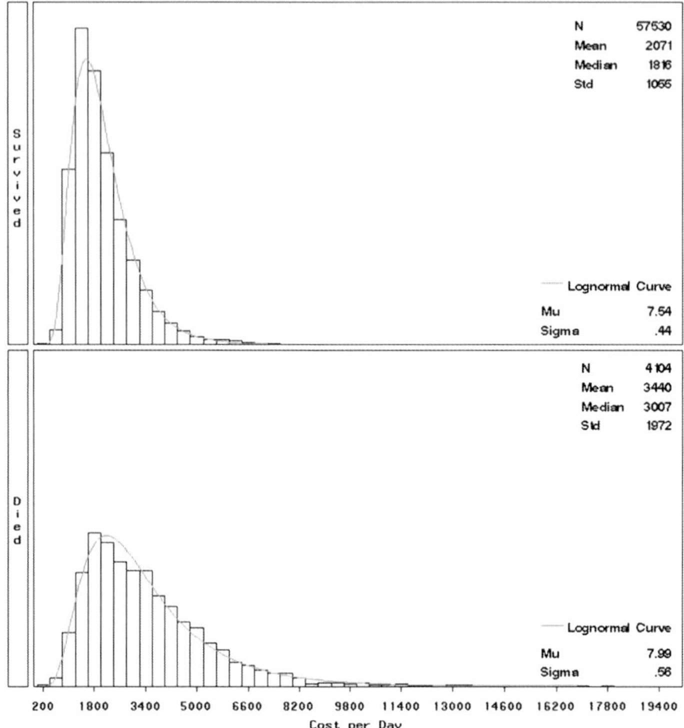

Fig. 22.1 Cost distributions among patients who recover from FN hospitalization (survive) and those with inpatient mortality (die)

with similar increase in FN hospitalization rates (p-value $= 0.002$) and all-cause hospitalizations [26].

High-Risk Versus Low-Risk Patients (Community Treatment, Antibiotic Use)

The most common standard care of FN is hospitalization for monitoring and treatment with broad-spectrum antibiotics, until neutrophil recovery and fever resolve (Fig. 22.2). In the last decade, two risk assessment models developed by Talcott et al. [27] and The Multinomial Association for Supportive Care in Cancer (MASCC) [28] have been validated [29] and have successfully assisted clinicians in identifying patients at low risk of developing complications, suggesting their FN can be managed in an outpatient settings. In a recent review, Carstensen et al. [30] compared the results of ten clinical trials evaluating the efficacy and safety of outpatient versus hospital-based therapy of low-risk FN in adult cancer patients and found both treatment strategies to be comparable and treatment response rate to be equal. To be eligible for outpatient treatment, a patient needs to not only have certain clinical characteristics (clinically stable, normal renal and hepatic function, expected duration of neutropenia less than 7 days, and no hospitalization-requiring comorbid)

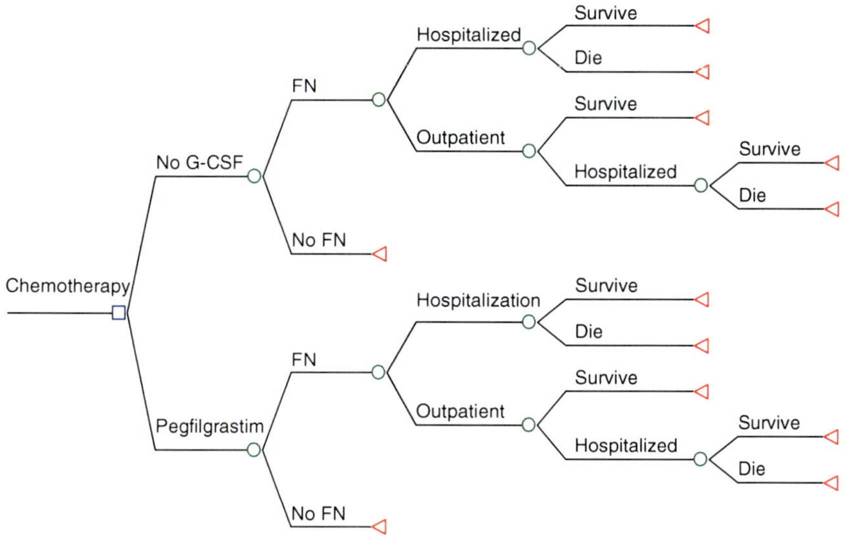

Fig. 22.2 An example of economic decision tree representing common treatment practice of febrile neutropenia (FN)

but also need to have a 24-h caregiver at home, have access to telephone or transportation, reside more than 30 min from treating center, and good compliance with previous outpatient treatment.

FN management in the outpatient settings holds the potential to improve treatment outcomes by decreasing the exposure of low-risk patients to hospital-related infections (hence, reduce morbidity and mortality) and reduce costs associated with hospitalization and use of antibiotics. A recent retrospective review [31] of 712 low-risk, solid tumor patients presenting to the ED with FN confirmed a significant reduction in costs; a group of low-risk outpatients were compared with a group of clinically similar low-risk inpatient who were ineligible for outpatient treatment. The mean cost of therapy among inpatients was significantly higher (p-value <0.001) than that of outpatient at $15,231 versus $7,772, respectively.

The use of G-CSFs has been shown to reduce the severity and duration of neutropenia, consequently may convert some patients to low-risk, outpatient eligible group. Cosler et al. [32] conducted a cost-minimization analysis to estimate the effect of outpatient treatment compared to traditional, inpatient treatment and found that the cost of FN episode was $13,355 for patients treated with no G-CSF, $8,677 for patients treated with G-CSFs and hospitalization, and $8,188 for patients treated with G-CSFs and risk stratification and outpatient management. These results indicate that the assumption of savings due to outpatient treatment was validated; however, that high-risk, hospitalized, patients still account for the majority of FN patients thus, the outpatient treatment option affected overall costs by relatively small amounts.

Productivity and Time Measures

Conducting a CE analysis from a societal perspective, as recommended by Gold et al. [6], requires estimating expenditures additional to those directly related to the medical treatment, for example, productivity and transportation costs. Such analysis is more inclusive and reflects a more accurate picture of the cost of treatment borne by society as a whole, but it may introduce more assumptions (and increase model uncertainty) into the economic model as such data are not always available. Cosler et al. [33] reported total indirect medical costs (including patient work loss, caregiver work loss, and caregiver payments) that totaled $3,835 per neutropenia episode.

Supportive cancer therapies such as G-CSFs can reduce the incidence of FN, but they may require additional medical visits. Treatment with filgrastim can require ten or more daily injections per chemotherapy cycle. Pegfilgrastim, however, is given only once per cycle and is estimated to generate less of a disruption in patient's life. In a survey of 189 adult cancer patients treated with prophylactic G-CSFs in 20 community-based oncology practices, Fortner et al. [34, 35] collected data on patient's time spent at the clinic, time spent traveling to and from the clinic, and the time affected by altering other activities (such as work) before and after the visit. The mean time spent on laboratory and treatment with filgrastim (each visit) and pegfilgrastim was comparable, at about 3 h. The mean time spent on physician and chemotherapy visit was 8 h.

In addition to the costs associated with travel to and from the clinic, as well as the costs associated with work-loss, other out-of-pocket expenses may be required, such as overnight accommodation, and often generate non-reimbursable costs [4]. Song et al. [36] examined the impact of FN on short-term disability (STD) days and time lost from work among cancer patients. They found that productivity lost was significantly higher (p-value $= 0.05$) among FN patients (mean $= $549, SD $= 1,005$) compared with non-FN patients (mean $= $394, SD $= 869$) and that FN patients had on average one additional STD day (p-value $= 0.046$).

Health Outcomes

Effect on Mortality

Patient survival remains the ultimate clinical measure of cancer treatment. The number of studies to evaluate the impact of G-CSFs on disease-free and overall survival is limited. The single study to report long-term survival from phase three study of filgrastim has limited generalizability as it was confined to de novo acute myeloid leukemia [37]. Among this patient population, after median follow-up of 7 years, there was a similar proportion of deaths in the filgrastim and placebo arms, no difference in median time to death (p-value $= 0.97$) or disease-free survival (p-value $= 0.52$).

While the reported mortality associated with FN in RCTs is relatively low, it is most likely due to the highly selected nature of patients eligible to participate in the trials and does not necessarily reflect mortality rate in the overall cancer population. In two studies of patients hospitalized for FN the overall mortality varied from 6.8% in one study [18] to 9.5% in the other [19]. Mortality rates were highest among patients with documented sepsis, pneumonia, and with other comorbidities of the lung, kidney, and liver [19].

Three recent meta-analyses estimated the effect of prophylactic use of G-CSFs on mortality. One meta-analysis [38] reported no significant difference between treatments in terms of short-term, all-cause, and infection-related mortality. However, this study included a very heterogeneous patient population (e.g., pediatric, adult, and elderly) and different cancer types (e.g., both solid and non-solid cancers) thus, may be masking any treatment effect in subpopulations. Two meta-analyses [39, 40], including RCTs from adult cancer patients, reported a 45% relative risk reduction in infection-related mortality for prophylactic G-CSF (p-value $= 0.018$) and 40% risk reduction in all-cause mortality during chemotherapy (p-value $= 0.002$).

Colony-Stimulating Factors Versus Reduction in Dose Intensity

Maintaining chemotherapy dose intensity and schedule is shown to be essential in achieving desired outcomes and long-term disease control [41, 42]. Reduction of standard-dose intensity (<85% of planned dose or >7 days delay in schedule) has been shown to increase the risk of disease recurrence and mortality in otherwise curable cancers. The use of G-CSFs has been shown to support and enable the administration of planned chemotherapy dose intensity and improve disease-free and overall survival in early-stage breast cancer and lung cancer [43, 44].

In a recent nationwide survey of 1,243 community-based oncology practices, data on 20,799 early-stage breast cancer patients were collected [45]. The study assessed the incidence and predictors of low-dose intensity in the entire study population, as those who received G-CSFs. The predictive factors for reduced relative dose intensity were age, body surface area, year of treatment, chemotherapy regimen, chemotherapy schedule (21 days vs 28 days), and primary colony stimulating factors (CSFs) prophylaxis. The odd ratio of patients receiving CSF to experience dose reduction was 0.733 (p-value $= 0.001$) compared to patients not treated with prophylactic CSFs. In a meta-analysis of four RCTs of solid cancers, Crawford et al. reported that the median average dose intensity was between 99 and 100% of the planned intensity in the G-CSF groups [46].

Quality of Life

Quality of Life and Side Effects

Randomized controlled trials found G-CSFs to have relatively mild side effects, with the most frequent reported adverse effect being mild-to-moderate skeletal pain (in about 25–35% of patients receiving pegfilgrastim and 26–42% of patents receiving filgrastim) [47, 48]. The limited data exploring the impact of G-CSFs on patient's quality of life have failed to demonstrate a significant difference between filgrastim and pegfilgrastim [49]. Other efforts to study the impact of neutropenia on quality of life or utilities using techniques such as standard gamble or time tradeoff [7] have resulted in preliminary data, as described in the following section.

Utility Measures

In health economics, utilities represent the patient's preference for a health state. When estimates collected directly from patients are not available, proxies (for example, relatives, caregivers, or clinicians) are used. Brown et al. [50] sought to estimate chemotherapy-related utilities of a patient with advanced breast cancer, regardless of specific chemotherapy regimen. Utilities were obtained from 30 oncology nurses from specialist cancer centers in the United Kingdom and from 150 nurses in four other Western European countries, using the standard gamble method. They report a mean utility value of 0.24 (SD $= 0.12$) for FN with hospitalization and a value of 0.48 for infection without hospitalization. Earlier study done by Launois et al. [51] also used oncology nurses ($n = 20$) as proxies and the standard gamble method. They reported utility values for neutropenia with hospitalization to be 0.47 and to be 0.66 without hospitalization.

Special Populations

Children

Pediatric cancer patients differ from adult patients because they are often treated with more intensive chemotherapy regimens and are therefore at higher risk for developing FN. The use of G-CSFs in the pediatric population has received less attention, resulting in considerable uncertainty about their role in improving treatment outcomes such as incidence of FN, documented infection, quality of life, or costs. Recent guidelines published by the American Society for Clinical Oncology (ASCO) suggest that the use of prophylactic G-CSFs is reasonable for pediatric patients with a likelihood of FN, with the exception of patient with acute lymphoblastic leukemia (ALL) where the risk of secondary myeloid leukemia or myelodysplastic syndrome is of concern [52]. In a retrospective analysis of longitudinal data from 115 hospitals in the United States, Basu et al. [53] documented a 3% mortality rate among children hospitalized with FN and a median LOS of 5 days (range 1–359 days).

Two meta-analyses [38, 54] of RCTs of children receiving G-CSFs report that patients receiving G-CSFs had lower rate of FN (RR about 0.8, p-value < 0.05), a decrease in documented infections (RR about 0.7, p-value < 0.05), a mean decrease of 3.5 days in duration of neutropenia, and decrease in LOS. The meta-analyses had conflicting results on the effect of duration of antibiotic use. These results suggest that the use of G-CSFs among appropriately selected pediatric population holds the potential for improved outcomes. However, like in other economic analyses involving pediatric population, one should carefully consider inclusion of other costs such as parents' time and productivity.

Elderly

About 50% of cancer population in the United States are older than 65 years of age [2], and this percent is expected to increase with the aging of the population. Older age is associated with higher risk of both short- and long-term complications, including FN, and other comorbidities and the use of supportive chemotherapy treatment is essential in maintaining chemotherapy dose schedule and quality of life. For these reasons, prophylactic G-CSF use is recommended for patients of older age, regardless of what the regimen neutropenia risk threshold is [52].

Once older patients develop FN, they are at higher risk of having prolonged hospitalizations than younger patients, often as a result of more sever complications (a study of NHL elderly population found a 3.9-day longer LOS for patients aged $\geq$ 65 years and a 5.13-day longer LOS for those not receiving early CSF [55]). These prolonged hospitalizations increase the cost of treating FN in the elderly, and are also more likely to result in treatment delays and dose reductions (hence, reduced treatment effectiveness) and changes in the individual's and his/her caregivers' daily routine [56].

Existing Cost-Effective Models for Colony-Stimulating Factors

Combined Costs and Effects – Are CSFs Cost-Effective?

The use of G-CSFs has been the subject of few economic analyses, where the various treatment options were compared. Clinical decision models have been utilized in such analyses for studying the tradeoff between the added cost of G-CSFs and improved health outcomes associated with the reduction in risk of neutropenia and FN. In most economic models, the use of clinical prediction tools to generate separate estimates of the costs and effects of high- and low-risk patients reflect actual clinical practice and improved cost-effective applications to "real-world" decisions.

Initial economic models for G-CSFs were primarily cost-minimization studies, where only direct medical costs (usually fixed estimates from a single institution) were included, and disease probabilities were based on one or very few RCTs available at the time [57, 58]. In these models, a baseline risk threshold for FN was assumed to be 40%, and the added cost of G-CSFs was offset by decreased number and duration of hospitalizations. In an economic literature review, Esser et al. [59] compared the results of 33 economic evaluations of prophylactic as well as therapeutic use of G-CSFs compared to no G-CSFs. The findings demonstrated the cost-saving potential of G-CSFs for standard-dose chemotherapy was limited, but after high-dose chemotherapy results indicated cost-saving in most studies.

The FDA's approval of pegfilgrastim in 2002 along with an increase in available RCTs of G-CSFs use and cost encouraged the initiation of more sophisticated economic models, where two or three treatment alternatives were compared and a range of costs, disease probabilities, and outcomes were considered simultaneously. In these analyses the baseline cost-effective threshold is usually bounded by a 95% confidence interval, representing the range of plausible CE values.

The first economic analysis of pegfilgrastim compared the prophylactic use of pegfilgrastim, filgrastim, and no G-CSFs during the first cycle of chemotherapy, when most patients receive full treatment dose. The study was based on data from hospital discharge records and incorporated both direct and indirect medical costs (e.g., time and productivity costs). Results showed that despite the high cost of pegfilgrastim it was both less costly and more effective (resulted in higher quality-adjusted life years) compared to both filgrastim and no-G-CSFs, with expected cost of $4,203 and 12.3 quality-adjusted days [21].

Lyman et al. compared the CE of pegfilgrastim versus 6-day filgrastim prophylaxis on early-stage breast cancer [60] and adults with non-Hodgkin's lymphoma receiving CHOP-21 [61]. The authors found that pegfilgrastim was cost-effective with ICER of $12,904/FN episode avoided, $14,415/QALY in the breast cancer population, and ICER of $2,167/FN episode avoided, and $6,190/QALY for non-Hodgkin's patients. Pegfilgrastim was found to be both cost-saving and more effective when filgrastim was used for 11 days in the breast-cancer population.

Comparing prophylaxis to secondary use (after an FN event) with pegfilgrastim, Ramsey et al. [62] reported that in women with early-stage breast cancer receiving chemotherapy regimens with $\geq$ 20% FN risk, the ICER was $48,000/FN episode avoided or $116,000/QALY (95% CI [$97,000/QALY-$135,000/QALY]). The model considered only direct medical costs, but simulated several chemotherapy cycles per patient and incorporated into a sensitivity analysis the option of reduction in chemotherapy dose intensity.

References

1. National Cancer Institute. Cancer Trend Progress Report-2007 Update. Available from: http://progressreport.cancer.gov/doc_detail.asp?pid=1&did=2007&chid=75&coid=726& mid=. Accessed 12 Jul 2009.
2. American Cancer Society. Cancer facts and figures 2009. Available from: http://www.cancer.org/downloads/STT/500809web.pdf. Accessed 12 Jul 2009.
3. Bach PB. Limits on Medicare's ability to control rising spending on cancer drugs. N Engl J Med. 2009;360(6):626–33.
4. Chang S, Long SR, Kutikova L, et al. Estimating the cost of cancer: results on the basis of claims data analyses for cancer patients diagnosed with seven types of cancer during 1999 to 2000. J Clin Oncol. 2004;22(17):3524–30.
5. Greenberg D, Earle C, Fang C-H, Eldar-Lissai A, Neumann PJ. When is cancer care cost-effective? A systematic overview of cost-utility analyses in oncology. J Natl Cancer Inst. 2010;102(2):82–8.

6. Gold MR, Siegel JE, Russell LB, Weinstein MC. Cost-effectiveness in health and medicine. New York, NY: Oxford University Press; 1996.

7. Drummond MF, Sculpher MJ, Torrance GW, O'brien BJ, Stoddart GL. Methods for the economic evaluation of health care programmes. New York, NY: Oxford Medical Publications; 2005.

8. Berger ML, Bingefors K, Hedblom EC, Pashos CL, Torrance GW. Health care cost, quality, and outcomes, ISPOR book of terms. New Jersey: International Society for Pharmacoeconomics and Outcomes Research; 2003.

9. Lyman GH, Kuderer NM. The economics of the colony-stimulating factors in the prevention and treatment of febrile neutropenia. Crit Rev Oncol Hematol. 2004;50(2):129–46.

10. Stone PW, Chapman RC, Sandberg EA, Liljas B, Neumann PJ. Measuring costs in cost-utility analyses: variations in the literature. Int J Technol Assess Health Care. 2000;6(1):111–24.

11. Greenberg D, Winkelmayer WC, Rosen AB, Neumann PJ, Palmer JA. Prevailing judgments about society's willingness to pay for a QALY: do they vary by country? Have they changed over time? Philadelphia, PA: International Society for Pharmacoeconomics and Outcomes Research (ISPOR); 2006.

12. Neumann PJ. Using cost-effectiveness analysis to improve health care: opportunities and barriers. New York, NYFord University Press; 2005.

13. Maher DW, Lieschke GJ, Green M, et al. Filgrastim in patients with chemotherapy-induced febrile neutropenia: a double-blind, placebo-controlled trial. Ann Intern Med. 1994;121: 492–501.

14. Vogel CL, Wojtukiewicz ZM, Carroll RR, et al. First and subsequent cycle use of pegfilgrastim prevents febrile neutropenia in patients with breast cancer: a multicenter, double-blind, placebo-controlled phase III study. J Clin Oncol. 2005;23(6):1178–84.

15. Crawford J, Ozer H, Stoller R, Johanson D, Lyman GH, et al. Reduction by granulocyte colony-stimulating factor of fever and neutropenia induced by chemotherapy in patients with small cell lung cancer. N Engl J Med. 1991;325:164–70.

16. Clark OAC, Lyman GH, Castro AA, Clark LGO, Djulbegovic B. Colony-stimulating factors for chemotherapy-induced febrile neutropenia: a meta-analysis of randomized controlled trials. J Clin Oncol. 2005;23(18):4198–214.

17. Centers for Medicare and Medicaid. Medicare Part B Drug Average Sales Price 2009 ASP Drug Pricing Files. Available from: http://www.cms.hhs.gov/apps/ama/license.asp?file=/McrPartBDrugAvgSalesPrice/downloads/July_2009_ASP_Pricing_File.zip. Accessed 18 Jul 2009.

18. Caggiano V, Weiss RV, Richert TS, Linde-Zwirble WT. Incidence, cost, and mortality of neutropenia hospitalization associated with chemotherapy. Cancer. 2005;103(9):1916–24.

19. Kuderer N, Dale D, Crawford J, Cosler L, Lyman G. The morbidity, mortality and cost of febrile neutropenia in cancer patients. Cancer. 2006;106(10):2258–66.

20. Cosler LE, Eldar-Lissai A, Culakova E, et al. Therapeutic use of granulocyte colony-stimulating factors for established febrile neutropenia: effect on costs from a hospital perspective. PharmacoEconomics. 2007;25(4):343–51.

21. Eldar-Lissai A, Cosler LE, Culakova E, Lyman GH. Economic analysis of prophylactic pegfilgrastim in adult cancer patients receiving chemotherapy. Value Health. 2008;11(2):172–9.

22. Courtney DM, Aldeen AZ, Gorman SM, et al. Cancer-associated neutropenic fever: clinical outcome and economic costs of emergency department care. Oncologist. 2007;12(8):1019–26.

23. Weycker D, Hackett J, Edelsberg JS, Oster G, Glass AG. Are shorter courses of filgrastim prophylaxis associated with increased risk of hospitalization? Ann Pharmacother. 2006;40(3):402–7.

24. Ip EJ, Lee-Ma A, Troxell LS, Chan J. Low-dose filgrastim in patients with breast cancer treated with docetaxel, doxorubicin, and cyclophosphamide. Am J Health Syst Pharm. 2008;65(16):1552–55.

25. Morrison VA, Wong M, Hershman D, Campos LT, Ding B, Observational MJ. Study of the prevalence of febrile neutropenia in patients who receive filgrastim or pegfilgrastim associated

with 3–4 weeks chemotherapy regimens in community oncology practices. J Manag Care Pharm. 2007;13(4):337–48.

26. Weycker D, Malin J, Kim J, et al. Risk of hospitalization for neutropenic complications of chemotherapy in patients with primary solid tumors receiving pegfilgrastim or filgrastim prophylaxis: a retrospective cohort study. Clin Ther. 2009;31(5):1069–81.

27. Talcott JA, Finberg R, Mayer RJ, The Medical GL. Course of cancer patients with fever and neutropenia: clinical identification of a low-risk subgroup at presentation. Arch Intern Med. 1988;148(12):2561–68.

28. Klastersky J, Paesmans M, Rubenstein EB, et al. The multinational association for supportive care in cancer risk index: a multinational scoring system for identifying low-risk febrile neutropenic cancer patients. J Clin Oncol. 2000;18(16):3038–51.

29. Uys A, Rapoport BL, Anderson R. Febrile neutropenia: a prospective study to validate the Multinational Association of Supportive Care of Cancer (MASCC) risk-index score. Support Care Cancer. 2004;8:555–60.

30. Carstensen M, Benn Sørensen J. Outpatient management of febrile neutropenia: time to revise the present treatment strategy. J Support Oncol. 2008;6(5):199–208.

31. Elting LS, Lu C, Escalante CP, et al. Outcomes and cost of outpatient or inpatient management of 712 patients with febrile neutropenia. J Clin Oncol. 2008;26(4):606–11.

32. Cosler LE, Sivasubramaniam V, Agboola O, Crawford J, Dale D, Lyman GH. Effect of outpatient treatment of febrile neutropenia on the risk threshold for the use of CSF in patients with cancer treated with chemotherapy. Value Health. 2005;8(1):47–52.

33. Cosler LE, Calhoun EA, Agboola O, Lyman GH. Effects of indirect and additional direct costs on the risk threshold for prophylaxis with colony-stimulating factors in patients at risk for severe neutropenia from cancer chemotherapy. Pharmacotherapy. 2004;24(4): 488–94.

34. Fortner B, Tauer K, Zhu L, et al. Medical visits for chemotherapy and chemotherapy-induced neutropenia: a survey of the impact on patient time and activities. BMC Cancer. 2004; 4(1):22.

35. Fortner BV, Okon TA, Zhu L, et al. Costs of human resources in delivering cancer chemotherapy and managing chemotherapy-induced neutropenia in community practice. Commun Oncol. 2004;1:23–8.

36. Song X, Fowler R, Ruiz K, Hurley D, Barron RL. Impact of neutropenic complications on short-term disability in patients with cancer receiving chemotherapy. J Med Econ. 2009;12(2):1–10.

37. Heil G, Hoelzer D, Sanz MA, et al. Long-term survival data from a phase 3 study of filgrastim as an adjunct to chemotherapy in adults with de novo acute myeloid leukemia. Leukemia. 2006;20(3):404–9.

38. Sung L, Nathan PC, Alibhai SMH, Tomlinson GA, Beyene J. Meta-analysis: effect of prophylactic hematopoietic colony-stimulating factors on mortality and outcomes of infection. Ann Intern Med. 2007;147(6):400–11.

39. Kuderer NM, Dale DC, Crawford J, Lyman GH. Impact of primary prophylaxis with granulocyte colony-stimulating factor on febrile neutropenia and mortality in adult cancer patients receiving chemotherapy: a systematic review. J Clin Oncol. 2007;25(21):3158–67.

40. Lyman GH, Kuderer NM, Djulbegovic B. Prophylactic granulocyte colony-stimulating factor in patients receiving dose-intensive cancer chemotherapy: a meta-analysis. Am J Med. 2002;112(5):406–11.

41. Budman D, Berry D, Cirrincione C, et al. Dose and dose intensity as determinants of outcome in the adjuvant treatment of breast cancer. The Cancer and Leukemia Group B. J. Natl. Cancer Inst. 1998;90(16):1205–11.

42. Kwak L, Halpern J, Olshen R, Horning S. Prognostic significance of actual dose intensity in diffuse large-cell lymphoma: results of a tree-structured survival analysis. J Clin Oncol. 1990;8(6):963–77.

43. Ellis GK, Livingston RB, Gralow JR, Green SJ, Thompson T. Dose-dense anthracycline-based chemotherapy for node-positive breast cancer. J Clin Oncol. 2002;20(17): 3637–43.

44. Thatcher N, Girling DJ, Hopwood P, Sambrook RJ, Qian W, Stephens RJ. Improving survival without reducing quality of life in small-cell lung cancer patients by increasing the dose-intensity of chemotherapy with granulocyte colony-stimulating factor support: results of a British medical research council multicenter randomized trial. J Clin Oncol. 2000;18(2): 395–404.

45. Lyman GH, Dale D, Crawford J. Incidence and predictors of low dose-intensity in adjuvant breast cancer chemotherapy: a nationwide study of community practices. J Clin Oncol. 2003;21(24):4524–31.

46. Crawford J, Green M, McGuire B, Combined SS. Analysis of average relative dose intensity in the chemotherapy of solid tumors with pegfilgrastim or filgrastim support. Support Cancer Ther. 2005;2(4):229–33.

47. Green MD, Koelbl H, Baselga J, et al. A randomized double-blind multicenter phase III study of fixed-dose single-administration pegfilgrastim versus daily filgrastim in patients receiving myelosuppressive chemotherapy. Ann Oncol. 2003;14(1):29–35.

48. Holmes FA, O'Shaughnessy JA, Vukelja S, et al. Blinded, randomized, multicenter study to evaluate single administration pegfilgrastim once per cycle versus daily filgrastim as an adjunct to chemotherapy in patients with high-risk stage II or stage III/IV breast cancer. J Clin Oncol. 2002;20(3):727–31.

49. Doorduijn JK, van der Holt B, van Imhoff GW, et al. CHOP compared with CHOP plus granulocyte colony-stimulating factor in elderly patients with aggressive non-Hodgkin's lymphoma. J Clin Oncol. 2003;21(16):3041–50.

50. Brown RE, Hutton J, Burrell A. Cost effective of treatment options in advanced breast cancer in the UK. PharmacoEconomics. 2001;19(11):1091–102.

51. Launois R, Reboul-Marty J, Henry B, Bonneterre J. A cost-utility of second-line chemotherapy in metastatic breast cancer. Docetaxel versus paclitaxel versus vinorelbine. PharmacoEconomics. 1996;11(5):492–97.

52. Smith TJ, Khatcheressian J, Lyman GH, et al. Update of recommendations for the use of white blood cell growth factors: an evidence-based clinical practice guideline. J Clin Oncol. 2006;24(19):3187–205.

53. Basu SK, Fernandez ID, Fisher SG, Asselin BL, Lyman GH. Length of stay and mortality associated with febrile neutropenia among children with cancer. J Clin Oncol. 2005;23(31):7958–66.

54. Wittman B, Horan J, Lyman GH. Prophylactic colony-stimulating factors in children receiving myelosuppressive chemotherapy: a meta-analysis of randomized controlled trials. Cancer Treat Rev. 2006;32(4):289–303.

55. Chrischilles E, Delgado DJ, Stolshek BS, Lawless G, Fridman M, Carter WB. Impact of age and colony-stimulating factor use on hospital length of stay for febrile neutropenia in chop-treated non-Hodgkin's lymphoma. Cancer Control. 2002;9:203–11.

56. Balducci L. Supportive care of elderly patients with cancer. Support Care Ther. 2005;2(4):225–8.

57. Lyman G, Lyman C, Sanderson R, Balducci L. Decision analysis of hematopoietic growth factor use in patients receiving cancer chemotherapy. J Natl Cancer Inst. 1993;85:488–93.

58. Lyman GH, Balducci L. A cost analysis of hematopoietic colony-stimulating factors. Oncology. 1995;9:85–91.

59. Esser M, Brunner H. Economic evaluations of granulocyte colony-stimulating factor: in the prevention and treatment of chemotherapy-induced neutropenia. ADIS International Limited, 2003.

60. Lyman GH, Lalla A, Barron RL, Dubois RW. Cost-effectiveness of pegfilgrastim versus filgrastim primary prophylaxis in women with early-stage breast cancer receiving chemotherapy in the United States. Clin Ther. 2009;31(5):1092–104.

61. Lyman GH, Lalla A, Barron RL, Dubois RW. Cost-effective of pegfilgrastim versus 6-day filgrastim primary prophylaxis in patients with non-Hodgkin's lymphoma receiving CHOP-21 in United States. Curr Med Res Opin. 2009;25(2):401–11.
62. Ramsey SD, Liu Z, Rob B, et al. Cost-effectiveness of primary versus secondary prophylaxis with pegfilgrastim in women with early-stage breast cancer receiving chemotherapy. Value Health. 2009;12(2):217–25.

Index

Note: The letters 'f' and 't' following locators refer to figures and tables respectively.